CLINICAL GUIDELINES IN CHILD HEALTH
Second Edition

Mary Virginia Graham
PhD, RNCS, ARNP

Constance R. Uphold
PhD, RNCS, ARNP

Family Nurse Practitioner Program
College of Nursing
University of Florida
Gainesville, Florida

1999
Barmarrae Books, Inc.
Gainesville, Florida

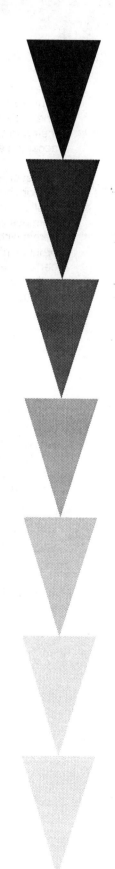

MESSAGE FROM THE AUTHORS AND PUBLISHER

Please keep in mind that medicine is an ever-changing science. As new research and clinical experience broaden our knowledge, changes in treatment including drug therapies are required. The authors and the publisher of this work have checked with sources believed to be reliable in their efforts to provide information that is complete and in accord with the standards of practice accepted at the time of publication.

However, in view of the possibility of human error or changes in medical sciences, neither the authors nor the publisher nor any other party who has been involved in the preparation or publication of this work are responsible for any errors or omissions or for the results obtained from use of such information. Readers are encouraged to confirm the information contained herein with other sources. For example, and in particular, readers are advised to consult the product information sheet included in the package of each drug they plan to administer to make certain that the information contained in this book is accurate and changes have not been made in the recommended dose or in the contraindications for administration. For medications that are administered infrequently, following this procedure is of critical importance.

First Edition 1994
Second Edition 1999

ISBN 0-9646151-4-2

Printed in the United States of America.

PREFACE

Since the publication of the first edition of <u>Clinical Guidelines in Child Health</u>, the field of primary care has become a major force in the health care system. An interdisciplinary array of health care clinicians including nurse practitioners, physician assistants, and physicians are playing a central role in the provision of comprehensive, personalized, cost-effective health care.

Like the previous edition, this edition was designed to help these clinicians quickly access up-to-date information regarding health supervision and commonly occurring primary care problems among children. The book contains the latest approaches to diagnosis, evaluation, and management in primary care. Diagnostic criteria and guidelines from national health advisory boards and authoritative sources are incorporated throughout.

The second edition of <u>Clinical Guidelines in Child Health</u> has been extensively updated and expanded with additional tables and illustrations to help the reader quickly locate information. Health supervision guidelines which focus on developmental assessment as well as approaches to behavioral problems are included. Twenty new topics including sleep problems, neonatal jaundice, head injury, and elbow pain have been added.

Each chapter has been reviewed by a practicing clinician with specialized knowledge and experience. We hope <u>Clinical Guidelines in Child Health</u> is a helpful reference and provides clinicians with valuable information to assist them in understanding and managing health problems of children.

Mary Virginia Graham
Constance R. Uphold

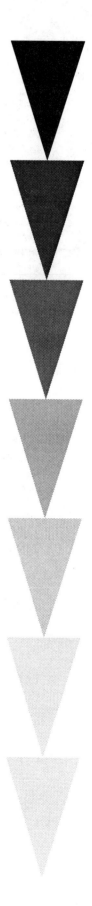

REVIEWERS

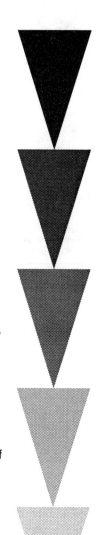

Yana Banks, MD
Pediatrician
Alachua County Health Department
Gainesville, Florida

M. Katherine Crabtree, DNSc, RNCS, ANP
Associate Professor
Primary Health Care Nurse Practitioner Specialty
Oregon Health Sciences University School of
    Nursing
Portland, Oregon

Jean E. DeMartinis, PhD, RNCS, ARNP
Assistant Professor
Director, Cardiac Health, Wellness &
    Rehabilitation Nursing Curriculum
Creighton University School of Nursing
Omaha, Nebraska

J. Jordan Goodman, PhD, RNCS, ARNP
Coordinator, Clinical Programs
Division of Endocrinology and Metabolism
University of Florida
Gainesville, Florida

Lori A. Graham, MN, RNCS, FNP
Graduate Student
University of Florida
Gainesville, Florida

Betsy Hernandez, MSN, RNCS, ARNP
Coordinator of Clinical Programs
Community Health and Family Medicine
University of Florida
Gainesville, Florida

Carol Massey Lavin, ARNP
Coordinator of Clinical Services
University of Florida Clinic at Fanning Springs
Gainesville, Florida

Donna J. Lilly, MSN, ARNP
Comprehensive Epilepsy Program
University of Florida
Gainesville, Florida

**Mary C. Schwartz Ryngaert, MSN,
RNCS, ARNP**
Pediatric Nurse Practitioner
The Kid's Health Team
Gainesville, Florida

**Nancy Hurley Pontes, MSN, RNCS,
FNP**
Doctoral Student
Columbia University School of Nursing
New York, New York

Cynthia S. Selleck, DSN, RNCS, ARNP
Associate Professor
Department of Family Medicine
University of South Florida
Tampa, Florida

Tish Smyer, DNSc, RN
Associate Professor
South Dakota State University College of
    Nursing
Brookings, South Dakota

**Paula J. Watt-Gilstrap, MS, RNCS,
FNP**
Program Manager for Nursing Programs
    and Services
Joseph F. Sullivan Center for Nursing
    and Wellness
Clemson University
Clemson, South Carolina

AUTHOR'S NOTE: We would like to thank **Gail Luparello** for her meticulous, creative work and dedication in the preparation of this text

To my children, Jay, Lori, and Robin, and to my mother, Cecile King.

M.V.G.

To my husband, Bill, our children, Lindsay and Nicholas, and to my parents, Charles and Myrtle Uphold.

C.R.U.

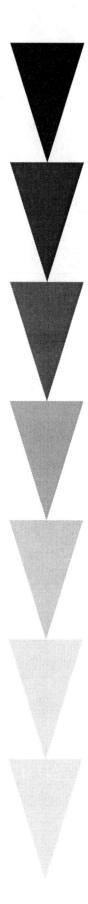

TABLE OF CONTENTS

Health Maintenance

CHILD HEALTH SUPERVISION

I.   Definition: Periodic evaluation of infants and children, and implementation of measures to promote health and detect unrecognized problems in asymptomatic infants and children

II.   **Neonates: Birth to One Month**

   A.   History
      1.   Obtain a complete history, including prenatal, birth history, nutrition, sleep, elimination patterns, and any illnesses since birth
      2.   Obtain family and social history (ask who lives in household, who provides care for infant, what the sleeping arrangements are for the infant, and if there are any smokers in the household)
      3.   Inquire about parental concerns
      4.   Observe parent-infant interaction (**Note**: To maximize the observation, have parent hold infant on lap; comment about the infant's social behavior and individuality)

   B.   Developmental Surveillance and Milestones
      1.   As part of the evaluation, perform a developmental assessment
      2.   Based on the milestones in the "Snapshot" below, ask appropriate history questions, and make appropriate observations to assess the neonate's development

---

A SNAPSHOT OF THE NEONATE

   ❖   Responds to sound by a state change
   ❖   Fixates on human face and follows with eyes (45 - 90°)
   ❖   Lifts head momentarily when prone
   ❖   Maintains position of flexion
   ❖   Sleeps for periods of 3-4 hours
   ❖   Can be comforted when crying by being held

   C.   Physical Examination
      1.   Measure and plot on growth chart the neonate's weight for age, length for age, weight for length, and head circumference; birth weight and length should also be charted (**Note**: National Center for Health Statistics [USDHHS] growth charts are recommended)
      2.   Share growth information with parent and determine if weight gain is appropriate (~1 oz/day)

EXAMINATION OF THE NEONATE

General:	The infant should be completely undressed. Observe for position of flexion and symmetrical movement of all extremities
Skin:	Observe color, hydration status, presence of lesions, evidence of trauma (always look for evidence of abuse)
Head:	Examine for symmetry, evidence of trauma, assess anterior and posterior fontanelles (expect anterior to be diamond-shaped and about 2-3 cm in diameter; posterior triangle-shaped and about 1 cm in diameter) **Remember:** Closure of anterior fontanelle varies (range is 7 to 19 months). Posterior fontanelle may not be palpable at birth, and is usually closed at about 3 months of age)
Eyes:	Observe for position, alignment, equality, obtain red reflex, elicit pupillary reflex. Assess the newborn's ability to fixate on and follow a human face (or interesting object such as small red ball) as a gross measure of vision. (**Remember:** Infant sees best at 10-12 inch range)
ENT:	Note position of ears (low set ears are associated with renal agenesis/chromosomal abnormalities). Visualize drums. Assess ability to alert toward a human voice or interesting sound (bell) as a gross measure of hearing. Test patency of nasal canals (occlude one and then the other nostril while baby sucks on pacifier). Visualization of throat beyond uvula is usually difficult unless baby is crying

(continued)

Mouth:	**Always** open baby's mouth to search for abnormalities. Insert gloved finger to feel for cleft palate. Check mouth for natal teeth, retention cysts, thrush
Chest/Car-diovascular:	Examine for rate (average rate is 140 in newborn), rhythm, and to detect murmurs. Palpate femoral pulses (which are weak or absent with coarctation of the aorta)
Lungs:	Observe respiratory pattern. Rate in newborns ranges from 30-60 per minute. Auscultate for bronchial breath sounds bilaterally (respiration is chiefly abdominal)
Abdomen:	Listen for bowel sounds. Palpate abdomen, checking for abdominal masses (including hernias), hepato-splenomegaly (liver may be palpated 2 cm below the costal margin; spleen should be nonpalpable). Inspect umbilical stump (cord should become dry in one week after birth, and fall off by the time baby is 14 days old)
Genitour-inary:	Males: Inspect penis for hypospadias or epispadias (in uncircumcised males, do not retract the prepuce more than is adequate for exam); palpate testicles. Females: Examine labia (labia minora usually prominent in infants); spread the labia and examine for imperforate hymen. Both genders: check for position and patency of anus
Musculo-skeletal:	Palpate for fractures of the clavicles; check for developmental hip dysplasia (rotate the thighs with the knees flexed)
Neuro-logical:	Elicit Moro's reflex (startle the infant by a clapping your hands--infant reacts by extending, then flexing, the arms, clenching the hands, and flexing the hips and knees). Note the cry (should be lusty). Evaluate muscle tone as infant is handled throughout the exam. Assess head control and head lag by grasping both hands and gently pulling the infant from a supine to an upright position. Check for grasp, rooting, and sucking reflexes

D. Diagnostic Tests: Metabolic and hemoglobinopathy screening as required by state (if not performed in hospital)

E. Immunizations: See RECOMMENDED CHILDHOOD IMMUNIZATION SCHEDULE, UNITED STATES, JAN-DEC 1999 table on page 19

F. Vitamin and Mineral Supplementation

Formula-fed term infants	**Require** no vitamin and mineral supplementation during first 6 months of life. Once solids are introduced at 6 months, formula combined with the solid food intake is sufficient after that period as well
Breast-fed infants	**Of well-nourished mothers** who have sufficient intake of Vitamin D and Vitamin B require no supplementation during this period. Human milk is low in Vitamins D and B; thus if maternal intake is low, infant may be at risk for deficiency. If there is adequate sunlight exposure, Vitamin D supplementation is not recommended. Best way to insure adequate Vitamin D intake of breast fed infant is to increase intake of this vitamin by the mother
Vegetarian females	**Who breast feed** are at risk of providing milk to infant that is low in Vitamin B_6 and B_{12} These females should supplement their diets with these vitamins in order for the infant to have adequate intake

G. Anticipatory Guidance

Injury and Illness Prevention: Advise parents as follows
- ❖ Use rear-facing infant car seat that is properly secured in the back seat of the vehicle (center of rear seat is the safest position)
- ❖ Never leave infant unattended
- ❖ Put baby to sleep on side or back ("Back to Sleep") without comforters or pillows
- ❖ Keep baby's environment smoke free
- ❖ Avoid overexposure to sun
- ❖ Recognize early signs of illness (see WHEN TO CALL THE HEALTH CARE PROVIDER in table on page 4)

Nutrition: Advise parents as follows

- ❖ Breast feeding: Counsel regarding appropriate frequency and duration of feeding, breast care, and maternal dietary requirements
- ❖ Bottle feeding: Counsel regarding amount and frequency of feeding, necessity of iron-fortified diet, formula preparation, and avoidance of bottle-propping
- ❖ **Remember:** Warn parent not to use microwave oven to heat formula
- ❖ See INFANT NUTRITION section for additional information relating to infant nutrition including **amount** and **frequency** of feedings

---

Oral health: Advise parent to never put infant to bed with bottle

---

Infant care: Advise parents as follows

- ❖ Normal sleep patterns and appropriate sleeping arrangements
- ❖ Bladder and bowel patterns
- ❖ Cord care (if cord still in place), care of circumcised and uncircumcised male
- ❖ Skin, nail care
- ❖ Importance of responding promptly to infant's crying; babies need to be held, cuddled
- ❖ How to console baby (demonstrate through role modeling if appropriate)
- ❖ How infant uses thumb sucking and pacifier in self-comforting
- ❖ Use of rectal thermometer (rectal temperature of 38.0 C/100.4 F or higher is a fever)
- ❖ When to call the health care provider

When To Call the Health Care Provider: Advise parent to call if the infant/child has

❖ Fever (Rectal temp of 100.4° F or higher)	❖ Poor feeding
❖ Vomiting, diarrhea, abdominal distention	❖ Irritability, lethargy
❖ Inconsolable crying	❖ Jaundice
❖ Skin rash, red eye	

III. **Infants: Ages 2, 4, 6, & 9 Months**

    A. History

        1. For initial visit, obtain a complete history including prenatal, birth, and family history

        2. For both initial and interval visits, obtain history related to nutrition, sleep, elimination patterns, growth and development, immunization status

        3. Obtain a social history on each visit including who lives in household, who provides care for the infant, what the sleeping arrangements are for the infant, and if there are any smokers in household

        4. Inquire about parental concerns

        5. Review any illnesses since birth

        6. Observe parent-infant interaction; have parent hold infant on lap; comment about infant's social behavior and individuality

    B. Developmental Surveillance and Milestones

        1. As part of the evaluation, perform a developmental assessment

        2. Based on the milestones in the "Snapshot" that follows, ask appropriate questions, and make appropriate observations during the history and examination to assess the infant's development

A SNAPSHOT OF 2, 4, 6, & 9 MONTH OLD		
Age Group	**Activities**	
2 Month Old	Coos and vocalizes reciprocally Smiles responsively; shows interest in visual/auditory stimuli	When prone, lifts head, neck, and upper chest with forearm support Some head control in upright position
4 Month Old	Babbles, coos, smiles, laughs, and squeals In prone position, raises body on hands Rolls from prone to supine Opens hands to grasp objects	Reaches for objects Controls head well Has spontaneous social smile May sleep for 6 hours
6 Month Old	Vocalizes single consonants ("dada") Rolls over both ways No head lag when pulled to sit Sits with support	Stands when placed and bears weight Starts to self-feed Transfers objects from hand to hand Usually has first tooth erupt
9 Months of Age	Responds to own name Understands a few words such as "no-no," "bye-bye" Babbles frequently, imitates vocalizations, and may say one or two words Crawls, creeps, moves forward by scooting Sits independently May pull to stand	Pokes with index finger Plays interactive games Feeds self with fingers Begins to use cup May sleep through night May show stranger anxiety

C. Physical Examination

    1. Measure and plot on growth chart the infant's weight for age, length for age, weight for length, and head circumference (**Note**: Infant should double birth weight by 5-6 months and triple birth weight by one year of age)

    2. Any infant whose weight gain is inappropriate (not following curve), whose weight is below the third percentile, and whose weight and length differ by more than 2 percentile lines requires further evaluation (**Note**: Infant should follow his/her own growth curve; serial [versus single measurements] allow clinician to determine if growth curve is being followed)

    3. Head-to-toe examination should be completed on each visit during this age period with a **special focus** on the following

Focus of Infant Exam
General appearance of the infant Muscle tone Hearing and visual tracking Red reflex and alignment of eyes Cardiac murmurs Presence of developmental hip dysplasia In males, descent of testes Evidence of abuse/neglect

    4. Provide developmental screening for all children (if possible) using the Denver II; refer any infant demonstrating a developmental delay for further evaluation

D. Diagnostic Tests:

Hemoglobin and/or hematocrit once between 6 and 9 months of age (AAP)

E. Immunizations: See RECOMMENDED CHILDHOOD IMMUNIZATION SCHEDULE, UNITED STATES, JAN-DEC 1999 on page 19

F.   Mineral and Fluoride Supplementation

MINERAL SUPPLEMENTATION	
For infants less than six months of age	See Vitamin and Mineral Supplementation on page 3 and follow those guidelines
Breast fed infants who are 6 months of age	**Require iron supplementation** in the form of iron-fortified cereal, 2 servings each day
Bottle fed infants who are 6 months of age	And who are receiving iron-fortified formula (which should be **all bottle fed infants**) do not require iron supplementation, but iron-fortified cereal is also fed to these infants beginning at six months of age

Once solids are introduced at 6 months, both breast milk and formula combined with the solid food intake is sufficient to meet all of the child's mineral and vitamin requirements with the possible exception of fluoride

Recommended daily doses of fluoride supplementation are contained in the table below (**Note**: Fluoride supplementation is no longer recommended for infants under 6 months of age)

FLUORIDE SUPPLEMENTATION RECOMMENDATIONS*			
Age	**Water Fluoride Content (in ppm)**		
	<0.3	**0.3-0.6**	**>0.6**
Birth to 6 months	0	0	0
6 months to 3 years	0.25	0	0
3 to 6 years	0.50	0.25	0
6 to 16 years	1.00	0.50	0

*Daily doses are given in milligrams
Adapted from American Academy of Pediatric Dentistry. (1994). Recommendations for preventive pediatric dental care. Pediatric Dentistry, 15(9), p. 39.

G.   Anticipatory Guidance

Injury and illness prevention: Advise parents as follows
- ❖ See Anticipatory Guidance on page 3 and counsel parents on all these points
- ❖ (**Note**: A front-facing child restraint seat may be used for children weighing more than 20 pounds, but must be secured in rear seat, preferably in the center position)
- ❖ Set hot water thermostat at less than 120°
- ❖ Keep toys with small parts, balloons, and plastic bags out of reach
- ❖ Keep dangerous objects/poisonous substances out of sight and reach
- ❖ Use safety locks on all cabinets; cover all electrical outlets with plastic covers
- ❖ Do not use infant walkers at any age; encourage use of expanding stair gates
- ❖ Keep Syrup of Ipecac on hand to use as directed by Poison Control Center (Keep PCC number near phone)
- ❖ Never leave infant unattended or alone with young siblings or pets
- ❖ Empty all buckets, tubs, or small pools immediately after use

Nutrition: Advise parents as follows
- ❖ See Nutrition on page 4 and counsel parents as appropriate regarding breast and bottle feeding
- ❖ Delay introduction of solids until 6 months of age (See INFANT NUTRITION section for more detailed information)
- ❖ At 6 months, encourage drinking from cup
- ❖ At 8-9 months, add chopped table foods while child is sitting at table with family so that child is completely transitioned from pureed to chopped foods by 12 months of age
- ❖ Limit juice to 4-6 ounces a day (child should get most of daily calories from food/milk, **not** juice)
- ❖ Avoid giving child peanuts, hot dogs, raisins, grapes, popcorn, large pieces of raw fruit/veggies to prevent aspiration/choking

Oral Health: Advise parents as follows

❖ Do not put infant to bed with a bottle containing formula or juice; (while water is acceptable, best to advise parent not to put baby to bed with a bottle at all)
❖ At 4 month visit, counsel parents regarding teething--what to expect and how to soothe painful gums
❖ As soon as teeth erupt (usually between 6 and 8 months), clean with a soft brush (see DENTAL HEALTH MAINTENANCE section for chronology of dentition in children)

Infant Care: Advise parents as follows

❖ Refer to Infant Care on page 4 and include those items in counseling
❖ Read books to, talk and sing to, and play music for infant to comfort and to encourage vocalizations
❖ Play social games such as pat-a-cake and peek-a-boo
❖ Establish a bedtime routine to discourage night awakening
❖ Provide baby with the same comfort objects (blanket, stuffed toy) so that he/she can console self at bedtime or in new situations
❖ Provide infant with age-appropriate toys
❖ Beginning at 6 months, provide opportunities for exploration of the environment
❖ Beginning at 6 months, set limits/discipline child using distraction, structure and routines
❖ Limit rules and enforce consistently

IV. **Toddlers: Ages 12, 15, & 18 Months**

   A. History
      1. For initial visit, obtain a complete history including prenatal, birth, and family history
      2. For both initial and interval visits, obtain history related to nutrition, sleep and elimination patterns, growth and development, immunization status, and illnesses since birth; ask about medications and allergies
      3. Obtain a social history on each visit including who lives in household, who provides care for the infant, what the sleeping arrangements are for the infant, and if there are any smokers in household
      4. Inquire about current concerns of parents
      5. Observe parent-child interaction

   B. Developmental Surveillance and Milestones
      1. As part of the evaluation (including both history and physical examination), perform a developmental assessment
      2. Based on the items in the "Snapshot" below, ask appropriate history questions, and make appropriate observations during the history and examination to assess the child's development

A SNAPSHOT OF 12, 15, & 18 MONTH OLD		
Age Group	**Activities**	
12 months	Pulls to stand, cruises Has vocabulary of 1-3 words, including "mama" and "dada"	May take few steps alone Uses precise pincer grasp; points with index finger, plays peek-a-boo
15 months	Walks well, stoops, climbs stairs Can point to one or more body parts Stacks two blocks	Feeds self with fingers Has vocabulary of 3-6 words
18 months	Walks quickly, runs stiffly, walks backwards Stacks 3-4 blocks Uses vocabulary of about 15 words	Points to some body parts May voice 2 or more wants Feeds self; uses spoon and drinks from cup

   C. Physical Examination
      1. Measure and plot on growth chart the child's weight for age, length for age, and weight for length, and head circumference
      2. By 12 months of age, birth weight should have tripled
      3. During the period from 12 months to 24 months, child, on average, should gain 4-6 pounds in weight and 3-5 inches in height
      4. Any child whose weight gain is inappropriate (not following curve), whose weight is below the third percentile, or whose weight and length (height) differ by more than 2 percentile lines requires further evaluation

5. Head-to-toe examination should be completed on each visit with special focus on the following

Focus of Exam	
General appearance of the child	Feet and gait once walking begins
Hearing and vision	Teeth for baby bottle caries
Red reflex and alignment of eyes	Evidence of abuse/neglect

D. Diagnostic Tests: Screening for lead poisoning

CDC recommends **universal** screening for lead poisoning in all children at ages 1 and 2 and all children 36-72 months of age who have **not** been previously screened **if** their risk for lead exposure is widespread

CDC recommends **targeted** screening for lead poisoning for children at ages 1 and 2, and children 36-72 months of age who have not previously been screened, if they meet one of the following criteria (as determined by local health department)
* Residence in a specific geographic area (e.g., a specified zip code)
* Membership in a high-risk group (e.g., Medicaid recipient)
* Answers to a personal-risk questionnaire indicating risk (see following table)

THE PERSONAL-RISK QUESTIONNAIRE

A basic personal-risk questionnaire:

✔ Does your child live in or regularly visit a house that was built before 1950? This question could apply to a facility such as a home day-care center or the home of a babysitter or relative
✔ Does your child live in or regularly visit a house built before 1978 with recent or ongoing renovations or remodeling (within the last 6 months)?
✔ Does your child have a sibling or playmate who has or did have lead poisoning?

Source: Centers for Disease Control and Prevention. (1997). Screening young children for lead poisoning: Guidance for state and local public health officials. Atlanta: Author.

E. Immunizations: See RECOMMENDED CHILDHOOD IMMUNIZATION SCHEDULE, UNITED STATES, JAN-DEC, 1999 table on page 19

F. Supplements: See FLUORIDE SUPPLEMENTATION RECOMMENDATIONS table on page 6

G. Anticipatory Guidance

Illness and Injury Prevention: Advise parents as follows

To Prevent MVA/Other Machine-Related Injuries:
❖ Switch to a toddler car seat and make sure it is properly secured, always in the rear seat
❖ Keep toddler away from moving machinery, lawn mowers, backing cars

To Prevent Burn/Scalding Injuries:
❖ Recheck the hot water heater to make certain the thermostat is <120°
❖ Test smoke detector frequently and change battery once a year
❖ Keep the toddler away from hot stoves, fireplaces, curling irons, space heaters
❖ Turn pot handles toward back of stove
❖ Ensure that electric outlets and appliances are inaccessible

To Prevent Accidental Ingestion/Poisoning:
❖ Keep all poisonous substances including medicines, alcohol, cleaning agents, paints, solvents out of the child's sight and reach
❖ Supervise the toddler constantly; do not expect young children to supervise toddler
❖ Keep Syrup of ipecac on hand to use as directed by Poison Control Center (Keep PCC number near phone)

To Prevent Drowning:
❖ Always supervise the toddler when around water (even if it is just a bucket of water)
❖ Ensure child wears a life vest if boating

(continued)

> **Illness and Injury Prevention:** Advise parents as follows (continued)
>
> **To Prevent Injury from Falls:**
> - ❖ Continue to use gates at top and bottom of stairs, safety devices on windows
> - ❖ Ensure that toddler wears a helmet when riding in a seat on an adult bike
>
> **To Prevent Illness/Disease:**
> - ❖ Keep the toddler's environment smoke free
> - ❖ Put sunscreen on toddler before he/she goes outdoors to play
>
> **To Prevent Other Injuries:**
> - ❖ Teach the child to use caution when approaching dogs
> - ❖ Get down on the floor and check for new hazards now that toddler is walking
> - ❖ Learn child CPR

> **Nutrition:** Advise parents as follows
> - ❖ Child should be sitting in highchair or booster seat eating table foods with the family
> - ❖ Give 2-3 nutritious snacks per day that are rich in complex carbohydrates, and limit sugary and high-fat snacks
> - ❖ Encourage toddler to feed self with hands at first, and then by using utensils as she/he progresses through toddlerhood
> - ❖ Let the toddler develop clear likes and dislikes and do not allow feeding to serve as focus of power struggles
> - ❖ Limit bottle use, avoid use of bottle in bed
> - ❖ Should be weaned from bottle/breast by about 18 months of age
> - ❖ Decrease in appetite is normal (growth slows compared with infancy)
> - ❖ May use whole cow's milk after 12 months of age (Absolutely no low fat milk until the child is ≥ 2 years of age)

> **Oral Health:** Advise parents as follows
> - ❖ Begin brushing child's teeth with a pea-sized amount of toothpaste containing fluoride
> - ❖ Initial dental referral is recommended anytime between 12 months of age and 3 years (AAP)

> **Child Care:** Advise parents as follows
> - ❖ Praise the toddler for good behavior
> - ❖ Encourage language development by reading books, singing songs
> - ❖ Encourage exploration of the environment
> - ❖ Reinforce self-care and self-expression
> - ❖ To promote a sense of competence, invite the toddler to make choices whenever possible
> - ❖ Encourage the toddler to play alone and with playmates, siblings, parents
> - ❖ Set limits and discipline toddlers through distraction, gentle restraint, removal from the situation, "time out," use of routines and structure
> - ❖ Limit the number of rules and enforce them consistently
> - ❖ Anticipate and avoid unnecessary conflicts; do not get into power struggle with child
> - ❖ Discipline the toddler so that he/she understands that hitting, biting are not allowed
> - ❖ Expect the toddler to sleep through night in own bed
> - ❖ Promote learning of self-quieting behaviors through provision of the same transitional object, such as blanket, stuffed animal so toddler can console self at bedtime and in new situations
> - ❖ Do not begin toilet training until child is ready (Dry for periods of about 2 hours, knows the difference between wet and dry and wants to be dry; can pull pants up and down, wants to learn, and can give a signal when voiding/bowel movement is imminent)
> - ❖ Limit television watching to less than one hour day
> - ❖ Anticipate that toddler may touch genitals

V. **Toddlers and Preschoolers: Ages 2 - 5 Years**

    A.   History
        1.   For initial visit, obtain a complete history including prenatal, birth, neonatal, and family history
        2.   For both initial and interval visits, obtain history related to nutrition, sleep, dental hygiene, elimination and sleep patterns, immunization status, relationship with family and playmates, play activities, discipline, child care arrangements, safety, and whether there are smokers in the household
        3.   Ask about parental concerns
        4.   Beginning at about age 4, ask children what questions or concerns they have about their health and bodies
        5.   Beginning at about age 4, screen for abuse and neglect by asking children open-ended questions about their own safety (see the following table)

```
+------------------------------------------------------------+
|                  Screening for Abuse                       |
|  ❖  Are you afraid of anyone?                              |
|  ❖  Does anyone ever hurt you?                             |
|  ❖  Does anyone make you keep secrets?                     |
|                                                            |
|  ❖  All positive responses should be followed up with more |
|     specific questions including, "What happened?" "When   |
|     did it happen?" and "Who did that?"                     |
+------------------------------------------------------------+
```

B. Developmental Surveillance and Milestones
    1. As part of the evaluation, perform a developmental assessment
    2. Based on the items in the "Snapshot" below, ask appropriate history questions, and make appropriate observations to assess the child's development

C. Physical Examination
    1. Measure and plot on growth chart the child's weight for age, height for age, weight-for-height, and head circumference (head circumference is routinely measured on the 2-year visit, but not on subsequent visits)
    2. Any child whose weight gain is inappropriate (not following curve), whose weight is below the third percentile, and whose weight and length differ by more than 2 percentile lines requires further evaluation

A SNAPSHOT OF 2, 3, 4, & 5 YEAR OLD

Age Group	Activities	
2 Year Old	Can go up and down stairs one step at a time Can kick ball Can stack 5-6 blocks Has vocabulary of at least 20 words	Uses two-word phrases Makes or imitates circular strokes with crayon Imitates adults Follows two-step commands
3 Year Old	Jumps in place, kicks a ball, balances on one foot Rides a tricycle Knows own name, age, and gender	Copies a circle and cross Has self-care skills (feeding/dressing) Shows early imaginative behavior
4 Year Old	Can sing a song Knows about things used at home (appliances) Draws a person with 3 parts	Distinguishes fantasy from reality Talks about daily activities Builds a tower of 10 blocks Throws overhand ball
5 Years of Age	Dresses self without help Knows address and phone number Can count on fingers Copies triangle or square	Draws a person with head, body, arms, and legs Recognizes most letters of alphabet Prints some letters Plays make-believe

    3. Head-to-toe examination should be completed on each visit during this age period
    4. Beginning with the 3 year old visit, **objective vision and hearing** screening are recommended
    5. Beginning with the 3 year old visit, **blood pressure** should be measured annually
    6. Always examine the child for evidence of abuse
    7. Provide developmental screening using the Denver II for all children (if possible) and refer any child demonstrating a developmental delay for further evaluation

D. Diagnostic Tests

```
+----------------------------------------------------------------------------------+
| Screening for elevated blood lead levels should be done according to CDC          |
|    recommendations for either universal or targeted screening (see IV.D. for      |
|    guidelines)                                                                     |
| Urinalysis is recommended at 5 years of age but can be done as early as the 4-year |
|    visit (AAP)                                                                      |
| TB skin testing (PPD) is recommended only in children in whom risk factors are     |
|    present                                                                          |
+----------------------------------------------------------------------------------+
```

E. Immunizations: See RECOMMENDED CHILDHOOD IMMUNIZATION SCHEDULE, UNITED STATES, JAN-DEC, 1999 table on page 19

F.   Supplements: See FLUORIDE SUPPLEMENTATION RECOMMENDATIONS table on page 6

G.   Anticipatory Guidance

Illness and Injury Prevention: Advise parents as follows

To Prevent MVA/Other Machine-Related Injuries:
❖ Continue to use an age-appropriate car safety seat or a properly secured booster until the child weighs 60 pounds or his head is higher than the back of the seat (check the law in your state--in Florida, safety seats must be used until child is 5 years of age); seat must be secured in rear seat of car
❖ Supervise all play near streets or driveways
❖ At age 4, teach the child pedestrian and neighborhood safety skills
❖ On entry to kindergarten (age 5) teach the child safety rules for getting to and from school; child should not cross street alone

To Prevent Burn/Scalding Injuries:
❖ Recheck the hot water heater to make certain the thermostat is <120°
❖ Test smoke detector frequently and change battery once a year
❖ Keep the child away from hot stoves, fireplaces, curling irons, space heaters, matches, lighters, or cigarettes
❖ Turn pot handles toward back of stove
❖ Ensure that electric outlets and appliances are inaccessible
❖ Beginning at age 4, conduct fire drills at home

To Prevent Accidental Ingestion/Poisoning:
❖ Keep all poisonous substances including medicines, alcohol, cleaning agents, paints, solvents out of the child's sight and reach
❖ Supervise the child constantly; do not expect young children to supervise preschooler
❖ Keep Syrup of Ipecac in the home to be used as directed by health care professional

To Prevent Drowning:
❖ Always supervise the child when in or near water
❖ Ensure child wears a life vest if boating
❖ At age 4, teach the child to swim but continue to supervise

To Prevent Injury from Falls:
❖ Until the child is at least 3, continue to use gates at top and bottom of stairs, safety devices on windows
❖ Ensure that child wears a helmet when riding in a seat on an adult bike; child should also wear a helmet when riding a tricycle or a bicycle

To Prevent Illness/Disease:
❖ Keep the child's environment smoke free
❖ Put sunscreen on child before he/she goes outdoors to play

To Prevent Other Injuries:
❖ Teach the child to use caution when approaching dogs
❖ Ensure that guns, if in the house, are locked up and that ammunition is stored separately
❖ At about age 2-3, teach child about body parts and good and bad touch
❖ Beginning at age 4 or 5, teach the child about safety rules for interacting with strangers

---

Nutrition: Advise parents as follows
❖ Serve the child meals with the family, with 2-3 nutritious snacks per day
❖ Enforce reasonable mealtime behavior, but do not force the child to eat
❖ Avoid engaging in struggles about eating
❖ See NUTRITION IN CHILDHOOD section for more counseling tips

---

Oral Health: Advise parents as follows
❖ Ensure that child's teeth are brushed twice a day with a pea-size amount of fluoridated toothpaste; parent should continue to brush child's teeth until child is about 5 years of age
❖ Learn how to prevent dental injuries and to handle dental emergencies such as loss or fracture of tooth
❖ Initial dental appointment should occur between 12 months and 3 years of age, with 3 years the preferred age (AAP)

Child Care to Promote Social Competence: Advise parents as follows
❖ Praise child for good behavior and accomplishments
❖ Model appropriate language and encourage language development by reading to child, singing with child, and communicating about what is happening
❖ Spend individual time with the child, playing, walking, talking together
❖ Beginning at about 3 years, encourage child to talk about preschool, friends, or observations
❖ Appreciate the child's inquisitive nature and do not limit his explorations

(continued)

- ❖ Promote physical activity in a safe environment
- ❖ In the 2 year old, encourage parallel play and do not expect shared play
- ❖ Provide opportunities for the 3 and 4 year old to socialize with other children in play groups, preschool
- ❖ By age 4, provide some type of structured learning environment for the child, whether Head Start, preschool, Sunday school
- ❖ Reinforce self-care and self-expression
- ❖ By age 4 or 5, encourage the child to express his/her feeling
- ❖ To promote feelings of competence and control, give child opportunities to make choices whenever possible
- ❖ Reinforce limits and appropriate behavior
- ❖ Use time out or remove source of conflict for unacceptable behavior
- ❖ By age 4 or 5, teach the child how to manage anger and resolve conflicts without violence
- ❖ By age 4 or 5, teach the child to respect authority
- ❖ Encourage self-quieting behaviors
- ❖ Promote toilet training when the child is ready
  - ★ Is dry for periods of 2 hours
  - ★ Wakes up from naps dry
  - ★ Knows the difference between wet and dry and prefers being dry
  - ★ Can pull pants up and down
  - ★ Wants to learn
  - ★ Can signal that needs to void or have bowel movement
- ❖ Limit television watching to less than 1 hour per day

VI. School-Age Children: Ages 6 - 10

A. History
1. For initial visit, obtain a complete history including prenatal, birth, neonatal, and family history
2. For both initial and interval visits, obtain history related to nutrition, sleep, dental hygiene, elimination and sleep patterns, immunization status, relationship with family and playmates, play activities, discipline, child care arrangements, safety, and whether there is a smoker in the household.
3. Ask about parental concerns
4. Discuss sexuality education issues with parents and with child
   a. Beginning at about age 8, ask if parent talks to child about sensitive subjects such as sex
   b. Ask if age-appropriate books relating to sexual education are available in the home for the child to read and ask questions about
   c. At about age 10, ask parent if menstruation has been discussed (girl) or wet dreams (boys); recommend that the topics be discussed now (if not already done)
   d. At age 10, assess the child's preparation for puberty and sexual development
      (1) Determine what the child already knows, and then provide additional information
      (2) Begin to teach the child that delaying sexual behavior is the surest form of protection against disease and pregnancy
      (3) Explore the child's understanding of sexually transmitted diseases, including AIDS
5. Ask child what questions or concerns he/she has about own health and body (**Note:** Beginning at about age 6, the child's role as historian should be fostered so that over the next few years, the parent's role as historian [except for birth history, past medical history, and family history] is relatively diminished as the child's role emerges)
6. Screen for abuse and neglect by asking child open-ended questions about his/her own safety (see following table)

Screening for Abuse
❖ Are you afraid of anyone?
❖ Does anyone ever hurt you?
❖ Does anyone make you keep secrets?
❖ All positive responses should be followed up with more specific questions including, "What happened?" "When did it happen?" and "Who did that?"

B. Developmental Surveillance and School Performance
1. Assessment of the child should include the following areas (**Ask the child**)
   a. **Family:** Ask "Who is in your family?" "How do you get along with your family?" "What kinds of things does your family do for fun?"
   b. **Friends:** Ask "Tell me who your friends are" "Do you have a best friend?" "What do you like to do with your friends?"
   c. **School:** Ask "What grade are you in at school?" "Who is your teacher?" "What do you like best about school?" "What don't you like about school?" (For child who is 8 or 9, "What are your grades?")
   d. **Activities:** Ask "What do you like to do for fun?" "Do you play any sports?"
2. Assessment of child should include the following areas (**Ask the parent**)
   a. **Family:** Ask "Have there been any major changes or stresses in your family since your last visit?" "How does (name) get along with his siblings?" "How are things going in the family?" "What are some of the things you do together as a family?"
   b. **Friends:** Ask "Does (name) have friends he likes to spend time with?" "What sorts of things do they do together?" "When (name) plays with other children, can he keep up with them?"
   c. **School:** Ask "How is (name) attendance at school?" "Does (name) seem to be able to follow the rules at school?" "Do you participate in school activities?" "Have you visited (name) classroom?"
   d. **Activities:** Ask "How does (name) spend her time outside of school [on weekends]?" "How much television does (name) watch each day?" "Does (name) participate in organized sports?" "Who takes (name) to practice and to games?"

C. Physical Examination
1. Measure and plot on growth chart the child's weight for age, height for age, and weight-for-height
2. Any child whose weight gain is inappropriate or whose weight and length differ by more than 2 percentile lines requires further evaluation
3. Head-to-toe examination should be completed on each visit during this age period
4. AAP physical examination screenings that are recommended during this age period in addition to measurements of height and weight are blood pressure and vision and hearing screening (both subjective and objective)
5. Some experts recommend screening for scoliosis during this age period (at age 8); orthopedic referral for curves greater than 15-20 degrees is recommended
6. As part of the complete physical examination, Tanner staging or Sexual Maturity Rating (SMR) should be completed to determine child's pubertal development (see PATTERN OF PUBERTAL DEVELOPMENT table and SEXUAL MATURITY STAGES in section on PRECOCIOUS PUBERTY)
7. Always examine the child for evidence of abuse

D. Diagnostic Tests: None recommended during this age period as part of routine screening; however, consult AAP's (1995) Recommendations for Preventive Pediatric Health Care (see in reference list for recommendations for screening of high-risk children)

E. Immunizations: See RECOMMENDED CHILDHOOD IMMUNIZATION SCHEDULE, UNITED STATES, JAN-DEC 1999 table on page 19

F. Supplements: See FLUORIDE SUPPLEMENTATION RECOMMENDATIONS table on page 6

G.   Anticipatory Guidance

Illness and Injury Prevention: Advise parents as follows

To Prevent MVA/Other Machine-Related Injuries:
❖   Continue to ensure that child wears a seat belt in the car at all times (Child should **not** ride in front seat because of risk of injury from air-bag deployment)
❖   Do not allow the child to operate a power lawn mower or electric tools
❖   Make certain child always wears a helmet when riding a bicycle and follows safety rules for riding bike and crossing street

To Prevent Burn/Scalding Injuries:
❖   Test the smoke detector frequently and change battery once a year
❖   Recheck the hot water heater to make certain the thermostat is <120°
❖   Instruct child what to do in case of fire; conduct fire drills at home

To Prevent Accidental Ingestion/Poisoning:
❖   Warn child about dangers of poisonous substances
❖   Keep all medications out of sight and reach of children; make sure that safety caps are used
❖   Keep Syrup of Ipecac in the home to be used as directed by health care professional; keep Poison Control Center telephone number by phone

To Prevent Drowning:
❖   Teach the child how to swim
❖   Reinforce safety rules for swimming pools and lakes (including wearing of life vest)
❖   Always supervise child when in or near water

To Prevent Injury from Falls:
❖   Discuss playground safety with child
❖   Make certain that helmet is worn when biking

To Prevent Illness/Disease:
❖   Keep the child's environment smoke free
❖   Teach the child how to put on sunscreen and make sure sunscreen is used before child goes outside in the sun for long periods of time

To Prevent Other Injuries:
❖   Anticipate providing less direct supervision as the child moves through this age period
❖   Anticipate that the child may make errors in judgment due to trying to imitate (and impress) peers
❖   Ensure that guns, if in the household, are locked up and that ammunition is stored separately
❖   Reinforce with child safety rules for interacting with strangers
❖   Make certain child is supervised before and after school in a safe environment
❖   Make sure child understands good touch and bad touch and what to do if someone tries to touch him/her in a "bad touch" way

---

Nutrition: See NUTRITION IN CHILDHOOD AND ADOLESCENCE

Oral Health: Advise child/parent as follow
❖   Brush teeth twice a day (parent should continue to supervise until confident child can do alone)
❖   Learn to floss teeth (by age 8)
❖   Learn how to prevent dental injuries and handle dental emergencies
❖   Schedule a dental appointment every 6 months
❖   As the permanent molars erupt, ensure that child is evaluated for application of dental sealants

---

Child Care to Promote Social Competence: Advise parents as follows
❖   Praise the child for cooperation and personal successes
❖   As the child moves through this age period, help him/her choose activities in which success is likely (Help child accept the reality that he/she will be better at some things than others)
❖   Encourage the child to express feelings and to talk with parent about school, friends, successes, and disappointments
❖   Encourage reading and hobbies such as collecting baseball cards, stamps, or making things
❖   Help the child learn how to get along with peers and help child learn how to follow group rules
❖   Promote physical activity in a safe environment
❖   Encourage self-discipline and impulse control; set limits and establish consequences for behavior that is not acceptable
❖   Expect the child to follow family rules such as those for bedtime, television viewing, and chores
❖   Teach the child to respect authority
❖   Ensure the child knows the difference between right and wrong
❖   As the child reaches 9 or 10 years of age, help him/her develop an ability to deal with peer pressure by suggesting strategies and role-playing with the child
❖   Teach the child how to constructively deal with conflict and anger in the family, at school, and in the neighborhood
❖   Provide personal space for the child at home, even if limited

VII. **Adolescence: 11 - 21 Years of Age (Early Adolescence is 11-14; Middle is 15-16; Late is 18-21)**

    A.   History
        1.   Determine your philosophy about seeing the adolescent (adolescent alone or with parent present for at least part of the visit) [As the adolescent transitions through this period, needs for privacy and confidentiality become increasingly important]
        2.   For initial visit, obtain a complete history including prenatal, birth, neonatal, and family history
        3.   For both initial and interval visits, obtain history related to nutrition, sleep, dental hygiene, elimination and sleep patterns, immunization status, relationship with family and playmates, play activities, discipline, child care arrangements and safety
        4.   Ask about parental concerns, particularly for the younger adolescent; once the child is independent from the family (age 18 in most circumstances) role of the family will become very individualized
        5.   Ask adolescent what questions or concerns he/she has about own health and body **(Note: By the time the child enters adolescence, he/she should be the primary historian with the parent supplying information about birth history, past medical history, and family history)**
        6.   Ask adolescent if he/she knows what to expect as body develops
            a.   At visits during Early Adolescence (11-14 years), ask the following questions
                (1)   "Has anyone talked with you about what to expect as your body develops?"
                (2)   "Have you read about changes in your body?"
                (3)   "Do you think you are developing pretty much like the rest of your friends?"
                (4)   "How do you feel about the way you look?"
            b.   At visits during Middle Adolescence (15-17 years), ask the following questions
                (1)   "How do you feel about the way you look?"
                (2)   "Do you think you have developed pretty much like the rest of your friends?"
        7.   Screen for abuse and neglect by asking adolescent open-ended questions about his/her own safety (see following table) **(Note:** These questions should be asked without the parent/care giver present)

Screening for Abuse

- ❖ Are you afraid of anyone?
- ❖ Does anyone ever hurt you?
- ❖ Does anyone make you keep secrets?

- ❖ All positive responses should be followed up with more specific questions including, "What happened?" "When did it happen?" and "Who did that?"

    B.   Developmental Surveillance and School Performance
        1.   Assessment of the adolescent should include the following areas (**Ask the adolescent**)
            a.   **Family:** Ask "Are you the youngest, oldest, or in the middle in your family?" "What is it like to the oldest (youngest or middle) child?" "Who are you closest to in the family?" "How do you get along with your family?" "What kinds of chores do you have around the house?" "How are you punished?"
            b.   **Friends:** Ask "Tell me who your friends are; do you have a best friend?" "What do you like to do with your friends?"
            c.   **Dating/Drug Use:** "Do you have a girlfriend (boyfriend)?" **Approach with a declaration such as** "Some teenagers your age have begun to be sexually active-- what are most of your friends doing about sexual activity?" "How are you and your (boyfriend/girlfriend) handling this?" "I know that drugs are common on school campuses--what drugs are common at your school?" "What drugs do your friends use?" "What drugs do you use?"
            d.   **School:** Ask "Tell me what happens to you on an average day at school?" "What is your favorite class?" "What grade are you in at school?" "Who is your favorite teacher?" "What makes him/her so special?" "Is yours a friendly or a not so friendly school?" "Who do you have to talk with if you are having a problem at school?" "What grades do you make?"
            e.   **Activities:** Ask "What do you like to do for fun?" "Do you play any sports?"

2. Assessment of adolescent should include the following areas (**Ask the parent** during the early-adolescent period [ages 11-14]); by middle adolescence (15-17), many adolescents may see the health care provider without the parent present [**Note**: This does not mean that the role of the parent in adolescence is unimportant; rather this is a time when child is transitioning to more independent role but reliance on parents as a valuable resource is very important]

   a. **Family:** Ask "Have their been any major changes or stresses in your family since your last visit?" "How does (name) get along with his siblings?" "How are things going in the family?" "What are some of the things you do together as a family?"

   b. **Friends:** Ask "Does (name) have friends she likes to spend time with?" "What sorts of things do they do together?"

   c. **Dating/Drugs:** Ask: "Has (name) started dating?" "What has (name) been taught at home or in school about sex (about drugs)?" "Do you think that smoking, drinking, or using drugs is a problem for anyone in your family?"

   d. **School:** Ask "How is (name) attendance at school?" "Does (name) seem to be able to follow the rules at school?" "Do you participate in school activities?" "Have you visited (name) classroom?"

   e. **Activities:** Ask "How does (name) spend her time outside of school [on weekends]?" "How much television does (name) watch each day?" "Does (name) participate in organized sports?" "Do you go to the games?"

3. Use of the HEADSS interview approach is also an excellent way to assess behavior (*H*ome, *E*ducation, *A*ctivities, *D*rugs, *S*ex, and *S*uicide)

HEADSS INTERVIEW APPROACH	
Home:	Ask questions such as those under Family above
Education:	Ask questions such as those under School above
Activities:	Ask questions such as those under Activities above
Drugs:	Ask questions such as those under Dating/Drugs above
Sex:	Ask questions such as those under Dating/Drugs above
Suicide:	Be direct. Ask: "Have you ever thought about killing yourself?"

C. Physical Examination

1. Measure height and weight and determine the body mass index (BMI); using the charts on the next page (Figure 1.1), determine if the adolescent needs further evaluation or counseling regarding his/her weight; blood pressure should be measured at each visit

2. Head-to-toe examination should be completed on each visit during this age period

   a. All sexually active females should receive a pap smear and screening for chlamydia

   b. All females should receive a pap smear at age 18 (regardless of sexual activity history)

3. During this age period, focus on scoliosis screening and assessment of skin for acne and other common dermatoses

4. Always look for evidence of abuse

5. As part of the complete physical examination, Tanner staging or Sexual Maturity Rating (SMR) should be completed to determine adolescent's pubertal development (see PATTERN OF PUBERTAL DEVELOPMENT table and SEXUAL MATURITY STAGES in section on PRECOCIOUS PUBERTY)

6. In males, evaluate for gynecomastia and examine for hernias

7. Vision and hearing screening should be completed at each visit

D. Diagnostic Tests

1. Urinalysis for both males and females, once between ages 11-21 (15 years is the preferred age) [AAP]

2. Hematocrit or hemoglobin for all menstruating adolescents, once between ages 11-21 (15 years is the preferred age) [AAP]

3. High risk adolescents may need additional screening (Refer to the AAP's (1995) Recommendations for Preventive Pediatric Health Care) [see reference list]

E. Immunizations: See RECOMMENDED CHILDHOOD IMMUNIZATION SCHEDULE, UNITED STATES, JAN-DEC, 1999 on page 19

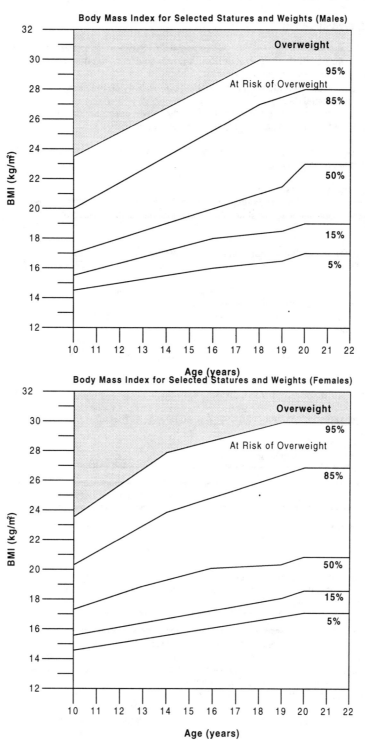

Figure 1.1. Body Mass Index: Age-Based and Gender-Specific Norms.

Source: Green, M. (Ed.). (1994). <u>Bright futures: Guidelines for health supervision of infants, children, and adolescents</u>. Arlington, VA: National Center for Education in Maternal and Child Health, p. 266.

F. Supplements: See FLUORIDE SUPPLEMENTATION RECOMMENDATIONS table on page 6 for adolescents ≤ 16 years of age. All females of childbearing age should receive a multivitamin with folic acid each day

G. Anticipatory Guidance

Illness and Injury Prevention: Advise adolescent regarding the following

To Prevent MVA/Other Machine-Related Injuries:
- ❖ Wear a seat belt in the car (**Accident**s are the leading cause of death in this age group, with deaths from MVAs the leading cause of accidental death)
- ❖ Never drink alcohol while driving and never ride with anyone who has been drinking
- ❖ Always wear a helmet when riding a motorcycle, ATV, or bicycle

To Prevent Burn Injuries:
- ❖ Test the smoke detector (or ask parent to) frequently and change battery once a year
- ❖ Continue to have fire drills at home
- ❖ Do not smoke

To Prevent Accidental Ingestion/Poisoning:
- ❖ Do not use drugs of any kind (most deaths from poisoning occur in young adult males)
- ❖ Do not drink alcohol until legal age in state is reached and then drink in moderation

To Prevent Drowning:
- ❖ Learn how to swim
- ❖ Do not drink alcohol or use drugs when boating or swimming
- ❖ Always wear a life vest when boating

To Prevent Injury from Falls:
- ❖ Wear appropriate safety gear at work and follow job safety procedures
- ❖ Make certain that helmet is worn when biking
- ❖ Wear protective sports gear such as mouth guard, face protector, or helmet when engaged in contact sports

To Prevent Illness/Disease:
- ❖ Avoid tobacco, illicit drug use, and underage drinking
- ❖ Use sunscreen to reduce risk of skin cancer and to decrease photoaging of skin

To Prevent Other Injuries:
- ❖ Avoid high noise levels, particularly in music headsets
- ❖ Do not carry or use a weapon of any kind (**Note**: Homicide is the 2nd leading cause of death in the 15-24 year old age group!)
- ❖ Learn techniques to protect yourself from physical, emotional, sexual abuse, including rape by either strangers or acquaintances
- ❖ Use care in interacting with strangers
- ❖ Avoid gangs and peers involved in unlawful activity

Nutrition: See NUTRITION IN CHILDHOOD AND ADOLESCENCE

Oral Health: Advise adolescent as follows
- ❖ Brush teeth twice a day with pea-size amount of fluorinated toothpaste, and floss daily
- ❖ Schedule a dental appointment every six months
- ❖ Ask the dentist how best to handle dental emergencies such as loss or fracture of tooth
- ❖ Ensure dentist evaluates permanent molars for application of dental sealants
- ❖ Do not smoke or use smokeless tobacco

Promoting Psychosocial Development: Advise adolescent as follows
- ❖ Take on new challenges to increase self-confidence; explore new roles without hurting yourself or others
- ❖ Continue to develop your sense of identity and learning about yourself--what you think, feel, believe in
- ❖ Accept who you are and enjoy both the child and adult in you
- ❖ Talk with a trusted adult or health care professional if you are sad or nervous, or feel that your life is not going right (**Note:** Suicide is the 3rd leading cause of death in the 15-24 year old age group!)
- ❖ Trust your own feelings as well as listening to the ideas of good friends and adults whose opinions you value
- ❖ Understand the importance of your spiritual and religious needs and try to fulfill them
- ❖ Learn to recognize and deal with stress

RECOMMENDED CHILDHOOD IMMUNIZATION SCHEDULE, UNITED STATES, JANUARY – DECEMBER 1999

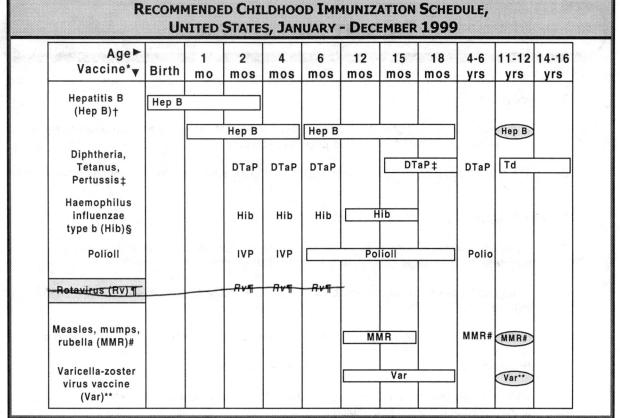

Age ▶ / Vaccine* ▼	Birth	1 mo	2 mos	4 mos	6 mos	12 mos	15 mos	18 mos	4-6 yrs	11-12 yrs	14-16 yrs
Hepatitis B (Hep B)†	Hep B										
		Hep B			Hep B					Hep B	
Diphtheria, Tetanus, Pertussis‡			DTaP	DTaP	DTaP		DTaP‡		DTaP	Td	
Haemophilus influenzae type b (Hib)§			Hib	Hib	Hib	Hib					
PolioII			IVP	IVP		PolioII			Polio		
Rotavirus (RV)¶			Rv¶	Rv¶	Rv¶						
Measles, mumps, rubella (MMR)#						MMR			MMR#	MMR#	
Varicella-zoster virus vaccine (Var)**						Var				Var**	

This schedule has been approved by the Advisory Committee on Immunization Practices (ACIP), the American Academy of Pediatrics and the American Academy of Family Physicians (AAFP). It indicates the recommended ages for routine administration of currently licensed childhood vaccines. Combination vaccines may be used whenever any components of the combination are indicated and its other components are not contraindicated. Providers should consult the manufacturers' package inserts for detailed recommendations.

*–Vaccines are listed under routinely recommended ages. Clear bars indicate range of recommended ages for immunization. Any dose not given at the recommended age should be given as a "catch-up" immunization at any subsequent visit when indicated and feasible. Shaded ovals indicate vaccines to be given if previously recommended doses were missed or given earlier than the recommended minimum age.

†–Infants born to hepatitis B surface antigen (HBsAG)-negative mothers should receive the second dose of hepatitis B vaccine at least one month after the first dose. The third dose should be administered at least four months after the first dose and at least two months after the second dose, but not before six months of age for infants. Infants born to HBsAg-positive mothers should receive hepatitis B vaccine and 0.5 mL hepatitis B immune globulin (HBIG) within 12 hours of birth at separate sites. The second dose is recommended at one to two months of age and the third dose at six months of age. Infants born to mothers wholse HBsAg status is unknown should receive hepatitis B vaccine within 12 hours of birth. Maternal blood should be drawn at the time of delivery to determine the mother's HBsAg status; if the HBsAg test is positive, the infant should receive HBIG as soon as possible (no later than one week of age). All children and adolescents (through 18 years of age) who have not been immunized against hepatitis B may begin the series during any visit. Special efforts should be made to immunize children who were born in or whose parents were born in areas of the world with moderate or high endemicity of hepatitis B virus infection.

‡–Diphtheria and tetanus toxoids and acellular pertussis vaccine (DTaP) is the preferred vaccine for all doses in the immunization series, including completion of the series in children who have received one or more doses of whole-cell diphtheria, tetanus, pertussis (DTP) vaccine. Whole-cell DTP is an acceptable alternative to DTaP. The fourth dose (DTP or DTaP) may be administered as early as 12 months of age, provided six months has elapsed since the third dose and if the child is unlikely to return at age 15 to 18 months. Tetanus and diphtheria toxoids (Td) is recommended at 11 to 12 years of age if at least five years has elapsed since the last dose of DTP, DTaP or DT. Subsequent routine Td boosters are recommended every 10 years.

§–Three Hib conjugate vaccines are licensed for infant use. If PRP-OMP (PedvaxHIB and COMVAX) is administered at two and four months of age, a dose at six months is not required. Because clinical studies in infants have demonstrated that using some combination products may induce a lower immune response to the Hib vaccine component, DTaP/Hib combination products should not be used for primary immunization in infants at two, four, or six months of age, unless it is approved by the U.S. Food and Drug Administration for these ages.

II–Two poliovirus vaccines currently are licensed in the United States: inactivated poliovirus vaccine (IPV) and oral poliovirus vaccine (OPV). The ACIP, AAP, and the AAFP now recommend that the first two doses of poliovirus vaccine should be IPV. The ACIP continues to recommend a sequential schedule of two doses of IPV administered at ages two and four months, followed by two doses of OPV at 12 to 18 months and four to six years. Use of IPV for all doses also is acceptable and is recommended for immunocompromised persons and their household contacts. OPV is no longer recommended for the first two doses of the schedule and is acceptable only for special circumstances such as: children of parents who do not accept the recommended number of injections, late initiation of immunization which would require an unacceptable number of injections, and imminent travel to polio-endemic areas. OPV remains the vaccine of choice for mass immunization campaigns to control outbreaks due to wild poliovirus.

¶–Rotavirus vaccine is shaded and italicized to indicate: 1) health care providers may required time and resources to incorporate this new vaccine into practice; and 2) the AAFP feels that the decision to use rotavirus vaccine should be made by the parent or guardian in consultation with their physician or other health care provider. The first dose of Rv vaccine should not be administered before six weeks of age, and the minimum interval between doses is three weeks. The Rv vaccine series should not be initiated at seven months of age or older, and all doses should be completed by the first birthday.

#–The second dose of MMR vaccine is recommended routinely at four to six years of age but may be administered during any visit, provided at least four weeks has elapsed since receipt of the first dose and that both doses are administered beginning at or after 12 months of age. Those who have not previously received the second dose should complete the schedule by the 11- to 12-year-old visit.

**–Var is recommended at any visit on or after the first birthday for susceptible children, i.e., those who lack a reliable history of chickenpox (as judged by a health care provider) and who have not been immunized. Susceptible persons 13 years of age or older should receive two doses, given at least four weeks apart.

This schedule is provided by the American Academy of Family Physicians only as an assistance for physicians making clinical decisions regarding the care of their patients. As such, they cannot substitute for the individual judgment brought to each clinical situation by the patient's family physician. As with all clinical reference resources, they reflect the best understanding of the science of medicine at the time of publication, but they should be used with the clear understanding that continued research may result in new knowledge and recommendations.

INFANT NUTRITION

I. The process of feeding

    A.   The process of feeding provides important opportunities for social interaction between parent and child; feeding is emotional as well as physical nourishment

    B.   The feeding situation is a good barometer of overall satisfaction in the relationship between infant and parent

II. Nutrient Requirements

    A.   Infancy is a period of very rapid growth and a high surface-area to volume ratio makes requirements for energy, protein, and water especially great

    B.   During first 3 months, infants gain about one ounce per day, slowing to a little less than that between ages 3-6 months

    C.   Full term infants require 110 to 120 Cal/kg and 150 to 180 mL of fluid per kilogram each day

    D.   Breast milk and infant formulas provide approximately 20 Cal/oz

    E.   Infants should be fed breast milk exclusively for the first six months of life, with iron-enriched solid foods added at 6 months to complement the breast milk diet

    F.   The American Academy of Pediatrics (AAP) recommends breast milk as the preferred source of feeding for almost all babies for at least the first year of life

    G.   Nutrient requirements during first 6 months of life can also be met by a commercially prepared formula if the mother is unable or unwilling to breastfeed

III. Breastfeeding

    A.   Benefits of breastfeeding
        1.   Breast milk is a better source of nutrition than infant formula, according to the AAP
        2.   Counsel parent that breast-fed infants develop fewer gastrointestinal infections, respiratory illnesses and allergic reactions than do formula-fed infants
        3.   Emphasize that breast milk contains no preservatives, is readily available, and is always the right temperature

    B.   Composition of human milk
        1.   Colostrum, produced during first few days after delivery, provides enzymes that promote gut maturation and facilitate digestion
        2.   Colostrum is high in protein mainly due to immunoglobulins and secretory IgA
        3.   Human milk has less protein than cow's milk and the protein is much more digestible; fat composition in human milk allows for excellent fat and calcium absorption; lactose is present in higher concentrations in human milk than in any other mammal
        4.   Breast milk is rich in vitamins A, C, and E, but low in vitamin D; breast milk of vegetarian females may be deficient in vitamins B_6 and B_{12} unless their diet is supplemented with these vitamins
        5.   Breast milk is low in iron, but the iron is so completely utilized that breast-fed babies need no iron supplementation until 6 months of age (iron-fortified cereals should be added at 6 months of age)
        6.   Breast milk is low in fluoride; however, fluoride supplementation is not recommended for infants under six months of age. Infants over 6 months of age may need fluoride supplements depending on their water supply

7. Advise lactating females to avoid all over-the-counter drugs and to remind health care provider that she is breastfeeding

C. Feeding schedule
1. Advise the mother to allow infant to nurse every 2-3 hours during the first weeks, and to decrease the number of feedings according to the infant's signals as the milk supply increases
2. Advise the mother that each feeding may take 30 minutes or more
3. Advise that the infant should nurse on the second side (after the first side is empty) until vigorous sucking subsides
4. Breastfed infants should have 6-8 wet diapers per day and may produce a soft, seedy, yellow stool after each feeding

D. Supplementary feeding
1. Advise using either expressed milk or formula for occasional supplementary feedings
2. Discourage offering the infant a bottle after breastfeeding
3. Encourage breastfeeding throughout the first year

E. Resources for Breastfeeding Information

Books
❖ Huggins, K. (1990). The Nursing Mothers's Companion. Harvard, MA: Harvard Common Press.
❖ Mason, D., & Ingersoll, D. (1986). Breastfeeding and the Working Mother. New York: St Martin's Press.
❖ Reukauf, D.M., & Trause, M.A. (1988). Commonsense Breastfeeding: A Practical Guide to the Pleasures, Problems, and Solutions. New York: Athenaeum.
❖ Lawrence, R.A. (1994). Breastfeeding: A Guide for the Medical Profession. St. Louis: Mosby
Pamphlets
❖ Childbirth Graphics, Ltd., P.O. Box 20540, Rochester, NY 14602.
   ✦ Danner, S.C., & Cerutti, E. Nursing Your Baby for the First Time.
   ✦ Danner, S.C., & Cerutti, E. Nursing Your Baby Beyond the First Days.
   ✦ Danner, S.C., & Cerutti, E. Expressing Breastmilk.

IV. Formula Feeding

A. Examples of commercially prepared formulas are Enfamil, Similac, and SMA. **Only iron-fortified formulas should be used!**
1. When using the iron-fortified versions of commercially prepared formula, no vitamin, mineral, or water supplementation are needed
2. Formulas come in 3 forms: powder, liquid concentrate, and ready-to-feed
3. Ready-to-feed is most expensive; powder is least expensive, but the hardest of the 3 to prepare
4. Instruct mother about preparation and refrigeration of formula
5. Formula taken from refrigerator does not need to be warmed before feeding
6. Warn against warming formula in microwave which can result in esophageal burns due to overheating
7. Bottle-fed infants should have 6-8 wet diapers per day and stools are typically tan to yellow in color, and are about the same consistency as peanut butter; may be less frequent than in breastfed infants

B. Feeding schedule: The following pattern is usually established:

Age (months)	Number of Feedings/Day (24 hours)	Ounces/Feeding
Birth-1	6-8	2-4
2-6	5-6	5-7
7-10	3-4	8
11-12	3-4	8

V. Whole Cow's Milk

    A. Not recommended for infants <12 months of age

    B. Low fat milk should not be given to infants <2 years of age

VI. Introduction of Solid Food

    A. Should be based on readiness of infant and **not before** 6 months of age

    B. Suggested ages and pattern for the introduction of semisolid food and table foods are contained in the table below

6 months	Cereals and fruits
7 months	Meats and vegetables
7-8 months	Egg yolks
8-9 months	Egg whites

    C. Suggest introduction of one food at a time, allowing the infant time to express acceptance or rejection of that food before introducing another

    D. Intake from formula between 6-12 months should be no more than 28-32 oz/day

    E. Fruit juice should be limited to 1-2 ounces per day and should not be used to quench thirst; instead, the infant who is thirsty should be offered water, not juice

NUTRITION IN CHILDHOOD AND ADOLESCENCE

I. **Toddlers and Preschoolers**: Counsel parents based on following

    A. During toddlerhood and the preschool years growth slows and appetite is often diminished

    B. Balance diet by week instead of day

    C. Generally children in the age group eat about 1 tbsp/year of age of each food served to family (e.g., 3 year old eats 3 tbsp of spaghetti and 3 tbsp of salad)

    D. Toddlers and preschoolers usually dislike casseroles and are very sensitive to colors and textures of food

II. **School-aged Children**: Counsel parents/child based on following

    A. Growth is steady during this time period and energy requirements are high

    B. Limit dietary fat to 30% or less of total calories. (Between 40-55% of calories in "fast food" meals come from fat)

    C. Lunches packed for school should contain variety, be low in sugar and fat, and high in complex carbohydrates
        1. Use whole-grain breads, bagels, and pita bread
        2. Avoid processed meats (bologna and salami) which are high in saturated fat and salt
        3. Use mustard instead of mayonnaise for a low-fat, low-calorie flavor booster

    D. Between-meal snacks are important and should consist of fresh fruits and vegetables; salt, simple sugars, and fats should be minimized

E.   Proper nutritional intake can be assured by offering child a variety of healthy foods, not by encouraging child to eat everything on his/her plate. **Remember!** Obesity is the major nutritional problem among children

III.   **Adolescents**: Counsel parents/teen based on the following

A.   Growth spurt during this time period requires increased calories, protein, carbohydrates, and fat

B.   During the year of the greatest rate of growth in height (about age 12 in girls and 14 in boys) about 2400 calories/day are required by females and 3000 by males

C.   Energy needs decline slightly after the growth spurt and by the end of puberty, about 200-300 fewer calories are needed, depending on activity level

D.   On average, about 25% of teen's calories come from snacks
   1.   Important to keep healthy snacks on hand in convenient forms
   2.   Examples are low-fat yogurt, rice cakes, sliced raw vegetables, fresh fruit, and low-fat cottage cheese

E.   There is an increased need for iron in both boys and girls: boys because of increase in muscle mass and blood volume; girls because of menstrual loss. The following foods should be encouraged:
   1.   Red meats (lean, of course) and green vegetables are good iron sources
   2.   Iron fortified cereals (drink orange juice with cereal and double or triple iron absorption)
   3.   Peanut butter and dried fruits are also important sources
   4.   Cook in cast iron skillet to increase iron content of food

F.   Vegetarian diets may not provide enough of some nutrients and counseling may be necessary to help vegetarians plan an adequate diet. Refer patient to a dietician for expert advice

G.   Prevalence of obesity is 11-15% during adolescence. Prevention is important; the following should be emphasized
   1.   Use baked or broiled foods, not fried
   2.   Use low fat dairy products
   3.   Avoid concentrated sugars

IV.   Instruct parents of children ≥5 years of age/adolescents in how to use the Food Guide Pyramid to put dietary guidelines into action (see Figure 1.2)

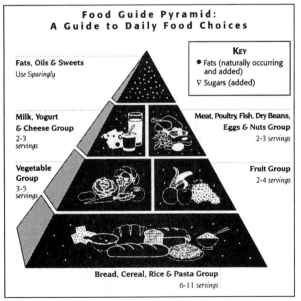

Figure 1.2. Food Guide Pyramid.

Source: US Department of Agriculture. Department of Health and Human Services. (1995). <u>Nutrition and you health: Dietary guidelines for Americans</u>. Washington, DC: Author, p. 4.

A. Most of the daily servings of food should be chosen from the food groups that are the largest in the picture and closest to the base of the pyramid

B. Most of the foods eaten each day should come from the grain products group (6-11 servings), the vegetable group (3-5 servings), and the fruit group (2-4 servings)

C. Only moderate amounts of foods should come from the milk group (2-3 servings) and meat and beans group (2-3 servings)

D. Foods high in fat and sugar should be used sparingly

WHAT'S IN A SERVING?		
Bread group	1 slice bread 1 oz ready-to-eat cereal	1/2 c cooked cereal, rice, or pasta
Fruit group	1 medium-sized piece of fruit or 1 melon wedge 1/2 c chopped, cooked, or canned fruit	3/4 c 100% fruit juice 1/4 c dried fruit
Vegetable group	1 c raw leafy vegetables 3/4 c vegetable juice	1/2 c other vegetables (cooked or raw)
Meat group	2-3 oz cooked lean meat, fish, or poultry 1-1 1/2 c of cooked dry beans	1 egg 2 tbsp peanut butter
Milk group	1 c milk or yogurt 1 1/2 oz natural cheese	2 oz processed cheese

V. Assist parents/adolescents to develop skills in eating healthy/ they must

A. Develop an awareness of current eating habits

B. Identify problem behaviors (eating high-calorie, high-fat foods that are low in nutritional value)

C. Learn ways to modify current eating habits; parents/adolescents should make a few, small permanent changes at a time, making additional changes only after previous changes are firmly in place

PREPARTICIPATION SPORTS EXAMINATION

I.   Definition: A sports-specific evaluation emphasizing recent injuries and/or any health condition affecting sports participation

II.   Overview of Evaluation

    A.   Objectives of evaluation
        1.   Help maintain the health and safety of athletes during both training and competition
        2.   Identify those athletes who need further conditioning, require further evaluation prior to clearance, or who require exclusion from a specific sport
        3.   Meet legal and insurance requirements

    B.   Timing of evaluation
        1.   Ideally, timing of the preparticipation examination should occur at least 6 weeks prior to preseason practice
        2.   Adequate time is needed to provide for conditioning, rehabilitation, or further evaluation, if needed

III. History

    A.   The history is the cornerstone of the evaluation and a thorough history will identify approximately 75% of problems affecting athletic participation
    B.   If possible, the athlete (and parents) should complete the history form prior to the examination, and the health care provider should review the history with the athlete at the time of the exam
    C.   Use a history form such as the one that follows which emphasizes the areas of greatest concern for sports participation

PREPARTICIPATION PHYSICAL EVALUATION

HISTORY	DATE OF EXAM _____

Name _____ Sex _____ Age _____ Date of birth _____

Grade _____ School _____ Sport(s) _____

Address_____ Phone _____

Personal health care provider _____

In case of emergency, contact

Name _____ Relationship _____ Phone (H) _____ (W) _____

Explain "Yes" answers below.
Circle questions you don't know the answers to.

	Yes	No
1. Have you had a medical illness or injury since your last check up or sports physical?	❏	❏
Do you have an ongoing or chronic illness?	❏	❏
2. Have you ever been hospitalized overnight?	❏	❏
3. Are you currently taking any prescription or nonprescription (over-the-counter) medications or pills or using an inhaler?	❏	❏
Have you ever taken any supplements or vitamins to help you gain or lose weight or improve your performance?	❏	❏
4. Do you have any allergies (for example, to pollen, medicine, food, or stinging insects)?	❏	❏
Have you ever had a rash or hives develop during or after exercise?	❏	❏
5. Have you ever passed out during or after exercise?	❏	❏
Have you ever been dizzy during or after exercise?	❏	❏
Have you ever had chest pain during or after exercise?	❏	❏
Do you get tired more quickly than your friends do during exercise?	❏	❏
Have you ever had racing of your heart or skipped heartbeats?	❏	❏
Have you had high blood pressure or high cholesterol?	❏	❏
Have you ever been told you have a heart murmur?	❏	❏
Has any family member or relative died of heart problems or of sudden death before age 50?	❏	❏
Have you had a severe viral infection (for example, myocarditis or mononucleosis) within the last month?	❏	❏
Has a physician ever denied or restricted your participation in sports for any heart problems?	❏	❏
6. Do you have any current skin problems (for example, itching, rashes, acne, warts, fungus, or blisters)?	❏	❏
7. Have you ever had a head injury or concussion?	❏	❏
Have you ever been knocked out, become unconscious, or lost your memory?	❏	❏
Have you ever had a seizure?	❏	❏
Do you have frequent or severe headaches?	❏	❏
Have you ever had numbness or tingling in your arms, hands, legs, or feet?	❏	❏
Have you ever had a stinger, burner, or pinched nerve?	❏	❏
8. Have you ever become ill from exercising in the heat?	❏	❏
9. Do you cough, wheeze, or have trouble breathing during or after activity?	❏	❏
Do you have asthma?	❏	❏
Do you have seasonal allergies that required medical treatment?	❏	❏

	Yes	No
10. Do you use any special protective or corrective equipment or devices that aren't usually used for your sport or position (for example, knee brace, special neck roll, foot orthotics, retainer on your teeth, hearing aid?	❏	❏
11. Have you had any problems with your eyes or vision?	❏	❏
12. Have you ever had a sprain, strain, or swelling after injury?	❏	❏
Have you broken or fractured any bones or dislocated any joints?	❏	❏
Have you had any other problems with pain or swelling in muscles, tendons, bones, or joints?	❏	❏
If yes, check appropriate box and explain below.		

❏ Head	❏ Elbow	❏ Hip
❏ Neck	❏ Forearm	❏ Thigh
❏ Back	❏ Wrist	❏ Knee
❏ Chest	❏ Hand	❏ Shin/calf
❏ Shoulder	❏ Finger	❏ Ankle
❏ Upper arm		❏ Foot

	Yes	No
13. Do you want to weigh more or less than you do now?	❏	❏
Do you lose weight regularly to meet weight requirements for your sport?	❏	❏
14. Do you feel stressed out?	❏	❏

15. Record dates of your most recent immunizations (shots) for:

Tetanus _____ Measles _____

Hepatitis B _____ Chickenpox _____

FEMALES ONLY

16. When was your first menstrual period? _____

When was your most recent menstrual period? _____

How much time do you usually have from the start of one period to the start of another? _____

How many periods have you had in the last year? _____

What was the longest time between periods in the last year? _____

Explain "Yes" answers here: _____

_____

_____

_____

_____

_____

_____

_____

_____

_____

_____

_____

Source: American Academy of Family Physicians. (1997). Preparticipation physical evaluation. New York: McGraw-Hill, p. 47. (Reprinted by permission)

I hereby state that, to the best of my knowledge, my answers to the above questions are complete and correct.

Signature of athlete _____ Signature of parent/guardian _____ Date _____

IV.   Physical Examination

A.   The physical exam is a screening tool emphasizing the areas of greatest concern in sports participation and areas identified in the history

B.   Use a physical examination form such as the one that follows which emphasizes the areas of greatest concern for sports participation

C.   Orthopedic screening deserves special attention. Use the general musculoskeletal screening examination that follows

PREPARTICIPATION PHYSICAL EVALUATION

PHYSICAL EXAMINATION

Name _____ Date of birth _____

Height _____ Weight_____ % Body fat (optional) _____ Pulse _____ BP ___/___ (___/___, ___/___)

Vision R 20/_____ L 20/_____   Corrected: Y   N   Pupils: Equal _____ Unequal _____

	NORMAL	ABNORMAL FINDINGS	INITIALS*
MEDICAL			
Appearance			
Eyes/Ears/Nose/Throat			
Lymph Nodes			
Heart			
Pulses			
Lungs			
Abdomen			
Genitalia (males only)			
Skin			
MUSCULOSKELETAL			
Neck			
Back			
Shoulder/arm			
Elbow/forearm			
Wrist/hand			
Hip/thigh			
Knee			
Leg/ankle			
Foot			

*Station-based examination only

❐   **Cleared**

❐   **Cleared after completing evaluation/rehabilitation for:** _____

_____

_____

❐   **Not cleared for:** _____ **Reason:** _____

Recommendations: _____

_____

_____

Name of health care provider (print/type) _____ **Date** _____

Address _____ **Phone** _____

Signature of health care provider _____

Source: American Academy of Family Physicians. (1997). Preparticipation physical evaluation. New York: McGraw-Hill, p. 48. (Reprinted by permission)

GENERAL MSK SCREENING EXAMINATION

Instructions	Observations
Stand facing examiner	Acromioclavicular joints, general habitus, symmetry of trunk, upper extremities
Look at ceiling, floor, over both shoulders; touch ears to shoulders	Cervical spine motion
Shrug shoulders (examiner resists)	Trapezius strength
Abduct shoulders 90° (examiner resists at 90°)	Deltoid strength
Full external rotation of arms	Shoulder range of motion
Flex and extend elbows	Elbow range of motion
Arms at sides, elbows 90° flexed; pronate and supinate wrists	Elbow and wrist range of motion
Spread fingers; make fist	Range of motion, hands and fingers
Tighten (contract) quadriceps; relax quadriceps	Symmetry and knee effusion; ankle effusion
"Duck walk" 4 steps (away from examiner with buttocks on heels)	Mobility of hip, knee and ankle; strength & balance
Back to examiner, bending forward at waist	Shoulder symmetry, scoliosis
Knees straight, touch toes	Scoliosis, hip motion, hamstring tightness
Raise up on toes, raise heels	Calf symmetry, leg strength

Adapted from American Academy of Family Physicians. (1997). Preparticipation physical evaluation. New York: McGraw-Hill.

V. Diagnostic Tests

    A.   Routine laboratory screening tests in asymptomatic athletes are not required

    B.   Findings from the health history or physical examination may indicate a need to arrange specific diagnostic test

VI. Plan/Management

    A.   Individuals with the following conditions may **not** participate in sports
        1.   **Carditis.** This condition may result in sudden death with exertion
        2.   **Fever.** Fever can increase cardiopulmonary effort, reduce exercise capacity, increase heat intolerance, and predispose to orthostatic hypotension during exercise
        3.   **Diarrhea.** Unless mild, diarrhea may increase the risk of dehydration and heat illness

    B.   Individuals with the following conditions **always require further evaluation** before clearance can be obtained; some sports may not be possible for some persons

CONDITIONS THAT REQUIRE FURTHER EVALUATION TO ASSESS THE SAFETY OF A GIVEN SPORT FOR A PARTICULAR ATHLETE

Cardiovascular Disorders	Hypertension Congenital heart disease Dysrhythmia	Mitral valve prolapse Heart murmur
Neurologic Disorders	Cerebral palsy Convulsive disorder, poorly controlled	History of serious head or spine trauma, severe of repeated concussions, or craniotomy
Respiratory Disorders	Pulmonary compromise, including CF	Acute upper respiratory infection
Hematologic Disorders	Bleeding disorders	Sickle cell disease

(continued)

CONDITIONS THAT REQUIRE FURTHER EVALUATION TO ASSESS THE SAFETY OF A GIVEN SPORT FOR A PARTICULAR ATHLETE (CONTINUED)		
Eyes	Loss of an eye	History of serious eye injury
Genitourinary	Absence of one kidney	
Musculoskeletal	Any MSK disorder	Atlantoaxial instability
Skin	Boils Herpes simplex Impetigo	Scabies Molluscum contagiosum
Gastrointestinal	Enlarged spleen	Enlarged liver
Behavioral	Obesity Anorexia nervosa	Bulimia nervosa

C.   Individuals with the following conditions should not be excluded from participation in sports solely on the basis of the condition

CONDITIONS NOT NECESSARILY PRECLUDING PARTICIPATION IN SPORTS	
Endocrine	Diabetes mellitus (with proper attention to diet, hydration, and insulin therapy)
Immunocompromised	HIV infection (all sports may be played so long as the person is able)
Genitourinary	Absence of one ovary Absent or undescended testicle
Respiratory	Asthma (with proper medication and education, only athletes with severe asthma will need to modify participation)
Hematologic	Sickle cell trait
Neurological	Convulsive disorder, well controlled (risk of convulsion during participation is minimal)

D.   A preparticipation clearance form such as the one that follows can be used to make recommendations regarding participation

PREPARTICIPATION PHYSICAL EVALUATION

CLEARANCE FORM

☐ **Cleared**

☐ **Cleared after completing evaluation/rehabilitation for:** _____

_____

_____

_____

☐ **Not cleared for:** _____   **Reason:** _____

Recommendations: _____

_____

_____

_____

Name of health care provider (print/type) _____ **Date** _____

Address _____ **Phone** _____

Signature of health care provider _____

Source: American Academy of Family Physicians. (1997). Preparticipation physical evaluation. New York: McGraw-Hill, p. 49. (Reprinted by permission)

E. Be aware of the medicolegal considerations when performing preparticipation physical evaluations
   1. Many athletes (and their parents) are unwilling to accept restrictions in sport participation
       a. A second medical opinion may be sought or an attorney may be retained
       b. Under the Rehabilitation Act of 1973, and the Americans with Disabilities Act of 1990, athletes may have the legal right to participate against medical advice
   2. Health care providers who recommend restricted participation or exclusion from a sport should consult with experts in the medical condition in question to assist in determining the risk to the athlete of participating in the desired sport
       a. This approach limits the likelihood that the athlete will be inappropriately excluded from the sport
       b. This approach also reassures the athlete and parents if restriction or exclusion is indeed the correct course
       c. Finally, such an approach provides liability protection for the health care provider who is making the recommendation

DENTAL HEALTH MAINTENANCE

I. Tooth Preservation is a Lifelong Process

   A. Maintaining good oral hygiene is important throughout life because poor oral hygiene can lead to gingival recession, increased tooth mobility, and eventual tooth loss

   B. Parents may cleanse the gums of infants by wrapping a piece of gauze around their finger and gently rubbing over gums and first teeth

   C. Generally, children are unable to clean their own teeth before the age of 7-8 years

II. Tooth Care Steps: Brushing and Flossing

   A. Brushing at margin of teeth and gums with a soft-textured, multi-tufted nylon bristle toothbrush is recommended after every meal or at least twice a day
       1. Recommend placing brush on gumline at a 45 degree angle, and then brushing gums and teeth with an elliptical motion
       2. Stress that thoroughness, rather than vigor, is the key
       3. For patients who have difficulty holding the toothbrush, suggest use of a sponge on adhesive tape to enlarge toothbrush handle diameter
       4. Use of fluorinated toothpaste in any age group speeds up remineralization, the process by which tooth enamel absorbs calcium and phosphorous
       5. Note: While some recent studies suggest that fluoride accumulated in bone over a lifetime may increase risk of hip fracture and osteoporosis in persons over 65, the data are conflicting, and intake of appropriate levels of fluoride do not appear to have this effect

   B. Flossing teeth after every meal can reduce plaque formation and may be even more important than brushing
       1. Explain that waxed or unwaxed products are equally effective
       2. For a better grip on dental floss, suggest use of a commercial dental floss holder

   C. For patients who cannot brush or floss after a meal, teach them to swish vigorously with a mouthful of water
       1. Swishing with water washes away food particles and reduces mouth bacteria by 30%
       2. In addition, swishing helps neutralize enamel-attaching acids

III. Dental Visits

A. Regular visits to a dentist for evaluation and oral health counseling should be scheduled at least once a year

B. Visits are to be initiated at 12 months of age even if significant problems are not evident

IV. Nutrition

A. Oral health is significantly influenced by diet

B. High sugar foods are to be discouraged in the diet
1. Advise patients to avoid foods that have a high sugar content, particularly ones that are sticky
2. Suitable between meal snacks are fresh fruits and vegetables which have a low caries potential index

V. Chronology of Dentition in Children and Adolescents

Primary Dentition	Age of Eruption (in months)	Age of Exfoliation (in years)
Upper (maxillary)		
Central incisor	7.5	6-7
Lateral incisor	9	7-8
Cuspid	18	10-11
First molar	14	9-11
Second molar	24	10-12
Lower (mandibular)		
Central incisor	6	6-7
Lateral incisor	7	7-8
Cuspid	16	9-12
First molar	12	9-11
Second molar	20	10-12

Permanent Dentition	Age of Eruption (in years)	
Upper (maxillary)		
Central incisor	7-8	
Lateral incisor	8-9	
Cuspid	11-12	
1st bicuspid	10-11	
2nd bicuspid	10-12	
1st molar	6-7	
2nd molar	12-13	
3rd molar	17-21	
Lower (mandibular)		
Central incisor	6-7	
Lateral incisor	7-8	
Cuspid	9-10	
1st bicuspid	10-12	
2nd bicuspid	11-12	
1st molar	6-7	
2nd molar	11-13	
3rd molar	17-21	

VI. Fluoride Supplementation

A. Fluoride supplements can result in reductions of 35-40% in incidence of tooth decay among children

B. Recommended fluoride dosage schedule (mg/day) based on concentrations of fluoride in drinking water is in table above under CHILD HEALTH SUPERVISION section

REFERENCES

American Academy of Pediatrics, Committee on Environmental Health. (1998). Screening for elevated blood lead levels. Pediatrics, 101, 1072-1077.

American Academy of Pediatrics, Committee on Infectious Diseases. (1999). Recommended childhood immunizations schedule, Jan-Dec 1999. Pediatrics, 103, 182-183.

Americans Academy of Pediatrics, Press Release. (1997, Dec). AAP releases new breast feeding recommendations. Elk Grove Village, IL: Author.

American Academy of Pediatric Dentistry. (1994). Recommendations for preventive pediatric dental care. Pediatric Dentistry, 15(7), 39.

American Academy of Family Physicians. (1997). Preparticipation physical evaluation. Minneapolis, MN: McGraw Hill.

American Academy of Pediatrics, Committee on Genetics. (1996). Newborn screening fact sheets. Pediatrics, 98, 473-477.

American Academy of Pediatrics, Committee on Infectious Diseases. (1997). Red book: Report of the committee on infectious diseases (24th ed.). Elk Grove Village, IL: Author.

American Academy of Pediatrics, Committee on Nutrition. (1998). Cholesterol in childhood. Pediatrics, 101, 141-147.

American Academy of Pediatrics, Committee on Practice and Ambulatory Medicine. (1995). Recommendations for preventive pediatric health care. Elk Grove Village, IL: Author.

American Dietetic Association. (1996). Complete food and nutrition guide. Minneapolis, MN: Chronimed Publishing.

Bedinghaus, J.M., & Melniknow, J. (1992). Promoting successful breast-feeding skills. American Family Physician, 45(3), 1309-1318.

Boyle, W.E., & Hoekelman, R.A. (1997). The pediatric history. In R.A. Hoekelman (Ed.), Pediatric primary care. St. Louis: Mosby.

Brangman, S.A. (1992). The mouth. In R.J. Ham & P.D. Sloan (Eds.), Primary care geriatrics: A case-based approach. St. Louis: Mosby.

Bromberg, D.I. (1997). Interviewing children. In R.A. Hoekelman (Ed.), Pediatric primary care. St. Louis: Mosby.

Cassamassimo, P. (1996). Bright futures in practice: Oral health. Arlington, VA: National Center for Education in Maternal Health.

Centers for Disease Control. (1997). Screening young children for lead poisoning. Guidance for state and local public health officials. Atlanta: Author.

Dixon, S.D., & Stein, M.T. (1992). Encounters with children: Pediatric behavior and development. St. Louis: Mosby.

Eiger, M.S. (1997). The feeding of infants and children. In R.A. Hoekelman (Ed.), Pediatric primary care. St. Louis: Mosby.

Berkowitz, R.J., & Den Besten, P.K. (1997). Prevention of dental caries. In R.A. Hoekelman (Ed.), Pediatric primary care. St. Louis: Mosby.

Gordon, S.R. (1990). Oral and dental problems. In R.W. Schrier (Ed.), Geriatric medicine. Philadelphia: Saunders.

Green, M. (Ed.). (1994). Bright futures: Guidelines for health supervision of infants, children, and adolescents. Arlington, VA: National Center for Education in Maternal and Child Health.

Grimm, K.C. (1999). The well-child visit. In R.A. Dershewitz (Ed.), Ambulatory pediatric care. Philadelphia: Lippincott.

Hergenroeder, A.C. (1997). The preparticipation sports examination. Pediatric Clinics of North America, 44, 1525-1540.

Igra, V., & Millstein, S.G. (1993). Current status and approaches to improving preventive services for adolescents. Journal of the American Medical Association, 269(11), 1408-1412.

Must, A. (1992). Long-term morbidity and mortality of overweight adolescents: A follow up of the Harvard growth study of 1922 to 1935. New England Journal of Medicine, 327, 1350-1355.

Pless, I.B., & Pless, C.E. (1997). Morbidity and mortality among the young. In R.A. Hoekelman (Ed.), Primary pediatric care. St. Louis: Mosby.

Snelling, A.M. (1997, Apr). A concise guide to nutrition counseling. Patient Care, 47-53.

Tigges, B.B. (1997). Infant formulas: Practical answers for common questions. Nurse Practitioner, 22(8), 70-87.

US Department of Agriculture, Department of Health and Human Services. (1995). Nutrition and your health: Dietary guidelines for Americans. Washington, DC: Author.

US Preventive Services Task Force. (1996). Guide to clinical preventive services (2nd ed.). Baltimore: Williams & Wilkins.

General

FEVER

I. Definition of fever: Traditionally defined as body temperature greater than 38.0°C (100.4°F) rectally, 37.8°C (100°F) orally, or 37.2°C (99°F) axillary; more recently defined as early morning body temperature (measured orally) ≥37.2° (≥99.0°) or a temperature of ≥37.8° (≥100°) (see table that follows for conversion of temperature)

CONVERSION OF TEMPERATURE		
37°C	=	98.6°F
38°C	=	100.4°F
39°C	=	102.2°F
40°C	=	104.0°F

A. Fever without localizing signs (source): unexplained fever of brief duration or lasting <5-7 days; source of acute febrile illness is not apparent after a careful history and physical examination (see FEVER WITHOUT LOCALIZING SOURCE section)

B. Fevers of unknown origin (FUO): fever persisting for 3 weeks, > 101°F and eluding one week of intensive diagnostic testing

II. Pathogenesis of Fever

A. Fever occurs when bacteria, viruses, toxins, or other agents are phagocytosed by leukocytes

B. Then, interluekin-1 and other chemical mediators (previously referred to as endogenous pyrogens) are produced and activate the production of prostaglandins

C. Prostaglandins act on the thermoregulatory mechanism in the hypothalamus and upwardly readjust the body's thermostat

D. Raising the hypothalamic set-point initiates the process of heat production and conservation by increasing metabolism, triggering peripheral vasoconstriction, and less frequently by triggering shivering which increases heat production from the muscles

E. Infection is the most common cause of fever in both adults and children; most infections are viral in etiology

F. Other causes include the following:
1. Hypersensitivity to drugs
2. Recent immunizations with certain vaccines
3. Vascular occlusive and/or inflammatory events such as deep vein thrombophlebitis, pulmonary emboli, or myocardial infarction
4. Acute hemolytic episodes associated with acute autoimmune hemolytic anemia or sickle cell anemia
5. Neoplasms
6. Collagen-vascular diseases
7. Central nervous system abnormalities

G. Occasionally, a patient may have a factitious fever or a high reading on the thermometer which was artificially produced by the patient for secondary gains

H. True fever must be differentiated from hyperthermia
1. Hyperthermia occurs when there is increased body temperature but no alteration in the hypothalamic set point

2. Hyperthermia may be due to increased metabolic heat (e.g., thyrotoxicosis), excessive environmental temperature (e.g., heat stroke), defective heat loss because of environmental conditions (e.g. high humidity, overdressing, sitting in unventilated, sunny car, exercise), or dermatologic disorder (e.g., ectodermal dysplasia)

III. Clinical Presentation

A. Fever, by itself, is not a illness; rather, a sign that the body is fighting an infection or reacting to a stimulus; normal temperatures are characterized by the following:
1. Temperature is usually highest around 6 pm and lowest around 6 am
2. Normal temperature deviations occur with physical activity, stress, ovulation, and environmental heat

B. Typical symptoms include malaise, fatigue, myalgias, and tachycardia (pulse rate is often elevated by about 10-15 beats per $1\,^{\circ}$C of fever)

C. Central nervous system symptoms may occur ranging from mild changes in alertness to delirium, particularly in the young children and chronically-ill patients

D. Children's normal temperature varies from adults
1. Infants tend to have higher normal temperatures than older children; infants often has subtle signs and symptoms: pallor, anorexia and irritability may be the only abnormalities present
2. Children will often have adaptive withdrawal or decreased activity and conversation, flushed cheeks, hot, dry skin, and an unusual glitter in their eyes
3. Febrile seizures may occur in children, particularly those children between the ages of 6 months and 5 years (see section on FEBRILE SEIZURES)

E. Although each $1\,^{\circ}$F raises the basal metabolic rate by 7%, most patients can tolerate fevers well with a few exceptions such as patients with underlying cardiac disease or chronically, debilitating diseases, immunocompromised patients, small infants, and the elderly who are at a greater risk for developing dehydration

F. Bacteremia, meningitis, and seizures are serious conditions related to fevers (see FEVER WITHOUT LOCALIZING SOURCE and FEBRILE SEIZURES sections)

IV. Diagnosis/Evaluation

A. History
1. Inquire about onset, duration, and pattern of fever; ascertain that patient or parents know how to correctly measure temperature; inquire about type of thermometer used
2. Ask parents if child is acting differently such as more irritable, more drowsy, or not playing as usual
3. Inquire about associated symptoms such as anorexia, chills, headache, nasal congestion, earache, sore throat, cough, abdominal pain, vomiting, diarrhea, painful urination
4. Explore hydration status by asking about amount of fluid intake and frequency and amount of fluid output
5. Ask about comfort level of patient
6. Explore possibilities of heat illness (heat stroke) or other types of environmental exposure
7. Ask whether patient started any new medications or had a recent immunization
8. Ask whether other household members are ill or have fevers
9. Inquire about recent travel, pet scratches, or exposure to ticks
10. Inquire about last dosage of an antipyretic and other self-treatment measures
11. In young children, always inquire about previous episodes of febrile seizures
12. Past medical history should include a list of medications currently being used, discussion of previous illnesses and diseases, particularly any cardiac or chronically debilitating disorders
13. A complete review of systems may be needed to uncover source of fever and to determine severity of debility due to elevated body temperature

B. Physical Examination
   1. Measure temperature
      a. Always confirm initial temperature measurement
         (1) Retake temperature before ordering diagnostic tests or prescribing treatment to reduce fever
         (2) Bundled infants need temperature measurement 30 minutes after undressing
      b. Rectal temperatures are gold standard as they are accurate, reproducible, and not affected by environmental factors; rectal temperatures are approximately 1° higher than oral temperatures and 2 to 2.5° higher than axillary temperatures
         (1) Do not use rectal thermometers in neutropenic patients for fear of rectal trauma
         (2) Lubricate thermometer and insert 3-6 cm; leave in place 1-3 minutes
      c. Oral temperatures are reliable with cooperative patient (age >5-6) but may vary with rapid breathing and recent ingestion of hot or cold fluids
         (1) Place thermometer on either side of posterior sublingual pocket
         (2) Leave in place 3 minutes
      d. The infrared ear thermometer estimates the temperature of the tympanic membrane (TM)
         (1) Improper placement and aiming, incomplete probe penetration into external ear canal, and obstruction/tortuosity of the external ear canal can lead to underestimating TM temperature
         (2) Tympanic thermometers should not be used to measure temperatures in children <3 years, and possibly up to 6 years
      e. Axillary measurements: Leave thermometer in dry axilla for 4 minutes
   2. Measure respiratory rate, pulse, and blood pressure
   3. Observe general appearance looking for subtle signs such as changes in alertness
   4. In young children, observe for playfulness, irritability, consolability, and response to overtures (e.g., smiling)
   5. In infants, assess the quality of the cry
   6. Observe skin for color, rashes, petechiae or purpura
   7. Assess for signs of dehydration such as skin turgor and capillary refill
   8. Assess neck for nuchal rigidity
   9. Check for lymphadenopathy
   10. Assess for swollen joints
   11. May need to do a <u>complete</u> physical examination to find localized infection such as otitis media, pharyngitis, sinusitis, meningitis, cervical adenitis, pneumonia, or urinary tract infection

C. Differential Diagnosis: See pathogenesis for ETIOLOGIES OF FEVER
   1. Febrile children with swollen joints, meningismus, labored respirations, dysuria, petechiae, lethargy, or dehydration should be carefully evaluated
   2. The height (unless extremely high) of the temperature, the duration of the fever, and whether the fever responds to antipyretics are usually not helpful in differentiating the cause
   3. Fevers almost always result in increases in pulse rates; absence of a pulse rate increase suggests factitious fever, mycoplasmal infection or typhoid fever
   4. It is important to differentiate true fever from hyperthermia
   5. Fever pattern provides clues to diagnosis:
      a. Continuous or sustained fever with slight remissions (not exceeding 2.0°F): lobar and gram-negative pneumonia, the rickettsioses, typhoid fever, CNS disorders
      b. Intermittent fever with wide fluctuations (usually normal or low in morning and peaking between 4:00 and 8:00 pm): localized pyogenic infections, bacterial endocarditis, malaria
      c. Intermittent fever with two daily peaks: salmonelloses, miliary tuberculosis, gonococcal and meningococcal endocarditis
      d. Sporadic episodes of fever or periods of normal temperature and recurrence of fever: cholangitis
      e. Weekly or longer periods of fever and equally long afebrile periods with repetition of cycle: Hodgkin's disease, brucellosis, occasionally tuberculosis

  f. Highest temperature elevation in early morning hours: occasionally in miliary tuberculosis, salmonelloses, hepatic abscess, bacterial endocarditis

  g. Sharply increased elevation of temperature with exacerbation of other clinical abnormalities occurs several hours after antibiotic treatment of syphilis, leptospirosis and tick-borne relapsing fever

 D. Diagnostic Tests: Recommended diagnostic tests depend on patient's age, clinical presentation, and previous medical history

  1. In the majority of cases, the history and physical examination will uncover likely causes of the fever and suggest selective diagnostic tests

  2. For patients who have a localized infection but also have 1 of the following: are <3 months of age, look toxic, have an extremely elevated temperature, are immunodeficient, or have an underlying chronic disease, consider ordering the following (also see table on Diagnostic Tests for Sepsis in section FEVER WITHOUT SOURCE)

   a. Urine analysis for specific gravity and the presence of ketones to determine hydration status

   b. CBC with differential and erythrocyte sedimentation rate (ESR) to determine likelihood of a bacterial etiology and/or blood cultures to rule out bacteremia and need for more aggressive treatments such as hospitalization and parenteral antimicrobial therapy

  3. Children less than 2 years without localizing signs (or a source for the fever) need further diagnostic tests (see section on FEVER WITHOUT LOCALIZING SOURCE)

  4. Fevers of unknown origin (FUO) require an extensive diagnostic evaluation.

V. Plan/Management

 A. Immediately transport the following patients to the hospital:
  1. Patients who are disoriented or delirious
  2. Patients with meningismus, petechiae or purpura

 B. Consider consultation and hospitalization for following patients:

  1. Any infant under 3 months of age needs special attention and in most cases hospitalization even if a source of the fever has been identified because of the risk of dehydration and other adverse reactions to elevated body temperatures. Also, these infants are at greater risk for sepsis, meningitis and pneumonia than other children. Remember that roseola or benign febrile seizures do not occur in infants less than 6 months of age

  2. Children between 3 months and 2 years old should not be treated on an outpatient basis without vigilant and special attention except if they have a localized, non-serious infection, are playful, drinking, voiding, and do not appear toxic. Children in this age group are more susceptible than older children to bacteremia and meningitis (see section on FEVERS WITHOUT LOCALIZING SOURCE)

  3. Patients with extremely elevated temperatures. In children bacteremia is more likely with fevers greater than 105°F. Even if a localized sign of infection is found such as otitis media, carefully consider the diagnosis of bacteremia in infants and young children with extremely high fevers

  4. Children who are lethargic and inconsolable

  5. Patients who are immunodeficient or have a history of cardiac or another serious disease

  6. Patients who are taking corticosteroid or immunosuppressive therapy

  7. Patients who have prosthetic devices

  8. IV drug abusers

  9. Patients who are dehydrated

  10. Any patient who appears toxic (rigors, hypotension, oliguria, CNS abnormalities, petechial rash, marked leukocytosis or leukopenia, cardiorespiratory distress, new significant cardiac murmurs)

  11. Any patient whose fever lasts longer than 7-10 days

 C. Treat cause of fever
  1. Antibiotics should be prescribed when there is an identified bacterial infection
  2. Also see section on FEVERS WITHOUT LOCALIZING SOURCE for treatment

D. Antipyretics: Controversy exists concerning when to treat a fever with antipyretics.
   1. Reasons for not treating a low-grade or moderate fever in an otherwise well patient include the following: Antipyretics do not alter the course or duration of disease; may mask the signs and symptoms of a serious disease and confuse the clinical picture; and can be potentially harmful in some patients (e.g., side effects, toxicity)
   2. However, most clinicians agree that antipyretics should be given in the following situations:
     a. When fevers are 103°F and higher
     b. In children with a history of febrile seizures
     c. In patients for whom side effects of fever may be harmful (e.g. patients with compensated cardiac disease and chronic debilitating disorders, patients who become dehydrated rapidly, patients who are alcoholics)
     d. Patients who are uncomfortable and unable to rest
   3. In hyperthermic states such as thyrotoxicosis, heat stroke and overdressing, the set point has not been changed and antipyretic medications are not effective because they act to lower set point
   4. The drug of choice is acetaminophen (Tylenol); Adolescents: 325-650 mg every 4-6, Children: 5-15 mg/kg/dose every 4-6 hours (See table that follows for doses by age and drug form); do not use in liver disease or transplant patients; strictly follow correct doses to prevent liver damage; maximum effect at 2 hours

ACETAMINOPHEN DOSAGES AND AVAILABLE FORMS FOR TREATMENT OF FEVERS

Age	Drops (80 mg/0.8 mL)	Elixir (160 mg/1 tsp)	Chewable Tablets (80 mg)	Adult Tablets (325 mg)
<4 mo	0.4 mL	---	---	---
4 mo - 1 yr	0.8 mL	½ tsp	---	---
1-2 yrs	1.2 mL	3/4 tsp	1 ½ tablets	---
2-3 yrs	1.6 mL	1 tsp	2 tablets	---
4-5 yrs	2.4 mL	1 ½ tsp	3 tablets	---
6-8 yrs	---	2 tsp	4 tablets	1 tablet
9-10 yrs	---	2 ½ tsp	5 tablets	1 ½ tablets
>10 yrs	---	---	8 tablets	2 tablets

   5. Aspirin (325-650 mg every 4-6 hours) should never be given to children and adolescents who have a fever because of the dangers of Reye syndrome
   6. Ibuprofen (Motrin) is another therapeutic option
     a. Dosage in adolescents is 400 mg every 6 hours
     b. In children with temperatures less than 102.5°F can give ibuprofen (Children's Motrin) 5 mg/kg/dose every 8 hours and 10 mg/kg/dose every 8 hours when temperatures are greater than or equal to 102.5°F. Available 50mg/1.25mL oral drops, 100 mg/5mL liquid OTC, and 50 mg chewable tablets
     c. Some clinicians recommend the following antipyretic schedule in children: Give acetaminophen every 4 hours, give ibuprofen if temperature is still elevated 1 hour after acetaminophen administration; however, never give ibuprofen more often than every 8 hours
     d. Overdose is rare and less toxic than salicylates and tylenol
     e. Avoid in patients with aspirin allergies, ulcers, renal insufficiency, and bleeding disorders
     f. Use cautiously because the long-term safety of administering ibuprofen in children has not been established, although a survey of 84,000 patients by Lesko & Mitchell (1995) found no association with medication and renal failure or significant bleeding; link to Reye Syndrome is uncertain

E.   Sponging may be performed but usually is unnecessary and may even be harmful because it can cause discomfort and chilling
    1.   If temperature is extremely high or if aggressive fever management is necessary such as a child with history of febrile seizures, sponge patient after giving antipyretic
    2.   Sponging is an important part of the management plan in the following cases: patients with severe liver disease who cannot take acetaminophen, neurologic problems in which temperature regulation mechanisms are abnormal, heat stroke, or in environments with excessive temperatures
    3.   When sponging, water should be lukewarm and should not cause the patient to shiver (colder temperatures are used for heat illness such as heat stroke)

F.   Patient Education
    1.   Teach parents the correct method to assess temperature
        a.   If child is less than 3 years, use a rectal or ear thermometer (less reliable)
        b.   If older than 3 years, child may be able to cooperate and use an oral thermometer
    2.   Reinforce when the parents should call a health care provider about an elevated temperature
        a.   Instruct parents to immediately have their children evaluated by a health care provider when there is delirium (disorientation or confusion), seizures, stiff neck, petechial or purpural rash, signs of dehydration (can teach how to assess capillary refill)
        b.   Call health care provider if child of any age has associated symptoms such as swollen joints, sore throat, earache, severe cough, is not eating/drinking well, is lethargic (doesn't maintain eye contact or engage in environmental stimuli), is inconsolable, is very restless during sleep
        c.   If child is 36 months or younger and has a fever greater than 100.4°F (38°C), call health care provider
        d.   For the older child, parents should call health care provider for fevers above 103°F (39.4°C)
    3.   Teach parents to avoid over-the-counter medications which may contain aspirin such as Pepto-Bismol when their children have fevers
    4.   Older children and adults should be taught to drink extra fluids; parents should be taught to offer their children fluids every 15-60 minutes depending on the child's condition
    5.   Parents of children should be taught when to administer antipyretics and the correct dosage of these medications
        a.   Parents often give lower than therapeutic doses
        b.   Remind parents that maximum temperature reduction takes 2-3 hours after antipyretic is given
    6.   Daily activities should be modified to provide for additional rest, light meals, and avoidance of strenuous activities depending on patient's condition
    7.   Adolescents should be taught to avoid overdressing when they have a fever; parents should be taught to avoid over bundling their febrile children
    8.   Tell patients to never use alcohol for sponging
    9.   Inform patients or parents that elevated temperatures are a normal body defense mechanism, not a disease; height of the temperature except when extremely high does not correlate well with serious diseases; assure everyone that there are almost always no adverse effects from fevers

G.   Follow Up
    1.   Variable and depends on age, diagnosis, and clinical presentation of patient as well as the amount of friend and family support available
    2.   For infants, young children, and chronically-ill patients consider scheduling return visit for following morning or have telephone contact within 24 hours to assess condition
    3.   Instruct patients to return for further evaluation if fever persists for more than 2 or 3 days

LYMPHADENOPATHY

I.   Definition: Lymph node enlargement

II. Pathogenesis

    A.   Following mechanisms result in lymphadenopathy
        1.   Proliferation in response to an antigen
        2.   Invasion of cells from cells outside the node such as malignant cells
        3.   Transformation of primary nodular tissue into neoplastic cells

    B.   Causes of generalized lymphadenopathy
        1.   Infections (most common cause)
            a.   Viral: Human immunodeficiency virus, mononucleosis, cytomegalovirus, hepatitis B, measles, rubella, rubeola
            b.   Bacterial: Group A. Streptococci, cat-scratch disease, secondary syphilis
            c.   Mycobacterial: atypical mycobacterial infection, miliary tuberculosis
            d.   Fungal: histoplasmosis
            e.   Protozoal: toxoplasmosis
        2.   Collagen vascular disorders: systemic lupus erythematosus, rheumatoid arthritis
        3.   Endocrine disorders: hyperthyroidism, hypopituitarism, hypoadrenocorticism
        4.   Neoplasms: leukemia, lymphoma, immunoblastic lymphadenopathy, metastases
        5.   Hypersensitivity states: serum sickness, drug reactions (phenytoin and less commonly: hydralazine, para-aminosalicylic acid, propylthiouracil, and allopurinol)
        6.   Miscellaneous: sarcoidosis, lipid storage disease, Kawasaki disease

    C.   Causes of localized lymphadenopathy: due to local infection, growth, or recent immunization in area drained by involved lymph node (also see table IV.B.1)
        1.   Anterior auricular: viral conjunctivitis, rubella, scalp infection
        2.   Submandibular or cervical (unilateral): buccal cavity infection, pharyngitis, nasopharyngeal tumor, thyroid malignancy
        3.   Cervical (bilateral): mononucleosis, sarcoidosis, toxoplasmosis, pharyngitis
        4.   Supraclavicular (right): pulmonary, mediastinal, and esophageal malignancies
        5.   Supraclavicular (left): malignancies (intra-abdominal, renal, testicular, ovarian)
        6.   Axillary: breast malignancy or infection, upper extremity infection
        7.   Epitrochlear: syphilis (bilateral), hand infection (unilateral)
        8.   Inguinal: syphilis, genital herpes, lymphogranuloma venereum, chancroid, lower extremity or local infection
        9.   Hilar adenopathy: sarcoidosis, fungal infection, lymphoma, bronchogenic carcinoma, tuberculosis
        10.   Any region: benign reactive hyperplasia, lymphomas, cat scratch disease, leukemia, sarcoidosis, malignancies

III. Clinical presentation: The following key factors are helpful in arriving at a diagnosis:

    A.   Generalized versus localized lymphadenopathy
        1.   Generalized adenopathy is due to systemic disease
        2.   Localized adenopathy is caused by either local infection, tumor, or systemic disease

    B.   Location of node (see PATHOGENESIS); supraclavicular node, often called "sentinel" node suggests Hodgkin's disease

    C.   Character of node
        1.   Size: a large node (>1 cm.) usually represents a specific pathology
        2.   Metastatic cancer: hard, painless, matted, fixed, often >3 cm.
        3.   Reactive: discrete, mobile, rubbery, and mildly tender
        4.   Lymphadenitis: tender, warm, red, fluctuant

5. Infection: firm, red, warm
6. Lymphoma, leukemia: firm or rubbery nodes

D. Age of patient
  1. In patients <30 years, most cases are benign and caused by infection
  2. Benign reactive hyperplasia or transient node enlargement from unknown causes occurs frequently in children and adolescents
  3. Palpable nodes in the anterior cervical triangle are common and usually normal
  4. Posterior cervical node enlargement in the older child and adolescent may be mononucleosis

E. Onset and duration
  1. Nodes of acute onset and duration are typically due to viral or pyogenic infection
  2. Chronicity suggests neoplastic disease, sarcoidosis, tuberculosis, and fungal infections although lymphadenitis may take several months to resolve

F. Rate of change: usually nodes that are rapidly growing are more pathologic than slow-growing nodes

G. Associated symptoms
  1. Low-grade fevers with night sweats and weight loss characterize lymphoma, HIV infection or tuberculosis
  2. Fatigue and weight loss suggest systemic infection, cancer, or connective tissue disease
  3. Hilar lymph node enlargement may cause compression of thoracic structures and result in cough, dyspnea, and wheezing

H. Associated signs
  1. Splenomegaly: mononucleosis, lymphoma, or leukemia
  2. Thyromegaly: hyperthyroidism
  3. Tender, warm, or enlarged joints: collagen vascular disease and leukemia
  4. Rash: viral exanthems, Kawasaki disease, collagen and vascular disease

I. Epidemiologic leads
  1. Recent exposure to cats is predisposing factor in cat-scratch disease
  2. History of multiple sexual partners and IV drug use may be associated with sexually transmitted disease or HIV infection
  3. Tick bite may be associated with Lyme disease
  4. Travel-related lymphadenopathy occurs

IV. Diagnosis/Evaluation

A. History
  1. Ask about onset, duration, and rate of growth of all palpable nodes
  2. Question about tenderness of node
  3. Ask about recent infections and trauma
  4. Inquire about systemic symptoms such as weight loss, night sweats, fatigue, and diarrhea
  5. Question about exposure to animals, travel to foreign countries, occupation, and explore other risk factors such as substance abuse and sexual exposure
  6. Ask about medications
  7. Explore past medical history and family history

B. Physical examination
  1. Assess all palpable nodes, noting size, localization, consistency, tenderness, warmth, and fixation (see table that follows)

PALPABLE LYMPH NODES AND LYMPHATIC DRAINAGE	
Node	**Drainage Area**
Occipital	Posterior scalp, neck
Mastoid	Mastoid area
Submental	Apex of tongue and lower lip
Submaxillary	Buccal cavity, tongue, cheek, lips
Cervical	Head, neck, and oropharynx
Axillary	Greater part of arm, shoulder, superficial anterior and lateral thoracic and upper abdominal wall
Supraclavicular	Right: Inferior neck and mediastinum Left: Inferior neck, mediastinum, and upper abdomen
Epitrochlear	Hand, forearm, and elbow
Inguinal	Leg and genitalia
Femoral	Leg
Popliteal	Posterior leg and knee

      a.   Normal, palpable nodes are discrete, freely mobile, and nontender
      b.   Normal size of nodes is < 1cm. with two exceptions:
          (1)   Inguinal nodes are normal up to 1.5 cm.
          (2)   Epitrochlear nodes are abnormal if >0.5 cm.
      c.   To assess for enlargement of supraclavicular node, have patient perform valsalva maneuver during palpation of supraclavicular fossa
  2.   For localized lymphadenopathy, carefully assess all body parts within the lymphatic drainage area (see preceding table)
  3.   For generalized lymphadenopathy a careful, comprehensive physical examination is needed

C.   Differential Diagnosis
  1.   Potential causes range from simple and benign to complicated and serious
  2.   For a large proportion of enlarged nodes, no specific cause is found (see pathogenesis for range of etiologies)
  3.   Persistent generalized lymphademopathy is defined as lymph node enlargement for at least 3 months in at least 2 extrainguinal sites; common causes are HIV infection, tuberculosis, syphilis, and lymphoma

D.   Diagnostic Tests (If benign cause of lymphadenopathy is suspected, close observation is indicated); when the diagnosis is uncertain, stepwise testing with the following tests is needed:
  1.   CBC
      a.   Atypical lymphocytes: mononucleosis or other viral syndromes
      b.   Increased granulocytes: bacterial infection
      c.   Increased eosinophils: hypersensitivity states
      d.   Decreased red blood cells and platelets: malignancy
  2.   Chest x-ray which will detect pulmonary disease and hilar adenopathy is needed for seriously ill patients and those with supraclavicular lymphadenopathy or respiratory complaints
  3.   Serologic tests
      a.   Monospot or Epstein-Barr virus: mononucleosis
      b.   VDRL: syphilis
      c.   HIV antibody: HIV infection
      d.   Antinuclear antibody and rheumatoid factor: collagen diseases
      e.   Other serologic tests: cytomegalovirus and toxoplasmosis infections
  4.   Tuberculin skin test for myobacterial disease

5. Cultures
    a. Throat for cervical adenopathy
    b. Urethral and cervical for inguinal adenopathy
    c. Aspirated lymph tissue for suspected fungal or mycobacterial infection
    d. Blood culture for suspected bacteremia
6. Lymph node biopsy provides a definitive diagnosis; indicated when simple testing fails to provide a diagnosis or for cases when cancer, tuberculosis or sarcoidosis are suspected
    a. The following characteristics suggest the need for an early biopsy:
        (1) Node > 2 cm
        (2) Abnormal chest x-ray
        (3) Enlarged supraclavicular node
        (4) Associated signs and symptoms of weight loss and hepatosplenomegaly
        (5) Absence of respiratory tract symptoms
    b. Nodes that remain constant in size for 4-8 weeks and those that fail to resolve in 8-12 weeks need a biopsy
    c. Consider biopsy sooner in patients with constitutional signs and symptoms and risk factors for malignancy
7. Ultrasound and computed tomography are sometimes helpful in differentiating lymphadenopathy from nonlymphatic enlargement
8. Bone marrow examination is needed for patients with severe anemia, neutropenia, thrombocytopenia or peripheral smear for malignant blast cells

V. Plan/Management

    A. Treatment depends on diagnosis; see sections on CERVICAL ADENITIS, KAWASAKI DISEASE, PHARYNGITIS, etc.

    B. Consider consultation for patients suspected of having serious disease or one of the following:
        1. Undiagnosed adenopathy lasting longer than 2 months
        2. Firm, matted, rapidly enlarging, nontender nodes
        3. Associated signs and symptoms such as night sweats, weight loss, bone pain, hepatosplenomegaly, fever of unknown etiology, and failure to thrive
        4. Associated complete cell count abnormality, positive PPD, or abnormal chest x-ray

    C. Follow Up
        1. Diagnosis will determine when patient should return for follow-up
        2. Patients with benign clinical history, unremarkable physical examination, and no constitutional signs and symptoms can be reevaluated in 3 weeks
        3. For other cases in which the cause of lymphadenopathy is uncertain, watchful waiting with follow up every 3-5 days for 2 weeks is appropriate

PAIN

I. Definition: Unpleasant sensory and emotional experience related to actual or potential tissue damage

II. Pathogenesis

    A. Peripheral stimulation occurs when free nerve endings or nociceptors found in various parts of body (i.e., skin, blood vessels, viscera, muscles) are stimulated and then action potentials are transmitted along afferent nerve fibers to the spinal cord

    B. Gate control theory further develops the pathophysiology of pain
        1. The perception of pain is an interplay between the nociceptive pain fibers and the nonociceptive or non-transmitting neurons that synapse in the spinal cord

2. Clinically, this is important because certain treatments such as acupuncture, topical irritants, and transcutaneous electrical nerve stimulation (TENS) can stimulate the large nonociceptive neurons and produce an analgesic effect

C. Pain-initiated processes as well as other information are carried through the ascending spinal cord pathways (particularly the spinothalamic tract) to the brain

D. In the brain, pain is perceived as a partial summation of two processes:
1. Positive feedback is the nociceptive stimulus which activates pain transmission
2. Negative feedback is the brain's modulatory network composed of the endogenous opiate system (opiate receptors, endorphins) which inhibits pain

E. Other neurotransmitter substances such as acetylcholine, dopamine, norepinephrine, and serotonin play a role in pain transmission as well

F. The brain also controls pain sensation through an organized descending or efferent pain transmission system

III. Clinical Presentation

A. Acute pain
1. Arises from injury, trauma, spasm or disease of body parts
2. Usually is short-lived and decreases as damaged area heals
3. Associated with hyperactivity of the sympathetic nervous system resulting in the following: tachycardia, tachypnea, elevated blood pressure, diaphoresis and dilated pupils

B. Chronic pain
1. Pain which lasts longer than 6 months and is rarely accompanied with hyperactivity of sympathetic nervous system
2. Can be characterized by its location
   a. Visceral locations (initiated in abdomen or thorax)
   b. Somatic pain (initiated in muscles and connective tissue)
   c. Neurologic causes (i.e., diabetic neuropathy)
3. Chronic pain typology:
   a. Pain that persists beyond the normal healing time for an acute injury
   b. Chronic disease pain
   c. Pain without identifiable organic cause
   d. Cancer pain
4. Symptoms of depression often accompany chronic pain

C. Pain in children is different than pain in adults; recent research suggests that the younger the person, the lower the pain threshold and the greater the sensitivity to pain

D. Level of cognitive development directly affects how the pediatric patient perceives and responds to pain
1. In infants and preverbal children, irritability, restlessness, poor feeding, excessive sweating, and sleep problems may be signs of pain
2. Preschool children do not understand that their pain is related to illness or injury, but instead, often believe pain is a form of punishment; children at this age become withdrawn, clingy, and quiet when in pain
3. School-age children may respond to pain with anxiety and aggressiveness
   a. Children at this age are fearful of bodily injury and may exaggerate minor bruises and injuries
   b. By age 7, when the child is in Piaget's concept of the origin of concrete thinking, understanding that pain is a result of injury or illness is possible
4. Children older than 10 years of age may be anxious and fear loss of control when they have pain

IV. Diagnosis/Evaluation

    A. History
        1. Mnemonic may be used to obtain patient's subjective description of pain
            a. P: palliative or precipitating factors such as stress, exertion
            b. Q: quality of pain such as sharpness, crushing, throbbing, burning
            c. R: region or radiation of pain
            d. S: subjective descriptions of severity of pain such as awakens at night or takes breath away
            e. T: temporal nature such as daytime, during meals; constant vs. intermittent
        2. May use a visual analog scale to quantify pain or ask patient to relate where pain falls on a line from zero (no pain) to 10 (worst pain ever experienced)
        3. In children use the "Faces" diagram/scale or for older children use Linear Analogue of "Faces" (see diagram from Beyer & Wells, 1989 in Harriet Lane Handbook)
        4. If the patient is a young child, ask parents to describe child's drinking pattern, activity level, amount of crying, and any unusual behaviors
        5. Inquire about drug use and its efficacy
        6. Ask about previous personal or family history of chronic pain
        7. Assess patient's level of functioning in all spheres of living such as family relationships, social relationships, employment, and hobbies to help determine secondary gains
        8. Complete review of systems to determine relationship of pain to other parts of body

    B. Physical Examination
        1. Assess vital signs
        2. Observe general appearance for signs of distress
        3. Observe patient's affect
        4. Inspect, palpate, percuss and auscultate, as appropriate, all areas and surrounding structures which patient perceives as painful

    C. Diagnostic tests are variable depending of patient's condition

    D. Differential Diagnosis
        1. Malingering for ongoing litigation or secondary gains
        2. Anxiety or depression

V. Plan/Management

    A. General principles of pain management
        1. For infants informal sensorimotor strategies such as swaddling, holding, rocking, and using pacifiers may be helpful
        2. For pediatric patients, it is important to provide a clear and realistic explanation of the problem and its treatment; allow parents to be present when a child must experience a painful procedure
        3. Cultivating a sense of control by the older child and adolescent over the pain is important in both acute and chronic situations
        4. Particularly in chronic situations, it is important to get the patient engaged in an active, productive life
        5. Essential to involve the patient's family and friends in the management plan

    B. Pharmacologic principles of treating pain
        1. Identify source of pain and treat as appropriate
        2. Use the least potent analgesic with the fewest side effects
        3. Give analgesics for adequate trial time and properly titrate the dose which means considering individual patient characteristics and needs
        4. Use analgesics on a regular dosing schedule and not on a "prn" basis which promotes anxiety and contributes to future drug dependence
        5. Prevent persistent pain and relieve breakthrough pain; Order rescue medication equivalent to half the standing dose to start on a prn basis
        6. Recognize and treat side effects; avoid excessive sedation

7. Use equianalgesic doses
8. Use appropriate route of administration
    a. Use oral medications, if possible, because of ease of administration and cost effectiveness
    b. NSAID, ketorolac (Toradol), is available in IM preparation
    c. Fentanyl (Duragesic) is available as a transdermal patch
    d. Morphine and hydromorphone are available as rectal suppositories
    e. Subcutaneous or intravenous administration of morphine and hydromorphone is sometimes needed; patient-controlled analgesia pumps can provide individualized pain relief
9. Watch for development of tolerance
10. For the pediatric patient, nonpharmacological approaches such as applying cold or warm compresses or hiding the injury with a Band-Aid may be helpful

C. The Three-Step Analgesic Ladder of the World Health Organization (see table that follows)
    1. Designed for chronic, cancer pain but can be used as a guide for all types of pain management
    2. Pharmacological management of pain in children is controversial
        a. Step approach is often recommended
        b. Children **<2months of age** who receive opioids **must be monitored in intensive care unit**

THREE-STEP ANALGESIC LADDER OF THE WORLD HEALTH ORGANIZATION		
Step	**Oral Medications**	**Regimen**
Step 1	Acetaminophen 324-650mg Q 4-6°; 5-15mg/kg/dose q 4-6° (children) Salicylates: aspirin 325-650 mg Q 4° (not recommended in children and adolescents with fevers) NSAIDS (dosage in next table) Tramadol 50-100mg Q 4-6° (not recommended <16 years)	Nonopioid ± adjuvant
If pain persists, maximize nonopioid and add step 2 opioid		
Step 2	Codeine 30-90 mg Q 4°; 0.5-1.2mg/kg Q 4° (children) dihydrocodeine 32 mg Q 4° hydrocodone 5-10 mg Q 4-6° } check dosage with pediatrician oxycodone 5 mg Q 6°	Opioid: mild-to-moderate pain +nonopioid ±adjuvant therapy
If pain persists at step 2, increase dose of opioid or change to step 3 opioid		
Step 3	Morphine IR 15-30 mg Q 4-6°; 0.1-0.2mg/kg Q 4-6° (children) oxycodone 7.5-10 mg Q 4-6° } check dosage with pediatrician hydromorphone 4 mg Q 4° fentanyl 50μg/hr Q 72°	Opioid: moderate-to-severe pain ±nonopioid ±adjuvant therapy

Adapted from WHO (1990). Cancer pain relief and palliative care: Report of WHO Expert Committee. WHO Technological Report Service, 804, 1-73.

D. Acetaminophen (Tylenol - APAP) is a nonnarcotic agent with antipyretic, analgesic effects; minimal anti-inflammatory effects
    1. Onset of 0.5-1 hour; duration 3-6 hours
    2. "Ceiling effect" exists, but many patients have greater pain relief from a single 1000 mg dose compared to single 560 mg dose
    3. Do not exceed 4 to 6 g per day to prevent liver damage
    4. In children, relatively small overdoses can cause liver damage and death (see section on FEVER for correct doses in children)
    5. Few adverse reactions; hepatotoxicity in overdose or in chronic alcoholics following therapeutic dosage

E. Acetylsalicylic acid (Aspirin - ASA) is a nonnarcotic agent with antipyretic, analgesic, and anti-inflammatory effects (see table on NSAIDs which follows) - <u>Never give aspirin when the child or adolescent has a viral infection or fever</u>
1. Onset within 0.5 hours; duration 3-6 hours
2. "Ceiling effect" exists such that single doses greater than 650 mg do not result in greater degree of pain relief
3. Stop taking drug at least one week before surgery; single therapeutic dose irreversibly inhibits platelet function for the 7-day lifetime of platelet
4. Adverse reactions include Reye syndrome, hypersensitivity reactions (asthmatic patients particularly), dyspepsia, indigestion, gastric ulcers, irreversible inhibition of platelet aggregation, tinnitus, renal effects, anemia
5. Monitor hematocrit, stool guaiac periodically; order plasma salicylate level determinations when patient is prescribed high dosages
6. Avoid in patients with asthma, thrombocytopenia, GI disorders

F. Other salicylic acid derivatives have a slower onset and longer duration than ASA, but are just as potent and cause fewer gastrointestinal and central nervous system side effects (See table on NSAIDs which follows)

G. Nonsteroidal anti-inflammatory drugs (NSAIDs), nonnarcotic agents, used for mild to moderate pain and have antipyretic, analgesic, and anti-inflammatory effects (See table which follows for dosing recommendations)
1. Useful for dental pain, rheumatoid arthritis, headaches, musculoskeletal pain, menstrual cramps, and bone pain with cancer
2. Major pathway of metabolism is hepatic
3. Patients have large variability in response to individual agents; switch to another NSAID/class if one agent is ineffective in an adequate trial
4. Before switching to another class of NSAIDs give an adequate trial of efficacy (1-2 weeks depending on half-life of drugs); instruct patient to continue to take drug at prescribed times even if pain stops
5. Always prescribe an adequate dosage (start with low dose and gradually increase to maximum dosage for patients in moderate pain)
6. Do not use combination of different NSAIDs
7. Side effects can occur: GI distress (take with meals to lessen this effect), fluid retention, peripheral edema, hepatic problems, renal disorders, and central nervous system effects such as dizziness and depression.
8. Be careful in prescribing if patient is on other drugs
9. Baseline tests for long-term therapy include hematocrit, liver function tests, urinalysis, blood urea nitrogen (BUN), serum creatinine; often these diagnostic tests are rechecked in first month after initiation and then at 6-month intervals
10. In young children, tolmetin (Tolectin), naproxen (Naprosyn), and ibuprofen (Children's Advil, Children's Motrin), are approved for use; IM preparation of ketorolac tromethamine (Toradol) now available for use in children

NONSTEROIDAL ANTI-INFLAMMATORY DRUGS (NSAIDS)			
Class & Agent	Half Life (hrs)	Tablet Size	Adolescent Dose
FENAMATES			
Meclofenamate Sodium (Meclomen)	2	50, 100	50-100 mg Q 4-6 hrs; max 400 mg
Mefenamic Acid (Ponstel)	2-4	250	Initial: 500 mg, then 250 mg QID; max use 1 week
INDOLES			
Indomethacin (Indocin)	4.5	25, 50	25 mg BID or TID; max 200 mg daily
Sulindac (Clinoril)	7.8	150, 200	150 mg BID; max 400 mg/day
Tolmetin sodium (Tolectin)*	1-1.5	200, 400, 600	400 mg TID; max 1800 mg/day
			(continued)

NONSTEROIDAL ANTI-INFLAMMATORY DRUGS (NSAIDS) (CONTINUED)

Class & Agent	Half Life (hrs)	Tablet Size	Adolescent Dose
NAPHTHYLKANONE			
Nabumetone (Relafen)	20-30	500, 750	1 g/day QD or BID; max 2 g/day
OXICAMS			
Piroxicam (Feldene)	30-86	10, 20	20 mg QD
PHENYLACETIC ACID			
Diclofenac sodium (Voltaren)	2	25, 50, 75, 100 ext. rel.	50-75 mg BID; max 200 mg/day 100 mg ext. rel. QD
PROPIONIC ACIDS			
Fenoprofen calcium (Nalfon)	2-3	200	200 mg Q 4-6 hrs
Flurbiprofen (Ansaid)	5.7	50, 100	50-100 mg TID
Ibuprofen (Motrin)†	1.8-2.5	200, 400, 600, 800	400-600 mg Q 4-6 hrs; max 3.2 g/day
Ketoprofen (Orudis)	2-4	12.5, 25, 50, 75	50-75 mg TID or QID; max 300 mg/day
Naproxen (Naprosyn)**	12-15	250, 375, 500	500 mg initially, followed by 250 mg Q 6-8 hrs
Naproxen sodium (Anaprox)	12-13	275, 550	550 mg initially, followed by 275 mg Q 6-8 hrs
PYRANOCARBOXYLIC ACID			
Etodolac (Lodine)	6-7	200, 300	200-400 mg Q 6-8 hrs; max 1200 mg/day
PYRAZOLES			
Phenylbutazone (Azolid, Butazolidin)	50-100	100	300-600 mg TID or QID; max 400 mg/day
SALICYLATES			
Acetylsalicylic acid (ASA)	0.25	varies	325-650 mg Q 4-6 hrs; max 5200 mg/day
Diflunisal (Dolobid)	8-12	250, 500	500-1000 mg initially, followed by 250-500 mg q 8-12 hrs
Choline magnesium trisalicylate(Trilisate)***	8-12	500, 750, 1000	500-1500 mg BID

†Ibuprofen (Children's Motrin, Children's Advil) >2yrs. 6-10 mg/kg Q 6-8 hours
*Tolmetin sodium (Tolectin): Children >2 yrs, 20 mg/kg/day in 3-4 divided doses.
**Naproxen (Naprosyn): Children >2 yrs, 2.5-5.0 mg/kg/dose TID or QID; max 15 mg/kg/day
***Choline magnesium trisalicylate (Trilisate):
    Children <37 kg, 50 mg/kg/day, in 2 divided doses
    Children >37 kg, 2.25 g/day, in 2 divided doses

11. In deciding which NSAID agent to prescribe consider the following:
    a. Mefenamic acid (Ponstel) is approved for primary dysmenorrhea
    b. Ketorolac tromethamine (Toradol) is injectable (IM) and has a longer duration, less drug abuse potential, less CNS side effects than morphine but similar potency of analgesia
    c. Consider type of dosing form
        (1) Liquids: ibuprofen, indomethacin, naproxen
        (2) Sustained release: diclofenac, indomethacin, ketoprofen, naproxen

H. Tramadol (Ultram), a central-acting analgesic, is sometimes used for treatment of mild-to-moderate pain; Particularly well suited when pain is not relieved by acetaminophen and the patient cannot tolerate NSAIDS and wishes to defer opioid therapy; not recommended for children <16 years

I. Step 2 should be initiated when the patient continues to have mild-to-moderate pain despite taking a nonopioid analgesia; the following should occur at this step:
    1. Maximize the dose of the nonopioid analgesia
    2. And, add a step 2 opioid analgesia

3. Step 2 opioids are restricted for the treatment of moderate pain because of their dose-limiting side effects or because they are prepared with fixed combinations of nonopioid analgesics (see table that follows for classification of controlled drugs)
    a. Codeine (CIII) is preferred drug; prescribe oral dose 1 mg/kg every 4 hours
    b. Hydrocodone (Lorcet, Lortab) (CIII) and oxycodone (Percocet) (CII) are limited because of their combinations with acetaminophen; for example, to not exceed 6 g of acetaminophen per day, adolescents cannot take more than 15 mg of these opioids

---

CONTROLLED DRUGS

CII: High potential for abuse which may lead to severe psychological or physical dependence. (Prescriptions must be written in ink or typewritten and signed by practitioner. Verbal prescriptions cannot be made.)

CIII: Use of these products may lead to moderate or low physical dependence or high psychological dependence. Prescriptions can be oral or written and may be redispensed.

CIV: These drugs have a low abuse potential, use may lead to limited physical or psychological dependence. Prescriptions may be oral or written and may be redispensed up to 5 times within 6 months.

CV: These drugs have a low abuse potential, may or may not require a prescription, and are subject to state and local regulation.

J. Step 3: If pain persists even when taking highest, safe dose of step 2 opioid, add a step 3 opioid to treat moderate to severe pain (respiratory depression is a serious, life-threatening problem in the pediatric population; particularly in children with pulmonary problems)
    1. Morphine is first line agent; Available in immediate release tablets, sustained release tablets (MS Contin) (CII), rectal suppository (Roxanol) (CII), liquid, injection, and intravenous
    2. Other choices
        a. Oxycodone (Oxycontin) (CII)
        b. Hydromorphone (Dilaudid) (CII)
        c. Fentanyl (Duragesic) (CII) transdermal patches can control pain for 72 hours
    3. Methadone (Dolophine) (CII) and levorphanol (Levo-Dromoran) are useful for severe pain, but because of long half-lives are not recommended for initial therapy

K. The following opioids are not recommended
    1. Meperidine (Demerol) has a short half-life and its metabolite, normeperidine, is toxic
    2. Propoxyphene (Darvon) has a long half-life and there is risk of accumulation of norpropoxyphene, a toxic metabolite,
    3. Mixed narcotic agonist-antagonists such as pentazocine (Talwin) (CIV), butorphanol (Stadol) (CIV), and buprenorphine (Buprenex) (CIV) cause less constipation and biliary spasmodic activity but have the tendency to cause psychotomimetic responses

L. Adjuvant analgesics
    1. Tricyclic antidepressants (TCAs) such as amitriptyline (Elavil) (most frequently used, but has most side effect) imipramine (Tofranil), desipramine (Norpramin), doxepin (Sinequan) are beneficial in certain circumstances:
        a. Have direct analgesic effects and may potentiate opiate analgesia
        b. Useful in treatment of pain due to nerve injury such as diabetic neuropathy
    2. Selective serotonin reuptake inhibitors (SSRIs) such as fluoxetine (Prozac) or sertraline (Zoloft) have fewer adverse effects than TCAs and may be beneficial
    3. Phenothiazines such as prochlorperazine (Compazine) 5-10 mg TID or QID (Children >2yrs.: 0.4 mg/kg/day in three or four divided doses) or promethazine (Phenergan) 25 mg BID (Children >2yrs: 0.1 mg/kg/dose Q 6 hours) are useful as antiemetics when used in combination with other pain medications

M. Nonpharmacologic modalities to treat pain include meditation, relaxation, distraction, exercise, massage, acupuncture, surgery (cordotomy), neuroablative blocks (chemical destruction of nerves), and nervous system stimulaters such as dorsal column stimulaters (DCS) and transcutaneous electrical nerve simulators (TENS)

N. Interdisciplinary pain management
1. Specialists in the fields of anesthesia, neurology, physical therapy, internal medicine, nursing, psychology, and physical therapy can combine their efforts in chronic pain centers
2. Goals of interdisciplinary pain management are to ease suffering and reduce patient's reliance on opiates through nonpharmacological methods such as biofeedback, visual imagery, and stress management

O. Follow up is variable depending on source of pain

WEIGHT LOSS, ACUTE

I. Definition: Loss of 3% to 5% of total body mass occurring in less than 30 days

II. Pathogenesis

A. Reduced food intake and/or anorexia can result in a calorie deficit from the following causes:
1. Psychological problems such as anorexia nervosa, depression, and anxiety
2. Physical and financial factors that limit eating food
   a. Poor dentition
   b. Immobility problems
   c. Dysphagia
3. Drug-related problems such as amphetamine abuse
4. Esophageal disease
5. Infections such as human immunodeficiency virus (HIV) infection, tuberculosis, fungal disease
6. Malignancy
7. Uremia
8. Hepatitis
9. Vitamin B deficiencies
10. Neurological disorders including trauma
11. Substance abuse and tobacco use
12. Competitive athletes (wrestlers) may intentionally lose weight

B. Calorie loss can occur because of malabsorption from the following conditions:
1. Crohn's disease
2. Pancreatic insufficiency
3. Cholestasis
4. Parasitic disease such as giardiasis
5. Blind loop syndrome
6. Food sensitivity in celiac disease
7. Lactose intolerance
8. Milk allergy in infants

C. Loss of fluids or dehydration from one of the following
1. Uncontrolled diabetes mellitus
2. Diabetes insipidous
3. Diarrhea
4. Vomiting

D. Accelerated metabolism can contribute to weight loss in the following conditions:
1. Hyperthyroidism
2. Pheochromocytoma
3. Fever
4. Malignancy
5. Tachypnea
6. Status epilepticus
7. Spastic states

III. Clinical presentation of common causes of weight loss

    A. Loss of fluids is the most common cause of acute weight loss in children

    B. Anorexia nervosa and bulimia nervosa occur mainly in adolescent and young adult females who have a body image disturbance and an intense fear of becoming obese (see EATING DISORDERS section)

    C. Patients with HIV infection often have chronic anorexia, nausea, vomiting, and diarrhea due to drugs or to infections of the hepatobiliary system

    D. Malignancies, particularly of the gastrointestinal tract, pancreas, and liver result in weight loss and may be present without major signs and symptoms

    E. Uremia often presents initially with anorexia and subsequent weight loss

    F. Uncontrolled diabetes mellitus has weight loss and increased food intake

    G. Hyperthyroidism or thyrotoxicosis is the most common endocrine disease: Patients often have increased appetite, food intake, and motor activity (see section on HYPERTHYROIDISM)

    H. In malabsorption syndrome, foul-smelling, bulky, greasy stools are typical

    I. Signs and symptoms of malnutrition may occur with any illness if there is a loss of 10 to 20% of normal body weight
        1. Typical complaints include fatigue, depressed immune function, increased susceptibility to infection, tendency for breakdown of skin, and changes in emotional stability such as irritability and apathy
        2. Laboratory tests: serum albumin <3.4g/dL and lymphocyte count <1,500

IV. Diagnosis/Evaluation

    A. History
        1. Carefully ascertain amount of weight loss; ask about change in clothing size if unable to elicit number of pounds lost
        2. Validate amount of weight loss from a family member or significant other
        3. Obtain a 24 hour daily food intake
        4. Determine whether patient has loss of appetite, normal appetite, or increased appetite; unappealing thought, appearance and/or odor of food occurs with malignancy, drugs, depression
        5. Ask about abnormal or bad taste in mouth (occurs in hepatitis, drugs, sinusitis, vitamin B deficiencies, zinc deficiency, psychological disorders)
        6. If decreased food intake is suspected, explore symptoms of depression, poor dentition, dysphagia, alcohol and drug use, pain, nausea, vomiting, fatigue, and symptoms of heart failure
        7. Question about chewing or swallowing difficulties (occurs in neurologic, dental, oral, esophageal or pulmonary diseases)
        8. If anorexia nervosa is suspected ask about eating habits, self-image and attitudes about weight control
        9. If malabsorption is suspected determine character of stools, signs of jaundice, easy bruising, sore tongue, and paresthesias
        10. If calories lost in stool or urine is suspected, inquire about polyuria, polydipsia, nausea, and character of the stools
        11. If accelerated metabolism is suspected inquire about fever, fatigue, melena, cough that has changed in character, and symptoms of hyperthyroidism such as tachycardia, nervousness, heat intolerance, menstrual disturbances, and palpitations
        12. Obtain history of tobacco dependence
        13. Question about alcohol and drug use; ask about participation in competitive sports
        14. Inquire about previous history of hepatitis exposure, renal disease, endocrine problems
        15. Determine family history, particularly noting any history of cancer in first-degree relatives

B. Physical Examination; assessment should focus on nutritional status as well as identification of the underlying cause of weight loss
1. Measure height and weight, comparing with previous measurements
   a. Unexplained losses of more than 5% of usual body weight over 6 months needs a systematic investigation
   b. Body weight measurement is not always a good indicator of weight loss; occasionally loss of body tissue is accompanied by equal gain in extracellular fluid such as ascites or edema; thus, it is important to observe face and limbs for loss of soft-tissue mass
2. Assess for orthostatic hypotension which accompanies dehydration and malnutrition
3. Observe general appearance for wasting such as sunken eyes, sallow complexion and hair loss and signs of depression such as inappropriate dress and dull affect
4. Observe skin for pallor, ecchymosis, and jaundice
5. Examine mouth for poor dentition, glossitis, and lesions
6. Palpate neck for thyromegaly and lymphadenopathy
7. Perform a complete cardiovascular examination
8. Auscultate the lungs
9. Inspect abdomen for shape, scars, and masses
10. Auscultate abdomen for bowel sounds
11. Palpate and percuss abdomen for tenderness, ascites, masses, and organomegaly
12. Perform a rectal examination
13. Assess extremities for edema, muscle wasting, and skin turgor
14. Assess position and vibratory senses
15. Assess deep tendon reflexes; check for prolonged relaxation phase of reflexes that often occurs with thyroid disorders

C. Differential Diagnosis
1. When weight loss occurs with increased food intake, consider diabetes, thyrotoxicosis, malabsorption, or possibly leukemia and lymphoma as the likely diagnosis
2. When food intake is normal or decreased, consider psychological problems, malignancy, infection, renal disease, or endocrine problems as the likely diagnosis

D. Diagnostic Tests
1. Diagnostic tests should be ordered based on the history and physical; an initial, recommended battery of tests includes three stool specimens for occult blood, CBC with differential, urinalysis, serum glucose, BUN, creatinine, albumin, and liver function tests and possibly chest x-ray and sedimentation rate
2. Order thyroid tests in patients who have not had reduced food intake with weight loss
3. For patients with decreased intake consider ordering a serum calcium, potassium, and blood urea nitrogen
4. If malnutrition is suspected, also order serum iron, transferrin, total iron-binding capacity, RBCs folate, B_{12}, and zinc levels
5. For patients with impaired absorption, a quantitative stool fat examination by means of a 72-hour stool collection or a breath test is definitive test; but screening for malabsorption can be performed with Sudan stain of stool for fat and serum tests for carotenoids and folic acid
6. Consider colonoscopy or flexible sigmoidoscopy, barium enema, upper endoscopy or upper gastrointestinal series with small bowel follow-through, abdominal ultrasonography, computerized tomography of the abdomen, or magnetic resonance imaging if concerns of abdominal malignancy exist
7. Order CBC and erythrocyte sedimentation rate if fever is present
8. Erythrocyte sedimentation rate, chest x-ray, and mammogram are recommended if concerns of other types of cancer exist
9. Consider serum amylase and lipase if pancreatic disorder is suspected
10. Stool for ova and parasites is ordered when giardia is suspected
11. To assess nutritional status consider the following: serum albumin concentration, grip strength, triceps skin-fold thickness, arm muscle circumference, total lymphocyte count, serum transferrin and transthyretin (prealbumin) concentrations

V. Plan/Management

    A.   Treat underlying cause of weight loss (i.e., treat depression with antidepressant medications or pancreatic insufficiency with oral pancreatic enzyme preparations)

    B.   Patient with weight loss of more than 10-20% is often hospitalized and has extensive diagnostic workup; referral to specialist is needed

    C.   Consultation with a dietician/nutritionist is beneficial

    D.   Symptomatic therapy includes the following:
        1.   Suggest patient eat small, frequent feedings (6 times per day) of foods with high-calorie density
        2.   Suggest dietary supplements such as Ensure (see section on HIV INFECTION for other supplements)
        3.   Consider ordering vitamin supplementation
        4.   For nausea, suggest salty foods, cool clear beverages, gelatin, popsickles; avoid sweet, greasy or high fat foods

    E.   Follow Up
        1.   Scheduling of subsequent visits will depend on underlying cause of weight loss
        2.   Encourage patient to keep daily record of food intake, activity level, and symptoms

REFERENCES

Agency for Health Care Policy and Research, Public Health Service, US Department of Health and Human Services (1993). Acute pain management in adults: Operative procedures. (AHCPR Pub. No. 92-0019). Rockville, MD: US Government Printing Office.

Amadio, P., Cummings, D.M., & Amadio, P. (1993). Nonsteroidal anti-inflammatory drugs: Tailoring therapy to achieve results and avoid toxicity. Postgraduate Medicine, 93, 73-96.

Armstrong, W.B., & Giglio, M.F. (1998). Is this lump in the neck anything to worry about: Postgraduate Medicine, 104(3), 63-78.

Asnes, R.S., & Asnes, J.D. (1999). Pain. In R.A. Dershewitz (Ed.), Ambulatory pediatric care (3rd ed.). Philadelphia: Lippincott-Raven.

Batmann, T.J. (1993). Pain management. In J.T. DiPiro, R.L. Talbert, P.E. Hayes, G.C. Yee, Gary R. Matzke, & L.M. Posey (Eds.), Pharmacotherapy: A pathophysiologic approach (2nd ed.). Norwalk, CT: Appleton & Lange.

Beyer, J.E., & Well, N. (1989). Multidimensional pain assessment of children. Pediatric Clinics of North America, 36, 387.

Bonadio, W.A. (1993). Defining fever and other aspects of body temperature in infants and children. Pediatric Annals, 22(8), 467-473.

Davis, A.E. (1996). Primary care management of chronic musculoskeletal pain. Nurse Practitioner, 21(8), 72-82.

Dershewitz, R.A. (1999). Fever. In R.A. Dershewitz (Ed.), Ambulatory pediatric care (3rd ed.). Philadelphia: Lippincott-Raven.

Dowd, T.R., & Stewart, F.M. (1994). Primary care approach to lymphadenopathy. Nurse Practitioner, 19(12), 36-44.

Ferrer, R. (1998). Lymphadenopathy: Differential diagnosis and evaluation. American Family Physician, 58, 1313-1320.

Goroll, A.H., May, L.A., & Mulley, A.G. Jr. (1995). Evaluation of weight loss. In A.H Goroll, L.A. May & A.G. Mulley, Jr. (Eds.), Primary care medicine. Philadelphia: Lippincott.

Graef, J.W. (1999). Acute weight loss. In R.A. Dershewitz (Ed.), Ambulatory pediatric care (3rd ed.). Philadelphia: Lippencott-Raven.

Greene, M.G. (1991). The Harriet Lane Handbook. St. Louis: Mosby.

Heizer, W.D. (1997). Weight loss. In L. Dornbrand, A.J. Hoole, & R.H. Fletcher (Eds.), Manual of clinical problems in adult ambulatory care. Philadelphia: Lippincott-Raven.

Lesko, S.M., & Mitchell, A.A. (1995). An assessment of the safety of pediatric ibuprofen: A practitioner-based randomized clinical trial. JAMA, 273, 929-933.

Levy, M.H. (1996). Pharmacologic treatment of cancer pain. <u>New England Journal of Medicine, 335,</u> 1124-1131.

Lipsky, M.S. (1996). Lymphadenopathy. In M.B. Mengel & L.P. Schwiebert (Eds.), <u>Ambulatory medicine: The primary care of families</u> (2nd ed.). Stamford, Conneticut: Appleton-Lange.

Mackowiak, P.A., Bartlett, J.G., Borden, E.C., Goldblum, S.E., Hasday, J.D., Munford, R.S., Nasraway, S.A., Stolley, P.d., & Woodward, T.E. (1997). Concepts of fever: Recent advances and lingering dogma. <u>Clinical Infectious Disease, 25,</u> 119-138.

Mauskop, A. (1998). Symptomatic care pending diagnosis: Pain. In R.E. Rakel (Ed.), <u>Conn's current therapy 1998</u>. Philadelphia: Saunders.

Polisson, R. (1996). Nonsteroidal anti-inflammatory drugs: practical and theoretical considerations in their selection. <u>American Journal of Medicine, 100</u> (suppl 2A), 2A-31S-2A-36S.

Simon, H.B. (1995). Evaluation of fever. In A.H. Goroll, L.A. May & A.G. Mulley, Jr. (Eds.), <u>Primary care medicine</u>. Philadelphia: Lippincott.

Simon, H.B. (1995). Evaluation of lymphadenopathy. In A.H. Goroll, L.A. May & A.G. Mulley, Jr. (Eds.), <u>Primary care medicine</u>. Philadelphia: Lippincott.

WHO (1990). Cancer pain relief and palliative care: Report of WHO expert committee. <u>WHO Technological Report Service, 804,</u> 1-73.

Wilson, D. W. (1995). Assessing and managing the febrile child. <u>Nurse Practitioner, 11</u>(20), 59-74.

Yaster, M., Kost-Byerly, S., & Maxwell, L.G. (1997). Management of acute pain in children. In R.A. Hoekelman (Ed.), <u>Primary pediatric care.</u> St. Louis: Mosby.

Behavioral Problems

ALCOHOL PROBLEMS

I. Definition: Problems caused by alcohol that may be acute or chronic, may range from mild to severe and vary in their response to treatment; problems exist on a continuum of increasing severity ranging from at-risk use to alcohol abuse to alcohol dependence

II. Pathogenesis

    A. Causes of alcohol problems are incompletely understood, but factors that contribute to teenage alcohol use are in the following table

FACTORS THAT CONTRIBUTE TO TEEN ALCOHOL USE
✔ A genetic predisposition supported by twin adoption studies
✔ Parental role models in terms of attitudes toward alcohol and drinking practices
✔ Style of parenting that is extreme (either very authoritarian or permissive)
✔ Peer pressure and desire for group acceptance

    B. Male gender is associated with a higher prevalence; heavy drinking may be inversely associated with age, income, and educational level

    C. The principal ingredient of all alcoholic beverages is ethanol with most beer and wine containing between 3% to 20% ethanol

III. Clinical Presentation

    A. Problem drinking is defined as having been drunk 6 or more times in past year or having problems in 3 or more of the following areas

CRITERIA FOR PROBLEM DRINKING
✔ Trouble with teacher/principal
✔ Trouble with police
✔ Criticism by dates/family
✔ Problems with friends
✔ Driving after drinking

    B. Alcohol abuse is the continued use of alcohol in spite of adverse consequences (UCR mnemonic--Use, followed by adverse Consequences, followed by Repetition). Consequences may be physical, social, or psychological (see CRITERIA FOR ALCOHOL ABUSE table)

CRITERIA FOR ALCOHOL ABUSE	
Pattern of alcohol use in which 1 (or more) of the following 4 criteria are present within a 12-month period	
Recurrent alcohol use resulting in	✔ Failure to fulfill major role obligations (home, work, school) ✔ Placing self and others in potentially hazardous situations (DUI) ✔ Legal problems (e.g., arrest for DUI)
Continued alcohol use despite	✔ Persistent or recurrent social/interpersonal problems due to effects of alcohol

Adapted from the American Psychiatric Association. (1994). Diagnostic and statistical manual of mental disorders (4th ed.). Washington, DC: Author.

    C. Binge drinking is the consumption of 5 or more consecutive drinks within the prior 2 weeks

D.   Alcohol dependence is a chronic disease characterized by impaired control over drinking, preoccupation with the drug alcohol, use of alcohol in spite of adverse consequences, and distortions in thinking, primarily denial (see CRITERIA FOR ALCOHOL DEPENDENCE table)

CRITERIA FOR ALCOHOL DEPENDENCE
Pattern of alcohol use in which 3 (or more) of the following 7 criteria are present within a 12 month period ✔ Physical tolerance (increased amounts are required for desired effect) ✔ Withdrawal symptoms when substance is discontinued ✔ Larger amounts of alcohol are used than intended ✔ Unsuccessful efforts to control use ✔ Much time and energy are spent in obtaining, using, and recovering from effects of alcohol ✔ Many social, work-related, and recreational activities are reduced because of alcohol use ✔ Continued use in spite of knowledge that alcohol causes physical and/or psychological problems

Adapted from the American Psychiatric Association. (1994). Diagnostic and statistical manual of mental disorders (4th ed.). Washington, DC: Author.

E.   Alcohol, the most widely used drug in the US, has been used by at least 80% of adolescents by 18 years of age

F.   Motor vehicle accidents resulting from driving under the influence of alcohol are the leading cause of death in the 15-24 year old age group

G.   Binge drinking is especially common among college students with half of all male and a third of all female students reporting heavy drinking at least once a month

H.   Frequent binge drinkers report numerous alcohol-related problems such as problems with school work, unsafe sex, and trouble with police

I.   Alcohol is a CNS depressant, but at low doses it has behavioral stimulant effects
   1.   In moderate doses, alcohol produces sedation, euphoria, decreased inhibitions, and problems with coordination
   2.   In higher doses, ataxia, slurred speech, poor judgment, and labile mood occur
   3.   Finally, heavy doses can result in loss of consciousness, respiratory failure, coma, and death

J.   Adolescent alcohol abusers are unlikely to experience consequences of prolonged alcohol use such as hepatitis, cirrhosis, and pancreatitis

IV.   Diagnosis/Evaluation

   A.   History
      1.   Keep in mind that the history (including interview and use of questionnaires) is by far more sensitive and specific than are physical exam and laboratory findings
      2.   All adolescents should be screened for alcohol problems. **Ask "Do you ever drink alcohol?"**
      3.   If patient **ever** drinks, ask quantity-frequency questions which deal with level of consumption, which can help distinguish moderate from at-risk drinking and identify binge drinking (see LEVEL OF CONSUMPTION and GENERAL EQUIVALENCIES OF ALCOHOLIC BEVERAGES tables)

LEVEL OF CONSUMPTION	
Frequency	How many days in a week do you usually have something to drink?
Quantity	On days that you drink, how many drinks do you have?
Maximum	What is the most you had to drink on any one day during the past month?
Last drink	When was your last drink? (Persons with a problem know exactly)

Adapted from Bower, K.T., & Severin, J.D. (1997). Alcohol and other drug-related problems. In D.J. Knesper, M.B. Riba, & T.L. Schwenk (Eds.), Primary care psychiatry. Philadelphia: Saunders.

GENERAL EQUIVALENCIES OF ALCOHOLIC BEVERAGES*

Hard liquor (80 proof spirits)

1 shot or highball ((1.5 ounces)	=	1 drink
1/2 pint of liquor	=	~5 drinks
1 pint of liquor	=	~10 drinks

Wine (11% to 12% alcohol)

1 glass of wine (5 ounces)	=	1 drink
1 bottle of wine (750 mL)	=	5 drinks

Beer (4% to 5% alcohol)

1 12-ounce bottle or can	=	1 drink
1 40-ounce container	=	~3 drinks
1 6-pack of beer	=	6 drinks

Wine Coolers (5% alcohol)

1 wine cooler (12 ounces)	=	1 drink

* One drink contains approximately 12 g of alcohol

4. Follow quantity-frequency questions with the CAGE questions. See THE CAGE QUESTIONNAIRE table

THE CAGE QUESTIONNAIRE

C	Have you ever felt you ought to **C**ut down on your drinking?
A	Have people **A**nnoyed you by criticizing your drinking?
G	Have you ever felt bad or **G**uilty about your drinking?
E	Have you ever had a drink the first thing in the morning (**E**ye opener) to steady your nerves or get rid of a hangover?
Scoring and Interpretation	Person receives one point for each positive answer. One "yes" answer indicates hazardous drinking and two or more "yes" answers indicates alcohol abuse or dependence

Source: Bush, B., Shaw, S., Cleary, P., Delbanco, T.L., & Aronson, M.D. (1987). Screening for alcohol abuse using the CAGE questionnaire. American Journal of Medicine, 82, 231-235.

5. Note that no consensus exists regarding optimal screening tools for use with adolescents; adolescents are less likely than adolescents to manifest physical dependence measured by the "E" in CAGE ("Have you ever had a drink first thing in the morning [**E**ye opener]...")
6. If patient answers "yes" to a CAGE question, prompt for more details
7. Patients who become angry and defensive with the CAGE questions have already responded positively to the second item in the questionnaire ("Have people Annoyed you by criticizing your drinking?")
8. If screening using quantity-frequency questions and CAGE questions indicates problems with alcohol, ask more specific questions based on criteria for alcohol abuse and criteria for alcohol dependence
9. Finally, carefully screen for use of other substances (high concomitant use of tobacco and other drugs by persons with alcohol problems)
10. Alternatives to the CAGE questionnaire are listed in SCREENING TESTS FOR ALCOHOL PROBLEMS table

SCREENING TESTS FOR ALCOHOL PROBLEMS		
Test	**Description**	**Source**
AUDIT (Alcohol Use Disorders Identification Test)	Excellent and simple 10-question, self-administered questionnaire that assesses both levels of consumption and related problems	Saunders, J.B., Aasland, O.G., Babor, T.F., & Unreal, N. (1993). Development of the Alcohol Use Disorders Identification Test (AUDIT): WHO collaborative project on early detection of persons with harmful alcohol consumption. Addiction: 88, 791-804
MAST (Michigan Alcoholism Screening Test)	Contains 24 items and there are several versions and scoring protocols available, including the simpler 13-item Short MAST	Hedlund, J.L., & Vieweg, B.W. (1984). The Michigan Alcoholism Screening Test (MAST): A comprehensive review. J. Operational Psychiatry: 15, 55-65
TACE	Contains 4 items and is based on the CAGE; for use with pregnant females	Russel, M., Martier, S.S., & Sokol, R.J., et al. (1994). Screening for pregnancy risk-drinking. Alcohol Clin Exp Res: 18, 1156-1161
TWEAK	Contains 5 items and is also for use with pregnant females	Ibid.
POSIT (Problem Oriented Screening Instrument for Teenagers)	Contains 16 items and is a subscale of a larger instrument	Rahdert, E.R. (1991). The adolescent assessment/referral manual. USDHHS Pub. No. (ADM) 91-1735. Available from the National Clearinghouse for Alcohol and Drug Information. Call (800) 729-6686

Adapted from Bower, K.T., & Severin, J.D. (1997). Alcohol and other drug-related problems. In D.J. Knesper, M.B. Riba, & T.L. Schwenk (Eds.), Primary care psychiatry. Philadelphia: Saunders.

B. Physical Examination
   1. Physical exam will most likely be normal; early manifestations of alcohol abuse/dependence are psychosocial, not physical. (**Note:** Physical findings such as skin changes, hepatomegaly, and gynecomastia are late manifestations of prolonged, heavy alcohol use and would be rare findings in the adolescent)
   2. Assess general appearance: weight loss, emaciated appearance are late findings in chronic alcoholism and are rarely, if ever, present in adolescents
   3. Examine skin for signs of chronic alcoholism (abnormal vascularization of the facial skin [spider angiomas] and jaundice when liver disease is present) [rare in adolescents]
   4. Perform abdominal exam for hepatomegaly and right upper quadrant tenderness (rare)
   5. Perform complete neurologic exam, including mental status exam, cranial nerves, gait, sensory, motor, reflexes, Romberg test
   6. During exam, note if patient smells of alcohol as alcohol on breath during primary care visit indicates that there is impaired control over drinking

C. Differential Diagnosis: Other mental disorders such as mood and anxiety disorders, psychosis, abuse of other psychoactive substances such as opiods, marijuana, hallucinogens, PCP, inhalants, and sedatives

D. Diagnostic Tests
   1. CBC (elevated mean corpuscular volume is a marker of excessive alcohol consumption; may be elevated due to other causes such as dietary deficiencies--B_{12}, folate--liver disease, smoking)
   2. Liver enzyme tests
      a. Gamma-glutamyl transpeptidase (GGT) is the most sensitive blood test for screening for detection of long-term heavy drinking; test lacks specificity as other causes of elevated GGT are such things as use of anticonvulsants, barbiturates, and from nonalcoholic liver disease
      b. Aspartate aminotransferase (AST) and alanine aminotransferase (ALT) have a low sensitivity for detecting alcohol problems; if elevations are suspected to be due to liver problems, advise abstinence and monitor over time to see if they decline. The enzymes are also released by muscle tissue and can be elevated by such events as intensive weight training; AST:ALT ratio can be helpful with a ratio of 2:1 suggestive of alcohol-induced liver disease

3. Carbohydrate-deficient transferrin can detect heavy drinking and may be useful for monitoring alcohol-dependent patients

V. Plan/Management

A. Plan is determined by the **identification** and **confirmation** that the patient has problems with alcohol and by his/her **willingness to change** behavior

B. **Identification** of problem-drinking is determined primarily from screening using the CAGE or POSIT and the Level of Consumption questions; the physical examination and the laboratory testing may provide additional evidence that a problem exists but in teens, abnormal findings are unlikely

C. **Confirming** the problem is based on the extent to which the patient meets the criteria for problem drinking, or for alcohol abuse or dependence and involves two important diagnostic issues
1. What happens when the patient uses alcohol? (adverse consequences), and
2. What happens when the patient tries to stop? (impaired control, tolerance and withdrawal)

D. Diagnostic Issues
1. **First diagnostic issue**. Assess problem areas first (adverse consequences) then link them to substance use. (Example: How are things going at home? At school? In your social life? and so on. As problems are introduced by the patient, be empathic, but ask patient "How do you think your use of alcohol fits in with this?")
2. **Second diagnostic issue**. Determine degree of **impaired control** by asking questions such as "Do you drink more than you intend to?" "Why do you think that happens?" "Do you ever make rules for your drinking?" "Are you able to follow those rules?" Assess **tolerance**. "Do you need more to get the same effect?" Ask about **withdrawal**. "Do you ever feel bad or sick when you try to stop drinking?"

E. **Motivation** for change on the patient's part is crucial to the success of any treatment plan. Appropriate questions to assess motivation are the following: "Are you concerned about your use of alcohol?" "Are you interested in changing?"; success of any intervention is dependent on the patient's willingness to participate in treatment goals

F. **Brief interventions have been demonstrated through research to be highly effective**
1. Can be conducted in the office for the following groups of patients: Problem drinkers who are not alcohol-dependent
2. Use the *FRAMES* acronym to guide the intervention

FRAMES FOR BRIEF INTERVENTIONS	
Feedback	related to screening tests, history, physical examination and laboratory findings should be provided as well as the implications of the findings (e.g., your liver enzyme GGT is increased to 128. The normal range for this enzyme is zero to 30 (show patient the lab report)
Responsibility	for changing alcohol use should be placed on the patient; success of treatment is up to patient
Advise	patient to cut down or abstain
Menu	of options should be presented to the patient in order to make the patient a partner in the decision-making process: Can attempt to stop on own; can attend AA meetings; can use self-help books
Empathic	approach is helpful
Self-efficacy	of the patient is encouraged by clinician's optimism relating to behavior change Advise the patient to make a change--stop drinking altogether or if controlled drinking is an option in your opinion, to limit drinking if patient is of legal age

Adapted from Miller, W.R., & Rollnick, S. (1991). Motivational interviewing: Preparing people to change addictive behavior. New York: Guilford Press.

G. For all patients with alcohol problems regardless of their pattern, abstinence for a minimum of two weeks is recommended at the beginning of the treatment regimen
1. Initial period of abstinence allows provider/patient to assess impact of alcohol on patient's overall health and functioning

2. Attainment of a two week period of abstinence appears to be related to patients reaching their ultimate goal, whether complete sobriety or controlled drinking
3. More intensive treatments are indicated for patients with alcohol dependence

H. Refer patient and family to self-help groups such as Alcoholics Anonymous (AA) for patients, Al-Anon for families. These groups are extremely effective in maintaining sobriety and helping patients and families to cope. Refer family even if patient declines to attend
   1. Alcoholics Anonymous, PO Box 459, Grand Central Station, New York, NY 10163, 212/686-1100
   2. Al-Anon Family Group Headquarters, Inc., 1600 Corporate Landing Parkway, Virginia Beach, VA 23454-5616, 1-800-356-9996

I. Familiarize yourself with AA in your community by attending an open meeting
   1. With patient's permission, ask for an AA volunteer who is willing to act as sponsor to meet with patient in your office
   2. Sponsor should be same gender as patient

J. Recommend self-help books for both patients and family members (see table below)

SELF-HELP BOOKS FOR ALCOHOL PROBLEMS	
For the patient (author of book is a woman, so particularly useful for female patients)	Knapp, C. (1991). Drinking: A love story. New York: Doubleday Delacorte Press
For the patient (emphasis is on lifestyle as well as behavioral change)	Washington, A., & Boundy, D. (1990). Willpower is not enough: Understanding and recovering from addictions of every kind. New York: Harper-Perennial
For parents of a patient with alcohol problems (written by former US Senator George McGovern)	McGovern, G. (1996). Terry: My daughter's life and death struggle with alcoholism. New York: Villard
For adult children of alcoholics and their risk issues	Black, C. (1981). It will never happen to me: Children of alcoholics as youngsters-adolescents-adults. New York: Ballantine

K. Some patients may benefit from treatment initiated in an inpatient or residential setting; criteria for treatment in this setting include presence of severe coexisting medical/psychiatric conditions, risk of harm to self or others, failure to respond to less intensive therapy

L. Be familiar with at least one specialized treatment facility in your area
   1. Feedback from patients will help you learn which programs in your area are most effective
   2. Referral for family therapy may be indicated when complex problems are present
   3. Inpatient drug treatment facilities for adolescents are unavailable in many areas

M. Pharmacologic adjuncts: Medications must be viewed as an adjunct to the process of recovery which is very time-consuming and difficult
   1. Disulfiram (Antabuse), 125-500 mg/day (available in 250 and 500 mg tabs)
      This medication may be used in adolescents >18 years who are motivated and who are involved with other modalities related to recovery. Must not be used until blood alcohol level is zero which is usually reached 24 hours after patient's last drink
      a. As with all medications, consult PDR regarding dosing and contraindications
      b. Liver function should be monitored at baseline, in 2-4 weeks, and then monthly for two months
      c. Counsel about avoidance of alcohol including OTCs with alcohol content while drug is being taken ; must abstain from alcohol for 14 days after stopping disulfiram therapy
      d. Potentially severe interactions with alcohol limit its widespread use
   2. Naltrexone (Revia), 50 mg/day (available in 50 mg scored tabs). Believed to blunt the pleasurable effects of alcohol; adolescent must be >18 years
      a. Indicated as adjunctive therapy for patients enrolled in residential alcohol treatment programs **only**

        b.   Drug is not used on an out-patient basis and is contraindicated in patients with hepatitis or liver failure

N.   Follow up is variable depending on type of treatment
1.   Patients for whom brief intervention is conducted: Follow up for two or more visits to monitor the patient's progress and assess need for additional approaches
2.   Patients who have been referred to alcohol treatment (either self-help groups or residential) should be followed for ongoing support; the natural course of alcohol problems includes remission as well as relapse

ATTENTION DEFICIT HYPERACTIVITY DISORDER

I.   Definition: Descriptive category for cluster of symptoms that include inattention, impulsivity, and motor hyperactivity that are more frequent and severe than seen in persons of the same developmental level; this disorder is usually first diagnosed in childhood but can persist into adulthood

II.   Pathogenesis

    A.   Causes are unknown

    B.   Probably encompasses several distinct disorders involving multiple genetic, neurological, temperamental, and environmental factors

    C.   Current research supports neurobiological factors as most prominent in the etiology

III.   Clinical Presentation

    A.   Once believed to largely resolve in childhood/adolescence, evidence now exists indicating that it can persist into adulthood. **Important**: Not an acquired disorder of adulthood

    B.   Estimated prevalence is between 3-9% with a male to female ratio of almost 10:1 during childhood; the male to female ratio is about even in adulthood

    C.   Presentation during preschool years
        1.   Most common time of onset
        2.   Child often described as "driven by motor"
        3.   Constant supervision required
        4.   Child-proofing house required beyond what is normally needed

    D.   Presentation during school age years
        1.   Usually presents soon after entry to school when cognitive/ behavioral abilities are challenged by teacher/situation expectations
        2.   Frequent teacher attention required to keep child "on task"
        3.   Child frequently disrupts classroom with motor activity (leaving desk without permission) impulsivity (talking out of turn)

    E.   Presentation during adolescence:
        1.   Almost without exception, adolescents with ADHD have **continuing** symptoms from childhood
        2.   Adolescent-onset ADHD is not a primary diagnosis but may occur secondary to a neurologic insult or to a psychiatric disorder
        3.   Regarding activity level, adolescents with ADHD are usually more active than other adolescents, but less active than they were as preadolescents
        4.   Low self-esteem from academic failure/social rejection becomes more of an issue during this age period

F.   **Hyperactivity is no longer a required diagnostic criterion for ADHD at any age**, and this is the most likely symptom to remit with age

G.   Diagnostic criteria for ADHD are contained in the following table
1.   Note there are **two** dimensions, inattention and hyperactivity/impulsivity, with behaviors specific to each dimension
2.   From these two dimensions, three subtypes are derived
a.   Predominantly inattentive type (criteria are met on inattention dimension, but **not** on the hyperactivity/impulsivity dimension)
b.   Predominantly hyperactive/impulsive type (criteria are met on hyperactive/ impulsive dimension but **not** on the inattention dimension)
c.   Combined type (criteria are met for both dimensions)

ADHD DIAGNOSTIC CRITERIA TABLE

Either 1 or 2

1. **Six or more symptoms of inattention have persisted for at least a 6 month period to the degree that is maladaptive and inconsistent with developmental level:**

Inattention-- The person **often**	➡ Fails to pay close attention to details resulting in careless mistakes
	➡ Has difficulty sustaining attention in activities (whether play or other tasks)
	➡ Does not seem to listen when being spoken to
	➡ Does not follow through on instructions and fails to complete schoolwork, chores, or duties in the workplace (not due to oppositional behavior or inability to understand directions)
	➡ Has difficulty with organization
	➡ Avoids, dislikes, or is reluctant to undertake activities that require sustained mental effort (such as schoolwork or homework)
	➡ Loses items necessary for tasks or activities
	➡ Becomes easily distracted by extraneous stimuli. Is forgetful in daily activities

2. **Six or more symptoms of hyperactivity-impulsivity have persisted for at least a 6 month period to a degree that is maladaptive and inconsistent with developmental level:**

Hyperactivity-- The person **often**	➡ Fidgets with hands or feet or squirms in seat
	➡ Leaves seat in situations where remaining in seat is expected
	➡ Runs or climbs excessively in situations in which it is inappropriate to do so (in adolescents or adults, this may be limited to subjective feelings of restlessness)
	➡ Has difficulty engaging in quiet play or leisure activities
	➡ Is "on the go" or seems driven by a motor
	➡ Talks excessively

Impulsivity-- The person **often**	➡ Blurts out answers before question has been asked
	➡ Has difficulty waiting turn
	➡ Interrupts or intrudes on others (butts into conversations or games)

In addition, the following must be true	➡ Some hyperactive-impulsive or inattentive behaviors were present **before** age 7 years
	➡ Some impairment from the symptoms is present in two or more settings (home, school or work)
	➡ Clear evidence of clinically significant impairment in social, academic, or work-related functioning must exist
	➡ Symptoms may not better be accounted for by another mental disorder (e.g., mood, anxiety, personality, psychotic)

Adapted from American Psychiatric Association. (1994). Diagnostic and statistical manual of mental disorders (4th ed.) Washington, DC: Author

---

IV.   Diagnosis/Evaluation

A.   History
1.   Focus of history taking is to determine whether patient meets the diagnostic criteria for ADHD as outlined above
2.   History must come from multiple sources with the two primary sources being parents and teachers
3.   Ask about age of onset and gather specific examples of child's behaviors according to the two dimensions -- inattention and hyperactivity/ impulsivity
4.   Determine if the symptoms have been present at least 6 months and establish that symptoms are present in two or more settings

5. In addition to parent/teacher/other report of characteristic behaviors, use of rating scales can also be helpful (see ADHD RATING SCALES table below)
6. Interview the child, particularly the child who is ≥5, as the child can provide insight into his/her feelings (may not provide accurate reports of behaviors, however)
7. Obtain social history, developmental history, past and present medical history, and **current medications**

ADHD RATING SCALES
Conners Rating Scales (versions for parent and for teacher) ADD Comprehensive Teacher's Rating Scale (ACTERS) [for teachers]
Source: Psychological Assessment Resources, Inc., Post Office Box 998, Odessa, FL 33556, 800/331-8378

B. Physical Examination
1. Complete neurologic exam including gait, muscular strength and tone, deep tendon reflexes, sensory responses
2. Vision and hearing to rule out sensory impairment
3. Results of the PE are usually negative

C. Differential Diagnosis
1. Anxiety (suspect if symptoms present in only one setting, e.g., home, but not at school)
2. Substance abuse (suspect if patient exhibits symptoms uncharacteristic of previous behavior)
3. Depression
4. Sensory impairment
5. Learning disability (children with comprehension difficulties often appear restless, inattentive)

D. Diagnostic Tests
1. Basic laboratory testing including a lead level, CBC with differential, and thyroid panel
2. No single neuropsychological test is diagnostic of ADHD; rating scales such as the ones listed in ADHD RATING SCALES table in section IV.A. can provide important data
3. When learning disabilities are suspected, a psychometric examination of the child's general cognitive abilities should be performed by the school (or by a private psychologist) at the parents' request

V. Plan/Management

A. A combination of psychosocial and pharmacologic management is usually beneficial

B. Psychosocial interventions most often involve behavior modification and environmental manipulation aimed at increasing appropriate and decreasing inappropriate behaviors
1. Successful programs require involvement of mental health counselor
2. Usually requires parents to work with counselor to learn techniques
3. Teachers often need additional support to implement these techniques

C. Social skills training within the school setting are also important as patients typically lack good social skills

D. General guidelines to provide to parent who are awaiting referral to a mental health counselor
1. A substantial commitment of time and energy by parent is required
2. A structured environment in which expectations are clear is the appropriate milieu
3. Regular and frequent exercise, a well-balanced diet, and good sleep hygiene are important; martial arts training may be very helpful
4. Limit rules to those that impact health and safety
5. Find tolerant baby-sitters for respite

E.   Management in school
    1.   Diagnostic testing is first step in order to determine proper classroom placement
    2.   Optimally, teachers, counselors, and school nurse can work together with child and parents to develop an effective educational plan

F.   The goal of pharmacologic management is to decrease motor activity, control impulsivity, and increase attention span
    1.   Pharmacologic management is indicated when there is clear evidence that a child's attentional difficulties affect school performance, present problems with social adjustment, or are associated with a behavioral disorder
    2.   Unless clearcut benefits are achieved, a medication should not be continued
    3.   Pharmacologic management should be undertaken only by experts in the diagnosis and treatment of ADHD
    4.   If referral to an expert is not possible, consultation with an expert is necessary prior to initiation of therapy to insure that the child is being appropriately treated
    5.   Stimulants are the first line of pharmacologic treatment for inattentive children and about 70% of patients respond to the first stimulant medication tried when the dose is titrated up to effective level
        a.   Methylphenidate (Ritalin) is given at 0.3 mg/kg/dose, and gradually increased (as necessary) to 0.6 mg/kg/dose 2-3 times/day (maximum 60 mg/day)
            (1)   Typical times of administration are 8 AM, noon, and a third dose at 4 PM if the duration of control provided by 2 doses is inadequate
            (2)   A usual starting dose of methylphenidate for elementary grade children is 5 mg in the AM and 5 mg at noon, with an additional dose after school if needed
            (3)   Whereas some authorities recommend a drug holiday (on weekend and vacations) to reduce tolerance to the drugs, others think that drug holidays can destabilize control [ADHD often creates problems and stress at home, e.g., inability to do chores, get along with siblings and playmates]
            (4)   Weekly follow up for several weeks is needed to monitor effectiveness and adjust dosage as necessary
        b.   Dextroamphetamine sulfate (Dexedrine supplied as 5 mg scored tabs, and Dexedrine spanules, supplied as 5, 10 mg sustained release caps) is also an effective stimulant. The recommended dose of dextroamphetamine is half that of methylphynidate
            (1)   Not recommended for children < 3 years of age
            (2)   For children 3-5, begin with 2.5 mg/day
            (3)   For children ≥6 years of age, begin with 5 mg/day
            (4)   Consult PDR for additional details on dosing, administration, drug interactions, and side effects
        c.   Another amphetamine with a slightly different chemical structure is Adderall, supplied as 5, 10 mg scored tabs
            (1)   Not recommended for children < 3 years of age
            (2)   Children 3-5 years, 2.5 mg/day, with dose given in AM
            (3)   Children 6 and older, starting dose is 5 mg/day; may need additional 1-2 doses at 4-6 hour intervals
            (4)   Consult PDR for additional details on dosing, administrations, drug interactions, and side effects
        d.   Main side effects of stimulants are anorexia, insomnia, irritability, and tics
        e.   Interactions of stimulant drugs with other medications can cause significant problems, particularly with anticonvulsive or other psychotropic medications
    6.   Tricyclic antidepressants such as desipramine (Norpramin) and imipramine (Tofranil) improve the symptoms in some children who do not respond to stimulants and their use should be considered as a second-line medication. **Sudden death** has occurred in children taking tricyclic antidepressants and **cardiac monitoring** is required; consult PDR for dosing

7. Alpha$_2$ agonists including clonidine (Catapres) and guanfacine (Tenex) reduce activity level, impulsiveness, and aggression and enhance attention only indirectly. May be used as an alternative to or an adjunctive treatment to stimulants. Should be avoided in children with pure inattention and **pulse and blood pressure must be monitored on a regular basis**. Consult PDR for clonidine and guanfacine dosing

G. Recommend resources for parents and patients from the following table

RESOURCES FOR PATIENTS WITH ADHD
Children and Adults with Attention Deficit Disorders (CHADD), National Headquarters, Suite 185, 1859 North Pine Island Road, Plantation, FL 33322, 1/800-233-4050
Attention Deficit Disorder Association, 4300 West Park Blvd., Plano, TX 75093
National Institute of Mental Health/IRIB, 5600 Fishers Lane, Room 7C-02, Rockville, MD 20857

H. Recommend readings for parents, patients, and teachers from the following table

READINGS FOR PARENTS, PATIENTS AND TEACHERS	
Taking Charge of ADHD: The Complete, Authoritative Guide for Parents by R.A. Barkley. Published by Guilford Press, New York, 1995	Basic book with comprehensive information for parents
The Time-Out Solution: A Parent's Guide for Handling Everyday Behavior Problems by L. Clark. Published by Contemporary Books, Chicago, 1989	Provides practical details on use of time-out as well as other ways to increase appropriate behavior
Driven to Distraction: Recognizing and Coping with Attention Deficit Disorder from Childhood Through Adulthood by E. Hallowell & J. Ratey. Published by Pantheon Books, New York, 1994	Especially good reference for diagnosis and treatment of ADHD in adults
ADHD: A Guide to Understanding and Helping Children with Attention Deficit Hyperactivity Disorder in School Settings by L. Braswell, M. Bloomquist, & S. Pederson. Published by the University of Minnesota, Department of Professional Development and Conference Services, Continuing Education and Extension, 315 Pillsbury Drive, SE, Minneapolis, MN 55455; 612/625-3502	An outstanding resource for teachers

I. Follow Up
1. Keep in mind that evaluation of children suspected of having ADHD is a very time-consuming process. Therefore, these patients are best managed in a specialized treatment center if one is available
2. Follow-up schedule is variable depending on whether patient is being managed in a specialty treatment center or in a primary care setting
3. For all patients on medications, very frequent monitoring for efficacy and for adverse events is essential

ENCOPRESIS

I. Definition: A chronic disorder in which young children have bowel movements in unacceptable sites (usually underwear) after age 4

II. Pathogenesis

    A. There are two types of encopresis: retentive in which there is involuntary leakage of fecal material from an impaction and nonretentive in which normal movements are passed into underwear

    B. In retentive encopresis, an impaction occurs when constipation has been present for about a week; pressure of the impaction dilates internal anal sphincter rendering it incompetent so that leakage of stool occurs due to gravity, exercise, or relaxation
        1. A small minority of children become impacted due to organic factors
        2. Most children in this category hold back stool because of fear of pain or because of control issues with parent

    C. In nonretentive encopresis, child has normal stool in underwear rather than in toilet
        1. Child is not constipated
        2. In preschoolers, a deliberate resistance to bowel training is likely cause
        3. In school-age child, reluctance to use public toilets or to leave enjoyable activity is likely cause

III. Clinical Presentation

    A. Varying degrees of disorder present in all cultures, though exact prevalence rates are unknown

    B. Children with retentive encopresis (most common type) have history of constipation and multiple daily soilings with liquid stool

    C. Children with nonretentive encopresis (affecting about 10-20% of children with encopresis) present with no history of constipation and have 1-2 normal stools per day

IV. Diagnosis/Evaluation

    A. History
        1. Distinguish between retentive and nonretentive encopresis by asking appropriate questions (See KEY QUESTIONS TO DISTINGUISH TYPES OF ENCOPRESIS table below)
        2. Take a complete dietary history including intake of dairy products, fruit juice, and fiber
        3. Inquire about pattern of toilet sitting--frequency during day and whether toilet sitting is voluntary or coerced by parent/teacher/day care provider
        4. Remember to talk to the child! Child should be a primary historian after about age 7 (except of course, in the areas of past medical history). What are child's perceptions of problem and parental responses to the problem?

KEY QUESTIONS TO DISTINGUISH TYPES OF ENCOPRESIS		
Question	**Retentive**	**Nonretentive**
Are there symptoms of constipation?	Yes	No
What is the frequency of soiling?	Many times/day	Once or twice/day
What is the stool size?	Small	Normal
What is the stool consistency?	Liquid	Normal
Is there a history of need for laxatives?	Yes	No
Does child experience pain with stooling?	Yes	No
Is there passage of huge stools that clog toilet?	Yes	No

B. Physical Examination
    1. Perform abdominal exam; in retentive soiling an abdominal mass most commonly involving the rectosigmoid area is usually palpable; mass is midline, suprapubic, irregular and mobile
    2. Inspect anus for hemorrhoids/anal tags, and **always** perform a rectal exam
        a. Rectum in all impacted children is dilated and packed with stool with a wet-clay consistency
        b. In nonretentive stooling, rectal exam should reveal either normal stool or nothing
        c. Inspect for skin staining and signs of chronic skin irritation in perianal area
    3. Do a neurologic exam to rule out any sensory or motor deficits

C. Differential Diagnosis
    1. Constipating medications or diet
    2. Hirschsprung disease
    3. Hypothyroidism

D. Diagnostic Tests
    1. Urinalysis for nitrites and leukocytes (impaction can cause partial bladder emptying and retention)
    2. Consider a plain-view x-ray of abdomen to detect retained stool

V. Plan/Treatment

    A. Management of retentive encopresis
        1. Counsel parent and child that holding back stool is the primary cause of soiling
        2. Removal of impaction is absolutely necessary if child is to maintain bowel control: Administer 2-3 sodium phosphate enemas over a 2 day period to remove impaction
        3. As soon as impaction is removed, long-term management of constipation should be begun with use of either mineral oil or lactulose for stool softening
            a. Mineral oil
                (1) Children: 1 ml/kg/dose BID (maximum 3 oz/day)
                (2) Adolescents: 60 ml/dose (maximum 4 oz/day)
            b. Mineral oil formulations that are more acceptable in terms of taste (also more expensive) are available (examples are Petrogalar and Kondremul)
            c. Lactulose (Cephulac10 g/15 mL syrup)
                (1) Children: 0.5 ml/kg/dose BID (maximum 1.5 oz/day)
                (2) Adolescents: 15 ml BID (maximum 2.5 oz/day)
            d. Aim of treatment with stool softeners is to enable child to produce 1-2 normal stools/day
        4. Use of stool softeners must continue for at least 3 months and perhaps 6 months or longer (child will need this much time to forget painful or stressful nature of hard stools)
        5. Medications need to be continued until there are no episodes of soiling for at least 1 month
        6. Child should sit on toilet for 10 minutes, 3 times/day after meals to take advantage of gastrocolic reflex; use of footstool for leverage may be helpful. Encourage parents to read to child while toilet sitting as this should not be an unpleasant experience
        7. Nonconstipating, high-fiber diet with good water intake is necessary to maintain soft stool
        8. All children with impaction require follow-up at 1 week after catharsis; about 30% are still impacted
            a. Repeat abdominal exam and the rectal exam
            b. If impaction is still present, have parent repeat the disimpaction process
        9. Advise parents to expect relapses
            a. If more than 48 hours pass without a BM, instruct parent to administer a laxative such as Senokot (>5 years, 10 ml syrup; adolescents, 15 ml syrup) or Dulcolax (>5 years, one 5 mg tab; adolescents, two 5 mg tabs)
            b. If soiling begins to recur, advise child/parent that rectum is full and impaction is returning; vigorous intervention is indicated (increasing dose of laxative, administration of a suppository or administration of enema is indicated) to restore normal stool patterns

B. Management of nonretentive encopresis
    1. Decreasing involvement of the parent in this problem (except for providing incentives to child) and increasing the responsibility of the child are **keys** to success
    2. Advise parents to discontinue any pressure on child regarding stooling (there should be no lectures, no reminders, no questions relating to toilet use, and absolutely NO PUNISHMENT for stooling in underwear)
    3. Advise parents to provide incentives for stooling in toilet (praise, hug, dining out at favorite fast-food place)
    4. Advise parents to not ignore soiling; parent should instruct child to immediately clean self up when soiling occurs; this should be a quick, impersonal interaction in which child is not made to feel ashamed of his behavior
    5. Medications are not indicated because stool retention is not the issue

C. Follow Up
    1. For both types of encopresis, continue to follow-up every 2 months for 6 months to evaluate progress
    2. Children who are severely resistant to intervention in the primary care setting or who have disturbed parent-child relationships need referral for specialized care

PRIMARY NOCTURNAL ENURESIS

I. Definition: Involuntary discharge of urine at night beyond the age of 5 years in girls and 6 years in boys

II. Pathogenesis

    A. Enuresis is considered to be multifactorial in etiology

    B. Various theories have been proposed to explain this disorder
        1. Developmental delay explanations have focused on a delay in adequate neuromuscular control
        2. Organic theories suggest disorders of the genitourinary and nervous systems; however, only about 3-4% of children with enuresis have organic pathology
        3. Psychological factors may have an impact on the expression of enuresis although the incidence of behavioral problems in enuretic children is difficult to determine
        4. Early sleep studies suggested that "disorder of arousal" may have role in enuresis but more recently, it has been concluded that sleep stage is unrelated to episodes of enuresis
        5. A lack of circadian rhythm in antidiuretic hormone secretion appears to play a major role in nocturnal enuresis
        6. Family history has an important role in development of enuresis with a 45% chance that a parent who was enuretic will have one or more children who is enuretic

III. Clinical Presentation

    A. Approximately 15% of all 5 year olds, 7% of 8 year olds, and 3% of 12 year olds have nocturnal enuresis with males predominating in all age groups

    B. Prevalence rates are highest among lower socioeconomic status (SES) groups, less educated groups, and those children who are institutionalized

    C. Fewer than 10% of all enuretics also wet in the daytime (diurnal enuresis)

    D. Primary enuresis exists when a child has never achieved consistent dryness

    E. Secondary enuresis exists when child has had a period of dryness for 3-5 months and then relapses; most children fall into this category

    F. About 10% of enuretic children will also be encopretic

IV.   Diagnosis/Evaluation

    A.   History
        1.   Determine if enuresis is primary or secondary, nocturnal or diurnal
        2.   Ask about onset, duration, severity (number of wet nights per week, for example 4/7)
        3.   Ask if either parent was enuretic as a child
        4.   Obtain prenatal, birth history including gestational age, birth weight; inquire about developmental milestones
        5.   Inquire about toilet training and how parent has managed the enuresis thus far
        6.   Review of systems should focus on genitourinary and nervous systems
        7.   Inquire about presence of encopresis
        8.   Determine attitudes of the parent toward the child and toward the problem by observing interactions with child and by listening to the content of their statements about the child and the problem
        9.   Remember to talk to the child! Child should be the primary historian after about age 7 (except, of course, in the area of past medical history). What are child's perceptions of problem and parental responses to the problem?

    B.   Physical Examination
        1.   Measure blood pressure, height, weight, and plot on growth chart (poor growth and/or elevated blood pressure suggest renal disease)
        2.   Examine genitals looking for major and minor anomalies
        3.   Perform neurological exam including gait, muscular strength and tone, deep tendon reflexes, sensory responses, and rectal sphincter tone
        4.   If possible, observe child voiding and note stream, ability to initiate and interrupt in midstream

    C.   Differential Diagnosis
        1.   Urinary tract infection
        2.   Genitourinary or neurologic anomalies

    D.   Diagnostic Tests
        1.   Urinalysis and urine culture
        2.   Complicated enuresis (severe voiding dysfunction, associated encopresis, urinary tract infection, and an abnormal neurologic exam) requires further study
            a.   Renal or bladder sonogram
            b.   Voiding cystourethrogram (VCUG)
            c.   Urodynamic measurement
            d.   Intravenous pyelogram

V.   Plan/Management

    A.   Supportive counseling should be provided to all families with an emphasis on the following:
        1.   Enuresis is a common problem with a spontaneous cure rate of approximately 15% a year after age 5
        2.   It is an involuntary process and the child has no control of the behavior; thus child should not be made to feel guilty, nor should parents punish the child
        3.   Acceptance of the behavior as an individual difference by parent and child is important and may hasten spontaneous resolution

    B.   In general, initiation of treatment for nocturnal enuresis is deferred until the child reaches 6 years of age because of the high spontaneous cure rates that occur with maturation (enuresis is very common among 5 year olds)

    C.   If the parents insist on more aggressive management or if the child's age appropriate activities with peers are compromised, some treatment modalities not involving pharmacologic approaches may be initiated as early as 5 years of age

D. For children ≥6 years of age, pharmacologic treatment is the most common approach to management of nocturnal enuresis
    1. Parents and child must understand that this is not a cure for the disorder but rather controls the symptoms
    2. Discontinuation of the medication usually results in the recurrence of enuresis, unless the child has reached the age at which he/she would have outgrown the problem without any therapy

E. The most commonly used pharmacologic treatment is desmopression (DDAVP), an effective and safe medication when used as directed; acts on the renal tubule to increase the absorption of filtered water, increasing urinary concentration and decreasing urinary volume; success rate reported to be 60 to 70%
    1. Available as a nasal spray and in tablet form (**Note:** Dosage is not titated by patient weight; there are conflicting reports regarding optimal dose which appears to vary according to the individual child)

Nasal spray	Children <6 years of age, not recommended Children ≥6 years, 20 micrograms (half of dose per nostril) at bedtime and may be increased gradually to 40 micrograms in order to achieve dryness [**Note:** Some children respond to as little as 10 micrograms]
Tablet form	Children <6 years of age, not recommended Children ≥6 years, 0.2 mg at bedtime; may be increased gradually to 0.6 mg in order to achieve dryness

    2. If there is good response to the drug, the program is maintained for several months and then the child is weaned off the DDAVP (using only every other night for several weeks and then stopping altogether)
    3. Caution parents that this medication, like others, must be used only as directed; daytime use can result in retention of water and subsequent dilutional hyponatremia

F. The tricyclic antidepressant imipramine (Tofranil) has been used extensively to treat enuresis but is **not commonly used today**. Initial dose is 25 mg for children 8-12 years of age and 50 mg for children over 12 years old, with the drug given 30 to 60 minutes before bedtime (maximum daily dose is 75 mg for children ≥12 years)
    1. Margin of safety between therapeutic and toxic doses is small
    2. **Caution must be used in prescribing this drug!** Consult PDR for details regarding dosing, adverse reactions, contraindications, and drug interactions

G. Use of a bed wetting alarm is probably the most effective therapy in treating enuresis in children ≥7 years, but most parents are not receptive to this therapy
    1. Uses a moisture activated sensor which attaches to child's underwear
    2. A small pin-on battery powered alarm awakens child
    3. Average of 60 days of treatment are needed to achieve success; relapses frequently occur but retreatment is usually successful
    4. Alarms are inexpensive ($40-$60) but are noisy, frequently awakening the entire household
    5. Devices commonly used include

WetStop by Palco Laboratories, 1595 Soquel Drive, Santa Cruz, CA 95065; 800/346-4488
Dry Night Training System by Fisher-Price
Nytone Enuretic Alarm by Nytone Medical Products, 2424 S. 900 West, Salt Lake City, UT 84119

H. Bladder training therapy is designed to increase child's bladder capacity through stretching
    1. Based on the observation that many enuretic children have decreased bladder capacity
    2. Children are instructed to try to avoid urinating for as long as possible during the day
    3. Parents should measure voiding volumes on a daily basis to monitor progress

4. Normal bladder volume can be estimated as one ounce per age in years plus 2 (**Example:** 6 year old = 6 ounces plus 2 = 8 ounces of bladder capacity, on average)
5. Limitations of the approach is that increased bladder capacity does not necessarily translate to nighttime dryness

I. Treatment failures and relapses are common, but a trial of 4-6 weeks should be given for an approach to have a fair chance of working

J. The presence of coexistent emotional problems and poor family interaction patterns suggests need for referral for counseling

K. Follow Up
1. In 2 weeks for patients on pharmacologic therapy to titrate dose, then monthly x 3 months
2. Important for provider to follow up at regular intervals to provide encouragement
3. The efficacy of all of the treatment modalities is enhanced by active involvement of the provider

EATING DISORDERS

I. Definition: Symptomatic disturbances of eating behavior unique to the developed world with anorexia nervosa (AN) and bulimia nervosa (BN) being the two major types

II. Pathogenesis

A. Eating disorders are best understood using a multidimensional model that encompasses biologic vulnerability, family issues, and societal pressure

B. Eating behavior is a complex integration of a person's attitude toward food and internal physiology resulting in individual concepts of hunger and satiety

C. Persons with AN tend to have perfectionistic, rigid, inflexible and conforming personalities

D. Impact of family functioning on persons with AN and BN is difficult to determine, but family dynamics can influence both the development and the persistence of the disorder

E. A thin, unrealistic body size is idealized in today's society and concepts of beauty are highly related to body size in the media

III. Clinical Presentation

A. Disordered eating represents a spectrum of behavior that is unique to the developed world and is overwhelmingly a disease of young females

B. Female-to-male ratio of eating disorders is approximately 10:1; of the two disorders, males are much more likely to have BN and overexercise is quite common

C. Because of the infrequency of this diagnosis in males, diagnosis and treatment may be more difficult

D. Using strict diagnostic criteria, the prevalence in the young female population, the group most often affected, is approximately 1% for AN and about 3% for bulimia

E. Using less stringent criteria, a much higher percentage of young females regularly engage in disordered eating including rigid dieting, binging, and purging, all behaviors that place them at risk for a number of sequelae

F. Increasing prevalence over the past few decades, particularly for BN due to both increased diagnosing and because of increased emphasis on thinness in the US

G. Diagnostic criteria for AN according to DSM-IV (1994) are contained in the following table

DIAGNOSTIC CRITERIA FOR ANOREXIA NERVOSA
➡ Refusal to maintain weight at or above a minimally normal weight for age and height (body weight is less than 85% of expected)
➡ Intense fear of weight gain even though underweight
➡ Amenorrhea (in postmenarcheal females)
➡ Severe body-image disturbance in which weight has undue influence on feelings of self-worth; denial that current low body weight is problematic
➡ Types of Anorexia Nervosa:
✱ Restricting Type: During current episode of AN, person has not regularly engaged in binge eating or purging behavior
✱ Binge-Eating/Purging Type: During current episode of AN, person has regularly engaged in binge eating or purging behavior

Adapted from American Psychiatric Association. (1994). Diagnostic and statistical manual of mental disorders (4th ed.) Washington, DC: Author

H. Diagnostic criteria for BN according to DSM-IV (1994) are contained in the following table

DIAGNOSTIC CRITERIA FOR BULIMIA NERVOSA
➡ Recurrent episodes of binge eating which includes **both** of the following
✱ Eating, in a discrete time period, an amount of food substantially larger than most people would consume in the same time period
✱ A sense of lack of control over eating during episode
➡ Recurrent inappropriate compensatory behavior to prevent weight gain such as laxative, diuretic, enema use, induced vomiting, fasting, excessive exercise
➡ The above two behaviors occur, on average, at least 2 times/week for 3 months
➡ Feelings of self-worth unduly influenced by weight
➡ Disturbance does not occur exclusively during episodes of AN
➡ Types of Bulimia Nervosa:
✱ Purging Type: During the current episode of BN, person has engaged in self-induced vomiting, laxative, diuretic, or enema use on a regularly basis
✱ Nonpurging Type: During the current episode of BN, person has used compensatory behaviors such as fasting or excessive exercise, but has not regularly engaged in self-induced vomiting, laxative, diuretic, or enema use

Adapted from American Psychiatric Association. (1994). Diagnostic and statistical manual of mental disorders (4th ed.) Washington, DC: Author

IV. Diagnosis/Evaluation

A. History
1. Obtain weight history including highest and lowest weights as adolescent, methods of losing weight, and how patient defines "ideal" weight
2. Through appropriate questioning, establish the presence or absence of criteria for eating disorders (see DIAGNOSTIC CRITERIA FOR ANOREXIA AND BULIMIA NERVOSA in the preceding tables)
3. If possible, obtain additional information from family/friends as patient may lack the capacity to accurately describe own behavior
4. Inquire about other behaviors that can support the presence of an eating disorder such as preference for eating alone, severely limited food preferences, unusual eating habits (ritualistic patterns)
5. Obtain a careful diet history, with a focus on overall caloric intake and intake of specific nutrients such as calcium
6. Obtain a complete menstrual history

7. Question about exercise patterns (overexercise believed to be especially prevalent in males with eating disorders)
8. Ask what medications have been used or are currently being used to induce weight loss

B. Physical Examination
1. Measure weight with the patient undressed and gowned; measure height and calculate BMI (See OBESITY section for calculation of BMI)
2. Measure blood pressure (resting and orthostatic hypotension are common) (see SYNCOPE section for DETERMINING ORTHOSTATIC HYPOTENSION table for details on assessment)
3. Perform complete physical examination observing for the stigmata of vomiting which includes parotid enlargement, soft palate lesions, dental erosions, calluses of the knuckles
4. Neurologic exam should include mental status, cranial nerves, motor and sensory systems, and cerebellar system

C. Differential Diagnosis
1. Numerous **medical conditions** can mimic presentation of eating disorders; however, persons with medical conditions that cause loss of appetite, weight loss, unexplained vomiting **lack the attitudinal features** of a primary eating disorder (obsession with thinness and body image distortion)
   a. Inflammatory bowel diseases (stool is often positive for blood, and erythrocyte sedimentation rate is increased in IBD, and usually subnormal in eating disorders)
   b. Thyroid disease (physical findings of hyperthyroidism are usually present and laboratory findings confirm the diagnosis)
   c. Diabetes mellitus (laboratory findings confirm the diagnosis)
   d. Central nervous system lesions and occult malignancies anywhere in the body (appropriate imaging studies)
   e. Chronic infections such as tuberculosis and acquired immunodeficiency
2. Psychiatric disorders can also present with decreased appetite and weight loss
   a. Mood disorders
   b. Obsessive-compulsive disorder
   c. Substance abuse
   d. Psychotic disorders

D. Diagnostic Tests
1. Initial laboratory evaluation should include CBC, serum electrolytes, calcium, magnesium, and phosphorous levels; electrocardiogram
2. Patients with atypical presentations should have laboratory evaluation based on history and physical in order to rule out other diagnoses
3. Serum amylase levels are elevated during active vomiting and return to normal within 72 hours after vomiting ceases (may be helpful in documenting presence of bulimia)

V. Plan/Treatment

A. Goals of treatment including restoring and maintaining normal weight, and management of physiologic and psychologic abnormalities; treatment at a speciality center is ideal

B. In-patient versus out-patient management depends on the severity of the condition as well as availability of local resources and insurance status of the patient
1. Patients with hemodynamic instability, significant hypovolemia, arrhythmias, congestive heart failure, cardiomyopathy must be hospitalized
2. Failure of appropriate out-patient treatment is also a criterion for hospitalization

C. Most out-patient treatment for patients with eating disorders is managed by a decentralized team, with patients seeing a variety of providers (including a psychotherapist and nutritionist) who communicate with each other about the progress of the patient

D. Cognitive behavioral treatment is the treatment of choice for eating disorders
1. Objective of cognitive techniques is to change faulty thought processes such as all-or-none thinking, judgmental thinking, and catastrophizing

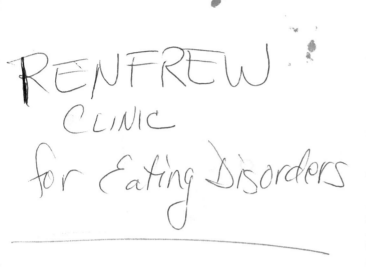

s are to break patterns of disordered eating through the
onitoring, meal regularity, and nutritional monitoring
nt component of treatment

onitor the medical aspects of the condition (weekly
[CBC, serum electrolytes, and serum amylase levels]);
professionals involved in care

'ale Avenue, Tulsa, OK 74136; 918/481-4044;

Park West, Suite 1R, New York, NY 10024; 212/501-8351;
n c . o r g

Disorders, Box 7, Highland Park, IL 60035; 847/831-3438

---

ers requires concerted efforts over a long time period
must be frequent in order to form therapeutic
supervision of health status
less frequent visits are appropriate; however, relapse is

on between all professionals involved in care is

D FAILURE TO THRIVE

ability to maintain the expected rate of growth over time

II. Pathogenesis

A. Immediate cause of failure to thrive is inadequate nutrition; ultimate cause is often difficult to determine

B. Organic causes include the following:
1. Inadequate caloric intake due to such conditions as cleft palate
2. Food assimilation defect due to conditions such as celiac disease
3. Loss of ingested calories such as occurs in chronic diarrhea or gastroesophageal reflux
4. Increased energy requirements due to conditions such as chronic infection, heart disease, or renal disease
5. Prenatal causes including intrauterine infection, maternal malnutrition, exposure to alcohol, drugs, or cigarettes during prenatal period

C. Nonorganic causes include the following:
1. Underfeeding the child due to improper mixing of formula (under dilution) or parental misconceptions about nutritional needs of the child; parent unintentionally fails to feed child enough to support growth
2. Economic and psychosocial factors, as well as child neglect and abuse also result in failure to thrive

D. Approximately 50% of cases of FTT admitted to tertiary care centers and almost all cases managed in primary care settings have nonorganic etiologies

III. Clinical Presentation

A. A common problem usually identified during the first three years of life with approximately **80% of cases in children less than 18 months of age**

B. Diagnostic criteria for failure to thrive are based on weight and height for age using National Center for Health Statistics (NCHS) growth charts; children below the fifth percentile for weight or with weight less than 80% of ideal (median) for age are considered to meet the criteria

C. Children whose slowed velocity of weight gain results in "crossing percentiles" (for example, dropping from 50th to 15th percentile for weight) may also be considered in the failure to thrive category. This is especially true after the child reaches 18-24 months of age, when changes in growth velocity are rarely physiologic

D. While weight is the major criterion, in more severe cases, linear growth and head circumference may be affected over time

E. Condition is seen in all socioeconomic levels, but incidence is particularly high among families living in poverty

F. Children with failure to thrive are at increased risk for developmental and behavioral problems in addition to growth problems

IV. Diagnosis/Evaluation

A. History
1. Obtain a detailed perinatal history including prenatal exposures to tobacco, alcohol and other drugs, gestational age, weight, length and head circumference at birth
2. Obtain detailed weight history including somatic measurements at every age since birth (obtain records from other agencies as needed)
3. Inquire about illnesses since birth, including vomiting, diarrhea, and the child's energy level
4. In order to determine if the child is receiving adequate calories, take a comprehensive feeding history, including type of formula/food, amount fed in 24 hour period, frequency of feeding, who feeds the child at each feeding, if the bottle is propped, and if there are any problems with sucking, swallowing, or regurgitation. **Important**: Caution should be used when interpreting a dietary history as parental guilt may lead to inaccuracies in reporting
5. In breast-fed infants, determine if there are any problems with milk supply, sore nipples, inadequate let-down reflex; ask mother about any ingestion of substances (alcohol, medications) that might affect the milk supply
6. Assess the development of the child to determine if age-appropriate
7. Determine if there is a family history of short stature or growth-retarding illnesses such as cystic fibrosis or malabsorption syndromes
8. Obtain a psychosocial history to determine family composition and functioning; look for strengths as well as risk factors

B. Physical Examination
1. Measure blood pressure to screen for acute or chronic renal disease
2. Carefully measure and plot weight (unclothed), length (recumbent under 2 years, standing height over age 2) , and head circumference (even in children >2 years). Plot weight for length. (Children with genetic short stature will have concordant weight and length)
3. Relate measurements to previous measurements to see pattern of growth; note if pattern of growth has been steady or if growth slowed at a specific point in time
4. Examine child for dysmorphic features, hypotonia, murmur, protuberant abdomen (associated with celiac disease, malabsorption, or cystic fibrosis), defects in soft and hard palate
5. Perform a neurologic examination, including an oral motor evaluation (suck, gag, and swallow reflexes), test cranial nerves, deep tendon reflexes, muscle strength, and passive and active muscle tone

Look for signs of abuse and poor hygiene during the exam
Perform a Denver II
If child still on breast/bottle feeding, observe mother feeding child (**Note: This is very important!**)

ential Diagnosis
Failure to thrive may be the result of a number of both organic and inorganic causes listed under Pathogenesis, above
Because birth weight and length are influenced to a greater degree by maternal size and intrauterine influences than by genetic factors, there are increases or decreases in growth velocity during the first 2 years of life to adjust for maternal factors and for genetic potential to be achieved. Therefore, some children experience a decrease in growth rate (a shift in height or weight of more than 25 percentile points) during the first 2 years of life. This may represent a physiologic adjustment, rather than true failure to thrive; in most of these cases, the growth rate does stabilize and follows a predictable pattern

stic Tests
Basic laboratory tests include CBC, lead and free erythrocyte protoporphyrin, urinalysis, urine cultures, stool for O&P, BUN, creatinine, serum electrolytes, TSH, T_4, liver enzymes, and a tuberculin test
Other tests to consider are skull, chest and long-bone x-rays, HIV screening and sweat est, bone age, and toxicology screen

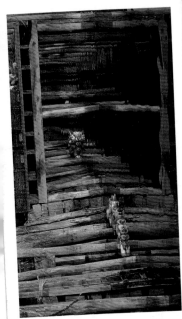

ent

nt to keep in mind that advocacy of the child must be maintained without becoming an
ry of the parents

ment and maintenance of an alliance with the family is of paramount importance

erlying organic disease is uncovered in H&P and diagnostic tests, refer immediately to st (WIC if eligible) for counseling on feeding techniques and high calorie diet. Caloric gher than normal is required for child to experience growth recovery (**Example:** Infants e year have nutritional requirements, on average, of 100 kcal/kg of body weight per day; intake of 150 kcal/kg/day may be needed in order to "catch up")

breastfeeding mothers to a certified lactation consultant for assessment and counseling

e parents are involved in treatment process in order to optimize treatment. A multi-
ry approach including nutritionist, visiting nurse, and social worker is needed for optimal
nent and follow up

F.   Children <3 years old should be referred to early intervention program. Children 4-5 years old should be referred to Head Start (to compensate for environmental deprivation) if eligible

G.   Any child who fails to responds after 2 months to intensive efforts at management should be referred for hospitalization or to a specialized clinic dealing with FTT

H.   Follow Up
1.   In 2 weeks for growth check and response to plan
2.   Then every 2-4 weeks until growth recovery is steadily progressing

OBESITY

I. Definition: Excessive accumulation of body fat

II. Pathogenesis

   A. The simplistic view that obesity is caused when energy intake exceeds expenditure fails to take into account other factors such as chronic stress which can affect metabolism through increasing cortisol secretion

   B. Multiple factors interact and contribute to development of obesity: a genetic predisposition combines with environmental factors to produce the disorder

   C. Identifiable exogenous causes of obesity are rare

III. Clinical Presentation

   A. According to the National Center for Health Statistics (NCHS), approximately one in five children in the US is overweight

   B. Prevalence of overweight has increased greatly over past 15 years in both genders of all ages and ethnic groups

   C. Body mass index (BMI) expressed as body weight in kilograms divided by the square of height in meters (kg/m^2) has recently been adopted as the standard obesity assessment in children; revised reference growth curves will soon be released by the NCHS [Until these reference growth curves are released, the definition of obesity as weight for height above the 95th percentile or weight greater than 120% of the median weight for a given height indicates obesity]
      1. BMI correlates with measures of body fatness in children and adolescents
      2. BMI also correlates with markers of secondary complications of obesity including blood pressure, lipids, and lipoproteins

   D. Whereas there is conflicting evidence linking obesity in infancy and childhood to adult obesity, obese adolescents are likely to remain obese as adults

IV. Diagnosis/Evaluation

   A. History
      1. Obtain prenatal history, weight milestones, growth pattern
      2. Obtain diet history to identify both foods eaten and patterns of eating

FOCUS OF DIET HISTORY IN OVERWEIGHT CHILD
Note: Questions about food consumption should be framed in a matter-of-fact, non-accusatory manner
✓ Ask parent (or child/adolescent) to describe the meals and snacks in a typical day ✓ Ask to estimate daily consumption of high-calorie and high-fat foods, such as chips, cookies, candy, granola bars; ask about high-calorie liquids such as soda, juice, whole milk ✓ Determine if meals prepared outside the home are important sources of high-calorie eating (from "take-out," fast-foods, school, day care, or with grandparents, etc.)

      3. Complete a psychosocial history, to detect emotional stresses at home or work/school which may be aggravating problem
      4. Determine amount and type of physical activity engaged in each week (estimate time spent in sedentary activities)

5. Ask about motivation for weight loss and types and results of past dieting
6. Obtain past medical history for orthopedic problems (most often hip or knee pain or limited range of motion), current medications

B. Physical Examination
1. Measure blood pressure, taking care to use the correct size cuff
2. To determine optimal weight, complete weight for height chart. Weight-for-height above the 95th percentile or weight greater than 120% of normal (i.e., 50th percentile for a given height) indicates obesity
3. Examination of the severely obese patient may be difficult (auscultation of the lungs and heart is compromised as is exam of the abdomen)
4. Skin over the neck may be hyperpigmented, thicker, and have a velvet appearance (acanthosis nigricans, associated with insulin resistance in obese adults, also occurs in children with NIDDM and in insulin-resistant children)
5. In adolescent females, observe for intertriginous dermatitis under breasts and abdominal panniculus
6. In adolescent males, examination of the genitalia may require that the prepubic fat tissue be lifted upward in order to visualize the penis which may be hidden by surrounding fat
7. Perform musculoskeletal exam for range of motion

C. Differential Diagnosis
1. Most obesity is the result of overeating; identifiable exogenous causes of obesity are rare
2. Major endocrine disorders that may manifest with obesity are the following:
   a. Pituitary and adrenal dysfunction (Hirsutism and truncal obesity occur in Cushing's syndrome and prominent violaceous striae should prompt an evaluation with a urine free cortisol or dexamethasone suppression test)
   b. Thyroid disease
   c. Polycystic ovarian disease
   d. Hypothalamic disease
3. Psychologic disorders (eating disorders, depression)

D. Diagnostic Tests: None are indicated unless history and physical examination suggest that obesity is secondary to a medical condition such as the ones listed under DIFFERENTIAL DIAGNOSIS in IV.C.

V. Plan/Management

A. Plan of care should be based on several underlying principles
1. Obesity is an important chronic medical problem that is treatable and this fact should be communicated to the child and the parents
2. Sensitive and compassionate care by the clinician is a critical part of any successful program
3. Time spent in understanding each family's particular circumstances is of paramount importance if the clinician is to support the child's and family's efforts

B. For a weight-management program to be successful, the parent (in the case of children) or adolescent must be ready to make changes; unsuccessful programs can diminish the child/adolescent's self-esteem, thereby jeopardizing future attempts to improve weight

C. A practical approach to assess readiness to make changes in diet and activity
1. Ask the patient and parents how concerned they are about the patient's weight
2. Ask if they believe weight loss is possible
3. Ask what practices they believe need to be changed
4. (**Note**: Families who are not ready to change may express a lack of concern about the child's obesity, may believe that obesity is inevitable, and are not interested in modification of eating or activity)

D. For patients/families who are ready to make changes, a program aimed at correcting obesity through healthy eating and activity patterns should be implemented

E. Experts recommend that children younger than 2 years of age be referred to a pediatric obesity center for management
   1. If such referral is not possible, focus should be on slowing excessive weight gain; weight reduction is inappropriate during this period
      a. Discourage feeding infant high calorie foods, such as puddings/desserts and limit juice to 4 ounces/day
      b. Advise parent to offer infant pacifier between feedings
      c. Children younger than 2 years of age should never be placed on reduced fat milk
      d. Refer to nutritionist for counseling (WIC if family is eligible)
   2. Monitor child's weight gain monthly to make certain child is gaining weight, but at an appropriate level

F. The initial step in management for all overweight children who are between 2 years and 7 years of age is to maintain baseline weight; prolonged weight maintenance allows for a gradual reduction in weight for height
   1. Beginning at age 2, it is acceptable to gradually reduce the amount of fat in the diet (Remember: Some fatty acids–linoleic and linolenic acid–are essential for growth and must be supplied by food)
   2. As children move though this age period, they can consume fewer calories from fat with nutrient-rich foods such as grain products, fruits, vegetables, and reduced fat dairy products supplying more of their caloric needs

G. For children older than 7 years of age, with weight for height greater than 120% of **average** (Note: **Average** weight is defined as the 50th percentile for a particular height), weight maintenance is the initial goal, and once that goal is achieved, additional changes in eating and activity to achieve actual weight loss of about 1 pound per month is appropriate
   1. By age 7, a child's pattern of eating should conform to the same dietary guidelines as older children and adults–limiting fat to no more than 30% of total calories, and saturated fat to no more than 10% of total calories
      a. The focus should be on consuming well-balanced, healthy meals
      b. The Food Guide Pyramid (See NUTRITION IN CHILDHOOD AND ADOLESCENCE section) is considered to be the most helpful guide to healthy eating
      c. Use of the Dietary Guidelines for Americans can also be helpful and these are summarized in the table that follows

DIETARY GUIDELINES FOR AMERICANS
* Eat a variety of foods that are low in calories and high in nutrients--check the Nutrition Facts Label
* Eat less fat and fewer high-fat foods
* Eat smaller portions and limit second helpings of foods high in fat and calories
* Eat more vegetables and fruits without fats and sugars added in preparation or at the table
* Eat pasta, rice, breads, and cereals without fats and sugars added in preparation or at the table
* Eat less sugars and fewer sweets (like candy, cookies, cakes, soda)
* Drink less or no alcohol

   2. Advise child/parents to do the following:
      a. Switch to skim milk and limit intake of hight fat foods such as butter, ice cream, cheese, salad dressings, and oil
      b. Avoid frequent consumption of high calorie snacks; some experts believe that no foods should be "forbidden," but that such high-calorie foods as candy, cookies, and chips should instead be eaten infrequently

H.   Encourage the development of parenting skills that promote successful management of obesity as outlined in the following table

---

PARENTING SKILLS THAT PROMOTE SUCCESSFUL TREATMENT OF OBESITY

* Find reasons to praise the child
* Use praise and correction that focuses on the child's behavior, not on the child (behavior can be good or bad, children are *always* good)
* Avoid the use of food as a reward; instead, use time and activities involving the parents or friends as a reward for desired behavior
* Establish daily family meals and snack times; parents determine what food is offered and child can decide whether to eat
* Offer only healthy options at meals and snacks–child can choose between apple and popcorn, not between cookie and apple
* Emphasize healthy eating and activities for the entire family, not just for the overweight child–all family members should eat the same diet and participate in energy expending activities
* Offer daily activities that involve a substantial expenditure of energy–child can choose between riding bike in park or going roller skating, not between doing a crafts project or riding bike in park
* Be consistent; don't unpredictably reward undesirable behavior by inconsistently giving in to the behavior

---

I.   Health care provider should assess parental success with these skills on each follow up visit in order to provide guidance and support

J.   Commercial programs such as Weight Watchers or Jenny Craig are not recommended for use by children

K.   Resources on nutrition and weight management are in the table below

---

RESOURCES ON NUTRITION AND WEIGHT MANAGEMENT

EatRight Lose Weight: Seven Simple Steps. Available from Oxmoor House, Inc., 800/884-3935

University of Alabama at Birmingham EatRight Nutrition Information Service Hot Line, 800/231-DIET for answers to nutrition questions

Weight-control Information Network (WIN) is a service of the National Institute of Diabetes and Digestive and Kidney Diseases. WIN assembles and disseminates information on weight control, obesity, and nutritional disorders to health professionals and the general public. Contact WIN at 1 WIN Way, Bethesda, MD 20892-3665; (800) 946-8098; http://www.niddk.nih.gov//NutritionDocs.html

The Food Guide Pyramid. US Department of Agriculture, Center for Nutrition Policy and Promotion, 1120 20th Street, NW, Suite 200, North Lobby, Washington, DC 20036; http://www.usda.gov/fcs/cnpp.htm

---

L.   Optimally, children and their families should be referred to a nutritionist for counseling

M.   Follow Up: Obesity represents a chronic disease; thus, frequent visits with continuous monitoring and feedback are required for success in assisting overweight children in attaining and maintaining a healthy weight

TOBACCO USE AND SMOKING CESSATION

I.   Definition: Destructive health behavior involving use of tobacco (cigarettes, chewing tobacco, and snuff)

II.   Pathogenesis

    A.   Tobacco smoke contains numerous substances which are toxic, mutagenic, or carcinogenic

    B.   In addition to harmful volatile substances such as carbon monoxide, the particulate phase of cigarette smoke contains nicotine and tars

    C.   The consequences of a product of combustion (smoke) being drawn into close contact with delicate pulmonary tissues are devastating

    D.   The etiology of tobacco dependence is multidimensional with physiological, psychological, and social/behavioral factors
        1.   Physiological factors include activation of the mesolimbic dopaminergic system ("reward circuit") and locus ceruleus (vigilance and arousal)
        2.   Psychological factors evolve from positive feedback provided by pleasurable sensations
        3.   Social/behavioral factors include the following: smoking becomes a habit or an automatic and intrinsic part of daily activities, and smoking can be used as a self-medication to reduce unpleasant sensations that occur with tobacco withdrawal or stress

III. Clinical Presentation

    A.   The number of adolescents who become daily smokers before the age of 18 increased by 73% from 1988 to 1996
        1.   Approximately 19% of all high school seniors smoke on a regular basis
        2.   Smokeless tobacco is used by about 20% of male high school seniors

    B.   Tobacco use is the most important cause of premature mortality, accounting for one out of every five deaths in the US
        1.   Among adolescents, short-term consequences of smoking include respiratory and nonrespiratory effects, addiction to nicotine, and associated risk of other drug use
        2.   Long-term consequences are based on the likelihood that most young persons who smoke regularly will continue to do so throughout adulthood

    C.   Smoking affects heath of nonsmokers
        1.   Children exposed to environmental tobacco have increased risk of premature births, low birth weights, growth disorders, sudden infant death syndrome, and upper respiratory tract infections
        2.   Each year about 3,000 nonsmoking adults die of lung cancer as a result of breathing second-hand smoke

    D.   Physiological tolerance develops gradually with an increase of a few cigarettes a day initially to several packs a day in several years

    E.   Withdrawal from nicotine includes symptoms of anxiety, irritability, craving, hunger, restlessness, decreased concentration, drowsiness, sleep disturbances, tremors, sweating, dizziness, headaches, and gastrointestinal disturbances such as constipation

IV.   Diagnosis/Evaluation

    A.   History
        1.   Inquire about smoking pattern such as number of years of smoking, how much tobacco is used, and depth of inhalation
        2.   Ask how long after awakening the first cigarette is smoked

3. Ask about past attempts at quitting including length of cigarette cessation, problems encountered, and reasons for relapse
4. Explore smoke-related symptoms such as cough, sputum production, shortness of breath, recurrent respiratory infections
5. Review family history and past medical history of tobacco-related diseases such as coronary heart disease, chronic obstructive pulmonary disease, and cancer

B. Physical Examination: Use the examination as an intervention, highlighting the damage that smoking can do to each body system which is assessed
1. Monitor vital signs, particularly blood pressure which adds an additional risk of heart disease if elevated
2. Examine ears, nose, sinuses, mouth, and pharynx, noting signs of inflammation due to irritation from tobacco
3. Perform complete exam of lungs
4. Perform complete exam of heart and peripheral vascular system

C. Diagnostic Tests
1. Consider spirometry
   a. If normal, stress the benefits of smoking cessation before damage occurs
   b. If abnormal, stress the importance of cessation before further damage occurs
2. Consider blood cholesterol levels to determine additional risk factors for heart disease

D. Differential Diagnosis: Tobacco use is a behavioral problem without a differential diagnosis

V. Plan/Management

A. Advise all smokers to stop
1. **Be clear**. In a straightforward manner tell the patient to stop smoking now
2. **Speak strongly**. Emphasize that quitting smoking is the single most important thing that patient can do for future health
3. **Personalize advice**: Point out reasons that smoking cessation will improve the personal health as well as the health of loved ones exposed to second-hand smoke. See GOOD REASONS FOR TEENS TO QUIT SMOKING in the table that follows

GOOD REASONS FOR TEENS TO QUIT SMOKING
☆ Cigarette smokers have a lower level of lung function than those persons who have never smoked
☆ Cigarette smoking causes heart disease and stroke in adults; studies have shown that early signs of these diseases can be found in adolescents who smoke
☆ Smoking hurts young people's physical fitness in terms of both performance and endurance--even among young people trained in competitive running
☆ On average, someone who smokes a pack or more of cigarettes each day lives 7 years less than someone who never smoked
☆ Smoking at an early age increases the risk of lung cancer
☆ Teenage smokers suffer from shortness of breath almost three times as often as teens who don't smoke
☆ Teenage smokers are more likely to have seen a doctor or other health professionals for an emotional or psychological complaint
☆ Teens who smoke are three times more likely than nonsmokers to use alcohol, eight times more likely to use marijuana, and 22 times more likely to use cocaine

Source: Office on Smoking and Health. Centers for Disease Control, www.cdc.gov/tobacco.

4. If patient unwilling to quit, **record plans** to manage the smoking status in the progress notes and list tobacco use in the problem list. For children who reside in households with smokers, **always** list "Exposure to passive smoke" in the problem list in child's chart. See following table, SOURCE FOR MATERIALS FOR SMOKING CESSATION INTERVENTIONS to obtain chart markers, stamps, labels, and educational/motivational materials

B.   Refer the patient for intensive smoking cessation programs
1.   Intensive programs are strongly correlated with success
2.   Intensive programs should consist of 4-7 sessions, each at least 20-30 minutes in length, lasting at least 2 weeks
3.   Counseling should offer problem solving and skills training as well as social support

C.   For patients who are unable/unwilling to enroll in an intensive program, assist patient with a quit plan (see ASSISTING THE PATIENT WITH A QUIT PLAN in table below)

ASSISTING THE PATIENT WITH A QUIT PLAN

Advise the smoker to:

➡   Set a quit date, ideally within 2 weeks
➡   Inform friends, family, and coworkers of plans to quit, and ask for support
➡   Remove cigarettes from home, car, and workplace and avoid smoking in these places
➡   Review previous quit attempts--what helped, what led to relapse
➡   Anticipate challenges, particularly during the critical first few weeks, including nicotine withdrawal

Give advice on successful quitting:

➡   Total abstinence is essential--not even a single puff
➡   Drinking alcohol is strongly associated with relapse
➡   Having other smokers in the household hinders successful quitting

Encourage use of nicotine replacement therapy:

➡   Both the nicotine patch and nicotine gum are effective pharmacotherapies for smoking cessation
➡   The nicotine patch may be easier to use than the gum in most clinical settings

Make culturally and educationally appropriate materials on cessation techniques readily available in your office

Source: Fiore, M.C., Bailey, W.C., Cohen, S.J., et al. (1996). Smoking cessation: Information for specialists. Clinical Practice Guideline. Quick Reference Guide for Smoking Cessation Specialists, No. 18. Rockville, MD: USDHHS, Public Health Service, Agency for Health Care Policy and Research and Centers for Disease Control and Prevention.

D.   Success is also enhanced by clinician-provided social support which communicates caring and concern by being open to the patient's fears and difficulties

E.   Clinician counseling even as brief as 3 minutes is effective; however, the more intense the treatment, the more effective it is in producing long-term abstinence

F.   Pharmacologic support for smoking cessation
1.   Every smoker should be offered nicotine replacement therapy (patch or gum) except when medically contraindicated (see SUGGESTIONS FOR THE CLINICAL USE OF THE NICOTINE PATCH/GUM in the tables that follow)
    a.   Use of nicotine replacement therapy with light smokers (10-15 cigarettes/day or less) has not been studied
    b.   If used with light smokers, or smokers weighing less than 100 pounds, a lower starting dose should be considered
2.   Nicotine nasal spray (Nicotrol NS) is also available and appears to be safe and effective for highly nicotine-dependent smokers (smoke > 20 cigarettes/day, smoke immediately upon awakening and report history of severe nicotine withdrawal symptoms)
    a.   Aqueous nasal spray containing 0.5 mg/spray
    b.   Usually 1-2 doses/hr with a maximum of 5 sprays/hr, 40 doses/day
    c.   May discontinue abruptly or tapered

    d.   Use for maximum of 3 months

    e.   Supplied as 1 bottle containing 10 mL (200 sprays) with metered spray pump

3.   Bupropion (Zyban) is a recent pharmacologic option for smoking cessation and is the only drug for this indication that is not nicotine based

    a.   Mechanism of action is unclear, but believed to affect noradrenergic and dopaminergic mechanisms in the brain which have been implicated as pathways of nicotine addiction

    b.   Available as a sustained-release tablet; dosage is 150 mg QD for 3 days and then BID (at least 8 hours between doses) for 7 to 12 weeks

    c.   Patient should be advised to stop smoking during the 2nd week of therapy

    d.   May be used with transdermal nicotine **(Patient must quit smoking when using transdermal nicotine)**

SUGGESTIONS FOR THE CLINICAL USE OF THE NICOTINE PATCH	
Patient Selection	Appropriate as a primary pharmacotherapy for smoking cessation Behavioral/educational support is recommended with this therapy
Precautions	***Pregnancy.*** Pregnant smokers should first be encouraged to attempt cessation without pharmacologic treatment. The nicotine patch should be used during pregnancy only if the benefits outweigh the risks. Similar factors should be considered in lactating females ***Cardiovascular Diseases.*** Nicotine patch should be used only after consideration of risks and benefits among particular cardiovascular patient groups: Those who are within 4 weeks of being post MI, who have arrhythmias, or who have worsening angina pectoris ***Skin Reactions.*** Up to 50% of patients using the nicotine patch have a local skin reaction. Less than 5% have a serious enough reaction to discontinue use

Dosage	Treatment of 8 weeks or less has been shown to be as efficacious as longer treatment periods. The following treatment schedules are suggested as reasonable for most smokers
	
	Brand — **Duration** — **Dosage**
	Nicoderm CQ (OTC), Habitrol — 4 weeks — 21 mg/24 hrs
	    then 2 weeks — 14 mg/24 hrs
	    then 2 weeks — 7 mg/24 hrs
	
	Prostep — 4 weeks — 22 mg/24 hrs
	    then 4 weeks — 11 mg/24 hrs
	
	Nicotrol (OTC) — 6 weeks — 15 mg/16 hrs

Prescribing Instructions	**No smoking** while on the patch. *Location.* At the start of each day, the patient should place a new patch on a relatively hairless location between the neck and the waist *Activities.* No restrictions while using the patch *Time.* Patches should be applied as soon as patients waken on their quit day

Adapted from Fiore, M.C., Bailey, W.C., Cohen, S.J., et al. (1996). Smoking cessation: Information for specialists. Clinical Practice Guideline. Quick Reference Guide for Smoking Cessation Specialists, No. 18. Rockville, MD: USDHHS, Public Health Service, Agency for Health Care Policy and Research and Centers for Disease Control and Prevention.

SUGGESTIONS FOR THE CLINICAL USE OF NICOTINE GUM	
Patient Selection	Appropriate as a primary pharmacotheraphy for smoking cessation. Behavioral/educational support is recommended with this therapy
Precautions	***Pregnancy.*** Pregnant smokers should first be encouraged to attempt cessation without pharmacologic treatment. Nicotine gum should be used during pregnancy only if the benefits outweigh the risks. Similar factors should be considered in lactating females ***Cardiovascular Diseases.*** Nicotine gum should be used only after consideration of risks and benefits among particular cardiovascular patient groups: Those who are within 4 weeks of being post MI, who have arrhythmias, or who have worsening angina pectoris ***Side Effects.*** Common side effects of nicotine chewing gum include mouth soreness, hiccups, dyspepsia and jaw ache. These effects can often be alleviated by correcting chewing technique

Dosage	Nicotine gum (Nicorette) is available in 2-mg and 4-mg (per piece) doses and is OTC Patients should be advised to use the 2-mg gum except in special circumstances
	    2-mg strength limit: 30 pieces per day
	    4-mg strength limit: 20 pieces per day

Prescribing Instructions	**No smoking** while on the gum *Chewing Technique.* Gum should be chewed slowly until a "peppery" taste emerges, then "parked" between the cheek and gum to facilitate nicotine absorption. Gum should be intermittently "chewed and parked" for about 30 minutes *Absorption.* Acidic beverages (e.g., coffee, juices, soft drinks) interfere with the buccal absorption of nicotine, so eating and drinking anything except water should be avoided for 15 minutes before and during chewing *Scheduling of Dose.* Instructions to chew the gum on a fixed schedule (at least one piece every one to two hours) for one to three months may be more beneficial than ad lib use *Duration of Therapy.* Should be tailored to fit the needs of each patient. Generally prescribed for several months (1-3)

Adapted from Fiore, M.C., Bailey, W.C., Cohen, S.J., et al. (1996). Smoking cessation: Information for specialists. Clinical Practice Guideline. Quick Reference Guide for Smoking Cessation Specialists, No. 18. Rockville, MD: USDHHS, Public Health Service, Agency for Health Care Policy and Research and Centers for Disease Control and Prevention.

G.   Follow Up
    1.   Schedule followup contact either in person or by telephone
    2.   Timing
        a.   First followup contact within 2 weeks of quit date, preferably during first week
        b.   Second contact within the first month
        c.   Further followup contacts as needed
    3.   Actions during followup visits
        a.   Congratulate success
        b.   If a relapse occurred, obtain recommitment to abstinence
        c.   Remind patient that lapse can be used as learning experience
        d.   Identify problems encountered and anticipate challenges in the immediate future
    4.   Preventing relapse
        a.   Congratulate, encourage, and stress importance of abstinence at every opportunity
        b.   Review benefits derived from cessation
        c.   Inquire about problems encountered and offer possible solutions
        d.   Anticipate problems or threats to maintaining abstinence

REFERENCES

American Academy of Child and Adolescent Psychiatry. (1997). Practice parameters for the assessment and treatment of children, adolescents, and adults with attention-deficit/hyperactivity disorder. Journal of American Academy of Child and Adolescent Psychiatry, 56 (Suppl. 10), 855-1215.

American Academy of Pediatrics, Committee on Drugs. (1996). Medication for children with attentional disorders. Pediatrics, 98, 301-304.

American Psychiatric Association. (1994). Diagnostic and statistical manual of mental disorders (4th ed.). Washington, DC: Author.

Aronne, L.J. (1998). Obesity. <u>Medical Clinics of North America, 82</u>, 161-182.

Barlow, S.E., & Dietz, W.H. (1998). Obesity evaluation and treatment: Expert committee recommendations. <u>Pediatrics, 102</u>(3), e29.

Barnes, H.N., & Samet, J.H. (1997). Brief interventions with substance-abusing patients. <u>Medical Clinics of North America, 81</u>, 867-880.

Bromberg, D.I. (1999). Enuresis. In R.A. Dershewitz (Ed.), <u>Ambulatory pediatric care</u>. Philadelphia: Lippincott.

Brower, K.J., & Severin, J.D. (1997). Alcohol and other drug-related problems. In D.J. Knesper, N.B. Riba, & T.L. Schwenk (Eds.), <u>Primary care psychiatry</u>. Philadelphia: Saunders.

Brownwell, K.D. (1998). Obesity management: A comprehensive plan. <u>American Journal of Managed Care, 4</u>(3), 126-132.

Bush, B., Shaw, S., Cleary, P.,Delbanco, T.L., & Aronson, M.D. (1987). Screening for alcohol abuse using the CAGE questionnaire. <u>American Journal of Medicine, 82</u>, 231-235.

Bussey, B.F., & Morgan, S.L. (1997). Obesity: Is there effective treatment now? <u>Consultant</u>, 2945-2957.

Carek, P.J., Sherer, J.T., & Carson, D.S. (1997). Management of obesity: Medical treatment options. <u>American Family Physician, 55</u>, 551-558.

Cohen, M.W. (1997). Enuresis. In R.A. Hoekelman (Ed.), <u>Primary pediatric care</u>. St. Louis: Mosby.

Fiore, M.C., Bailey, W.C., & Cohen, S.J., et al. (1996). Smoking cessation: Information for specialists. <u>Clinical Practice Guideline. Quick Reference Guide for Smoking Cessation Specialists.</u> Rockville, MD: USDHHS, Public health Service, Agency for Health Care Policy and Research and Centers for Disease Control and Prevention.

Gahagan, S., & Holmes, R. (1998). A stepwise approach to evaluation of undernutrition and failure to thrive. <u>Pediatric Clinics of North America, 45</u>, 169-188.

Gimpel, G.A., Warzak, W.J., Kuhn, B.R., & Walburn, J.N. (1998). Clinical perspectives in primary nocturnal enuresis. <u>Clinical Pediatrics, 37</u>, 23-30.

Glynn, T.J., & Manley, M.W. (1991). <u>How to help your patients stop smoking: A National Cancer Institute manual for physicians</u>. Bethesda, MD: NIH Publication No. 92-3064.

Larson, D. (1997). Smoking cessation: Counseling your patients. <u>Clinician Reviews, 7</u>, 57-80.

Miller, W.R., & Rollnick, S. (1991). <u>Motivational interviewing: Preparing people to change addictive behavior</u>. New York: Guilford Press.

National Institute on Alcohol Abuse and Alcoholism. (1995). <u>The physicians' guide to helping patients with alcohol problems</u> (NIH Publication No. 95-3769). Washington, DC: US Government Printing Office.

Neinstein, L.S. (1996). <u>Adolescent health care: A practical guide</u>. Baltimore: Williams & Wilkins.

Nemethy, M. (1997). Attention deficit/hyperactivity disorder. <u>Advance for Nurse Practitioners</u>, 22-29.

O'Connor, P.G., & Schottenfeld, R.S. (1998). Patients with alcohol problems. <u>New England Journal of Medicine, 338</u>, 592-602.

Rosen, D.S., & Demitrack, M.A. (1997). Eating disorders and disordered eating. In D.J. Knesper, N.B. Riba, & T.L. Schwenk (Eds.), <u>Primary care psychiatry</u>. Philadelphia: Saunders

Rosenbaum, M., Leibel, R.L., & Hirsch, J. (1997). Obesity. <u>New England Journal of Medicine, 337</u>, 396-405.

Schmitt, B.D. (1997). Encopresis. In R.A. Hoekelman (Ed.), <u>Primary pediatric care</u>. St. Louis: Mosby.

Schteingart, D.E., Edwards, G.J., & Starkman, M.N. (1997). Obesity. In D.J. Knesper, N.B. Riba, & T.L. Schwenk (Eds.), <u>Primary care psychiatry</u>. Philadelphia: Saunders

Smith, T.A, House, R.F., Croghan, I.T., Gauvin, T.R. (1996). Nicotine patch therapy in adolescent smokers. <u>Pediatrics, 98</u>, 659-667.

Smith, M., Pomerlau, O.F., & Wadland, W. (1997). Nicotine and smoking. In D.J. Knesper, N.B. Riba, & T.L. Schwenk (Eds.), <u>Primary care psychiatry</u>. Philadelphia: Saunders.

Taylor, M.E. (1997). Evaluation and management of attention-deficit hyperactivity disorder. <u>American Family Physician, 55</u>, 887-901.

Tan, G., & Schneider, S.C. (1997). Attention-deficit hyperactivity disorder: Pharmacotherapy and beyond. <u>Postgraduate Medicine,</u> <u>101</u>, 201-210.

US Department of Health & Human Services. (1995). <u>Nutrition and your health: Dietary guidelines for Americans</u>. Washington, DC: Author.

Wan, J., & Greenfield, S. (1997). Enuresis and common voiding abnormalities. <u>Pediatric Clinics of North America, 44,</u> 1117-1131.

Wiseman, C.V., Harris, W.A., & Halmi, K.A. (1998). Eating disorders. <u>Medical Clinics of North America, 82</u>, 145-160.

Wolraich, M.L., & Baumgaetel, A. (1997). The practical aspects of diagnosing and managing children with attention deficit hyperactivity disorder. <u>Clinical Pediatrics</u>, 497-504.

CHAPTER 4

Mental Health

DOMESTIC VIOLENCE:
CHILD ABUSE AND NEGLECT

I. Definition: Any physical or mental nonaccidental injury to a child; any failure to provide a child with adequate food, clothing, shelter, supervision, and care

II. Pathogenesis

    A. There are no single set of factors that produce neglectful and abusive parents

    B. There do appear to be some common themes in parental behavior that is abusive and neglectful and these are listed here:
        1. Often, parent was victim of abuse him/herself
        2. Increased family stress is correlated with abuse in many cases
        3. Low income is associated with increased rates of neglect and abuse
        4. Some psychiatric conditions in parents are related to abuse and neglect
        5. Alcohol and drug abuse are associated with high rates of neglect and abuse
        6. Characteristics of the child such as male gender, being fussy as an infant, being slow to develop, and being handicapped increase rates of abuse and neglect

III. Clinical Presentation

    A. More than 600,000 cases of physical abuse are reported in the US each year, and there are at least 1000 deaths among children each year caused by abuse

    B. Surveys of adults indicate that approximately 30% of girls and 20% of boys are sexually assaulted by the age of 18 years

    C. An estimated 1.3 to 1.5 million cases of child neglect are reported each year

    D. Physical indicators of abuse:
        1. Retinal hemorrhages (shaken baby syndrome), unexplained fractures, burns, bruises, welts, bald spots, human bite marks
        2. Bruises or bleeding in external genitalia
        3. Vague complaints such as abdominal pain and sleep disturbances

    E. Behavioral indicators of abuse:
        1. Withdrawn, clothing worn is inappropriate to season and may be worn to cover injuries; history of being a runaway
        2. Role reversal (overly concerned for siblings); sudden school difficulties, habit disorders (sucking, rocking), peer problems, isolation
        3. Sexual display/acting out, excessive or public masturbation, promiscuity

    F. Physical indicators of neglect:
        1. Abandonment, inappropriate dress, poor hygiene, unattended medical needs
        2. Undernutrition or failure to thrive

    G. Behavioral indicators of neglect:
        1. Often tardy or absent from school; school dropout (adolescent)
        2. Listless, withdrawn, substance abuse

IV. Diagnosis/Evaluation

    A. History
        1. Obtain social history including information about parents, care takers, family functioning
        2. Screening for abuse and neglect should be part of every health supervision visit
            a. Parents should be asked routine questions about current family stressors, discipline, child behavior, and home safety

   b. Children should be asked open-ended questions about their own safety using questions in the table that follows

---

Screening for Abuse

❖ Are you afraid of anyone?
❖ Does anyone ever hurt you?
❖ Does anyone make you keep secrets?
❖ Children older than 10 should be interviewed in private, without the parent present

❖ All positive responses are followed up with more specific questions including "What happened?" "When did it happen?" and "Who did that?"

---

  3. If physical injury is present, ask detailed questions including "When did it happen, how did it happen, and who did it?"
   a. Long interval between injury and seeking help is red flag
   b. Story that is inconsistent, contradictory, or fails to adequately explain injury is a red flag
   c. Important to keep in mind that many injuries are accidental
  4. Important to get history in child's own words, using child's vocabulary, and if appropriate, using an anatomically correct doll to help clarify what the child is describing
  5. If behavioral problems are evident, ask appropriate questions to determine etiology
  6. Question about child's past or present medical or behavioral problems in the following areas:
   a. Difficulties with pregnancy, labor, delivery, or neonatal period
   b. Feeding difficulties or problems with toilet training
   c. Behavioral problems, especially of recent onset
   d. Previous trauma, ingestions, or frequent visits for vague complaints
   e. Enuresis or encopresis
  7. History should be carefully recorded as it may be part of court case; stories that change over time are suggestive of abuse -- thus statements made as part of the initial disclosure take on added significance

B. Physical Examination
  1. Measure height and weight; record on growth chart, comparing it to norms and the child's own growth curve (undernutrition may be a sign of neglect)
  2. Observe child's behavior during exam for fearfulness, listlessness, and withdrawn behavior
  3. Inspect skin for hygiene, burns, bruises, bites, and lacerations
   a. Use measuring tape and record on anatomic diagrams on chart
   b. Injuries from accidental trauma generally occur on extensor surfaces; trauma to other areas deserve more evaluation
  4. Examine head focusing on any patchy hair loss, battle's sign (bruising over mastoid process behind ears) raccoon eyes, and blood behind the tympanic membranes
  5. Observe eyes for retinal hemorrhages
  6. Examine abdomen for signs of injury. Note: Cutaneous signs of abdominal injury are rare. Blunt trauma to abdomen can cause serious injury difficult to detect with physical exam alone
  7. Examine genitalia for injury. Note: The majority of children who have been sexually abused have no detectable genital injury
  8. If child <6 years of age, perform Denver II

C. Differential Diagnosis
  1. Unintended injury
  2. Poverty resulting in poor clothing/hygiene

D. Diagnostic Tests
  1. History and physical exam dictate tests
  2. Sexual abuse requires meticulous collection of laboratory and forensic evidence, and its description is beyond the scope of this book (Consult your state health department or social service agency for requirements in your state.)

V.   Plan/Treatment

   A.   Goal of management in cases of suspected abuse and neglect is protection of the child from
        further harm, identification of risks and how these might be dealt with, and compliance with legal
        reporting requirements

   B.   In cases where severe injury or serious threat of further abuse is present, child must be removed
        from the situation and immediate legal intervention must be sought

   C.   In most cases of suspected abuse or neglect, child can be left in the care of the parent/guardian
        while an investigation takes place
        1.   All states require that health care providers (as well as teachers and child care providers)
             report suspected cases of abuse and neglect
        2.   Suspicion, not certainty of child abuse and neglect is what mandates reporting
        3.   Immunity from liability is provided for all reports made in good faith, even if the abuse is
             not confirmed through investigation
        4.   The National Child Abuse Hot-Line number is 1-800-422-4453 and can be used by anyone
             needing more information about reporting mechanisms and requirements

   D.   Explain to parent that you are required by law to report your concerns to the state's child
        protection agency; many states also require that health care providers file a written report within a
        specified time period

   E.   Once the report has been made, the child protection agency is responsible for investigating the
        case
        1.   The goals of child protective services are to keep the child safe and to identify solutions to
             problems that jeopardize child safety
        2.   If possible, the family unit is preserved and the child is removed from the family as a last
             resort

   F.   Documentation is critical in all cases of suspected abuse and neglect; when possible, consult
        with an expert in child abuse and neglect

   G.   National family violence resources are listed in the following table

NATIONAL FAMILY VIOLENCE RESOURCES
✦ National Domestic Violence Hot Line: 800/799-SAFE (TDD hearing impaired: 800/787-3224)
✦ National Resource Center on Domestic Violence: 800/537-2238
✦ Department of Justice Response Center: 800/421-6770
✦ Division of violence prevention of the Centers for Disease Control and Prevention: 770/488-4646
✦ Family Violence and Sexual Assault Institute: 903/534-5100
✦ National Center for Assault Prevention: 908/369-8972
✦ National Coalition Against Domestic Violence: 303/839-1852
✦ National Council on Child Abuse and Family Violence: 800/222-2000
✦ National Institute for Violence Prevention: 508/833-0731

   H.   Follow Up: Primary care providers have a responsibility to follow up closely on all cases of abuse
        and neglect involving children

GRIEF

I.   Definition: A variable but normal response to loss, deprivation, injury, illness, or disenfranchisement

II.   Pathogenesis

    A.   A full depressive syndrome that is a normal reaction to loss

    B.   Persons with uncomplicated bereavement regard the feeling of depressed mood as normal and transitory

III. Clinical Presentation

    A.   Feelings of depression and associated symptoms of poor appetite, weight loss, and insomnia following loss are usually present

    B.   Feelings of guilt, if present, are usually related to things done or not done at time of death by the survivor (if the loss is via death)

    C.   Approximately 80% of persons are markedly improved in 10 weeks after the loss

    D.   Morbid preoccupation with feelings of worthlessness and prolonged functional impairment indicate abnormal grieving and the development of major depression

    E.   By age 18, approximately 4% of US children will experience death of a parent, one of the most stressful life events

    F.   Children usually show affective, cognitive, and behavioral symptoms during the first year of bereavement

    G.   Children under age 6 who have lost a parent are likely to have difficulty with separation from the surviving parent, to be very fearful and to demonstrate increased dependency needs; those older than 6 experience symptoms of anger, aggression, depression, and problems with discipline

IV.   Diagnosis/Evaluation

    A.   History
        1.   Determine when loss occurred, how child is accepting and coping with loss
        2.   Prior experience with child/family is crucial in making an assessment of adjustment
        3.   Ask about functional status (if able to carry out usual activities)
        4.   Ask about presence of support system
        5.   Determine if child is able to mourn
        6.   Determine if child is experiencing despair to the level of self-harm

    B.   Physical Examination: Not indicated

    C.   Differential Diagnosis: Major depressive disorder

    D.   Diagnostic Tests: None indicated

V.   Plan/Management

    A.   Differentiating between children/families who are experiencing a normal grief process and those who exhibit significant pathology requiring referral to a mental health provider is an important first step in management

1. Continued preoccupation with feelings of worthlessness, marked functional impairment that is prolonged, and significant psychomotor retardation suggest a major depressive episode
2. Bereavement that is unduly severe or prolonged indicates the need for management by a mental health provider

B. Interventions for acute grief
  1. Encourage child to mourn, and to express grief in ways that are consistent with his/her particular personality (children, like adults, mourn differently). Message to child should be "You have the right to mourn"
  2. Children typically need frequent, brief discussions of the loss rather than a few long discussions (advise parents regarding this)
  3. Encourage family and small group of people who knew deceased to talk about him/her in presence of the grieving child
  4. Parents should not lie to child, but should use the term "death" when appropriate
     a. By age 4-5, child can understand a brief explanation about how the deceased person died
     b. Child's questions should be answered at that time and later as they arise
     c. Children should attend and be involved in funeral activities
  5. Emphasize that grief is normal, and the goal is not to get rid of it as quickly as possible
  6. Recognize that your presence is the most important comfort you have to offer. Avoid the pressure to provide your own philosophy of death and loss (or to talk about your own losses). Don't worry about what to say; being present and listening are what the patient needs, not your advice. Message should be, "I care"
  7. Accept child's grief for loss that conventional society may not acknowledge as very important (such as loss of pet)
  8. Recognize that providers are not equally capable of intervening effectively in situations of acute loss

C. **Return to routines**: Children do much better if their normal routine is re-established quickly; thus, they should return to normal routines as soon as is practical (no more than 2 weeks between death and return to school and other activities)

D. **Physical exercise**: Recommend daily exercise which can be very beneficial in dealing with depression

E. **Support groups**: Some children and families benefit from sharing with a group; others do not; prior knowledge about family functioning should guide referral

F. Patient or family with significant preexistent psychopathology cannot be expected to adjust in the same way as healthy persons and should be referred for counseling

H. Children's books relating to death and grieving which may be helpful to children are in the table below:

CHILDREN'S BOOKS RELATING TO DEATH AND GRIEVING	
Author	**Book**
Blackburn, Lynn	Timothy Duck
Buchanan-Smith, Doris	A Taste of Blackberries
Carrick, Carol	The Accident
Conley, B.H.	Butterflies, Grandpa and Me
Fassler, Joan	My Grandpa Died Today
Viorst, Judith	The Tenth Good Thing About Barney

I. Follow Up: Frequently by telephone/mail over the period of acute grief during first few weeks; can offer checkup during the first nine months, depending on mourner's wishes or needs. Beware of delayed grief reaction. These reactions may occur close to anniversary of a death (anniversary reaction)

REFERENCES

American Psychiatric Association. (1994). <u>Diagnostic and statistical manual of mental disorders</u> (4th ed.). Washington, DC: Author.

Brummel-Smith, K., Rubenstein, L.Z., & Whitehouse, P.J. (1998, May). A practical guide to screening and assessment. <u>Patient Care</u>, 31-67.

Buckman, R., Lipkin, M., Dourkes, B.M., & Tolle, S.W. (1997, June). Strategies and skills for breaking bad news. <u>Patient Care</u>, 61-72.

Christophersen, E.R. (1999). Death in the family. In R.A. Dershewitz (Ed.), <u>Ambulatory pediatric care</u>. Philadelphia: Lippincott-Raven.

Eyler, A.E., Cohen, M., & Kershaw, M.O. (1997). Domestic violence and abuse. In D.J. Knesper, M.B. Riba, & T.L. Schwenk (Eds.), <u>Primary care psychiatry</u>. Philadelphia: Saunders.

Jaudes, P.E. (1999). Child maltreatment. In R.A. Dershewitz (Ed.), <u>Ambulatory pediatric care</u>. Philadelphia: Lippincott-Raven.

Neufeld, B. (1996). SAFE questions: Overcoming barriers to the detection of domestic violence. <u>American Family Physician, 53</u> (8), 2575-2580.

Weisman, A. (1998). The patient with acute grief. In T.A. Stern, J.B. Herman, & P.L. Slavin (Eds.), <u>The MGH guide to psychiatry in primary care</u>. New York: McGraw-Hill.

Wells, B.G., DiPiro, J.T., Schwinghammer, T.L., & Hamilton, C.W. (1998). <u>Pharmacotherapy handbook</u>. Stanford, CT: Appleton & Lange.

CHAPTER 5

Metabolic and Endocrine Problems

Diabetes Mellitus
Table: Diagnostic Criteria for Diabetes Mellitus
Table: Screening Criteria
Table: Definitions of Abnormalities in Albumin Excretion
Table: Glycemic Control
Table: Guidelines for Calculating Calorie Requirements
Table: Various Human Insulin Preparations
Table: Common Insulin Regimens
Table: Adjusting Insulin Therapy
Table: Tips on Insulin Therapy
Table: Patient Education - Insulin Therapy

Dyslipidemia
Table: Coronary Heart Disease Risk Factors Other than LDL Cholesterol
Table: Example of Foods in Step I and Step II Diets
Table: Summary of Bile Acid Sequestrants

Hyperthyroidism

Hypothyroidism

Gynecomastia

Precocious Puberty
Table: Pattern of Pubertal Development
Table: Sexual Maturity Stages in Girls
Table: Sexual Maturity Stages in Boys

Delayed Puberty

DIABETES MELLITUS

I. Definition: Group of metabolic diseases characterized by hyperglycemia from defects in insulin secretion, insulin action, or both

II. Pathogenesis; etiologic classification of diabetes mellitus (DM)

   A. Type 1 [formerly known as insulin-dependent (IDDM), or juvenile-onset diabetes] due to β-cell destruction which usually results in absolute insulin deficiency; can be either of the following forms:
      1. Immune-mediated
      2. Idiopathic

   B. Type 2 [formerly known as non-insulin dependent type (NIDDM) or adult-onset diabetes] is relatively rare in children
      1. Occasionally occurs in adolescents from susceptible genetic backgrounds
      2. Characterized by resistance to the action of insulin; also, may have impairment of insulin secretion
      3. Some obese adolescents may have this type

   C. Other specific types of diabetes
      1. Genetic defects in β-cell function
      2. Genetic defects in insulin action
      3. Diseases of the exocrine pancreas (pancreatitis, trauma, infection, pancreatectomy, and pancreatic carcinoma)
      4. Endocrinopathies such as acromegaly, Cushing's syndrome, pheochromocytoma
      5. Drug or chemical-induced diabetes (thiazide diuretics, steroids, phenytoin, nicotinic acid, thyroid hormones, α-interferon)
      6. Infections such as congenital rubella or cytomegalovirus
      7. Uncommon forms of immune-mediated diabetes ("stiff man" syndrome and anti-insulin receptor antibodies)
      8. Other genetic syndromes such as Down's syndrome, Klinefelter's syndrome and Turner's syndrome

III. Clinical Presentation

   A. Criteria for diagnosing diabetes mellitus in children and adolescents (see following table)

DIAGNOSTIC CRITERIA FOR DIABETES MELLITUS*

✔ Symptoms of diabetes (polydipsia, polyuria, and weight loss) plus casual plasma glucose concentration ≥200 mg/dl (11.1 mmol/l); "casual" is any time of day without regard to time since last meal
   OR
✔ Fasting plasma glucose (FPG) ≥126 mg/dl (7.0 mmol/l); "fasting" is no caloric intake for at least 8 hours
   OR
✔ 2 hour plasma glucose ≥200 mg/dl during a oral glucose tolerance tests (OGTT); OGTT should be performed using a glucose load containing the equivalent of 75-g anhydrous glucose (in children, use 1.75 g/kg to maximum of 75-g glucose load)

---

*These criteria should be confirmed by repeat testing on a different day except in the case of unequivocal hyperglycemia with acute metabolic decompensation

Adapted from American Diabetic Association. (1998). Report of the Expert Committee on the diagnosis and classification of diabetes mellitus. Diabetes Care, 21,(Supp. 1), S5-S19

   B. Criteria for diagnosing impaired fasting glucose (IFG) or IGT, respectively: FBG ≥110 mg/dL (6.1 mmol/l) and < 126 mg/dl (7.0 mmol/l) or 2-hour glucose ≥140 (7.8 mmol/l) and <200 mg/dL (11.1 mmol/l)

C. Type 1 diabetes
1. Occurs in approximately 10% of all persons diagnosed with diabetes
2. Usually appears with acute onset of symptoms: polydipsia, polyphagia, polyuria, weight loss, blurred vision, and frequent infections such as dermatologic fungal infections
3. After the initial presentation of symptoms, the newly diagnosed patient often undergoes a "honeymoon" period or remission phase which may last from several months to 2 years
4. Ketoacidosis may develop in children who are not identified in early stages of disease; symptoms in severe cases include dehydration, Kussmaul respirations, fruity or acetone odor to breath, and impaired consciousness
5. Can occur at any age (rarely after age 30) with highest incidence between ages 10-14 years
   a. Morbidity and mortality is greater in the very young child; be alert when a small infant has persistent vomiting and lethargy because of high risk of rapid progressive to severe dehydration
   b. In the young child, the diagnosis may be missed; failure to grow and gain weight are important warning signs of diabetes in this age group
   c. Most children have the classic symptoms as well as fatigue, weakness, and listlessness
   d. Nocturnal enuresis may occur in a previously toilet-trained child; an infant may need his/her diaper changed constantly
   e. Prior to age 6 or 7, children lack the cognitive capacity to recognize hypoglycemic symptoms
   f. Children have more infections and sick days than adults which complicates their care

D. Type 2 diabetes
1. Gradual onset and slow progression of symptoms
2. Fatigue is a common symptom
3. Ketoacidosis rarely occurs except in times of stress, illness or infection

E. Macrovascular and microvascular complications include the following
1. Retinopathy is the leading cause of new adult blindness in U.S.
   a. Background retinopathy or nonproliferative retinopathy involves microaneurysms and dot hemorrhages but does not impair vision unless it involves the macula
   b. Retinopathy often develops 7 years before clinical diagnosis is made
   c. Occurs in almost every patient who has had diabetes for 10-20 years or more
   d. Proliferative retinopathy can lead to blindness and involves neovascularization (new vessels develop) with retinal detachment and vitreous hemorrhages; occurs in 60-70%% of patients with Type 1 and 30% of patients with Type 2 diabetes
2. Nephropathy
   a. Develops in 35-45% of patients with Type 1 and 20% with Type 2
   b. Progresses from the development of microalbuminuria to overt proteinuria and finally to end-stage renal disease(ESRD) (this process may take as long as 23 years); diabetes is the most common single cause of ESRD in U.S.
3. Neuropathy
   a. Most common manifestation is a peripheral, symmetric sensorimotor neuropathy which is usually only minimally uncomfortable
   b. A minority of patients have painful peripheral neuropathy with lancinating or burning pain
   c. Autonomic neuropathy may affect gastric or intestinal motility, erectile function, bladder function, cardiac function, and vascular tone
4. Cardiovascular Disease: Diabetes is a major risk factor
5. Other complications include an increased prevalence of infections, cognitive impairment, and contractures of digits (Hammer toes)

IV. Diagnosis/Evaluation

A. History
1. To establish the diagnosis, explore the following:
    a. Symptoms such as fatigue and complications associated with diabetes
    b. To uncover polyuria in children, inquire about bedwetting, nocturia, number of diapers used, or whether the child frequently leaves the classroom to urinate
    c. Explore family history of diabetes and other endocrine problems
    d. With children, ask about neonatal history including the weight and condition of the child at birth, and whether complications occurred during the mother's pregnancy or at the time of labor and delivery
    e. Ask about attention span and school performance
2. In patients who are already diagnosed, inquire about the following:
    a. Frequency, severity, and cause of hypoglycemia or ketoacidosis
    b. Symptoms and treatments of chronic eye, kidney, nerve, genitourinary (including sexual), bladder, gastrointestinal function, heart, peripheral vascular, foot, and cerebrovascular complications
    c. Prior or current infections
    d. Previous and current pharmacological, nutritional, and self-management treatment plans
    e. Patterns and results of glucose monitoring
    f. Dietary habits (especially amount of carbohydrates such as juices), nutritional status, and weight history; growth and development
    g. Amount, intensity, and frequency of exercise
    h. In adolescents, risk factors for atherosclerosis such as smoking, hypertension, obesity
    i. Psychological, sociological and economic factors that may impact on management plan

B. Physical Examination
1. Measure height and weight (and compare to norms)
2. During peripubertal period, determine sexual maturation stages
3. Determine vital signs including orthostatic blood pressure measurements
4. Examine skin including sites of previous insulin administration if applicable
5. In adolescents, perform a thorough ophthalmoscopic examination (best done with dilation)
6. Perform a thorough mouth and dental examination
7. Palpate thyroid
8. Perform complete cardiac examination
9. Palpate and auscultate pulses
10. Perform abdominal examination; check for liver enlargement
11. Assess hand and wrist mobility, checking for contractures
12. Carefully examine feet
13. Particularly in adolescents, perform complete neurological exam
14. May need to do a complete physical exam to exclude any sources of occult infection

C. Differential Diagnosis
1. Glucosuria without hyperglycemia occurs in benign renal glucosuria or in renal tubular disease
2. Diabetes insipidus presents with polyuria and polydipsia but not hyperglycemia
3. Transient hyperglycemia is present when patients have severe stress from trauma, burns or infection or are on glucocorticoids
4. Salicylate intoxication mimics ketoacidosis
5. Children with inborn errors of metabolism may present with modest hyperglycemia and acidosis
6. Intercurrent illness may cause stress-induced hyperglycemia

D. Diagnostic Tests
   1. <u>Screening tests</u> to detect diabetes in asymptomatic, undiagnosed individuals (see table); American Diabetic Association recommends the following:

SCREENING CRITERIA

✦ Testing should be considered in all individuals ≥45 years and, if normal, it should be repeated at 3-year intervals
✦ Testing should be considered at a younger age or be performed more frequently in individuals who
- are obese (≥120% desirable body weight or a BMI ≥ 27 kg/m^2)
- have a first-degree relative with diabetes
- are members of a high-risk ethnic population (e.g., African-American, Hispanic-American, Native American, Asian-American, Pacific Islander)
- have delivered a baby weighing >9 lb or have been diagnosed with GDM
- are hypertensive (≥140/90)
- have an HDL cholesterol level ≤ 35 mg/dl (0.90 mmol/l) and/or a triglyceride level ≥250 mg/dl (2.82 mmol/l)
- on previous testing, had IGT or IFG

✦ Fasting Plasma Glucose (FPG) is test of choice (fast for 8 hours prior to test)
✦ If FPG is ≥126 mg/dl, repeat test on different day to confirm diagnosis

Adapted from American Diabetic Association. (1998). Report of the Expert Committee on the diagnosis and classification of diabetes mellitus. <u>Diabetes Care, 21,</u>(Supp. 1), S5-S19

      a. Random plasma glucose measurements can be made when food or drink has been ingested within 3 hours preceding test; ≥200 mg/dL is considered a positive screening test and the diagnosis of diabetes should be confirmed with an additional test, preferably a fasting plasma glucose (FPG) test
      b. Screening for autoantibodies related to type 1 diabetes is not recommended outside the context of research studies
      c. Consider screening lean new-onset diabetic patients for type 1 diabetes by measuring postprandial serum C peptide

   2. Tests to determine the <u>degree of glycemic control</u>
      a. Glycosylated hemoglobin (HbA_1 or HbA_1C)
         (1) Reflects mean glucose levels for the preceding 2-3 months
         (2) Order at least every 6 months for well-controlled patients
         (3) Order more often (every 3 months) in diabetics with poor control, when beginning new therapies, or young children
         (4) Levels <7.5% indicate good diabetic control in adolescents
         (5) For children, the normal range is 5.4 to 7.4%
         (6) Falsely elevated levels may occur in presence of uremia, alcoholism, and aspirin use
      b. Glycated serum protein indicates glycemic control in a short period of time and needs to be performed monthly; currently this test is not recommended

   3. Tests helpful in defining <u>associated complications and risk factors</u>:
      a. Order fasting lipid profile: total cholesterol, high-density lipoprotein (HDL) cholesterol, low density lipoprotein (LDL) cholesterol, and triglycerides
         (1) Order when diabetes is first diagnosed in patients >2 years
         (2) In patients whose values fall within acceptable risk levels, repeat tests every 5 years; see section on DYSLIPIDEMIA for monitoring in children with abnormal levels
      b. Order annual serum creatinine if proteinuria is present in children
      c. Order annual urinalysis: ketones, glucose, protein, sediment
         (1) If protein is positive, a quantitative measure should be performed
         (2) If protein is negative a test for the presence of microalbuminuria is necessary (see IV.D.3.d), which immediately follows
      d. Testing for microalbuminuria
         (1) Because microalbuminuria rarely occurs with short duration of type 1 diabetes or before puberty, individuals with type 1 diabetes should begin testing with puberty and after 5 years duration
        (2) Because of marked day-to-day variability in albumin excretion, at least two of three collections measured in a 3- to 6-month period should show elevated levels before arriving at a diagnosis of microalbuminuria

(3) Testing for microalbuminuria can be performed by 3 methods
  (a) Measurement of the albumin-to-creatinine ratio in a random, spot collection
  (b) 24 hour collection with serum creatinine which allows for simultaneous measurement of creatinine clearance
  (c) Timed collection such as 4 hours or overnight
(4) Microalbuminuria and clinical albuminuria is defined in following table

DEFINITIONS OF ABNORMALITIES IN ALBUMIN EXCRETION			
Category	24-h Collection	Timed Collection	Spot Collection
Normal	<30 mg/24 h	<20 μg/min	< 30 μg/mg creatinine
Microalbuminuria	30-300 mg/24 h	20-200 μg/min	30-300 μg/mg creatinine
Clinical albuminuria	>300 mg/24 h	>200 μg/min	>300 μg/mg creatinine

Two of three specimens collected within a 3- to 6-month period should be abnormal before considering a patient to have crossed one of these diagnostic threshholds. Exercise within 24 hours of infection, fever, congestive heart failure, marked hyperglycemia, and marked hypertension may elevate urinary albumin excretion over baseline values

Adapted from American Diabetes Association. (1998). Diabetic nephropathy. Diabetes Care, 21, (Supp. 1), S50-S53.

  e. Order T_4 and thyroid stimulating hormone annually
  f. Some, but not all authorities, also suggest regular serum BUN and CBC tests
4. Diabetic ketoacidosis presents with reduced plasma bicarbonate, reduced blood pH, increased anion gap, and hyperlipidemia; hyperkalemia often occurs with significant metabolic acidosis

V. Plan/Management

  A. The Diabetes Control and Complications Trial (DCCT), a long-term, multi-center trial, found that type 1 diabetics with tight glycemic control of their plasma glucose had a significant reduction in their risk for developing diabetic retinopathy, nephropathy, and neuropathy when compared with the standard treatment groups
    1. Degree of tight glycemic control must be individualized and balanced with the risk of developing hypoglycemia; tight glycemic control is contraindicated in infants <2 years old and used very cautiously in children <7 years of age due to the risk of injuring the developing brain
    2. Goals of glycemic control are shown in the following the table

GLYCEMIC CONTROL			
Measurement	Nondiabetic	Goal	Additional action suggested*
Preprandial glucose (mg/dl)**	<110	80-120	<80 or >140
Bedtime glucose (mg/dl)**	<120	100-140	<100 or >160
Glycosylated hemoglobin	<6	<7	>8

*Additional action must be individualized. Actions may be referral to endocrinologist, change in medications, self-management education, etc.
**Measurement of capillary blood glucose

Adapted from American Diabetic Association. (1998). Standards of medical care for patients with diabetes mellitus. Diabetes Care, 21, (Supp. 1), S23-S31.

  B. Hospitalization is recommended for all children who are newly diagnosed with and without ketoacidosis

  C. All diabetic patients benefit from medical nutritional therapy (MNT), exercise, and extensive patient education
    1. Type 1 diabetics also require insulin therapy
    2. Type 2 diabetics may be controlled with diet and exercise alone, however, oral antidiabetic agents and, in some cases, insulin may be needed for blood glucose control

D.   Patient education is essential; education must be integrated with all aspects of the plan (also, see patient education in each of the following sections)
1.   Discuss basic pathophysiology of diabetes
2.   Explain long-term complications of diabetes, emphasizing that recent research indicates that these complications can be prevented or delayed when blood glucose is well controlled
3.   Encourage patient to wear Medic-Alert tags

E.   Nutritional recommendations: Diet is an important aspect of the treatment plan and collaboration or referral to a dietician is beneficial
1.   Currently, there is no one "diabetic" diet or meal plan; medical nutrition therapy (MNT) should be individualized
2.   Patients with Type 1 diabetes:
   a.   Cannot be treated with diet alone
   b.   Monitor blood glucose levels and adjust insulin based on the amount of food usually consumed; individuals on intensified insulin programs can make adjustments in rapid or lispro insulin to cover carbohydrate content of meals and/or snacks and for deviations from typical eating and exercising habits
   c.   Plan meals to provide the amount of calories and nutrients that are expected to be metabolized when insulin is administered
      (1)   Keep timing and amount of calories and nutrients in meals the same each day
      (2)   Have a consistent, daily pattern of exercise and physical activity (may need supplemental snacks before and after exercise; may need to alter insulin dosage before activity)
   d.   Carbohydrate counting in which the patient takes insulin based on the amount of insulin consumed for a meal may be effective; approximately 1 unit of insulin will cover 10-15 grams of carbohydrate consumed
   e.   Patients of various ages have different caloric needs (see table)

GUIDELINES FOR CALCULATING CALORIE REQUIREMENTS		
Age	**Gender**	**Calories**
0-12 years	Male & Female	1000 calories plus 100 calories per year of age
12-15 years	Female Male	1500-2000 calories plus 100 calories per year over 12 2000-2500 calories plus 200 calories per year over 12
15-20 years	Female Male	13-15 calories/pound desired body weight 15-18 calories/pound desired body weight

Adapted from Bode, B.W., Davidson, P.C., & Steed, R.D. (1997). In J.S. Skyler. Diabetes Dek: Professional Edition. Infodek: Atlanta.

   f.   Younger children have difficulty following strict meal plans; 3 meals and 3 snacks daily are typically recommended
   g.   Older children often omit the mid-morning snack and add the calories derived from this snack to their breakfast or lunch; bedtime snack should never be missed
3.   Patients with type 2 diabetes can often improve blood glucose levels by moderate weight loss (5-9 kg or 10-20 lb) and hypocaloric diets (250-500 calories less than average daily intake as calculated from diet history) **alone**; spacing of meals throughout day and regular exercise can also improve control
4.   Dietary recommendations include the following
   a.   Carbohydrates should make up approximately 50-60% of the total calories; unrefined carbohydrates and fiber should be eaten whenever possible
   b.   Protein intake should be the recommended dietary allowance for Americans or about 10-20% of daily calories (in children protein intake should be sufficient for optimal growth)
   c.   Total fat should comprise <30% of total calories with saturated fats restricted to <10% of total calories and cholesterol <300 mg/day; unsaturated fats should replace saturated fats

d.　Patients can use nutritive and nonnutritive sweeteners
　　　e.　Balance in salt is needed with upper limit of 3000 mg/day but recognizing that sodium restriction may lead to electrolyte imbalance

F.　Exercise positively affects the levels of blood glucose; for patients on insulin therapy, the following guidelines are helpful
　　　1.　Avoid exercising at times when insulin is at its peak action
　　　2.　Monitor blood glucose before and after exercise to identify when changes in insulin or food intake are necessary and to learn glycemic response to different exercise conditions
　　　3.　Avoid exercise if FPG levels are <80 mg/dl or >250 mg/dl and ketosis is present or if glucose levels are >300 mg/dl, regardless of whether ketosis is present
　　　4.　Ingest added carbohydrates if glucose levels are <100 mg/dl
　　　5.　Eat added carbohydrates as needed to avoid hypoglycemia; keep carbohydrate-based food readily available during and after exercise; in general, one serving of carbohydrates increases plasma glucose about 40 points
　　　6.　Avoid exercising extremities in which insulin has recently been injected

G.　Insulin therapy: Goals of normalized glycohemoglobin must be balanced with risks of hypoglycemia
　　　1.　Consider type of insulin to use
　　　　　a.　If patients are on beef or pork insulin, do not switch if they are well-controlled
　　　　　b.　Newly diagnosed diabetics should be on human insulin because of its lower incidence of insulin allergy, resistance, and lipoatrophy (see following table for brand names of human insulin)
　　　2.　Use U-100 insulin
　　　3.　Consider onset, peak, and duration of various insulin preparations (see following table)

VARIOUS HUMAN INSULIN PREPARATIONS			
Type	Onset (hours)	Peak (hours)	Duration (hours)
Rapid acting analog			
Humalog (Lispro)	<0.25	1	3.5-4.5
Short acting			
Humulin R	0.5	2.4	6-8
Novolin R	0.5	2.5-5	8
Velosulin BR	0.5	1-3	8
Intermediate acting			
Humulin N (NPH)	1-2	6-12	18-24
Novolin N (NPH)	1.5	4-12	24
Humulin L (lente)	1-3	6-12	18-24
Novolin L (lente)	2.5	7-15	22
Long acting			
Humulin U (Ultralente)	4-6	8-20	24-48
Premixed: Insulin isophane suspension (NPH)/regular insulin (R)*			
Humulin 70/30	0.5	2-12	24
Humulin 50/50	0.5	3-5	24
Novolin 70/30	0.5	2-12	24

*Do Not use premixed with Type 1 diabetics as it severely limits flexibility

　　　4.　Special considerations of insulin therapy in children and adolescents
　　　　　a.　Initiating insulin (pubertal patients and those physically inactive and overweight should receive upper end of the following dosage ranges)
　　　　　　　(1)　For nonketoacidotic children begin with 0.25-0.5 units/kg/day of insulin
　　　　　　　(2)　For ketoacidotic children start with 0.5-0.75 units/kg/day
　　　　　b.　Established diabetics require 1.0 units/kg/day
　　　　　c.　The adolescent may need 1.25-1.50 units/kg/day during the pubertal growth spurt

d. Adjust insulin levels to meet target blood glucose ranges
   (1) Preschool child should be in the range of 90 to 140 mg/dl preprandially and 90-200 postprandially
   (2) School-aged children should be in the range of 80 to 120 mg/dl preprandially and 80 to 180 postprandially
e. Typically, children are given a twice-daily injection of intermediate-acting and short-acting insulins (see following table on COMMON INSULIN REGIMENS); adolescents seem to benefit from the 3-injection regimen
f. Because of the danger of hypoglycemia to the developing brain, cautiously lower blood glucose in young children
g. About 1/3 of children under 3 years of age, develop hypoglycemia at nighttime on split/BID dosing regime which can lead to cognitive and neurological deficits; instruct parents to occasionally check blood glucose at 3 AM and if low, reduce evening dose of insulin by 10% every few days until control is reached
h. Humalog (lispro) insulin is not FDA approved for children <12 years, but some experts recommend that it is beneficial, particularly for toddlers and adolescents who have difficulty adhering to a strict mealtime routine
i. In adolescent, consider an eating disorder if glycosolated hemoglobin levels are >12%; adolescents may intentionally miss doses to lose weight

5. Honeymoon phase: after initial therapy is instituted this phase occurs and may last 12-18 months; insulins dosages may be reduced to 0.2-0.5 units/kg/day (important to tell patients about this phase to prevent false beliefs that the diabetes is partially cured)
6. Determine the pattern or regimen of insulin therapy (see following table)

COMMON INSULIN REGIMENS

Regimen	Dosing	Comments
2-Injection -or- Split/Mix	2/3s of total daily dosing in am 1/3 of total daily dosing in pm - then - AM - 2/3 NPH + 1/3 regular or lispro[†] PM - 1/2 NPH + 1/2 regular or lispro[†]	✦Best in Type 2 and early Type 1 ✦Disadvantages: poor peaking of noon insulin & excess insulin at night (to resolve this problem, limit noon meal and eat a bedtime snack)
3-Injection	Of total daily dose: AM* -40% NPH & 15% regular or lispro[†] PM** -15% regular or lispro[†] Bedtime -30% NPH	✦Advantage: Less risk of nighttime hypoglycemia & better control of dawn phenomenon or persistent AM hyperglycemia ✦Disadvantages: poor peaking of insulin at noon (to resolve, limit noon meal)
4-Injection or Prandial/Basal	Of total daily dose: Before each meal (Prandial insulin) -20-25% regular or lispro[†] At bedtime (Basal insulin) - 25-40% NPH, lente, or ultralente	✦Requires committed patient and care-provider, with frequent self-blood-glucose monitoring ✦Disadvantage: No more than 5 hours can transpire between meals ✦Advantage: Clear relationship between insulin dose and glucose level
Continuous Subcutaneous Insulin Infusion -or- Insulin Pump Therapy	-Continually delivers regular insulin or lispro[†] -Provides both basal insulin release and adjustable pre-meal bolus release	✦Not used in children; older adolescents who are conscientious may benefit from this therapy ✦Indications: Inability to control glucose with 2 or more injections; recurrent, major hypoglycemia due to hypoglycemic unawareness, loss of counter-regulatory mechanisms or variable absorption of modified insulins ✦Prerequisites: Patient must have intellectual & emotional abilities for self-care ✦Advantages: Closely resembles endogenous insulin release; results in more predictable insulin absorption and fewer dosage errors ✦Disadvantages: Expensive; blood glucose must be monitored 4 times/day

* AM is before breakfast: regular insulin should be taken 30-45 minutes before breakfast and lispro should be taken 15 minutes before breakfast
**PM is before evening meal or supper
[†]Lispro is often more convenient for patients because it can be injected immediately before meals and can lessen the likelihood of late post-prandial hypoglycemia and nocturnal hypoglycemia but is more expensive and needs more intensive monitoring than regular insulin

Adapted from Mengel, M.B. (1996). Diabetes mellitus. In M.B. Mengel & L.P. Schwiebert (Eds.), Ambulatory Medicine (2nd ed.), pp. 412-419. Stamford, CT: Appleton & Lange.

7. Adjusting insulin is based on daily blood glucose levels and on peak effect of a given insulin dose (patients should record their blood glucose and insulin doses with comments on a flow sheet)
   a. Calculating adjustments: Adjustments should be made by 20% increments or decrements; for example, 1 unit for doses of 5 units or 2 units for doses of 10 units
   b. Downward adjustments should be made the day following a "below range blood glucose" to avoid repeat hypoglycemia
   c. Upward adjustments should be delayed for 2 days to establish a pattern
   d. Consider timing and type of insulin when making adjustments (see following table):

ADJUSTING INSULIN THERAPY	
Insulin	**Affected Blood Glucose Value**
AM* Intermediate	Post-lunch Pre-supper
AM* Regular	Post-breakfast Pre-lunch
PM** Intermediate	Early morning
PM** Regular	Bedtime
Bedtime Intermediate	Early morning

*AM is before breakfast
**PM is before evening meal or supper

8. Tips on administering insulin therapy (see following table)

TIPS ON INSULIN THERAPY

★ Insulin should approximate the natural release of insulin by the beta cell
★ Administer Insulin to provide a basal amount in 40-50% of total daily dose as well as peaks after each meal
★ One time a day insulin therapy is **not** sufficient for patients with Type 1 diabetes
★ Be careful in adjusting insulin with type 1 diabetics; they are very sensitive to adjustments because they have no endogenous insulin secretion
★ Consider giving PM NPH at bedtime to reduce early morning hyperglycemia
★ Use NPH when there is a need to mix with another type of insulin
★ Consider the following when blood glucose is not controlled with insulin: malignant insulin resistance, occult infection, noncompliance, poor coping skills

9. Patient education concerning the administering, storage, and disposal of insulin is essential (see following table)

PATIENT EDUCATION - INSULIN THERAPY

● Insulin in use can be kept at room temperature, for one month only, to limit local irritation at injection site; unopened insulin should be refrigerated
● When mixing insulins, the clear, short-acting insulin should be drawn into syringe first
● Syringes can be prefilled and stored in a vertical position in the refrigerator for 3 weeks (do not allow if using Lispro)
● Usually, the insulin should be given 30-60 minutes before eating; lispro should be given 15 minutes before eating
● Subcutaneously inject insulin into upper arm, anterior and lateral aspects of thigh, the buttocks and abdomen (with exception of a circle with a 2-inch radius around the navel); Do not rotate to different anatomical sites, but do make injections in different areas of one anatomical site
● Dispose syringes in resistant disposal container and contact local public health unit or local trash-disposal authority for appropriate disposal provisions
● Proper procedure of syringe reuse involves cleaning needle after use and putting in refrigerator (only teach patients who have good cognitive and psychomotor functioning)
● Syringe alternatives such as jet injectors, pen-like devices, and insulin-containing cartridges are usually expensive but may be more convenient and improve technique of insulin injection

H. Self-monitoring of blood glucose has replaced urine testing as a method to assess glucose control; however, Type 1 patients need to check urine for ketones whenever their blood glucose level is >300 mg/dL, during illness, stress, pregnancy or when symptoms of ketoacidosis such as nausea, vomiting, or abdominal pain are present

    1. Frequent monitoring is essential when patients are on intensive insulin therapy or insulin pump therapy; monitor blood glucose before meals, at bedtime and occasionally in the middle of night

    2. Less frequent monitoring may be appropriate for some patients, but even these patients should adhere to the following recommendations:

        a. When medications are altered:

            (1) Patient should check blood glucose before each meal, at bedtime, and 2-4 in AM for 3 days

            (2) Next 7 days, blood glucose can be checked before breakfast and dinner

        b. After glucose is initially controlled, monitoring can be once a day at different times

        c. When glucose is stabilized, check 2-4 times per week at different times

I. Contingency plan for managing hypoglycemia episodes

    1. Teach patient and family the signs and symptoms of hypoglycemia such as shakiness, sweating, restlessness, hunger, headache, confusion, or seizures

    2. Instruct older children and adolescents to carry 10-15 g of oral glucose (2 glucose tablets, 5 lifesavers, or 4 oz. of orange juice) to eat in case of a hypoglycemic reaction

    3. Family or friends should be instructed in administering a subcutaneous or intramuscular injection of glucagon if patient is unresponsive or unable to swallow

        a. Adolescent dose: 1 mg

        b. Children <5 years: 0.25-0.5 mg; Children 5-10 years: 0.5-1 mg

    4. After consciousness is regained, patient should ingest oral carbohydrates to prevent further hypoglycemia

    5. Encourage patient to carry medical identification

J. Managing diabetes when the patient is ill; difficult to predict if blood glucose will increase or decrease during sickness; teach patients the following:

    1. Continue to take usual dose of insulin or oral agent

    2. Perform blood-glucose monitoring several times a day as well as check urine for ketones (twice a day)

    3. If patients are able to drink, increase intake of non-caloric fluids

    4. Drink small continuous amounts of sugar-containing liquids such as Gatorade or Coke in conjunction with the readings from their self-monitoring if they are vomiting or nauseated

    5. Call health care provider in following circumstances

        a. Inability to drink fluids

        b. Blood glucose is >240 mg/dl and urine is positive for ketones

K. Management of associated problems and complications. Growing recognition that tight glycemic control prevents or delays many of the following problems

    1. Diabetic ketoacidosis and hyperosmolar coma usually require referral to an endocrinologist

        a. Encourage fluid intake to prevent dehydration

        b. Initial workup: electrolytes, urinalysis, serum ketones, CBC, ECG, chest x-ray

        c. Treatment is usually insulin, fluids, and potassium replacement

    2. Diabetic retinopathy: Refer to ophthalmologist; laser therapy and vitrectomy have been effective

    3. Nephropathy may occur in adolescence

        a. Patients with microalbuminuria will likely progress to clinical albuminuria (≥300 mg/24 hours) and decreasing glomerular filtration rate (GFR) over a period of years; once clinical albuminuria appears, the risk of end-stage renal failure is high

        b. Achieving normoglycemia and lowering blood pressure have proven to delay progression of nephropathy

            (1) Consider prescribing a angiotensin-converting enzyme (ACE) inhibitor to all type 1 patients with microalbuminuria even if they are normotensive;

            (2) Periodically monitor potassium levels to detect an adverse drug reaction of hyperkalemia

(3) Periodically monitor urine albumin to document the effect of treatment and to detect the rare case of adverse effects of drug therapy

    c. Protein restriction should be initiated when GFR starts to fall; meal plans should be developed by a registered dietician

    d. Refer to a subspecialist in diabetic renal disease when GFR falls to <70 ml • min^{-1} • 1.73 m^{-2}, when serum creatinine is greater than 2.0 mg/dl, or there is hypertension or hyperkalemia

    e. Phosphate lowering therapies may be helpful

4. <u>Cardiovascular disease</u>: Efforts to reduce risk factors and delay further progression of the disease should be started in childhood

5. <u>Hypertension</u> should be treated with goal to reduce arterial blood pressure to below 130/85 mm Hg

    a. Persistent hypertension is often a manifestation of diabetic nephropathy

    b. As for other hypertensive patients, lifestyle modification should be initially employed

    c. ACE inhibitor is often drug of first choice and is preferred for patients with diabetic nephropathy; angiotensin II receptor blockers are alternative medications

L. Referrals and health maintenance plan

1. Eye examination: Patients >9 years who have had diagnosis for 3-5 years should have annual comprehensive examinations by an ophthalmologist or optometrist

2. Consult with podiatry services as needed

3. Referral to dentist and dental hygienist is often indicated

4. Annual influenza vaccine is recommended

M. Current research

1. Prophylactic therapies to prevent the development of clinical type 1 diabetes

2. Administration of humalog (lispro) after meals to enable patients to adjust insulin requirements based on how much food was eaten

N. Follow Up: Scheduling of return visits will depend on degree of glucose control, changes in therapeutic regime, and presence of illnesses or complications of diabetes

1. Patients beginning insulin or who are making a major change in their insulin program need frequent contact with the health team, possibly daily, until control is achieved and risk of hypoglycemia is low

2. After control is achieved, see patient and family in 4 weeks, and thereafter every 2-3 months

3. Increase visits if patients are involved in intensive insulin therapy, not meeting glycemic or blood pressure goals, or there is evidence of progression in microvascular or macrovascular complications

DYSLIPIDEMIA

I. Definition: Elevation of one of or more of the following: cholesterol, cholesterol esters, phospholipids, or triglycerides

II. Pathogenesis

A. Pathophysiology

1. An elevated cholesterol level is an independent and significant risk factor for coronary heart disease (CHD)

2. Blood cholesterol levels are regulated by lipoproteins or "carriers" which are a combination of lipids (fats) and proteins.

3. High-density lipoproteins (HDL), major carriers, are thought to prevent or delay atherogenesis because of their low fat content and their probable role in carrying lipids away from blood vessels to the liver for degradation
4. The other major carrier, low density lipoproteins (LDL), are considered harmful lipoproteins because they help to keep cholesterol in the blood vessels, forming fatty deposits.

B. Etiology
1. Primary hyperlipidemia occurs in individuals with specific inherited traits that result in defects in lipid metabolism or transport
2. Several secondary factors can contribute to hyperlipidemia
   a. Obesity
   b. Low activity levels
   c. High dietary fat, cholesterol, and calorie intake
   d. Endocrine disorders such as diabetes mellitus, Cushing's syndrome, hypothyroidism, lipodystrophies, anorexia nervosa, acute intermittent porphyria
   e. Renal disorders such as uremia and nephrotic syndrome,
   f. Hepatic disorders such as primary biliary cirrhosis, acute hepatitis, hepatoma
   g. Immunologic disorders such as systemic lupus erythematosus
   h. Stress
   i. Medications such as thiazide diuretics, loop diuretics, beta-blockers without intrinsic sympathomimetic activity, progestin, and glucocorticoids
   j. Alcohol

III. Clinical Presentation: Most patients are asymptomatic, but some individuals may have the following:

A. Vascular problems are the most frequent adverse clinical sequelae
1. In the most severe forms of hyperlipidemia which are due to specific inherited traits, cholesterol levels can reach as high as 1200 mg/dL and these patients develop coronary heart disease (CHD) in childhood and usually die before age 30
2. In contrast, many patients with other types of hyperlipidemia, do not develop symptoms of CHD until they are in their 60s or 70s
3. No research has documented that expensive, lengthy interventions to lower cholesterol levels in children are more efficacious in lowering coronary artery disease than shorter, less-costly interventions which are begun during adulthood

B. Except for children and adolescents with the severe form of dyslipidemia, other manifestations do not usually occur; older patients with severe dyslipidemia may present with the following:
1. Dermatological manifestations can occur: Xanthomas which are cutaneous or subcutaneous papules, plagues or nodules may develop in the tendons, extensor surfaces of the extremities, buttocks, knees, skin folds, scars, and eyelids
2. Gastrointestinal problems may develop, particularly with hypertriglyceridemia
   a. Severe abdominal pain which is often associated with pancreatitis can occur
   b. Hepatomegaly or splenomegaly may be present
   c. Less severe symptoms include mild pain, nausea, vomiting and diarrhea
3. Other clinical manifestations include premature arcus cornea, aortic stenosis, Achilles tendinitis, hyperinsulinemia, hyperuricemia, arthritis, and possibly cholelithiasis

IV. Diagnosis/Evaluation

A. History
1. Ask about previous or present cardiovascular disease
2. Inquire about presence or absence of CHD risk factors (see list of risk factors in table below)

CORONARY HEART DISEASE RISK FACTORS OTHER THAN LOW-DENSITY LIPOPROTEIN CHOLESTEROL

Positive
- Family history of premature CHD
- Smoking
- Hypertension
- HDL cholesterol <35 mg/dL (0.9 mmol/L)
- Diabetes

Negative
- HDL Cholesterol ≥60 mg/dL (1.6 mmol/L)

3. Explore past medical history including pancreatitis, renal disease, liver disease, vascular disease, diabetes mellitus, and hypothyroidism
4. Inquire about family history of premature cardiovascular disease or lipid disorders
5. Complete a medication history particularly asking about anabolic steroids, oral contraceptives, and anticonvulsants which can elevate cholesterol levels
6. Explore amount of alcohol consumption
7. Inquire about typical diet over a 24-hour period
8. Determine amount and intensity of physical activity
9. Ask about occurrence of xanthomas and abdominal pain
10. If female, ask about menstrual history

B. Physical Examination
1. Measure blood pressure
2. Measure height and weight
3. Observe skin for cutaneous xanthomas
4. Palpate thyroid
5. Perform a complete heart and vascular exam
6. Perform a complete abdominal exam; assess for hepatomegaly and splenomegaly

C. Differential Diagnosis: Rule out all secondary causes listed under pathogenesis

D. Diagnostic Tests (plan/management describes these screening tests again):
1. Selectively screen children >2 years of age in the following groups:
   a. Children whose parents or grandparents have a history of coronary of peripheral vascular disease before the age of 55 years; lipoprotein analysis is recommended
   b. Children whose parents have blood cholesterol levels ≥240 mg/dL: Screen for total blood cholesterol level
      (1) If child's total blood cholesterol level is ≥200 mg/dL, obtain lipoprotein analysis
      (2) If child's total cholesterol level is borderline (170-199 mg/dL), repeat and average results; if the average of these two total cholesterol levels is >170 mg/dL perform lipoprotein analysis
   c. Children and adolescents with several risk factors for future coronary heart disease whose family history cannot be accurately determined: Screening is at the discretion of the health care provider and involves total blood cholesterol level and then lipoprotein if needed
2. Lipoprotein analysis includes the following:
   a. Measurement of fasting levels of total cholesterol, total triglyceride, and HDL cholesterol
   b. From the values above, LDL cholesterol is calculated: LDL cholesterol = (Total cholesterol - HDL cholesterol) - (triglycerides/5)
3. Results from lipoprotein analysis will determine when patient needs further diagnostic testing (see section on Plan/Management V.B.)

V.   Plan/Management

A.   Recommendations for primary prevention of hyperlipidemia in children
      1.   No restriction of fat or cholesterol for infants <2 years of age; skim or low-fat milk is not recommended in the first 2 years of life
      2.   After age 2, children and adolescents should gradually assume a healthy diet by eating a wide variety of foods and caloric intake should be adequate for growth and development to reach or maintain desirable body weights
      3.   Children and adolescents (2-18 years) should have the following pattern of nutrient intake: saturated fatty acids <10% of total calories; total fat over several days of ≤30% of total calories and no less than 20% of total calories, and dietary cholesterol <300 mg per day
      4.   Selectively screen "at risk" children >2 years of age (see Section IV. Diagnostic Tests for recommended screening procedures)
      5.   Efforts should be made to identify and eliminate risk factors for coronary heart disease
      6.   Encourage children at any age to have an active life-style with strenuous exercise and the avoidance of tobacco

B.   Management plan for children >2 years of age who were selectively screened because of parental history of hyperlipidemia, family history of coronary artery disease (CAD), and several risk factors for CAD (see section IV.D. Diagnostic Tests); Refer children <2 years of age to a specialist
      1.   Children who have acceptable LDL cholesterol level (LDL-C <110 mg/dL) need routine care (counseling about prudent diet, elimination of risk factors and maintaining a healthy life style) and repeat lipoprotein analysis every 5 years
      2.   For children who have borderline LDL cholesterol (LDL-C 110-129 mg/dL) offer advice about risk factors for cardiovascular disease, begin Step-One diet and other risk factor interventions; re-evaluate lipid profile in one year (see V.D. for dietary therapy and table on following page)
      3.   For children who have high LDL cholesterol (LDL-C ≥130 mg/dL) examine for secondary causes (thyroid, liver, and renal disorders) and familial disorders, screen all family members, begin Step-One diet, and then, Step-Two diet if necessary
      4.   Consider drug therapy only after consulting lipid specialist
            a.   Consider drug therapy in children >10 years of age after an adequate trial of diet therapy (6-12 months) whose LDL cholesterol level remains >190 mg/dL or whose LDL cholesterol remains ≥160 mg/dL and there is a family history of premature cardiovascular disease or two or more risk factors
            b.   The recommended drugs are bile acid sequestrants because they have documented efficacy and are relatively free of adverse effects in children; other medications are not recommended for routine use except in consultation with a lipid specialist (see V.E. for discussion of bile acid sequestrants)

C.   Treatment of triglyceridemia in children: Refer any child with triglyceride levels >300 mg/L to a lipid specialist: Nonpharmacologic therapy as weight reduction in overweight patients and increased physical activity is recommended

D.   Dietary therapy occurs in 2 steps, Step I and Step II diets, and is aimed at reducing intake of saturated fatty acids, cholesterol and at promoting weight loss in overweight patients by eliminating excess total calories and increasing physical activity (see following table on foods to eat and avoid in diet therapy)
      1.   Step I Diet should be prescribed and explained; involves intake of the following:
            a.   Saturated fat: 8-10% of total calories
            b.   Total fat: 30% or less of total calories
            c.   <300 mg of cholesterol per day
      2.   Step II Diet or intensive dietary therapy (often dietician is consulted or implements the diet therapy); involves intake of the following:
            a.   Saturated fat intake: <7% of calories
            b.   Cholesterol: <200 mg per day
            c.   Weight reduction of overweight patients and increased physical activity should be encouraged

EXAMPLE OF FOODS IN STEP I AND STEP II DIETS

Food group	Foods to eat	Foods to avoid
Lean meat, poultry and fish (≤6 oz a day)	Beef, pork, lamb–lean cuts, well-trimmed Poultry, without skin Fish, shellfish	Beef–regular, ground beef, fatty cuts, spare ribs, organ meats Fried fish and chicken Regular luncheon meat
Eggs (step 1: ≤4 yolks per week; step II: ≤2 yolks per week)	Egg whites, cholesterol-free egg substitute	Egg yolks
Low-fat dairy products (2 to 3 servings a day)	Milk–skim, 1/2% or 1% low-fat milk Nonfat or low-fat yogurt, cottage cheese, coffee creamer, sour cream	Whole milk, 2% low-fat milk, imitation milk Whole-milk yogurt Regular cheese & cottage cheese Ice cream Cream, half & half
Fats and oils (≤6 to 8 teaspoons a day)	Unsaturated oils–safflower, sunflower, corn, soybean, canola, olive, peanut Soft margarine Salad dressings–made from unsaturated oils, fat-free or low-fat Seeds and nuts, peanut butter Cocoa powder	Coconut oil, palm oil Butter, lard, shortening, bacon fat, hard margarine Salad dressings–made with egg yolk, cheese, whole milk, sour cream Coconut Milk chocolate
Breads and cereals (≤6 servings a day)	Whole grain breads, English muffins, bagels Oat, wheat, corn, and multigrain cereals, pasta, rice, dry beans and peas Low-fat crackers Homemade baked goods containing unsaturated oils, skim or 1% milk, egg substitute	Croissants, breads in which eggs, fat, or butter are major ingredients Most granolas High-fat crackers
Soups	Low-fat and reduced-sodium varieties	Soups containing whole milk, cream, meat fat, poultry fat
Vegetables (3 to 5 servings a day)	Fresh, frozen, or canned vegetables without added fat or sauce	Fried vegetables or those with butter, cheese, or cream sauce
Fruits (2 to 4 servings a day)	Fresh, frozen, canned, or dried fruits	Fried fruit or fruit with cream sauce
Sweets and modified-fat desserts	Frozen yogurt, sherbet, sorbet, ice milk, popsicles Cookies, cake, pie, pudding prepared with egg substitute, skim, or 1% milk, unsaturated oils	Commercially baked goods.

Adapted from National Cholesterol Education Program. (1993). Second report for the Expert Panel on Detection, Evaluation, and Treatment of High Blood Cholesterol in Adults (adult treatment panel II). Bethesda, MD: National Cholesterol Education Program, National Institutes of Health, National Heart, Lung, and Blood Institute.

E.   Bile acid sequestrants; valuable in patients with moderately elevated LDL cholesterol, in patients with hepatic disease, and when medications are needed in children and adolescents (see following table)

SUMMARY OF BILE ACID SEQUESTRANTS	
Doses of available drugs	
Cholestyramine (Questran Light)	Start 1 packet mixed with fluid or food 1-2 times/day; max. 4-6 packets in 2-3 divided doses*
Colestipol (Colestid tablets)	Start 2 g with adequate fluids 1-2 times/day; increase by 2 g 1-2 times/day at 1-2 months intervals; max. 16 g/day*
Major use	To lower LDL cholesterol
Contraindications	Familial dysbetalipoproteinemia Triglycerides >500 mg/dL
Use with caution	Triglycerides >200 mg/dL
Major adverse effects	Gastrointestinal complaints Decreased absorption of other drugs (take other meds at least one hour before or four to six hours after the sequestrants) Pancreatitis in patients with hypertriglyceridemia
Comments	To reduce GI complaints suggest the following: *Take medicine slowly, reducing amount of swallowed air *Increase fluid and fiber intake and drink with pulpier liquids such as orange juice *May combine with psyllium hydrophilic mucilloid such as Metamucil

*Consult specialist for dosage in children <18 years

Adapted from National Cholesterol Education Program. (1997). Cholesterol lowering in the patient with coronary heart disease. National Institutes of Health, National Heart, Lung, and Blood Institute, NIH Publication No. 97-3794.

F. Future therapeutic modalities
  1. Lifibrol is a lipid-lowering agent under investigation
  2. Gene therapy may be a future modality for patients with genetic disorders such as familial hypercholesterolemia
  3. Plasmapharesis in which the patient's plasma is replaced with salt-free human albumin is a potential therapy for patients with severe dyslipidemia
  4. Surgery such as partial ileal bypass, portacaval shunt, or liver transplantation shows promise for patients with severe dyslipidemia who do not respond to other treatments

G. Follow up is based on results of screening cholesterol levels and if needed, subsequent lipoprotein analysis; patients on drug therapy should be reevaluated at 6-8 weeks with frequent follow-up appointments

HYPERTHYROIDISM

I. Definition: Condition that results when tissues are exposed to an excess of thyroid hormone; clinical manifestation is termed thyrotoxicosis

II. Pathogenesis: Typically, results from the uncontrolled secretion or release of thyroid hormones, thyroxine (T_4) and triiodothyronine (T_3) into the blood stream; hyperthyroidism in childhood is rare and accounts for <5% of all cases

  A. Congenital hyperthyroidism or neonatal thyrotoxicosis occurs almost exclusively in infants of mothers with Graves' disease

  B. Acquired hyperthyroidism is most often due to Graves' disease and is most likely to appear in childhood at ages 12-14 years

  C. Other causes of hyperthyroidism are uncommon

III. Clinical Presentation

    A. Congenital hyperthyroidism
       1. The disease may last several weeks to over 6 months
       2. Disease can be life-threatening
       3. Infants frequently have low birth weight, failure to gain weight despite hyperphagia, microcephaly, irritability, hyperactivity, tachycardia, tachypnea, prominent eyes and thyroid enlargement
       4. Other symptoms include vomiting, diarrhea, hepatosplenomegaly, jaundice, thrombocytopenia and cardiac failure

    B. Graves' Disease
       1. Condition is 8 times more common in females than males
       2. Often has a insidious onset; patients may be asymptomatic for months
       3. Disease is often self-limited, lasting 1-2 years
       4. Patients typically have one or more of the following complaints:
          a. Nervousness which manifests as irritability, inability to concentrate, emotional lability, or insomnia
          b. Weight loss may be present even though appetite is often increased
          c. Bowel movements tend to increase
          d. Heat intolerance is a common symptom
          e. Palpitations may be a troublesome, intermittent complaint
       5. The following are signs:
          a. Hair may be fine and silky; thinning of hair may occur
          b. Nails may develop onycholysis (irregular separation of the nail plate from the nail bed near its distal end), psoriasis (ridges in nail), or onychomycosis (thickening and yellowing of nail)
          c. Skin may have diffuse hyperpigmentation, particularly over the extensor surfaces of the elbows, knees, and small joints
          d. Dermopathy may occur and is thickening of the skin on the legs (pretibial area) or less frequently on the foot, back, hands or face
          e. Eye changes include the following:
            (1) Ophthalmopathy and exophthalmus is caused by the hypertrophy of the eye muscles coupled with increased connective tissue in the orbit; may cause diplopia, difficulty converging eyes, trouble in preforming extreme movements of gaze, and in rare cases, blindness
            (2) Lid lag may be present
            (3) Lid retraction with increased scleral visibility above and below the iris often gives the patient the appearance of "staring"
          f. Thyroid may be visibly or palpably enlarged; thrill can sometimes be palpated or bruit can sometimes be auscultated
          g. May have widespread lymphadenopathy and at times, splenomegaly
          h. Postural tremor, particularly of the hands, is commonly found

    C. Thyroid storm is a life-threatening syndrome that may occur with decompensated hyperthyroidism
       1. Stressful events such as trauma and infection often precipitate an episode
       2. Symptoms such as nausea, vomiting, and abdominal pain may precede the storm
       3. Patient often is agitated, confused, delirious, psychotic, or comatose with high fever and diaphoresis
       4. Tachycardia is always present; tachyarrhythmias may occur

IV. Diagnosis/Evaluation

    A. History
       1. A complete review of systems is needed because symptoms may be subtle and involve every system of the body
       2. Inquire about changes in weight; in children, always ask about growth and development
       3. Obtain a complete medication history

4. Inquire about previous endocrine problems and autoimmune diseases in patient's past medical history or family history

5. Ask about behavioral problems and/or performance in school

B. Physical Examination
1. Observe general appearance, paying particular attention to signs of nervousness or hyperactivity
2. Measure blood pressure, resting pulse, temperature and weight
3. Inspect and palpate skin, noting pigmentation pattern, moistness, and turgor
4. Inspect hair for texture and thickness, nails for ridges, discoloration or splitting
5. Examine fingers and toes for thickening or acropachy
6. Examine eyes, noting exophthalmos, lid lag, and/or extraocular movements
7. Test visual acuity
8. Assess for lymphadenopathy
9. Observe the neck and palpate the thyroid, noting thrills, nodules, diffuse enlargement, firmness, and tenderness; measure size (see section on HYPOTHYROIDISM)
10. Auscultate thyroid for bruits
11. Palpate for lymphadenopathy and splenomegaly
12. Auscultate the heart, noting murmurs and rate and rhythm
13. Assess the abdomen for splenomegaly
14. Do a complete neuromuscular exam, noting fast relaxation of tendon reflexes
15. Evaluate for tremor (can place piece of paper on outstretched hand to observe for movement of paper with slight tremors)
16. Test muscular strength; focusing on signs of proximal muscle weakness
17. Assess lower extremities, noting pretibial myxedema

C. Differential Diagnosis
1. Neoplasm is often suspected due to weight loss and weakness that typically accompanies hyperthyroidism
2. Psychological problems such as panic disorder and depression
3. Suppressed TSH and elevated T_4 levels occur in conditions not associated with hyperthyroidism; glucocorticoids, severe illness, and pituitary dysfunction may result in suppressed TSH in the absence of hyperthyroidism
4. Other diseases associated with hypermetabolism such as leukemia, severe anemia, and chronic infections

D. Diagnostic Tests
1. Order sensitive assay for thyroid-stimulating hormone (TSH) (expected value should be lower than normal or undetectable); with widespread availability of third-generation ultra-sensitive TSH assays, this test is the most important
2. Usual recommendation is to also order a free T_4, which measures unbound thyroxine in serum, to confirm diagnosis (expected values should be higher than normal); the alternative, second-line test, a total T_4, can be altered with estrogen and pregnancy
3. If free T_4 levels are normal, order T_3 level because approximately 5% of hyperthyroid patients have normal T_4 levels
4. Consider ordering 24-hour radioiodine uptake (RAIU)
5. Thyroid autoantibodies including TSH receptor antibody (TSI or TRab): not ordered routinely except in selected cases such as pregnancy

V. Plan/Management:

A. Treatment of congenital hyperthyroidism (refer to pediatric endocrinologist)
1. Needs immediate treatment to prevent dangerous sequelae to nervous system
2. Therapy often consists of a combination of Lugol's solution, propylthiouracil, and propranolol

B. Children and adolescents with hyperthyroidism are usually referred to endocrinologist initially

C. Radioactive iodine (Sodium iodide, I^{131}, Iodotope) is treatment of choice for most adolescents who have Graves' disease and severe symptoms of thyrotoxicosis with multinodular goiter and single hyperfunctioning adenoma; increasingly recommended by specialists for children as well
   1. Many experts recommend an ablative dose of radioactive iodine whereas some prefer to try to render the patient euthyroid with smaller doses
   2. Radioactive iodine works slowly; most patients become euthyroid or hypothyroid in 8-26 weeks

D. Antithyroid drugs, propylthiouracil (PTU) and methimazole (Tapazole), were used extensively in the past; today these drugs are used temporarily to regress the thyroid sufficiently for thyroid ablation with either radioiodine or surgery or, less frequently, as a first-line treatment
   1. Drugs will control excessive production of thyroid hormone, but about half of patients will have a remission if no other treatment is instituted
   2. Often the preferred initial treatment for children, patients scheduled for surgery, and patients with mild disease
   3. One of the following drugs are usually prescribed:
      a. Methimazole (Tapazole) is often first choice because it is long-acting; initial adolescent dosage is 20-30 mg BID or TID (available in 5 and 10 mg tablets); when patient is euthyroid use maintenance therapy of 5-10 mg QD or BID; Children's initial dose: 0.5 to 1.0 mg/kg/day divided in 3 doses
      b. Propylthiouracil (PTU) has the most rapid onset with initial adolescent dosage of 100-150 mg every 8 hours (available in 50 mg tablets); when patient is euthyroid use maintenance therapy of 50-100 mg BID; Children's initial dose is 5-10 mg/kg/day in three divided doses
   4. May need to give both these drugs at higher dosages if patient is severely ill
   5. It takes 4-6 weeks for patients taking methimazole and 6-12 weeks for patients taking PTU to reach euthyroid state; monitor with thyroid tests every 6 weeks
   6. Patients usually remain on drugs for 1-2 years, then drug is gradually withdrawn with the hope of permanent remission
   7. Consider prescribing levothyroxine sodium (Synthroid) after the patient becomes euthryoid
   8. Instruct patient to call provider if severe sore mouth, sore throat or fever develop (signs of agranulocytosis, a rare side effect of both drugs)
   9. Order WBC count before initiating therapy and then periodically during the first 3 months of treatment; however, agranulocytosis occurs so rapidly that periodic monitoring is not considered cost-effective by some experts
   10. A transient rash may occur; symptomatically treat with an antihistamine

E. Adjunctive therapy:
   1. β-blockers may be initiated before or in conjunction with radioactive iodine therapy
      a. Provide symptomatic relief, stabilize the patient with all types of hyperthyroidism and reduce the signs and symptoms of thyrotoxicosis
      b. Propranolol (Inderal LA) or atenolol (Tenormin) may be prescribed. Consult specialist for treating children and adolescents
   2. Gradually, discontinue adjunctive therapy as soon as patient is euthyroid

F. Patient education
   1. Recommend a supplemental multivitamin; additional calcium and vitamin D may rebuild bone density lost during period of hyperthyroidism; remind patients that increased thyroid hormone is a risk factor for osteoporosis
   2. Successful treatment of hyperthyroidism may be followed by serious depression; warn patient and family of this potential risk and frequently monitor mental health

G. Surgical therapy is a less frequently considered option due to potential complications such as hypoparathyroidism and vocal cord paralysis

H. Thyroid storm, a medical emergency, requires prompt therapy and referral
   1. Antithyroid drugs are often recommended and coadministered with corticosteroids, beta-adrenergic blockers and iopanoic acid (Telepaque)
   2. Other supportive measures include fluids, nutritional support and electrolyte corrections

I. Follow Up (plan follow up with endocrinologist)
1. Patients treated with radioactive iodine
   a. Order free T_4 levels every 4-8 weeks until patient becomes euthyroid or hypothyroid and thyroid hormone replacement is needed
   b. Once patients are stable, schedule visits at 3 months, then 6 months, and then annually
2. Patients on antithyroid drugs
   a. Free T_4 level should be measured after a month of treatment and every 2-3 months thereafter
   b. Order WBC after several weeks of therapy and after any changes in drug doses
   c. Order liver enzymes every 3-6 months when patient is stable
3. Patients on ß-adrenergic antagonists should be initially followed every 1-3 months, and then periodically depending on symptoms
4. Patients who are not treated with medications should be followed periodically based on their diagnosis and clinical presentation (i.e., every 3-12 months)

HYPOTHYROIDISM

I. Definition: Condition in which serum thyroid hormone levels are not sufficient to maintain normal intracellular hormone levels

II. Pathogenesis

A. Congenital hypothyroidism
   1. Permanent primary hypothyroidism is due to one of the following:
      a. Most common cause is irreversible failure of thyroid gland to produce sufficient thyroid hormone; cause is an ectopic thyroid gland which failed to migrate properly during fetal development
      b. Second most common cause is hypoplasia or aplasia of the thyroid gland
      c. Third most common cause is dyshormonogenesis or an inborn error of thyroid hormone synthesis, secretion or utilization
   2. Another type is transient primary hypothyroidism related to maternal iodine deficiency, fetal or neonatal exposure to iodine, maternal antithyroid drugs, or maternal antibodies
   3. Permanent secondary hypothyroidism can also occur and is usually associated with congenital hypopituitarism

B. Juvenile acquired hypothyroidism
   1. Primary hypothyroidism is the most common form
      a. Most likely an autoimmune disease
      b. Often occurs as sequel to Hashimoto's thyroiditis (also called chronic thyroiditis)
      c. May occur at any age, even during first year of life
   2. Post-therapeutic hypothyroidism is the second most common form and occurs after treatment with one of the following:
      a. Radioactive iodine
      b. Surgery or a thyroidectomy
      c. Thioamide drugs
   3. Transient hypothyroidism is often associated with acute or subacute thyroiditis which may have a viral etiology
   4. Less common causes include iodine ingestion, neck irradiation, and certain medications such as lithium or para-aminosalicylic acid
   5. Hypothyroidism can occur with a malfunctioning of the hypothalamic-pituitary axis as a result of deficient secretion of thyroid releasing hormone (TRH) from the hypothalamus or lack of secretion of thyroid stimulating hormone (TSH) from the pituitary

III. Clinical Presentation

A. Newborns with congenital hypothyroidism often have the following:
    1. Clinical symptoms may appear in the first 2 weeks, but some infants are asymptomatic for the first month
    2. At first only subtle abnormalities present such as persistent jaundice (bilirubin >10 mg/dl after 3 days of age), temperature instability, hypoactivity, poor feeding, and delayed first stooling
    3. Later, the classic signs and symptoms are present and include thickened tongue, coarse facies, facial edema, hirsute forehead, umbilical hernia, combination of lethargy and irritability, delayed growth, short extremities, persistently open posterior fontanelle, and large anterior fontanelle; irreversible mental changes may occur before these symptoms become manifest
    4. Infants who are treated for congenital hypothyroidism from the early months usually have normal intellectual function and linear growth; when therapy is begun after the first three months of age there is an increased risk or mental retardation

B. Severity of acquired hypothyroidism is contingent on the duration and extent of hormone deficiency; symptoms range from vague and subtle symptoms to severe, multisystem problems associated with myxedema
    1. Early symptoms have an insidious onset and consist of fatigue, dry skin, slight weight gain, cold intolerance, constipation, and heavy menses
    2. As disease progresses, following symptoms present: very dry skin, yellow skin, coarse hair, hair loss of lateral eyebrows, slight alopecia, hoarseness, continued weight gain, slight impairment in mental activity, depression, and hypersomnia
    3. Myxedematous changes occur in later stage with thickened, scaly and "doughy" skin, enlarged tongue, muscle weakness, joint complaints, hearing impairment, bradycardia, possibly cardiac enlargement, pleural effusion and ascites
    4. Children have the following additional manifestations: poor growth and development, decreased activity level, delayed dentition, skeletal maturation delay and limb length reduction which leads to increased upper to lower segment ratio, delayed puberty; mental retardation does not occur
    5. Myxedema coma is an infrequent sequelae of long-standing disease
        a. Uncommon in children and is precipitated by intercurrent illness
        b. Symptoms, in addition to obtundation or coma, include hypothermia, bradycardia, respiratory failure, and possibly, cardiovascular collapse

C. Patients with Hashimoto's thyroiditis have variable symptoms
    1. Frequently, the patient experiences transient hyperthyroidism and later becomes hypothyroid, but some may remain euthyroid; in rare cases, the patient may change from hypothyroid to euthyroid or hyperthyroid
    2. Thyroid may be atrophic, normal-sized, or enlarged

D. In "subclinical" hypothyroidism, patients have nonspecific complaints, normal levels of serum thyroid hormone but an elevation of TSH; may have an enlarged thyroid

E. With malfunctioning of the hypothalamic-pituitary axis, there may be loss of axillary and pubic hair, amenorrhea, and postural hypotension; low levels of TSH and T_4 will be present

F. The following groups of individuals are at high risk for developing hypothyroidism
    1. Newborns
    2. Patients with a strong family history of thyroid disease
    3. New mothers in the postpartal period
    4. Individuals with autoimmune diseases (e.g., Addison's disease)

IV.   Diagnosis/Evaluation

    A.   History
        1.   A complete review of systems is needed because symptoms are subtle and may involve every system of the body
        2.   Ask about pain and swelling or enlargement in the neck
        3.   Ask about history of radiation to the neck
        4.   Inquire about previous endocrine problems in past or family medical history
        5.   Obtain a complete medication history
        6.   In adolescent females, determine date, characteristics, and duration of last menstrual period
        7.   If patient was previously diagnosed with thyroid disease, ascertain past symptoms, treatments, and responses

    B.   Physical Examination
        1.   Observe overall appearance, noting slow movements and dull facies
        2.   Measure height and weight; plot on growth chart, comparing with past measurements
        3.   Measure blood pressure, resting pulse, temperature and weight
        4.   Inspect head for coarseness and thinning of hair, thinning of eyebrows, thickened tongue
        5.   Assess for lymphadenopathy
        6.   Inspect the neck; fully extend neck and observe from front and side; observe for prominences and scars (evidence of previous surgery)
        7.   Palpate neck and thyroid for the following:
            a.   Tenderness
            b.   Consistency (i.e., firmness, fluctuance)
            c.   Measure size of gland
            d.   Note whether there is a focal nodule or diffuse growth
            e.   The easiest method to palpate infant's thyroid is to place the infant prone with the neck extended
        8.   Auscultate thyroid for bruits
        9.   Determine point of maximal impulse (PMI) as an indirect method for uncovering dilation and hypertrophy of the heart
        10.   Auscultate heart, noting rate, rhythm, and murmurs
        11.   Do a complete lung exam
        12.   Palpate for splenomegaly
        13.   Auscultate the abdomen, noting bowel sounds which may be diminished in hypothyroidism
        14.   Perform a complete neurological exam; tendon reflexes may have a brisk contraction and a prolonged relaxation period in hypothyroidism

    C.   Differential Diagnosis: The following conditions mimic certain characteristics of hypothyroidism
        1.   Ischemic heart disease
        2.   Nephrotic syndrome
        3.   Cirrhosis

    D.   Diagnostic Tests
        1.   Screening for congenital hypothyroidism
            a.   Newborn screening is done in all U.S. states; the following are three different methods of screening that are used in the U.S. (each method has advantages and disadvantages):
                (1)   Initial T_4 level with TSH determination only if the T_4 level is abnormally low
                (2)   Initial TSH level only; can be falsely elevated if obtained within first 24 hours after birth
                (3)   Both initial T_4 level and TSH level obtained
            b.   The most desirable time for testing is 2 to 6 days of age
            c.   Neonates with normal thyroid tests can develop hypothyroidism during the first weeks of life; retest all infants who present with symptoms of hypothyroidism
        2.   Screen for thyroid disease in the following individuals:
            a.   All symptomatic individuals
            b.   Children with Down syndrome should be retested at age 3 months
            c.   Past history of medically or surgically treated thyroid disease (screen annually)

      d.   Past history of receiving supervoltage x-ray therapy to neck for nonthyroid cancer

      e.   Patients with other autoimmune diseases and those with cognitive dysfunction, unexplained depression and hypercholesterolemia

      f.   Patients on lithium therapy

      g.   Patients with type 1 diabetes; 10% of these patients develop hypothyroidism in their lifetime; obtain sensitive TSH levels at regular intervals particularly if a goiter develops

      h.   Consider screening for patients with menstrual irregularities and a family history of thyroid disease

3.   Diagnostic testing for acquired hypothyroidism includes the following: (all tests may be normal in patients with chronic thyroiditis)

      a.   Order a sensitive thyroid-stimulating hormone (TSH) assay (most labs now use the sensitive third-generation assay) which is the most cost-effective test for assessing thyroid function

          (1)   TSH is elevated in hypothyroidism

          (2)   If serum TSH is normal, there is no need for additional thyroid tests as 98% of the time T_4 is normal when TSH is normal

      b.   Order free T_4 assay in following circumstances

          (1)   When TSH is elevated, a low free T_4 level will confirm the diagnosis of acquired hypothyroidism

          (2)   When hypothyroidism secondary to pituitary or hypothalamic failure is suspected

               (a)   TSH may be normal, low, or mildly elevated with secondary hypothyroidism; (TSH does not rise proportionally to low T_4)

               (b)   Further evaluation is needed with results suggesting secondary hypothyroidism: neuroradiologic studies, measurement of serum prolactin, and assessment of pituitary-adrenal and pituitary-gonadal function

      c.   If autoimmune thyroiditis is suspected, order either antimicrosomal antibody (anti-TPO antibody) which is test or choice or antithyroglobulin antibody; positive in 95% of patients with Hashimoto's thyroiditis

      d.   Thyroid scan or sonogram may be needed to evaluate suspicious structural thyroid abnormalities

      e.   The free thyroxine index provides an indirect estimate of free T_4 and is rarely ordered today

4.   Consider ordering the following:

      a.   Serum electrolytes, blood urea nitrogen, creatinine, glucose, calcium, PO_4, and albumin levels

      b.   Urine pregnancy test in adolescent females

      c.   Urinalysis to detect proteinuria

      d.   Lipid studies for hyperlipidemia which often occurs with hypothyroidism

V.   Plan/Management

    A.   Treatment of congenital hypothyroidism

        1.   Consult pediatric endocrinologist immediately to prevent or minimize the adverse effects that can occur to the developing nervous system

        2.   Pharmacological treatment is levothyroxine

        3.   Educate parents concerning the etiology of the disease, impact of early diagnosis and treatment in preventing mental retardation, importance of periodic follow-up care, and the manner of administering thyroxine

    B.   Consult specialist when patient is myxedemic, has significant cardiac disease, has secondary hypothyroidism, or is chronically ill or hospitalized with abnormal thyroid function tests

    C.   For acquired hyperthyroidism endocrinologist referral is recommended initially; pharmacological treatment with levothyroxine (Levothroid, Levoxine, Synthroid, Euthyrox) is recommended first-line therapy for acquired hypothyroidism; do not switch brands as there may be variability in potency among brands

1. Full dose of brand Levothroid is 100-125 micrograms (0.1-0.125 mg) per day, which may be started in otherwise healthy older adolescents; increase by 25 micrograms QD every 2-3 weeks based on clinical condition and laboratory values; average dose is 125 micrograms (0.125 mg) QD and maximum dose is 300 micrograms (0.30 mg)
2. In children, dosage should be titrated upward with dosages of the following;
   a. Under 6 months: 8-10 micrograms/kg/day
   b. 6 months - 1 year: 6-8 micrograms/kg/day
   c. 1-5 years: 5-6 micrograms/kg/day
   d. Over 6 years: 4-5 micrograms/kg/day
3. Continually monitor response to medication
   a. TSH assay which should be ordered every 4-6 weeks until concentration is normalized (Keep in mind that TSH levels may remain elevated for several months despite effective treatment; rapid increase in medication based on TSH levels should be avoided because of the risk of thyrotoxicosis or excessive thyroid hormones)
   b. Ask patient about symptoms of thyrotoxicity such as tachycardia, nervousness, tremor and evaluate with diagnostic tests
      (1) If hyperthyroidism is confirmed the current dose of levothyroxine should be withheld for one week and restarted at a lower dose
      (2) Some patients remain asymptomatic even with elevated free T_4 and/or TSH abnormalities; these patients should have dose reduced until TSH concentration is normalized to prevent development of osteoporosis which may occur with levothyroxine overreplacement
   c. Signs and symptoms of hypothyroidism should improve within 2 weeks and resolve within 3-6 months
   d. Need careful monitoring of growth and development and diagnostic tests (TSH and T_4) in children who begin drug treatment; these children may have school and behavioral problems due decreased attention spans and increased activity; parents and teachers need to be warned about this possibility
4. Maintenance treatment is lowest dosage required to maintain euthyroidism with a nonelevated serum TSH and a normal or slightly elevated T_4
5. Drug interactions
   a. Drugs such as cholestyramine, ferrous sulfate, sucralfate, and aluminum hydroxide antacids may interfere with levothyroxine absorption from the stomach; space levothyroxine at least 4 hours from these medications
   b. May need to increase dose of levothyroxine when used with phenytoin, carbamazepine, and rifampin

D. Liothyronine sodium (Cytomel) replaces T_3: used in only rare circumstances as an alternative medication

E. Follow Up
   1. Congenital hypothyroidism
      a. Order free T_4 and TSH every month for first 6 months; every other month between 6 and 12 months, and then, every 3 months
      b. Assess bone age at start of therapy and at age 1 year
   2. Acquired hypothyroidism
      a. When beginning medication therapy, patient's therapeutic response should be monitored every 4-6 weeks until TSH is normalized
      b. After medication dosage is stabilized, schedule visits every 6-12 months and order serum TSH assays
      c. If drug dosage is changed, patient should return to care provider in 2-3 months for repeat TSH
      d. Values within normal limits imply adequate treatment
      e. Undetectable TSH levels suggest overtreatment and medications should be decreased
      f. TSH >20 μU/L indicates undertreatment or noncompliance; after ascertaining that patient is taking medication, increase dose

GYNECOMASTIA

I. Definition: Proliferation of glandular component of male breast

II. Pathogenesis: Due to an imbalance between serum estrogen and androgen levels with an excess of estrogens resulting in breast duct proliferation

    A. Physiologic causes
        1. In neonatal period may have palpable breast tissue due to transplacental passage of estrogens
        2. Breast enlargement in puberty is associated with lower free testosterone levels and excessive levels of estrogen created by peripheral conversion of adrenal androgens

    B. Pathological causes
        1. Tumor: testicular, adrenal, pituitary, breast, lung,
        2. Chronic diseases: liver disease, renal disease and dialysis, pulmonary disease, nervous system damage
        3. Malnutrition
        4. Hyperthyroidism or hypothyroidism
        5. Adrenal disorders
        6. Primary gonadal failure
        7. Secondary hypogonadism
        8. Enzymatic defects of testosterone production
        9. Androgen-insensitivity syndromes
        10. Drugs such as hormones, anti-infectives (e.g., isoniazid, ketoconazole, metronidazole), antiulcer drugs, cardiovascular drugs (e.g., digoxin, verapamil, captopril, spironolacone), psychoactive agents (e.g., diazepam, tricyclic antidepressants, phenothiazines), drugs of abuse (e.g., alcohol, amphetamines, heroin, marijuana), and phenytoin and penicillamine
        11. Idiopathic gynecomastia
        12. Familial gynecomastia

    C. The most common causes are idiopathic gynecomastia (approximately 25%), gynecomastia due to puberty (approximately 25%), drugs (approximately 10-20%), cirrhosis or malnutrition (approximately 8%) and primary hypogonadism (8%).

    D. The following are risk factors for developing gynecomastia: Klinefelter's syndrome, obesity, testicular failure, recovery from prolonged severe illness associated with malnutrition and weight loss, positive family history, Peutz-Jeghers syndrome, and male pseudohermaphroditism

III. Clinical Presentation

    A. Physiological
        1. Occurs in most newborn males during the first 3 weeks of life with resolution by time infant is 4 months old
        2. In puberty, gynecomastia is characterized by the following:
            a. High prevalence; occurs in approximately 49-65% of pubertal boys
            b. Average age at onset is between 12-14 years
            c. Usually occurs during Tanner stages II, III, or IV
            d. More common in obese boys due to excessive conversion of androgens to estrogens in the adipose tissue
            e. Has 3 different types
                (1) Type I is characterized by 1 or more subareolar nodules which are freely movable
                (2) Type II presents with nodules beneath areola but extending beyond areolar perimeter
                (3) Type III resembles breast development of sexual maturity rating 3 in the female

      f.   Transitory tenderness is common in Types I and II
      g.   Breasts are of a firm, rubbery consistency in Types I and II, whereas in Type III consistency is similar to female breast
      h.   There is an absence of ulceration or nipple retraction
      i.   Often unilateral but may progress to bilateral disease
      j.   Enlargement resolves spontaneously in several months to 2 years except if there was greater than 2 cm of palpable tissue in the first year (will never fully regress)
      k.   Patients' testes are normal in size and volume for Tanner stage and no other physical abnormalities are present

B.   Pathological
    1.   Tumors
      a.   Suspect a neoplasm in children < 10 years who have gynecomastia
      b.   Risk of breast cancer in males is proportional to the amount of breast tissue present; increased risk in patients with substantial gynecomastia
    2.   Familial gynecomastia may be an X-linked recessive or sex-linked autosomal dominant trait
    3.   Patients with other pathological causes present with variable signs and symptoms

IV.   Diagnosis/Evaluation

A.   History
    1.   Carefully determine the age of onset of gynecomastia, and its course and duration
    2.   Ask about pain and discharge from breast
    3.   Ask whether the breast(s) is(are) growing or shrinking
    4.   Explore the relationship of breast enlargement to other pubertal events
    5.   Ascertain the pattern and timing of pubertal events
    6.   Inquire about medication history
    7.   Inquire about alcohol use and illegal drug use
    8.   Obtain a complete nutrition history
    9.   Determine whether patient is active in athletics and/or lifts weights to identify breast enlargement due to pectoral muscle hypertrophy
    10.   Inquire about family history of breast enlargement
    11.   Inquire about previous medical history including liver, renal, pulmonary, nervous, adrenal, pituitary and endocrine disorders
    12.   Inquire about any recent weight loss or gain
    13.   Explore the impact of the gynecomastia on the patient's lifestyle and self-image

B.   Physical Examination
    1.   Obtain measurements of height, weight, and arm span
    2.   Assess general health and observe for evidence of feminization such as lack of male hair distribution and a eunuchoid body habitus
    3.   With patient lying supine, grasp breast between thumb and forefinger and gently bring the 2 fingers toward the nipple; a disk-like mound of tissue is often felt with gynecomastia
      a.   Measure dimensions of glandular tissue and areolae
      b.   Note consistency, tenderness, and mobility of any lesion or mass; squeeze nipple and note any discharge
    4.   Palpate for axillary lymphadenopathy
    5.   Check for signs of thyroid hormone excess such as thyromegaly, tachycardia, and diaphoresis
    6.   Check for signs of liver dysfunction such as hepatomegaly, jaundice and skin changes.
    7.   Deeply palpate upper abdomen for tumor of the adrenal glands or kidney
    8.   Determine Tanner staging of sexual development
    9.   Perform complete testicular examination
      a.   Measure size of testes (small, firm testes are characteristic of Klinefelter's syndrome)
      b.   Palpate for masses or tumor

C. Differential Diagnosis: Gynecomastia may be a normal physiologic phenomenon or a result of a pathologic condition
  1. Pseudogynecomastia presents with smooth, fatty enlargement of breasts without glandular proliferation; more common in obese males
  2. Breast cancer is characterized by a unilateral, hard or firm, mass which is fixed to the underlying tissues and may be associated with dimpling of the skin, retraction or crusting of the nipple, nipple discharge or bleeding, or axillary lymphadenopathy.
  3. Neurofibromas, lipomas, and dermoid cysts are other breast masses that may present like gynecomastia

D. Diagnostic Tests: Ordered on the basis of patient's clinical presentation
  1. Laboratory tests are usually not needed if patient has signs and symptoms of pubertal gynecomastia (see preceding clinical presentation)
  2. When the following characteristics exist, there is a need for further evaluation:
     a. Breast development that has occurred in prepubertal boy without genital changes
     b. Males with genital abnormalities such as small testes with penile enlargement, hypospadias, or incomplete testicular descent
     c. Gynecomastia that persists beyond 2 years or is unusually prominent
     d. Males >18 years with recent onset of enlarging and tender breasts
     e. Males who have physical abnormalities without a known etiology
     f. Breast masses which are large (>4 cm in diameter)
  3. Consider the following workup for the above mentioned group of males who need further evaluation (Consultation with a specialist is often recommended)
     a. Serum β-hCG level (may be elevated in carcinomas)
     b. Serum estradiol (may be elevated in interstitial-cell tumors and feminizing adrenal tumors)
     c. Luteinizing hormone (LH) and testosterone to detect testicular failure, increased primary estrogen production and carcinomas
     d. Dehydroepiandrosterone (may be abnormal in adrenal diseases)
     e. Prolactin (may be elevated in pituitary tumors)
     f. Thermography and testicular ultrasound should be considered when patient has a suspected testicular tumor
     g. Chest film to screen for pulmonary tumors and metastatic lesions
     h. Thyroid or liver function tests, if indicated
     i. BUN and creatinine, if indicated
     j. Chromosomal karyotype (if both testes small)
  4. Order mammogram or fine-needle aspiration biopsy if breast enlargement is not characteristic of typical gynecomastia

V. Plan/Management

A. Consider consultation with an endocrinologist in the following situations: any male with physical abnormalities, prepubertal and pubertal males whose breast development has occurred without genital changes, breast enlargement which persists (>2 years) or is >2-4 cm, males older than 18 years of age

B. If the patient has pubertal gynecomastia reassurance should be given that the condition is physiological and transient in nature

C. Postpubertal males who have had a thorough negative evaluation will also need assurance that the breast enlargement is not pathological

D. Males that have residual fibrous tissue may benefit from referral to a surgeon if they are embarrassed or emotionally distressed by the breast enlargement

E. Medical approaches to treating gynecomastia have included use of antiestrogens (i.e., clomiphene, tamoxifen), testosterone, nonaromatizable androgens, and danazol in pubertal boys

F. Follow Up: Males with pubertal gynecomastia should be re-evaluated every 3-6 months

PRECOCIOUS PUBERTY

I. Definition: Onset of puberty before the age of 8 in females and before the age of 9 years in males

    A. Isosexual precocity is advanced sexual development appropriate to the phenotype of the child

    B. Heterosexual precocity is advanced sexual development at a variance with the phenotype of the child

II. Pathogenesis

    A. Central or true isosexual precocious puberty results from stimulation of the hypothalamic-pituitary axis with gonadotropin secretion and resultant sex steroid secretion
        1. May be classified as constitutional in some early-school-age children who are actually in the lower range of normal on the distribution curve; usually these children have a family history of early puberty
        2. Often there is no abnormal organic cause (idiopathic); 90% of female cases and 50% of male cases are idiopathic
        3. Other causes are central nervous system (CNS) abnormalities such as the following:
            a. Congenital anomalies
            b. Benign or malignant tumors in the hypothalamus region
            c. Head trauma
            d. Infections such as encephalitis, meningitis or brain abscess
            e. Syndromes such as neurofibromatosis or tuberous sclerosis
        4. Severe hypothyroidism may also cause abnormal development

    B. Pseudo-precocious isosexual puberty occurs independent of the stimulation of the hypothalamic-pituitary axis with elevated sex hormones but low gonadotropins
        1. In females, possible causes are ingestion of oral contraceptives or other estrogen-containing agents, estrogen-producing tumors of the ovary and adrenal glands, gonadotropin-producing tumors, and McCune-Albright syndrome
        2. In males, possible causes are abuse of androgenic agents, untreated congenital adrenal hyperplasia, adrenal tumors, testicular tumors, and familial Leydig cell hyperplasia

    C. Heterosexual precocious puberty has the following etiologies:
        1. In females, ovarian abnormalities, adrenal problems such as tumors or congenital adrenal hyperplasia, and adrenal enzyme deficiencies are likely causes
        2. In males, adrenal tumors, estrogen-producing teratomas, neurofibromatosis, and iatrogenic factors are possible factors

    D. Variations of pubertal development occur frequently and are related to the following factors:
        1. Premature thelarche or premature breast development often has no known causative factor but may be a result of ovarian cysts or ingestion of exogenous estrogens such as birth control pills
        2. Premature adrenarche of premature development of sexual hair is often due to organic abnormalities such as adrenal hyperplasia, adrenal tumors, gonadal tumors, and possible central nervous system abnormalities

III. Clinical Presentation

    A. Most girls have idiopathic central precocious puberty whereas boys have an identifiable cause of precocity such as tumor, congenital adrenal hyperplasia, or familial gonadotropin-independent precocity

    B. Children with central isosexual precocious puberty have the following characteristics:
        1. Complete sexual development (pubic hair, axillary hair, breasts and phallus)
        2. Pattern of progression of pubertal events is normal

3. Potential to be fertile due to production of mature sperm or ova
4. Accelerated linear growth and advanced bone age is typical; at first child is tall for age, but owing to premature closure of epiphyses, smallness of stature is usually the end result
5. Pubertal levels of luteinizing hormone (LH), follicle stimulating hormone (FSH), and sex steroids
6. Common symptoms are emotional lability, high energy levels and increased appetite
7. Girls may have white vaginal secretion (leukorrhea) and/or vaginal bleeding due to menarche
8. Patients with precocity due to central nervous system abnormalities have neurological symptoms and signs such as headache, visual impairments, and seizures

C. In pseudo-precocious isosexual puberty, children have the following characteristics:
1. Elevated sexual hormones but low gonadotropins
2. Infertility due to immature sperm or ova
3. Clinical presentation is variable and will depend on the causative factor
   a. For example, in males, enlargement of one testes may indicate a testicular tumor
   b. For example, in females, a palpable mass on bimanual examination may indicate an ovarian tumor

D. Heterosexual precocious puberty
1. Occurs mainly in the newborns
2. Results in virilization in females and feminization in males

E. Variations of puberty have the following characteristics:
1. Girls with thelarche have enlarged breasts usually without nipple and alveolar development
   a. Commonly occurs in girls between 2 months and 4 years of age
   b. Enlarged breasts often regress within several months to a year
   c. There are no others signs of premature pubertal development and no linear growth acceleration
2. Children with adrenarche have development of sexual hair which gradually increases
   a. Usually occurs between 5-8 years of age
   b. Most common in African-American or Hispanic girls
   c. Typically, children have no or slightly accelerated growth and slightly advanced bone age
   d. Some children have mild neurologic problems

IV. Diagnosis/Evaluation

A. History
1. Carefully explore the pattern and times of pubertal changes (compare with following table)

PATTERN OF PUBERTAL DEVELOPMENT		
	Mean Age (years)	
Sign	Females	Males
Breast buds	11	
Enlargement of testes		11
Pubic hair	11	13
Maximum linear growth rate	12	14
Menses	12	
Axillary hair	13	15
Facial hair		16+

2. Ask about associated symptoms such as headaches, changes in vision, changes in appetite, thirst, vaginal discharge, vaginal spotting, menses, hot flashes, seizures, mood lability

3. Ask about past medical history, particularly, past central nervous system infections and abnormalities, thyroid problems, adrenal disorders, and gonadal disorders
4. Ask at what age grandparents, parents, and other siblings experienced first pubertal changes
5. Inquire about family history of accelerated height
6. Inquire about ingestion of sex steroids and oral contraceptives
7. Inquire about quality of family and peer relationships
8. Ask about school performance; inquire about aggressive behaviors

B. Physical Examination
   1. Measure for height (standing and sitting) and weight, plot on growth chart and compare with previous measurements
   2. Observe skin for facial sebaceous glands, café au lait markings, neurofibromatosis lesions, or lesions of McCune-Albright syndrome (one or more large brown macules with irregular borders)
   3. Palpate thyroid for enlargement or tenderness
   4. Check for axillary hair and odor
   5. Check for amount of breast tissue and whether the nipples and areolas are enlarging and thinning
   6. Perform a complete abdominal and rectal exam
   7. In females, consider performing pelvic and speculum examinations
      a. Depending on the age of and clinical condition of the child, external examination of the genitalia may be all that is necessary
      b. If speculum and bimanual exams are done, note uterine and ovarian size and look for evidence of maturation such as pink and dull vagina following estrogenization or developing fullness of the labia minora (normal uterus measures 1-2 cm and the ovaries measure 0.5-1.0 cm until puberty)
   8. In males, measure length and width of stretched penis
   9. In males, perform testicular exam, noting size and evidence of masses
   10. Perform a complete neurological exam
   11. Assess for sexual maturity stages or Tanner stages (see table which follows)

SEXUAL MATURITY STAGES IN GIRLS	
Stage	Breasts
1	Preadolescent - only papilla is elevated above level of chest wall
2	Breast budding - Breast and papilla elevated as small mound, increased diameter of areola
3	Continued breast and areola enlargement, no contour separation
4	Areola and papilla form secondary mound
5	Mature - Nipple projects, areola is part of general breast contour
	Pubic Hair
1	Preadolescent - None or vellous hair in pubis area
2	Sparse, straight, lightly pigmented along medial border of labia
3	Darker, coarser, curlier and in increased amount
4	Abundant but has not spread to medial surface of thighs
5	Adult feminine, inverse triangle, spread to medial surface of thighs

SEXUAL MATURITY STAGES IN BOYS	
Stage	**Penis, Testes, and Scrotum**
1	Preadolescent - all are size and proportion seen in early childhood (testes 1 cm)
2	Slight enlargement, with alteration in color (more reddened) and texture of scrotum (testes 2.0-3.2 cm)
3	Further growth and enlargement (testes 3.3-4.0 cm)
4	Penis significantly enlarged in length and circumference; further development of glans; enlargement of testes and scrotum with darkening of scrotal skin (testes 4.1-4.9 cm)
5	Genitalia of adult size (testes 5.0 cm)
	Pubic Hair
1	Preadolescent - None or vellous hair in pubis area
2	Sparse, straight, lightly pigmented at base of penis
3	Darker, coarser, curlier and in increased amount
4	Abundant but less quantity than adult type
5	Adult distribution, spread to medial surface of thighs

Adapted from Tanner, J.M. (1962). Growth at Adolescence. Oxford: Blackwell Scientific Publications.

C. Differential Diagnosis: Aimed at distinguishing idiopathic precocity from those conditions which have correctable and possibly life-threatening causes

D. Diagnostic Tests: Tests to order are dependent on what is uncovered in history and physical exam
   1. Consider measurement of luteinizing hormone (LH), follicle-stimulating hormone (FSH), human chorionic gonadotropin levels, gonadal steroid levels, and estradiol levels to determine whether precocity is central or pseudo-precocious
   2. An easy way to determine whether a girl is in active puberty is a vaginal smear obtained by cotton swab and fixed immediately to assess estrogen effect (vaginal cells change from immature parabasal cells toward intermediate and finally superficial squamous cells under the influence of estrogen)
   3. A GnRH stimulation test is helpful in determining whether the patient has central or peripheral precocious puberty
   4. Consider tests to determine bone age (radiographs of the nondominant hand and writs)
   5. Consider computed tomography (CT) or magnetic resonance imaging (MRI) of the head if CNS abnormality is suspected; studies have found that small CNS tumors were present in children believed to have idiopathic precocity
   6. Abdominal CT, MRI, or ultrasound should be considered if ovarian cysts/tumors, testicular tumors or adrenal gland tumors or abnormalities are suspected
   7. Consider ordering urinary 17-ketosteroids and plasma dehydroepiandrosterone and its sulfate in boys with premature adrenarche
   8. For premature thelarche, consider ordering plasma FSH, LH, and estradiol and an ultrasound to rule out ovarian cyst
   9. For premature adrenarche, consider 17-hydroxyprogesterone, androstenedione, and testosterone
   10. Consider ordering thyroid stimulating hormone (TSH) levels

V. Plan/Management

A. Cases which involve organic abnormalities are usually referred to an endocrinologist

B. True isosexual precocity which is idiopathic may be treated in the following way with consultation an endocrinologist
   1. Observe child for 3-12 months to determine whether status is changing
   2. If condition remains unchanged, continue to observe

3.   When sexual maturation is progressing:
    a.   Typical treatments involve the following medications to suppress the hypothalamic-pituitary-gonadal axis: GnRH agonist therapy is usually the treatment of choice and is available in subcutaneous and nasal formulations; medroxyprogesterone acetate (progestational steroid), danazol (androgen) or cyproterone acetate (antiandrogen) are other pharmacological therapies that may be beneficial
    b.   Investigational agent, testolactone, has been used in girls
    c.   Antifungal drug, ketoconazole, has been used in males

C.   Medical treatment of peripheral precocious puberty depends on the etiology and includes medroxyprogesterone acetate, testolactone, ketoconazole, cyproterone acetate, and spironolactone

D.   Treatment of premature thelarche and adrenarche
    1.   If all organic causes have been eliminated, no treatments are necessary
    2.   Close follow up is essential as both conditions are clinically indistinguishable from the early stages of precocious puberty

E.   Patient education and counseling is extremely important

F.   Follow Up
    1.   Confer with endocrinologist about frequency of follow-up visits for children with precocity due to organic causes
    2.   Children with idiopathic isosexual precocious puberty or premature thelarche or adrenarche should be re-evaluated at least every 3-6 months

DELAYED PUBERTY

I.   Definition: Absence of breast budding by age 13.4 in females or lack of testicular enlargement by age 13.7 in males as well as arrest in pubertal maturation

II.   Pathogenesis: is due to failure at any point along the hypothalamic-pituitary-gonadal axis and is associated with one of the following factors:

A.   Constitutional delayed puberty
    1.   Involves slow maturation but with secretion of appropriate amounts of hormones
    2.   Heredity probably plays an important role

B.   Gonadotropin-releasing hormone (GnRH) secretion can be inhibited by functional causes such as the following:
    1.   Inadequate nutrition or poor eating habits
    2.   Chronic diseases such as Crohn's disease or celiac disease
    3.   Environmental stress
    4.   Intensive athletic training or exercise
    5.   Hypothyroidism
    6.   Drugs such as opiates

C.   The ability of the hypothalamus to secrete GnRH may cause delayed puberty and be related to the following factors:
    1.   Brain tumors
    2.   Central nervous system infections
    3.   Congenital brain defects

D. The pituitary may not be able to respond to the GnRH with gonadotropin production from the following causes:
   1. Pituitary tumor
   2. Pituitary adenoma

E. The gonads may be unable to respond to the luteinizing hormone (LH) and follicle-stimulating hormone (FSH) for the following reasons:
   1. Gonadal dysgenesis in association with abnormalities of sex chromosomes (Turner syndrome)
   2. Orchitis or oophoritis
   3. Radiation or chemotherapy

III. Clinical Presentation

A. Criteria used to determine pubertal delay in females
   1. Breast stage 1 (see SEXUAL MATURITY STAGE IN GIRLS in Precocious Puberty section) persisting beyond age 13.4 or pubic hair stage 1 beyond age 14.1
   2. Greater than 5 years elapsing between initiation of breast growth and menarche
   3. Failure to menstruate beyond age 16

B. Criteria used to determine a pubertal delay in males
   1. Genital stage 1 persisting beyond age 13.7 or pubic hair stage persisting beyond age 15.1
   2. More than 5 years elapsing from initiation to completion of genital growth

C. Delayed puberty is more common in males

D. Constitutional Delay
   1. Most common type; 90-95% of delayed puberty is constitutional
   2. Frequently, children with this delay have been slow growers throughout their childhood with growth curves below the third percentile
   3. Final, adult height is often shorter than average
   4. Patient has negative review of systems, normal diagnostic tests, normal physical exam, but bone age is slightly delayed

E. Other types of delayed puberty will have abnormal physical findings (e.g., gynecomastia in a male with a gonadal disorder or abnormal cranial nerve function in a child with gonadotropin deficiency) and abnormal diagnostic tests (e.g., low testosterone response to hCG in gonadotropin deficiency)

IV. Diagnosis/Evaluation

A. History
   1. Ask about onset and pattern of pubertal changes
   2. Obtain a neonatal history which includes previous maternal miscarriages and congenital lymphedema (Turner syndrome)
   3. Gather a thorough medical history including history of chronic disease, congenital anomalies, previous surgery, radiation exposure, chemotherapy, or drug use
   4. Pay particular attention in the review of systems to weight changes, dieting, stress, exercise, athletics, gastrointestinal symptoms, neurologic complaints, and symptoms common with thyroid disorders
   5. Ask about family history of infertility and endocrine disorders
   6. Inquire about heights of parents, siblings, grandparents
   7. Inquire about age of menarche in mother and adolescent sisters
   8. Explore quality of family and peer relationships
   9. Ask about school performance

B. Physical Examination
   1. Observe for general body habitus to determine nutritional status
   2. Measure height, weight, and plot on growth chart, noting pattern in relationship to previous measurements

3. Check thyroid for nodules and enlargement
4. Measure dimensions of areolae and any glandular breast tissue
5. Perform a complete chest exam to eliminate any chronic lung problems
6. Perform a complete heart exam, noting evidence of congenital heart disease
7. Palpate for liver and spleen enlargement
8. In males, measure testicular length, width, midshaft diameter, and stretched length of penis
9. In females, assess estrogen effect on external genitalia (pale, pink vaginal mucosa with white discharge indicates estrogen exposure)
10. Speculum and bimanual pelvic exams are not always necessary in the initial evaluation of girls with delayed sexual development but should be done in the girl who has normal pubertal development but delayed menarche
11. Note any evidence of heterosexual development such as clitoromegaly or hirsutism in females or gynecomastia in males
12. Perform a complete neurological exam to eliminate intracranial abnormalities
13. Determine sexual maturity rating

C. Differential Diagnosis
1. Constitutional delayed puberty is common but is a diagnosis of exclusion; all correctable and organic causes must be ruled-out
2. A child whose delayed puberty is associated with nutritional deficiency due to an eating disorder or a chronic disease will show a greater decline in weight gain than height, whereas in children with pubertal delay due to endocrine factors, there is a greater slowing of linear growth than weight

D. Diagnostic Tests
1. Order complete blood count and erythrocyte sedimentation rate (screen for chronic disease)
2. Order LH, FSH, dehydroepiandrosterone sulfate, and testosterone or estradiol levels (elevated levels are suggestive of primary gonadal failure)
3. Consider test for bone age (delayed bone age will be seen in adolescents with hypopituitarism, hypothyroidism, chronic illness, and constitutional delay in puberty; normal bone age is seen in patients with Turner's syndrome)
4. Consider thyroid function tests
5. Consider lateral skull x-ray to rule out CNS disorders
6. Other tests are necessary in some workups:
   a. Karyotype to rule out Turner's syndrome
   b. Growth hormone measurements to determine whether a growth hormone deficiency exists
   c. HCG test to rule out hypogonadotropic hypogonadism
   d. Prolactin level, computerized tomography (CT) and magnetic resonance imaging (MRI) to rule out central nervous system abnormality

V. Plan/Management

A. Children with pubertal delay who have abnormal physical findings or diagnostic tests are usually referred to an endocrinologist

B. Treatment of constitutional pubertal delay
1. Usually no treatment is necessary, but close follow up and monitoring is essential
2. In boys with constitutional delay and severe psychological problems, injections of human chorionic gonadotropin or testosterone can be used to initiate secondary sexual development

C. Counseling and education are integral parts of the plan

D. Follow up of constitutional pubertal delay is at least every 6 months

REFERENCES

Adlin, V. (1998). Subclinical hypothyroidism: Deciding when to treat. <u>American Family Physician, 57,</u> 776-780.

American Academy of Pediatrics. (1992). Statement on cholesterol. <u>Pediatrics, 90,</u> 467-472

American Academy of Pediatrics. (1993). Newborn screening for congenital hypothyroidism: Recommended guidelines. <u>Pediatrics, 91,</u> 1203-1209.

American Academy of Pediatrics. Committee on Nutrition. (1998). Cholesterol in childhood. <u>Pediatrics, 101,</u> 141-147.

American Academy of Pediatrics. Sections on Endocrinology and Ophthalmology. (1998). Screening for retinopathy in the pediatric patient with type 1 diabetes mellitus. <u>Pediatrics, 101,</u> 313-314.

American Association of Clinical Endocrinologist and the American College of Endocrinology. (1995). AACE clinical practice guidelines for the evaluation and treatment of hyperthyroidism and hypothyroidism. <u>Endocrine Practice, 1,</u> 56-62.

American Diabetes Association. (1993). Implications of the diabetes control and complications trial. <u>Diabetes Care, 16</u>(11), 1517-1520.

American Diabetes Association. (1995). <u>Intensive diabetes management.</u> Alexandria, VA.: Author.

American Diabetes Association. (1998). Diabetes mellitus and exercise. <u>Diabetes Care, 21</u> (Supp. 1), S40-S44.

American Diabetes Association. (1998). Diabetic nephropathy. <u>Diabetes Care, 21</u> (Supp. 1), S50-S53.

American Diabetes Association. (1998). Insulin Administration. <u>Diabetes Care, 21</u> (Supp. 1), S72-S75.

American Diabetes Association. (1998). Nutrition recommendations and principles for people with diabetes mellitus. <u>Diabetes Care, 21</u> (Supp. 1), S32-S35.

American Diabetes Association. (1998). Report of the Expert Committee on the diagnosis and classification of diabetes mellitus. <u>Diabetes Care, 21</u> (Supp. 1), S5-S19..

American Diabetes Association. (1998). Standards of medical care for patients with diabetes mellitus. <u>Diabetes Care, 21</u> (Supp. 1), S54-S55.

American Diabetes Association. (1998). Tests of glycemia in diabetes. <u>Diabetes Care, 21</u> (Supp. 1), S69-S71.

Bauer, D.C., & Brown, A.N. (1996). Sensitive thyrotropin and free thyroxine testing in outpatients. <u>Archives of Internal Medicine, 156,</u> 2333-2337.

Begany, T., Braverman, L.E., Dworkin, H.J., & Macindoe II, J.H. (1998). When to screen, when to treat thyroid disease. <u>JAAPA, 11</u> (4), 72-87.

Biro, F.M. (1999). Gynecomastia. In R.A. Dershewitz (Ed.), <u>Ambulatory pediatric care</u> (3rd ed.). Philadelphia: Lippincott-Raven.

Bode, B.W., Davidson, P.C., & Steed, R.D. (1997). How to control and manage diabetes mellitus. In J.S. Skyler (Ed.), <u>Diabetes Dek: Professional Edition,</u> Atlanta: Infodek

Braunstein, G.D. (1993). Gynecomastia. <u>The New England Journal of Medicine, 328,</u> 490-495.

Cheffer, N.D., & Brady, M.A. (1996). Endocrine and metabolic diseases. In C.E. Burns, N. Barber, M.A. Brady, & A.M. Dunn (Eds.). <u>Pediatric primary care: A handbook for nurse practitioners.</u> Saunders: Philadelphia.

Einhorn, D. (1997). Advances in managing insulin-dependent diabetes. <u>Family Practice Recertification, 19</u> (2), 13-34.

Foley, T.P. (1997). Hypothyroidism. In R.A. Hoekelman (Ed.). <u>Primary pediatric care.</u> Mosby: St. Louis.

Hennessey, J.V. (1996). Diagnosis and management of thyrotoxicosis. <u>American Family Physician, 54,</u> 1315-1324.

Hoeg, J.M. (1994). Familial hypercholesterolemia: What the zebra can teach us about the horse? <u>JAMA, 271,</u> 543-546.

Jacobs, M.B. (1991). Gynecomastia: A bothersome but readily treatable problem. <u>Postgraduate Medicine, 89,</u> 191-193.

Krieger, D.R., Nathan, D.M., Schade, D.S., & Trubo, R. (1998). Insulin: Recent developments and common quandaries. <u>Patient Care, 32</u> (3), 71-88.

Lee, P.A. (1994). Advances in the management of precocious puberty. Clinical Pediatrics, 54-61

Levitsky, L.L. (1999). Diabetes mellitus. In R.A. Dershewitz (Ed.), Ambulatory pediatric care (3rd ed.). Philadelphia: Lippincott-Raven.

Linder, B. (1997). Improving diabetic control with a new insulin analog. Contemporary Pediatrics, 14 (10), 52-73.

Mansfield, M.J. (1999). Delayed puberty. In R.A. Dershewitz (Ed.), Ambulatory pediatric care (3rd ed.). Philadelphia: Lippincott-Raven.

Mansfield, M.J. (1999). Precocious puberty. In R.A. Dershewitz (Ed.), Ambulatory pediatric care (3rd ed.). Philadelphia: Lippincott-Raven.

Mengel, M.B. (1996). Diabetes mellitus. In M.B. Mengel & L.P. Schwiebert (Eds.), Ambulatory medicine (2nd ed). Stamford, CT: Appleton & Lange.

Nathan, D.M. (1993). Long-term complications of diabetes mellitus. The New England Journal of Medicine, 328, 1676-1683.

National Cholesterol Education Program. (1993). Summary of the second report of the national cholesterol education program (NCEP) expert panel on detection, evaluation, and treatment of high blood cholesterol in adults (adult treatment panel II). Journal of American Medical Association, 269, 3015-3023.

National Cholesterol Education Program. (1997). Cholesterol lowering in the patient with coronary heart disease. National Institutes of Health. National Heart, Lung, and Blood Institute. NIH Publ. #97-3794.

National Institute of Health Consensus Development Panel on Triglyceride, High-Density Lipoprotein, and Coronary Heart Disease. (1993). Triglyceride, high-density lipoprotein, and coronary heart disease. Journal of American Medical Association, 269, 505-510.

Neuman, J.F. (1997). Evaluation and treatment of gynecomastia. American Family Physician, 55, 1835-1844.

Revak-Lutz, R. (1997). Diabetes mellitus. Class outline at College of Nursing, University of Florida.

Schilling, J.S. (1997). Hyperthyroidism: Diagnosis and management of Graves' disease. Nurse Practitioner, 22, (6), 72-95,

Singer, P.A., Cooper, D.S., Levy, E.G., Ladenson, P.W., Braverman, L.E., Daniels, G., Greenspan, F.S., McDougall, I.R., & Nicolai, T.F. (1995). Treatment guidelines for patients with hyperthyroidism and hypothyroidism. JAMA, 273, 808-812,

Stone, N.J. (1996). Lipid management: Current diet and drug treatment options. American Journal of Medicine, 101 (suppl 4A), 4A-40S-4A-48S.

Styne, D.M. (1997). New aspects in the diagnosis and treatment of pubertal disorders. Pediatric Clinics of North America, 44, 505-529.

Tamborlane, W.V., & Ahern, J. (1997). Implications and results of the diabetes control and complications trial. Pediatric Clinics of North America, 44, 285-299.

Tanner, J.M. (1962). Growth at adolescence. Oxford: Blackwell Scientific Publications.

Wallace, K., & Hofmann, M.T. (1998). Thyroid dysfunction: How to manage overt and subclinical disease in older patients. Geriatrics, 53 (4), 32-41.

Wiczyk, H.P. (1998). Recognizing thyroid disease. The Female Patient, 23(3), 9-22.

Infectious Disease

CAT SCRATCH DISEASE

I.   Definition: Infection causing unilateral regional adenitis usually due to scratch of a cat

II. Pathogenesis

   A. *Bartonella henselae* (previously *Rochalimaea)* is the causative pathogen in most cases

   B. Pathogen enters the body through a break in the skin, usually caused by the scratch of a cat (usually cats are immature and not ill); dogs, monkeys, and fleas are other possible transmitters of infection

   C. Period of communicability unknown; not directly transmitted from person to person

III. Clinical Presentation

   A. Most cases (80%) are persons <20 years

   B. Clinical diagnosis of cat scratch disease (CSD) is based on the presence of 3 out of 4 of the following criteria:
       1. History of animal (usually cat) contact, with presence of a scratch or inoculation lesion of the eye, skin, or mucous membrane
       2. Positive cat scratch disease skin test
       3. Regional lymphadenopathy (predominant sign) with normal laboratory results for other causes of lymphadenopathy (see section on LYMPHADENOPATHY)
       4. Biopsied lymph node has characteristic histopathologic features

   C. Natural history:
       1. Cat scratch occurs and produces a primary cutaneous lesion 7-12 days later; lesion typically begins as a macule, progresses to a papule then to a vesicle
       2. Regional lymph node enlargement typically follows lesion in 1-2 weeks
           a. Node is usually singular, measuring between 1.5-5.0 cm
           b. Area around affected node is usually tender, warm, erythematous and indurated

   D. In most cases, the illness is self-limited with minimal malaise, headaches, and generalized aching; approximately 30% of cases have fever and mild systemic symptoms

   E. Lymphadenopathy usually regresses within 2-4 months, but may persist for more than a year

   F. Occasionally, Parinauds' oculoglandular syndrome develops
       1. Soft granuloma or polyp develops on palpebral conjunctiva
       2. Preauricular lymphadenopathy is usually present
       3. Patient typically does not recall cat scratch or bite; hypothesized that pathogen is transmitted in saliva left on cat's fur; patient pets cat, rubs eye, and transmits organism to conjunctiva

   G. Other rare complications include encephalitis, splenomegaly, and hepatic granulomata

IV. Diagnosis/Evaluation

   A. History
       1. Ask about onset and duration of all symptoms
       2. Determine whether patient lives in household with a cat (particularly kitten) or other animals
       3. Carefully determine whether patient saw scratch or bite of any animal
       4. Specifically ask whether any skin lesion was noticed within the last 2-3 months
       5. Ask about symptoms which typically accompany CSD such as low-grade fever and aching

6. Ask about symptoms which are related to other illnesses that present with lymphadenopathy such as pharyngitis (mononucleosis), weight loss and fatigue (malignancy), exanthem (Kawasaki disease), cough (tuberculosis), ear pain (otitis media), facial tenderness (sinusitis), mouth pain (dental abscess)
7. Inquire about symptoms which would denote complications of CSD such as abdominal pain, neurological complaints, conjunctivitis

B. Physical Examination
1. Obtain vital signs, noting temperature
2. Carefully examine skin for inoculation lesion which may be hidden in the interdigital webs of fingers, eyelids, or scalp
3. Observe skin for exanthem
4. Palpate all areas where lymph nodes are present, noting any node enlargement, erythema, or tenderness (see section on LYMPHADENOPATHY)
5. If a node is enlarged, assess the area that the node drains for signs of infection
6. Inspect eyes for signs of conjunctivitis
7. Do a complete head, ears, eyes, nose, and throat exam to rule out infection
8. Auscultate heart and lungs
9. Palpate abdomen for organomegaly, masses and tenderness
10. Perform a neurological examination to rule out complications

C. Diagnostic Tests: usually no tests are needed
1. Indirect fluorescent antibody test for detection of serum antibody to antigens of *Bartonella* species is sometimes helpful (available through the Centers for Disease Control and Prevention)
2. A newer test, enzyme immunoassay, may be more accurate in detecting the antibody
3. Polymerase chain reaction assays are available in some commercial laboratories
4. A cat scratch antigen skin test was used in past but is no longer recommended
5. A stain (Warthin-Starry silver impregnation stain) can be used to identify the pathogen if lymph node, skin, or conjunctival tissue is available
6. Biopsy of the node may be necessary when malignancy is suspected

D. Differential Diagnosis: Involved lymph node in CSD is usually tender whereas nodes are usually nontender in noninfectious diseases (see sections on LYMPHADENOPATHY and CERVICAL ADENITIS for further discussion)

V. Plan/Management

A. Management is usually symptomatic; complete resolution occurs without medications in 2-4 months
1. Prescribe analgesics for pain (see section on PAIN MANAGEMENT)
2. Recommend application of local heat to affected nodes
3. Limitation of vigorous activity is advised to prevent trauma to the node

B. Antibiotic therapy may be beneficial in immunosuppressed patients and other patients who are severely ill but is NOT recommended for healthy patients
1. Intramuscular gentamicin (Garamycin), oral trimethoprim-sulfamethoxazole (Bactrim), ciprofloxacin (Cipro) or rifampin (Rifadin) are possible choices
2. Therapy is discontinued when enlarged node has decreased in size (about 10 mm), the patient has no systemic symptoms and has been afebrile for at least one week

C. Node aspiration is done when nodes are tender and fluctuant; excision of the node is usually unnecessary but is curative and can relieve symptoms

D. Patient Education
1. Animals do not need to be destroyed or removed from the house
2. No person-to-person transmission so patients do not need to be isolated
3. Instruct patients to always thoroughly cleanse animal scratches and bites to prevent CSD

4. Persons with immune deficiencies should avoid contact with cats that scratch or bite
5. Recommend control of fleas as patients who own flea-infested kittens have greatly increased risk for disease

E. Follow Up: None needed if patient's condition remains stable

FEVER WITHOUT SOURCE (OR LOCALIZING SIGN) IN CHILDREN 0-36 MONTHS OF AGE

I. Definitions

A. Fever without source (FWS): unexplained fever (>38°C or >100.4°F) of brief duration or lasting <5-7 days; source of acute febrile illness is not apparent after a careful history and physical examination (see section on FEVER for table to convert temperatures)

B. Other important definitions:
1. Occult bacteremia: presence of viable bacteria in circulating blood not manifest or detectable by clinical methods alone
2. Sepsis: presence of pathogenic microorganisms or their toxins in blood or other tissues
3. Lethargy: level of consciousness characterized by poor or absent eye contact or the failure of the child to recognize parents or to interact with persons or objects in the environment
4. Toxic: clinical presentation congruent with the sepsis syndrome (see table that follows for signs)

SIGNS OF A TOXIC INFANT OR CHILD
➡ Altered level of consciousness
➡ Abnormal breathing
✱ Slow or rapid rate
✱ Irregular rate
✱ Stridor
✱ Prolonged expiration
✱ Grunting
✱ Nasal flaring
✱ Chest retractions
✱ Paradoxic or abdominal breathing
➡ Rapid pulse rate
➡ Elevated temperature
➡ Skin abnormalities
✱ Petechiae
✱ Central cyanosis
✱ Pallor
➡ Head bobbing
➡ Delayed capillary refill
➡ Poor muscle tone

II. Pathogenesis

A. Many cases resolve spontaneously with unknown etiology

B. Occult bacteremia and underlying sepsis are serious disorders which are always a paramount concern in children with unexplained fevers; common pathogens in these disorders are the following:
1. *Streptococcus pneumoniae* (most common)
2. *Haemophilus influenzae*, type b (second most common)

3. Third common bacterium is *Neisseria meningitidis*
4. Less common pathogens include *Salmonellae, Group A streptococcus, Staphylococcus aureus*, gram-negative enterics

C. Urinary tract infections are present in about 7% of male infants less than 6 months and 8% of female infants less than 12 months who have a fever without a source

D. Other less frequent causes are chronic disorders such as juvenile rheumatoid arthritis, drug reactions, allergic or hypersensitivity disorders, heat illnesses, or Kawasaki syndrome

E. In some cases, the health care provider is unable to find the source of fever until later in the course of the infection such as occurs with roseola, cytomegalovirus infection, typhus, and typhoid fever; these infectious diseases have long prodromal periods in which fever may be the only presenting symptom

III. Clinical Presentation

A. Signs and symptoms will depend on causative agent of fever

B. Important to remember: the clinical presentation of children who have a fever without a source due to a viral infection may be similar in appearance to those with occult bacteremia or a more serious bacterial infection

C. Occult bacteremia has a variable presentation and course
1. Typically, the higher the child's fever, the younger the age, and the more elevated the WBC count, the greater the risk for bacteremia
2. Occult bacteremia can occur in children with otitis media
3. The majority of children recover completely from occult bacteremia, but 25% of the children develop meningitis, significant soft tissue infection, osteomyelitis, septic arthritis, or have persistent bacteremia

D. The probability of having a serious bacterial infection varies with age and clinical presentation
1. Toxic-appearing infants less than 12 weeks have a 17% probability of having a serious bacterial infection which includes 11% probability of bacteremia and 4% probability of meningitis
2. The probability of serious bacterial infection in non-toxic-appearing febrile infants <12 weeks is 8.6% which includes a 2% probability of bacteremia and a 1% probability of meningitis
3. The mean probability of having bacteremia is 4.3% in children 3 to 36 months of age with a fever >39°C

IV. Diagnosis/Evaluation

A. History
1. Inquire about onset, duration, and pattern of fever
2. Ask about associated signs and symptoms (usually need a complete review of systems)
3. Ascertain severity of condition by asking about level of alertness, hydration status, and comfort level
4. Always ask about illnesses or fevers in other household members
5. Ask about immunization status
6. Inquire about exposure to animals
7. Explore possibilities of heat illness (heat stroke) or other types of environmental exposure
8. Inquire about recent immunizations, transfusions, risk factors for HIV infection
9. Inquire about last doses of antipyretic and other self-treatment measures
10. Ask about previous episodes of febrile seizures
11. Complete a thorough birth history, past medical history, and family history
12. Explore child's social situation and home environment, assess availability of transportation, telephone, thermometer, and whether parents are reliable and if heat and water are adequate

B. Physical Examination; most fevers without source **necessitate a complete physical examination** to uncover focal and generalized infections (remember that roseola rarely occurs in infants <6 months of age)
   1. Carefully measure rectal temperature; axillary and tympanic measurements can be variable and unreliable
   2. Assess vital signs (see following table for normal heart and respiratory rates)

| | | Heart Rate (beats per minute) | |
Age	Range of Respiratory Rate (breaths per minute)	Average	Range
Term - Newborn	40-60	140	90-170
One month	30-50	135	110-180
Six months	25-35	135	110-180
One year	20-30	120	80-160
Two years	20-30	110	80-130
Three years	20-30	105	80-120

AGE-SPECIFIC PULSE AND RESPIRATORY RATES IN CHILDREN AND INFANTS

Adapted from Daaleman, T.P. (1996). Fever without source in infants and young children. American Family Physician, 54, 2503-2512.

   3. Observation is critical; the Yale Observation Scale is helpful in quantifying observations (see following table)

YALE OBSERVATION SCALE

Observation Item	Normal = 1	Moderate Impairment = 3	Severe Impairment = 5
Quality of cry	Strong or none	Whimper or sob	Weak or moaning or high-pitched
Reaction to parent stimulation	Cries briefly or appears content and not crying	Cries on and off	Persistent cry or hardly responds
State variation	If awake, stays awake or if asleep, awakens quickly	Eyes close briefly when awake or awakens with prolonged stimulation	No arousal and falls asleep
Color	Pink	Pale extremities or acrocyanosis	Pale or cyanotic or mottled or ashen
Hydration	Skin and eyes normal and moist membranes	Skin and eyes normal; mouth slightly dry	Skin doughy or tented and dry mucous membranes and/or sunken eyes
Responds to social overtures	Smiles or alerts consistently ($\leq$ 2 mo)	Smiles or alerts briefly ($\leq$ 2 mo)	No smile, anxious, dull, expressionless; no alerting to social overtures ($\leq$ 2 mo)

A total score of less than 11 signifies a less than 3% probability of serious illness.
A total score of 11-15 signifies a 26% probability of serious illness.
A total score of greater than 15 signifies a greater than 92% probability of serious illness.

Adapted from McCarthy, P.L., Sharpe, M.R., Spiesel, Z., et al. (1982). Observation scales to identify serious illness in febrile children. Pediatrics, 70, 802-809.

   4. Determine capillary refill time
   5. Assess neck for nuchal rigidity (remember that infants <90 days old do not exhibit meningeal signs even if they have meningitis)
   6. Inspect the eyes for conjunctivitis (a sign of Kawasaki disease)
   7. Carefully examine the ears, nose, sinuses, and pharynx for focal signs of infection
   8. Check for localized and generalized lymphadenopathy
   9. Complete exam of the lungs and heart is needed
   10. Assess for suprapubic tenderness and costovertebral angle tenderness
   11. In males, note whether the child is uncircumcised which is a predisposing factor for urinary tract infections (UTI)
   12. A complete exam of the musculoskeletal and neurological systems is important to rule out arthritis, osteomyelitis, and meningitis

C. Differential Diagnosis
    1. Any young child with a FWS should be evaluated for a serious bacterial infection such as sepsis, bacteremia, and meningitis. Be highly suspicious of the diagnosis of a serious bacterial infection in the following circumstances:
        a. Child <28 days old
        b. A fever greater than 102°F (38.9°C)
    2. To help formulate a diagnosis it is important to determine if the child is at low or high risk for a serious bacterial infection (see following table)

CRITERIA FOR FEBRILE INFANTS AT LOW RISK FOR SERIOUS BACTERIAL INFECTION	
Clinical Criteria	**Laboratory Criteria**
History: * No previous hospitalizations * No chronic illness * No previous antibiotic therapy Physical Examination: * No toxic appearance * No focal bacterial infection (except otitis media) * Normal activity, hydration, and perfusion Social Situation: * Parents/care giver mature and reliable * Transportation available * Thermometer and telephone in home * Travel time to care facility <30 minutes	White Blood Cell Count: * 5,000-15,000 per mm^3 Band cell count * <1,500 per mm^3 Urinalysis * <5 WBCs per high-power field or normal gram-stained smear Stool * <5 WBCS per high-power field

Adapted from Barraff, L.J., Bass, J.W., Fleisher, G. R., et al. 1993. Practice guideline for management of infants and children 0 to 36 months of age with fever without source. Pediatrics, 92, 1-12.

    3. Differentiate fevers of unknown origin (FUO) which are undiagnosed fevers lasting >10 days from fevers without source; FUO may be due to infections, neoplasms, and collagen inflammatory diseases
    4. The **sole diagnosis of otitis media or pharyngitis in an infant with a temperature greater than 102°F (38.9°C) should be questioned**

D. Diagnostic Tests
    1. Must balance between need to exclude presence of bacteremia and other serious bacterial diseases with the indiscriminate use of costly, uncomfortable, and frightening diagnostic procedures
    2. To partially determine whether child is in low risk or high risk group for serious bacterial infections order the following laboratory screening tests: CBC with differential, urinalysis, stool smear if child has diarrhea, chest-x-ray if child has tachypnea or rales
    3. Children at high risk for serious bacterial infection (see preceding table to differentiate low risk vs. high risk children in IV.C.2), children with high fevers, immunocompromised children, and children <28 days old should have an evaluation for sepsis, bacteremia, and meningitis (see following table)

DIAGNOSTIC TESTS FOR SEPSIS, BACTEREMIA, AND MENINGITIS EVALUATION
Cultures - cerebrospinal fluid, blood, urine* Complete blood cell with differential count Examination of cerebrospinal fluid for cells, glucose, and protein Chest x-ray if child is tachypneic, has cough, or shows signs of respiratory distress Culture of stool if child has diarrhea (Some authorities also recommend erythrocyte sedimentation rate, Group B strep antigen detection obtained from urine and   CSF, arterial blood gas, C-reactive protein, serum calcium, haptoglobin, fibrinogen)

*Urine cultures should be obtained by catheter or suprapubic aspiration

Adapted from Barraff, L.J., Bass, J.W., Fleisher, G.R., et al. 1993. Practice guideline for management of infants and children 0-36 months of age with fever without source. Pediatrics, 92, 1-12.

4. Additional diagnostic tests for low risk children are dependent on age, clinical presentation, and social situation, etc.; additional tests to order are discussed in V. PLAN/MANAGEMENT

V. Plan/Management: Consider consultation with specialist for any child <36 months with FWS

A. All of the following children should be hospitalized, given parenteral antibiotic therapy and have an evaluation for sepsis and meningitis (see table SEPSIS AND MENINGITIS EVALUATION under Diagnostic Tests IV.D.3):
   1. **All infants 28 days** or less regardless of appearance or risk status
   2. All toxic-appearing infants and children
   3. All children NOT meeting low risk criteria for serious bacterial infection
   4. Immunocompromised children
   5. Consider hospitalization in other children who have high fevers and/or abnormal laboratory tests

B. Nontoxic appearing infants aged 28-90 days should be carefully evaluated to determine if they are in low-risk group; low risk infants in this age group can be managed on an outpatient basis if close followup is ensured. One of the following two approaches is recommended
   1. Approach one
      a. Order cultures of blood, urine, cerebrospinal fluid, possibly stool (order if child has bloody diarrhea)
      b. While waiting for culture results, administer intramuscular ceftriaxone (Rocephin) 50 mg/kg/day
      c. Recheck in 18-24 hours, at which time a second injection of ceftriaxone can be given or admit child to hospital if condition worsens
      d. See **Section V.B.3.** for further treatment if culture results are abnormal
   2. Approach two
      a. Order urine culture
      b. Provide careful observation
      c. Re-evaluate in 24 hours; if condition deteriorates patient should be admitted for sepsis evaluation and parenteral antibiotics
      d. See **Section V.B.3.c.** for further treatment if urine culture is abnormal
   3. Additional treatment may be needed after results of cultures are available for infants aged 28-90 days who are low-risk for occult bacteremia
      a. Most infants whose blood or lumbar cultures are positive should be admitted to hospital for parenteral antimicrobial therapy
      b. Afebrile, non-toxic-appearing infants with bacteremia caused by *Streptococcus pneumoniae* and who appear normal at recheck can be treated with second injection of ceftriaxone and 10-day course of oral amoxicillin (40 mg/kg/day in three divided doses) or penicillin (50 mg/kg/day in four divided doses) as an outpatient if careful followup can be maintained
      c. Afebrile, non-toxic-appearing infants with urinary tract infection without bacteremia can be treated with 10-day course of oral antibiotics (see section on URINARY TRACT INFECTION)
      d. Infants with otitis media without bacteremia should receive appropriate oral antimicrobial therapy (see section OTITIS MEDIA)
   4. Fever management: Administer acetaminophen (Tylenol) 5-15 mg/kg/dose every 4-6 hours (see section on FEVER)

C. For non-toxic appearing children 3 months of age (>90 days) to 36 months of age with fever ≥39°C, without underlying host defense deficiency and who are in the low risk group:
   1. Order following diagnostic tests:
      a. Urine culture for the following:
         (1) Males <6 months of age
         (2) Females <2 years of age
      b. Stool culture if blood or mucus in stool or ≥5WBCs/hpf in stool smear
      c. Chest x-ray for children with dypsnea, tachypnea, rales, or decreased breath sounds

d. Blood culture: either of following approaches are acceptable
(1) Approach one: all children with temperature ≥39°C
(2) Approach two: Temperature ≥39°C and WBC≥15,000
2. Empiric antibiotic therapy (prior to obtaining culture results) is usually prescribed but either of following approaches are acceptable [empiric antibiotic therapy is ceftriaxone (Rocephin) IM or some authorities suggest oral amoxicillin clavulanate (Augmentin), trimethoprim sulfamethoxazole (Septra) or erythromycin sulfisoxazole (Pediazole]
a. Approach one: prescribe to all children with temperature ≥39°C
b. Approach two: prescribe to only children whose temperature is ≥39°C and WBC≥15,000
3. Administer acetaminophen (Tylenol)
4. Recheck patient in 12-24 hours
5. Check cultures in 24-72 hours
a. If clinical condition deteriorates at any time or if *N. meningitidis* or *H. influenzae* are in blood cultures, hospitalize child
b. Children with blood culture positive for *S. pneumoniae* who are afebrile and well appearing can be treated as outpatients with second injection of ceftriaxone and 10-day course of penicillin or amoxicillin
c. Afebrile, non-toxic-appearing children with urinary tract infection without bacteremia can be treated with 10-day course of oral antibiotics (see section on URINARY TRACT INFECTIONS)
d. Children with otitis media without bacteremia should receive appropriate oral antimicrobial therapy (see section OTITIS MEDIA)

D. Teach the parents of any child with FWS to frequently assess child for signs of increasing fever (measure rectal temperature at least every 4 hours), respiratory distress, skin mottling, rash, cyanosis, nuchal rigidity, dehydration, and changes in level of alertness; any deterioration in condition necessitates an emergency room visit

E. Close follow-up is essential
1. Open telephone communication should be established during the night
2. Schedule return visit the following morning for reevaluation
3. Check cultures in 24-72 hours and reevaluate plan
4. See V. Plan/Management for additional follow-up based on age and risk

FIFTH DISEASE (ERYTHEMA INFECTIOSUM)

I. Definition: Mild viral disease with an erythematous eruption

II. Pathogenesis

A. Causal agent is human parvovirus B19

B. Mode of transmission probably is through contact with infected respiratory secretions or blood

C. Incubation period
1. 4-14 days from acquisition of infection to onset of initial symptoms
2. Rash and joint symptoms present 2-3 weeks after infection

D. Period of communicability: Greatest before onset of rash; probably not communicable after onset of rash; patients with aplastic crises are contagious from before the onset of symptoms and at least through the week after onset

III. Clinical Presentation

    A. Parvovirus B19 infections are ubiquitous and cases can occur as a community outbreak or sporadically
        1. Outbreaks frequently occur in elementary or junior high schools
        2. Secondary spread to susceptible household members is common

    B. >50% of adults have serologic evidence of past infection and are not susceptible to reinfection whereas only 5-10% of young children are immune

    C. Approximately 20% of all persons are asymptomatic

    D. First manifestation is typically a rash which usually appears without fever or other symptoms; in some cases there may be a prodrome with fever, headache, conjunctivitis, coryza, and pharyngitis

    E. Rash is characteristic
        1. First erupts as a bright, erythematous rash on cheeks and forehead with circumoral pallor
        2. A maculopapular rash on the proximal extremities occurs the following day
        3. Rash gradually spreads to trunk and distal extremities leaving a lacelike appearance as it clears; this stage lasts 2-4 days
        4. In third stage, rash appears transiently when skin is traumatized by pressure, sunlight, or extremes of hot and cold

    F. Infection during pregnancy can result in fetal hydrops and death (risk of fetal death is <10% after proven maternal infection in first half of pregnancy and less in second half)

IV. Diagnosis/Evaluation

    A. History
        1. Question about degree, onset and duration of fever or prodromal symptoms
        2. Ask patient to describe progression of rash
        3. Ask whether rash becomes more visible when patient is in sunlight or becomes overheated
        4. Determine whether there are other accompanying symptoms
        5. Determine whether other family or household members have similar symptoms
        6. Inquire about symptoms which would denote complications such as joint pain and stiffness
        7. Determine medication use
        8. Inquire about present and past health history of patient and other household members; specifically question about immunosuppression and pregnancy in females

    B. Physical Examination
        1. Measure vital signs
        2. Assess general appearance
        3. Carefully inspect skin, apply pressure to skin noting whether rash becomes more visible
        4. To rule out other viral exanthems may need to perform a complete head, eyes, ears, nose, throat and mouth exam
        5. Assess neck for nuchal rigidity and adenopathy
        6. Auscultate heart and lungs
        7. Assess joints for tenderness, swelling, and range of motion

    C. Differential Diagnosis: "Slapped cheek" appearance, lacy rash, and transient nature of rash with heat, cold and pressure is characteristic of fifth disease

D. Diagnostic Tests
   1. No tests are needed unless diagnosis is uncertain or when treating immunosuppressed patients or pregnant females
   2. Assay for serum B19-specific IgM antibody is available for confirming infection within the past several months; serum IgG antibody indicates previous infection and immunity
   3. Other tests are investigational such as the nucleic acid hybridization assay or polymerase chain reaction assay

V. Plan/Management

   A. Treatment is symptomatic for healthy persons; usually the condition is benign and self-limited

   B. Patients with aplastic crisis may need blood transfusion

   C. For immunosuppressed patients with chronic infection, intravenous immunoglobulin therapy is effective

   D. Control procedures
      1. Precautions for pregnant females:
         a. Routine exclusion from the workplace where disease is occurring is not recommended due to the high prevalence of B19, the low incidence of ill effects on fetus, and the fact that avoidance of child care or teaching classrooms can only reduce but not eliminate the risk of exposure
         b. Explanation of the relatively low potential risk and option of serologic testing should be given to pregnant females who have been in contact with patients in the incubation period of disease or who were in aplastic crisis; fetal ultrasound can be offered to assess damage to the fetus
      2. Children with fifth disease may attend child care or school as they are not contagious
      3. Good hand washing and disposal of facial tissues containing respiratory secretions lessen transmission of infection

   E. Follow Up: None needed unless complications develop

INFLUENZA

I. Definition: Acute viral disease of the respiratory tract

II. Pathogenesis

   A. Causal agent is influenza virus of 3 antigenic types (A, B, and C)

   B. Mode of transmission: Spread from person to person by direct contact, by large droplet infection, or by articles recently contaminated with nasopharyngeal secretions; during an outbreak, airborne transmission by small-particle aerosols may occur

   C. Incubation period: Short, ranges from 1-3 days

   D. Period of communicability is probably from 3-5 days from clinical onset; patients are most infectious in the first 24 hours before onset of symptoms and during the period of peak symptoms; viral shedding in nasal secretions usually stops within 7 days of onset of infection

III.   Clinical Presentation

   A.   Influenza virus infection occurs in epidemics which last approximately 5-6 weeks and may be associated with attack rates as high as 10-20% of the population

   B.   Reason for continuing problems with epidemic influenza is the phenomenon of antigenic variation in which there are alterations in the structure of antigens, leading to variants which the general population has little or no resistance against

   C.   Characterized by abrupt onset of fever, malaise, diffuse myalgia, headache, and nonproductive cough; later, sore throat, nasal congestion, and cough become more prominent
          1.   Unlike other common respiratory infections, severe malaise may linger for several days
          2.   Cough is usually the most frequent and troublesome symptom and may be associated with substernal discomfort
          3.   Symptoms usually last about 3-4 days, but cough and malaise may persist for 1-2 weeks

   D.   Gastrointestinal tract manifestations such as nausea, vomiting and diarrhea occur in children, but are less common in adults

   E.   Influenza can affect metabolism of certain medications such as theophylline and result in toxicity from high serum concentrations

   F.   Complications include primary influenza pneumonia, secondary bacterial pneumonia, myositis (calf tenderness, refusal to walk in children), and central nervous system problems; Reye syndrome is associated primarily with influenza B

IV.   Diagnosis/Evaluation

   A.   History
          1.   Inquire about onset and duration of symptoms, specifically question about myalgia and malaise which occur with influenza, but may not be present in other respiratory infections
          2.   To ascertain that patient does not have complications associated with influenza, ask about chest pain, hemoptysis, severe muscle pain, and central nervous system manifestations such as confusion
          3.   Determine whether household members or close contacts of patient are ill
          4.   Determine history of previous influenza vaccinations
          5.   Obtain a medication history, especially ask about use of theophylline

   B.   Physical Examination
          1.   Observe general appearance for lassitude and distress
          2.   Measure vital signs
          3.   Assess hydration status
          4.   Perform complete eyes, ears, nose, and throat examination
          5.   Palpate sinuses for tenderness
          6.   Examine neck for nuchal rigidity and cervical adenopathy
          7.   Auscultate heart
          8.   Perform complete lung exam
          9.   Abdominal exam and neurological exam should also be considered in patients with severe cases

   C.   Differential Diagnosis
          1.   Other viral illnesses
          2.   Pneumonia

   D.   Diagnostic Tests
          1.   Epidemiologic data are usually sufficient to make diagnosis in uncomplicated cases (in other words, when it is known that a certain influenza type is prevalent in a community, most persons with acute febrile, respiratory symptoms, and myalgia can safely be assumed to have influenza)

2. Consider cultures of nasopharyngeal secretions; must collect within the first 72 hours of illness
3. Change in antibody titer between acute and convalescent sera using complement fixation, hemagglutination inhibition, neutralization, or enzyme immunoassay tests can help confirm diagnosis retrospectively
4. Consider CBC and urinalysis

V. Plan/Management

A. Two antiviral agents, amantadine and rimantadine, diminish the severity and shorten the course of influenza A but not influenza B; only amantadine is approved for treatment in BOTH children and adolescents (see following table on DOSAGE FOR AMANTADINE AND RIMANTADINE TREATMENT)
   1. Consider antiviral treatment for unvaccinated patients with severe disease or those with underlying medical problems which may increase their risk for severe or complicated influenza infection
   2. Start therapy as soon as possible after onset of symptoms
   3. Duration of therapy: 2-5 days or for 24-48 hours after patient becomes asymptomatic; immunocompromised patients may require longer course
   4. Children <14 years: Only amantadine is approved for treatment; be cautious in children with epilepsy who have increased risk of seizures when taking amantadine
   5. Adolescents may be prescribed either amantadine or rimantadine; choice of antiviral depends on the following two factors
      a. Incidence of CNS-related adverse effects is higher when amantadine is used; adverse effects more common in patients with seizure disorders, psychiatric disorders, elderly, and patients with renal insufficiency
      b. Some experts recommend rimantadine in patients with mild to moderate renal insufficiency

DOSAGE FOR AMANTADINE AND RIMANTADINE TREATMENTS			
Antiviral agent	1-9 years of age	10-13 years of age	14-64 years of age
Amantadine* (Symmetrel)	5 mg/kg/day in 2 divided doses[†]; Max. 150 mg/day	100 mg BID[§]	100 mg BID
Rimantadine[¶] (Flumadine)	Not recommended	Not recommended	100 mg BID

* Check drug package insert when administering amantadine to persons with creatinine clearance ≤10 mL/min
[†] 5 mg/kg of amantadine or rimantadine syrup = 1 tsp/22 pounds
[§] Children aged ≥10 years who weigh <40 kg: prescribe amantadine 5 mg/kg/day
[¶] Reduce dose to 100 mg/day for persons with severe hepatic dysfunction or those with creatinine clearance ≤10 mL/min. Cautiously monitor persons with less severe hepatic or renal dysfunction taking >100 mg/day

Adapted from CDC: Prevention and control of influenza: Recommendations of the Advisory Committee on Immunization Practices. MMWR, 46(No. RR-9), 1-25

B. Other supportive measures may be needed depending on clinical presentation
   1. Treatment of fever and myalgia; especially important in young children because the fever of influenza can precipitate febrile seizures
      a. **Children and adolescents should not receive salicylates because of increased risk of developing Reye syndrome**
      b. Recommend acetaminophen or ibuprofen (see section on FEVER for doses)
   2. Treatment of cough if patient cannot sleep or rest (encourage patient to use only at bedtime)
      a. Suggest dextromethorphan polistrex (Delsym): Adolescents 10 mL every 12 hours; not recommended in children under 2 years; children 2-5 years, 2.5 mL; children 6-12 years, 5 mL (both every 12 hours)
      b. Alternatively, prescribe cough suppressants which include codeine

C. Patient Education
   1. Recommend rest and increased fluids
   2. Encourage cessation of smoking in household
   3. Teach patient to return to clinic if chest pain, dyspnea, hemoptysis, wheezing, increased temperature, agitation, behavioral changes, or confusion occur
   4. Instruct patient who is taking amantadine to be cautious of concurrent medications that affect the central nervous system such as antihistamines and anticholinergic drugs

D. Control Measures
1. Consider influenza vaccine for certain groups of individuals (see following table, TARGET GROUPS FOR INFLUENZA VACCINE)
2. Administer influenza vaccine in the fall (optimal time is October to mid-November), before the start of the influenza season (see following table DOSE AND SCHEDULE OF INFLUENZA VACCINE for administration of vaccine)
    a. Annual vaccination is recommended
    b. Do **not** administer vaccination to persons known to have anaphylactic hypersensitivity to eggs without consulting an expert in infectious disease
    c. Do **not** vaccinate adults with acute afebrile illnesses until their symptoms have abated; minor illnesses with or without fever should not contraindicate use of vaccine in children

---

TARGET GROUPS FOR INFLUENZA VACCINE

Groups at Increased Risk for Influenza-Related Complications

➡ Persons greater than or equal to 65 years of age

➡ Residents of nursing homes or chronic-care facilities

➡ Adults and children with chronic disorders of the pulmonary or cardiovascular system, including children with asthma

➡ Adults and children who have chronic metabolic diseases, renal dysfunction, hemoglobinopathies or immunosuppression (including immunosuppression caused by medications)

➡ Children and adolescents (6 months-18 years) who are receiving long-term aspirin therapy and might be at risk for developing Reye syndrome after influenza

➡ Females who will be in the second or third trimester of pregnancy during the influenza season

Groups That Can Transmit Influenza to Persons at High Risk

➡ Health care providers in both hospitals and outpatient settings

➡ Employees of nursing homes and chronic-care facilities who have contact with residents

➡ Providers of home care to persons at high risk

➡ Household members (including children) of persons in high risk groups including high risk infants

Special Groups

➡ Persons with HIV infection: vaccine effective in persons with mild AIDS-related symptoms and high CD4+ T-lymphocyte counts

➡ Breast-feeding is <u>not</u> contraindicated for vaccination

➡ Persons traveling to foreign countries: risk of exposure to influenza varies depending on season and destination; if persons traveling were not vaccinated the previous fall or winter, encourage vaccine

➡ General population: administer to any person who wishes to receive; especially encourage persons who provide community services and students or other persons living in institutional settings

Adapted from American Academy of Pediatrics. (1997). Summaries of infectious diseases. In Peter, G. (Ed.). <u>1997 Red Book: Report of the committee on infectious diseases</u> (24th ed.). Elk Grove Village, IL: Author

---

DOSE AND SCHEDULE FOR INFLUENZA VACCINE *[†]

Age Group	Product	Dosage	# Doses
6-35 months	Split virus only	0.25 mL	1-2[§]
3-8 years	Split virus only	0.50 mL	1-2[§]
9-12 years	Split virus only	0.50 mL	1
>12 years	Whole or split virus	0.50 mL	1

* The recommended site of vaccination is the deltoid muscle for adolescents and older children. The preferred site for infants and young children is the anterolateral aspect of the thigh
[†] Dosages are those recommended in recent years; refer to product circular each year for correct dosage
[§]Two doses given at least 1 month apart are recommended for children <9 years who are receiving vaccine for the first time

Adapted from American Academy of Pediatrics. (1997). Summaries of infectious diseases. In Peter, G. (Ed.). <u>1997 Red Book: Report of the committee on infectious diseases</u> (24th ed.). Elk Grove Village, IL: Author

E. Chemoprophylaxis with rimantadine or amantadine is an alternative method of protecting patients against influenza (see following table for PERSONS FOR WHOM CHEMOPROPHYLAXIS IS INDICATED)

    1. Chemoprophylaxis is not a substitute for vaccination; vaccination is preferred for prevention of influenza

    2. Chemoprophylaxis in vaccinated persons may provide additional protection and does not interfere with the immune response

    3. For maximal effectiveness of prophylaxis, drug must be taken each day for duration of influenza activity in community; to be cost effective, prophylaxis should only be prescribed during period of peak influenza activity

---

PERSONS FOR WHOM CHEMOPROPHYLAXIS IS INDICATED

➡ Persons at high risk who were vaccinated after circulation of influenza A in the community has begun; chemoprophylaxis is helpful during the interval before a vaccine response or 2 weeks after the recommended vaccine schedule has been completed

➡ Unimmunized persons who provide care to high-risk individuals

➡ Immunodeficient persons whose antibody response to vaccine is likely to be poor

➡ High-risk persons for whom vaccine is contraindicated

➡ May also administer chemoprophylaxis to any healthy person over age 1 year for whom the prevention of influenza is considered particularly desirable; these persons should also be immunized

Adapted from American Academy of Pediatrics. (1997). Summaries of infectious diseases. In Peter, G. (Ed.). 1997 Red Book: Report of the committee on infectious diseases (24th ed.). Elk Grove Village, IL: Author

---

    4. Prophylactic doses

       a. Children 1-9 years and children <40 kg: Amantadine 5 mg/kg/day in 1-2 doses*

       b. Children 10-13 years who weigh ≥40 kg: Amantadine 100 mg BID*

       c. Children ≥14 years and adults <65 years: 100 mg BID of either amantadine or rimantadine**

       d. Adults ≥65 years: ≤100 mg/day of amantadine or 100 or 200 mg/day of rimantadine** (reduce dose of amantadine in elderly who experience side effects when taking 200 mg/day)

       e. *Alternative and acceptable dosage for children who weigh >40 kg and adults is 100 mg/day in 1 or 2 divided doses

       f. **for persons with severe hepatic dysfunction or those with creatinine clearance ≤10 mL/min, reduce dose of rimantadine to 100 mg/day

F. Follow Up

    1. No follow up needed if symptoms resolve within one week

    2. Reevaluate if symptoms persist beyond 7-10 days

KAWASAKI DISEASE

I. Definition: Generalized vasculitis which is often referred to as mucocutaneous lymph node syndrome

II. Pathogenesis: Unknown etiology, but the following causative factors have been hypothesized

    A. Infection caused by rickettsiae, viruses (Epstein-Barr virus and retrovirus) and bacteria (*Group A Streptococcus*, other streptococci, and *propionibacteria*)

    B. Disease may be related to living near bodies of water or exposure to house dust mites or recently shampooed carpets

III.   Clinical Presentation

A.   Leading cause of acquired heart disease in children in the US

B.   Approximately 80% of cases occur in children less than 5 years of age; majority of affected children are under 2 years of age

C.   Highest incidence is in children of Asian ancestry

D.   The following clinical criteria are available to assist in formulating the diagnosis (see table that follows)

DIAGNOSTIC CRITERIA (PRINCIPAL CLINICAL FINDINGS) OF KAWASAKI DISEASE*

Fever of at least 5 days duration[†]

Presence of 4 of the following principal features:

➡   Changes in extremities

➡   Polymorphous exanthem

➡   Bilateral conjunctival injection

➡   Changes in the lips and oral cavity

➡   Cervical lymphadenopathy

Exclusion of other diseases with similar findings (see DIFFERENTIAL DIAGNOSIS)

*Patients (usually infants) with fever and <4 principal features can be diagnosed with atypical Kawasaki disease when coronary artery disease is detected by 2-dimensional echocardiogram or coronary angiography.

[†]Many experts believe that, in the presence of classic features, the diagnosis of Kawasaki disease can be made by experienced practitioners before the fifth day of fever.

Adapted from Dajani, A.S., et al. (1993). Diagnosis and therapy of Kawasaki disease in children. Circulation, 87, 1776-1780

E.   Fever is one of the prominent symptoms, lasting 1-2 weeks or longer despite the use of antibiotics and the standard dose of antipyretics

F.   Within 3 days of fever other characteristic signs appear:
1.   Swollen, indurated, erythematous, and tender palms of the hands and soles of the feet
2.   Polymorphous, erythematous rash involving the entire body and accentuated in the perineal region
3.   Cervical lymphadenopathy which is usually unilateral and involves at least one node that is greater than 1.5 cm in diameter
4.   Other signs include bilateral conjunctival injection, cracking of lips, strawberry tongue, erythema of the oropharyngeal mucosa and mouth ulcerations

G.   Approximately by the sixth day of illness, patient has drying, cracking, and fissuring of lips, followed by periungual desquamation and peeling of palms and soles during second to third week; in the last phase of disease the patient may have deep transverse grooves across the nails or Beau's lines

H.   Cardiac problems occur in the acute phase of the disease and are the primary cause of morbidity and mortality
1.   Coronary aneurysms occur in approximately 20% of untreated patients
2.   Pericardial effusion occurs in about 30% of cases
3.   Another common cardiac manifestation is myocarditis
4.   Myocardial infarction is the major cause of death

I.   Noncardiac problems are also associated with Kawasaki disease
1.   Arthritis and arthralgias
2.   Diarrhea, vomiting and abdominal pain are frequent manifestations
3.   Other presentations include mild obstructive jaundice, liver and gallbladder problems, and aseptic meningitis
4.   A prodrome of cough, rhinorrhea, otitis media or pulmonary infiltrates often occurs

J. Course of disease: Without treatment, mean duration of fever is 12 days; other symptoms and complications resolve by 6-8 weeks of onset of illness, although myocardial infarction and sudden death can occur months to years later; in the US the mortality rate is less than 0.5%

K. Ayptical Kawasaki is often misdiagnosed; criteria for diagnosis are two of the principal features and a coronary artery aneurysm
    1. Most common in infants <1 year who have a greater chance of coronary artery aneurysm and other complications
    2. Severe, life-threatening thrombocytopenia has been reported

IV. Diagnosis/Evaluation

A. History
    1. Inquire about onset and duration of symptoms
    2. Ask about occurrence, pattern, and degree of fever and effectiveness of self-care measures to reduce fever
    3. Explore possible associated symptoms such a rash, swollen and tender hands and feet, mouth lesions, conjunctivitis, upper respiratory complaints, gastrointestinal disturbances, arthralgias, and chest pain
    4. Inquire about previous streptococcal infection
    5. Inquire about exposure to infectious agents
    6. Complete a thorough medication history
    7. Carefully determine whether patient is up-to-date with all immunizations

B. Physical Examination
    1. Quickly assess whether patient is in distress or has signs of dehydration such as decreased capillary refill, poor skin turgor, and dry mucous membranes
    2. Measure vital signs, carefully determine temperature
    3. Inspect skin for exanthems
    4. Perform a complete eye examination
    5. Assess ears, nose and throat for signs of infection
    6. Carefully assess neck for lymphadenopathy and nuchal rigidity
    7. Perform complete heart and cardiovascular exams
    8. Auscultate the lungs
    9. Palpate abdomen for organomegaly and tenderness
    10. Assess the joints for swelling, erythema, and tenderness
    11. In males, check for testicular swelling

C. Diagnostic Tests: Diagnosis is based primarily on clinical presentation
    1. No specific tests are available but consider ordering the following:
        a. CBC (typically will have increased neutrophils)
        b. Erythrocyte sedimentation rate (ESR) (almost universally elevated) or C-reactive protein (almost universally elevated)
        c. Platelet count (elevated after the first week of onset of illness)
        d. Urinalysis (proteinuria and sterile pyuria are typical)
        e. Serum transaminases (usually elevated)
    2. Order a baseline echocardiogram, followed by subsequent echocardiograms at 3 and 8 weeks after onset of illness; additional echocardiograms will depend on degree of coronary artery involvement

D. Differential Diagnosis
    1. Rubeola
    2. Scarlet fever
    3. Other febrile viral exanthemas
    4. Drug reactions
    5. Stevens-Johnson syndrome
    6. Lyme disease
    7. Rocky Mountain spotted fever
    8. Scalded skin syndrome
    9. Toxic shock syndrome

10. Juvenile rheumatoid arthritis
11. Leptospirosis
12. Mercury poisoning
13. Infectious mononucleosis

V. Plan/Management: Treatment consists of supportive care, detection of coronary artery disease, and anti-inflammatory therapy

A. Consult specialist and arrange hospitalization for patients with suspected Kawasaki disease; patients are usually followed by a cardiologist

B. Therapy should begin when diagnosis is established or strongly suspected; treat with the following two agents in the first 10 days of illness:
1. Intravenous gamma globulin (2 gm/kg as single infusion over 12 hours); some children do not respond to first dose and retreatment with second infusion is needed
2. Aspirin 80-100 mg/kg/day orally in 4 divided doses until patient is afebrile (some experts recommend for first 14 days); then reduce dose to 3-5 mg/kg orally once a day for up to 6-8 weeks (continue indefinitely if there are coronary artery abnormalities)

C. Do not administer varicella vaccine for at least 5 months and measles vaccine for 11 months after gamma globulin therapy; other immunizations should be given at routine times; to reduce risks of Reye syndrome administer influenza vaccine yearly in patients 6 months to 18 years of age

D. Education
1. Due to risk of Reye syndrome in patients with influenza or varicella receiving salicylates, instruct parents whose children are receiving aspirin to contact health care provider immediately if child develops symptoms or is exposed to either disease
2. Teach parents and patients, if applicable, about the signs and symptoms of possible complications such as arthralgias, chest pain, and palpitations
3. Explain that Kawasaki disease is not spread from person-to-person contact so there is no need to preventively treat family members

E. Follow Up
1. Patients should be examined frequently during the first 2 months of onset of illness to detect arrhythmias, heart failure, valvular problems and myocarditis
2. Echocardiogram should be ordered at time of diagnosis, 3 weeks after onset, and then 8 weeks later
3. See Dajani (1997) "Guidelines for long-term management of patients with Kawasaki Disease" for specific follow-up management of patients with varying risk levels of myocardial ischemia

LYME DISEASE

I. Definition: Infection caused by *Borrelia burgdorferi*, a member of the family of spirochetes or corkscrew-shaped bacteria

II. Pathogenesis

A. Ticks transmit disease to humans during the nymph stage when they are small in size and are likely to feed unnoticed on individuals for 2 or more days

B. Small mammals, particularly rodents, are important hosts of ticks and critical for maintenance of *B. burgdorferi* in nature; deer are hosts for the adult tick

154

C. Adult ticks are less likely to transmit disease because they are readily noticed and removed; transmission of the disease is unlikely if tick attachment is less than 48 hours.

D. Incubation period is 3-31days (typically 7-14 days); late manifestations occur several months to more than one year later

III. Clinical Presentation

A. Incidence of Lyme disease is increasing and there has been an expansion of the affected geographic area; leading vector-borne disease in U.S.

B. Highest incidence in the US occurs in the northeast from Massachusetts to Maryland, north-central states, especially Wisconsin and Minnesota, and the west coast, particularly northern California

C. Most human infections occur between the months of April and October in U.S.

D. Less than 50% of all patients with Lyme disease remember receiving a tick bite

E. Case definition for the national surveillance of Lyme disease
1. Individual with erythema migrans
2. Individual with at least one manifestation and laboratory confirmation of infection

F. First stage is called early localized and is characterized by the following:
1. Erythema migrans (EM) is a lesion that starts as a red macule or papule at the site of a recent tick bite and enlarges over days or weeks to form a large, round lesion, often with central clearing
   a. Lesion must measure at least 5 cm to be considered EM
   b. Lesion varies in size, shape and may be vesicular or necrotic in the center
2. Fever, malaise, headache, neck stiffness and arthralgia may occur with rash; these symptoms may be intermittent over several weeks

G. Second stage is called early disseminated disease and presents as the following:
1. Characteristic rash, multiple erythema migrans, develops 3 to 5 weeks after tick bite and appears as annular erythematous lesions which are smaller but similar to primary lesion; occurs in about 50% of patients
2. Other common manifestations: Palsies of cranial nerves, meningitis, conjunctivitis and systemic symptoms such as arthralgia, myalgia, headache, and fatigue; carditis is a rare occurrence

H. Third stage is called late disease and signs and symptoms in this stage may not present until months or years after tick bite; characterized by following:
1. Recurrent arthritis which is pauciarticular and affects large joints, particularly the knees
2. Central nervous system manifestations such a encephalopathology and neuropathy may also occur

IV. Diagnosis/Evaluation

A. History
1. Ask about possible exposure to tick bites such as recent camping trip, frequent yard work, pets who are outside in vegetation
2. Ask patient to describe the duration, characteristics, and course of any skin lesion
3. Question about fatigue, headache, fever, myalgias after outdoor exposure
4. Inquire about late manifestations such as arthritis and nervous system and cardiac problems

B. Physical Examination
1. Carefully inspect the skin
2. Palpate for lymphadenopathy
3. Perform a thorough cardiac exam
4. Inspect joints for swelling, tenderness or erythema
5. Perform a neurological examination

C. Differential Diagnosis
1. Rheumatoid arthritis
2. Meningitis/encephalitis
3. Viral syndrome
4. Tularemia
5. Acute rheumatic fever
6. Systemic lupus erythematosus
7. Rocky Mountain spotted fever
8. Bell's palsy
9. Reiter syndrome

D. Diagnostic Tests
1. Patients presenting with rash resembling erythema migrans or with arthritis, or who have a history of characteristic rash, and a previous tick bite should have empiric antibiotic therapy; no diagnostic tests are needed
2. For patients who do not meet the above criteria in IV.d.1, but who have objective clinical signs and who live in a community in which Lyme disease is present or who have a pre-test probability of 20% should undergo a two-test protocol:
   a. First, order an enzyme-linked immunosorbent assay (ELISA) or an immunofluorescence assay; these tests often have false positive results
   b. Follow with a Western blot for specimens found to be indeterminant; positive test increases likelihood that patient has Lyme disease whereas negative test rules out disease
3. Patients with singular symptoms of arthralgias, myalgia, headache, fatigue or palpitations have a low chance of having Lyme disease and should not be tested
4. Other diagnostic tests are not usually ordered but may be beneficial:
   a. In patients with suspected primary erythema migrans, skin culture with a saline-lavage needle aspiration and a 2-mm punch biopsy of the leading edge of lesion successfully obtains causative organism in 60%-80% of cases
   b. Changes in antibody levels in paired acute-phase and convalescent-phase serum samples may help diagnose disease, but published data are not yet available to determine the clinical utility of this approach

V. Plan/Management

A. Treat the following patients with antibiotics (see following table on Recommended Therapy)
1. Patients with erythema migrans or a history of this lesion and a positive history of tick bite
2. Patients with pre-test probability of ≥20% who have positive results from two-test protocol (ELISA or immunofluorescence assay and Western blot)

B. Do not treat patients whose only evidence of Lyme disease is a positive immunologic test; the risks of empiric antibiotic treatment outweigh the benefits

RECOMMENDED TREATMENT

Disease Category	Drug/Duration	Adolescent Dosage	Pediatric Dosage
Early Localized Disease*	Doxycycline (Vibramycin) 14-21 days	100 mg BID	Not recommended <8 years of age
	Amoxicillin (Amoxil) 14-21 days	250-500 TID	25-50mg/kg/day divided into 3 doses
Early Disseminated and Late Disease			
➡ Multiple erythema migrans	Same as early disease except duration is 21 days		
➡ Isolated facial palsy	Same as early disease, except duration is 21-28 days[†‡]		
➡ Arthritis	Same as early disease except duration is 28 days		
➡ Persistent or recurrent arthritis[§] ➡ Carditis ➡ Meningitis or Encephalitis	Ceftriaxone (Rocephin) IV or IM for 14-21 days OR Penicillin G IV for 14-21 days	2 g QD or 1 g BID 20 million units in 4 divided doses	75-100 mg/kg QD (maximum, 2 g/day) OR 300,000 U/kg/day given in divided doses every 4 hours (maximum 20 mil. U/day)

*Cefuroxime axetil and erythromycin are alternative drugs for patients allergic to penicillin
[†]Do not give corticosteroids
[‡]Antibiotics do not affect resolution of nerve palsy; purpose is to prevent late disease
[§]Considered persistent when there is objective evidence of synovitis for at least 2 months after treatment is initiated.
 Some experts use a second course of an oral agent before using an IV antibiotic

Adapted from American Academy of Pediatrics. (1997). Summaries of infectious diseases. In Peter, G. (Ed.). 1997 Red Book: Report of the committee on infectious diseases (24th ed.). Elk Grove Village, IL: Author

C.   For patients without objective clinical signs, antimicrobial prophylaxis after a tick bite is not recommended because of the low rate of transmission and fact that transmission requires 24-48 hours of tick attachment; consult specialist in certain cases such as when patient is pregnant or when patient has been exposed to long duration of feeding by tick as evidenced by removal of an engorged tick

D.   Prevention: Teach patient the following:
1.   Remove leaves and clear brush and tall grass from around houses and at the edges of gardens
2.   Avoid tick-infested areas in the late spring and summer months
3.   Always inspect body carefully after being outdoors
4.   Daily inspect pets and remove ticks
5.   Wear lightly colored clothing so that ticks can be seen more easily
6.   Prevent ticks from getting under clothing; tuck pant legs into socks or tape area where pants and socks meet, and tuck shirt into pants
7.   Wear a hat and long-sleeved shirt
8.   Avoid overhanging grass and brush by walking in the center of trails
9.   Spray permethrin on clothing or treat clothes with permethrin which kills ticks on contact and prevents tick attachment
10. Spray insect repellent containing N,N-diethyl-m-toluamide (DEET) on all exposed skin other than face, hands and abraded skin (must reapply every 1-2 hours); use DEET sparingly because of rare reports of serious neurologic complications after use (wash treated skin with soap and water after being outdoors)

11. Remove clothing and wash and dry it in high temperature after outdoor exposure
12. Remove attached ticks with tweezers; pull tick straight back with a slow steady force; disinfect skin before and after tick is removed; do not use nail polish, alcohol, or matches to remove

E. Follow Up
1. Patients treated with oral antibiotics should be reevaluated at the end of treatment
2. Patients with more severe symptoms should be seen more frequently based on their clinical condition

INFECTIOUS MONONUCLEOSIS

I. Definition: Acute viral syndrome with classic triad of fever, pharyngitis, and adenopathy

II. Pathogenesis

A. Causal agent is the Epstein-Barr virus (EBV)

B. Spread person-to-person by the oropharyngeal route (via saliva); rarely via blood transfusion

C. Incubation period is from 30 to 50 days

D. Period of communicability is indeterminant but may be prolonged
1. Pharyngeal excretion may persist for many months or more after illness
2. Asymptomatic carriage is common

III. Clinical Presentation

A. Common infection in college-age individuals and adolescents living in group settings such as educational institutions; in infants and young children, the disease is frequently unrecognized and generally mild

B. Spectrum of disease is variable; patients may be asymptomatic or suffer from fatal infection

C. Common signs and symptoms include the classic triad of fever, exudative pharyngitis, adenopathy (particularly posterior cervical), as well as fatigue, eyelid edema, headache, pain behind eyes, and a palatal petechial rash

D. Atypical lymphocytosis and abnormal liver function tests often accompanies disease

E. Splenic enlargement may occur; usually resolves within the first month of the illness

F. Duration of the illness is variable with the average, uncomplicated illness lasting 3-4 weeks

G. Complications occur more often in patients under 10 or over 50 years of age and include central nervous system (CNS) disorders such as aseptic meningitis, encephalitis and the Guillain-Barré syndrome; rare complications include splenic rupture, thrombocytopenia, agranulocytosis, myocarditis, hemolytic anemia

H. The definition of "chronic" infectious mononucleosis is still controversial

IV.   Diagnosis/Evaluation

    A.   History
       1.   Ask about onset of symptoms
       2.   Ascertain that patient does not have trouble breathing or severe swallowing difficulty
       3.   Question about severe headaches, weakness, and confusion (CNS complications of mononucleosis)
       4.   Ask about fever, sore throat, malaise, rash
       5.   Question about recent history of exposure to others with mononucleosis

    B.   Physical Examination
       1.   Observe general appearance
       2.   Measure vital signs
       3.   Observe skin for exanthems
       4.   Perform a complete ears, nose, and throat examination
       5.   Auscultate the heart
       6.   Auscultate the lungs, making certain that the patient does not have upper airway obstruction from enlarged tonsils and lymphoid tissue
       7.   Palpate abdomen for organomegaly
       8.   Perform a neurological examination to rule out CNS complications

    C.   Differential Diagnosis
       1.   Streptococcal or viral pharyngitis (posterior cervical adenopathy and splenomegaly help distinguish pharyngitis of infectious mononucleosis from other types of pharyngitis)
       2.   Viral syndromes
       3.   Hepatitis
       4.   Cytomegalovirus infection
       5.   Toxoplasma infection
       6.   Secondary syphilis

    D.   Diagnostic Tests
       1.   Order complete blood count with differential: Absolute lymphocytosis in which more than 10% of cells are atypical is characteristic
       2.   Order Mono test or nonspecific tests for heterophil antibody (Monospot, Paul-Bunnell test, and slide agglutination reaction are most widely available)
          a.   Often negative in children younger than 4 years but will identify 90% of cases in older children and adults
          b.   Early in the course of this illness, some patients who are infected may have a negative Mono test because the level of antibodies in the blood has not reached sufficient levels; if patient continues to have symptoms repeat Mono test in 7-10 days
          c.   A positive result may remain positive for up to a year after the initial illness
       3.   Consider obtaining throat swab and perform rapid strep test. If the rapid strep test is negative (3-30% of patients with mononucleosis also have streptococcal infection) send a throat culture
       4.   Consider ordering liver function tests
       5.   EBV antibody seroconversion test is usually not performed in uncomplicated cases but may be needed in adults without heterophile antibodies or who have a negative monospot test and there is a suspicion of mononucleosis

V.   Plan/Management

    A.   Patients with uncomplicated acute mononucleosis require only symptomatic therapy
       1.   Most authorities advise NOT to treat uncomplicated mononucleosis with corticosteroid therapy or acyclovir
       2.   Pain medication and warm salt water gargles may help the discomfort of the sore throat

B. If patient has concomitant streptococcal pharyngitis treat with erythromycin (E-Mycin): For adolescents, prescribe 250 mg QID for 10 days; for children prescribe erythromycin (Eryped) 30-50 mg/kg/day in 4 divided doses for 10 days. Available as suspension, 200 mg/5 mL or 400 mg/5 mL. (Do not prescribe ampicillin or amoxicillin-containing agents because they frequently cause a rash; infrequently, penicillin can also cause a rash)

C. For patients with more severe symptoms, consult specialist and consider the following:
   1. Corticosteroid therapy may be useful for treating some complications such as obstructive tonsillar enlargement, autoimmune hemolytic anemia, thrombocytopenia, aplastic anemia, encephalitis, myocarditis, pericarditis, and massive splenomegaly; prescribe prednisone 1mg/kg per day orally for 7 days and then taper
   2. Acyclovir in combination with corticosteroids has been recommended but the clinical benefits have not been demonstrated except in HIV-infected patients with hairy leukoplakia

D. Patient Education
   1. Contact sports, heavy lifting, and strenuous activity should be avoided for at least one month or until resolution of splenomegaly because an enlarged spleen is susceptible to rupture
   2. Help patient plan a realistic schedule of rest with modification of work and/or school responsibilities depending on patient's condition
   3. Increased fluid intake may be beneficial
   4. Patient does not need to be isolated from others, but to prevent spread of disease teach the following: good hand washing technique, avoidance of sharing eating or drinking utensils with others, avoidance of kissing or sharing oral secretions
   5. Remind patient to avoid alcohol consumption for at least a month to decrease the work of the liver
   6. Instruct patient with a recent history of mononucleosis to avoid donating blood
   7. Tell patient to avoid ampicillin or amoxicillin during course of disease as a drug-related rash may develop
   8. Instruct patient to immediately report pain in left upper area of abdomen or in shoulder as this could be a sign of splenic rupture
   9. Inform patient that recovery is typically in 2 to 4 weeks, but that some patients have a slow recovery of 2 to 3 months

E. Follow Up: Every 1-2 weeks until symptoms resolve

RHEUMATIC FEVER

I. Definition: Inflammatory, multisystem disease that occurs 1-5 weeks to 6 months after group A streptococcal pharyngitis

II. Pathogenesis

A. One widely-held theory is that antibodies that react with *Streptococcus* cross-react with human cardiac myocytes (carditis), cartilage (arthritis), and thalamic and subthalamic nuclei of the central nervous system (chorea)

B. Another theory suggests that hereditary plays a role whereby individuals who develop acute rheumatic fever (ARF) have a particular immune response to *Streptococcus*

III. Clinical Presentation

    A. Although the frequency and severity of acute rheumatic fever (ARF) have decreased in the U.S. in the last century, rheumatic heart disease remains the leading cause of cardiac death in individuals between 5 and 24 years of age

    B. The initial, nonspecific group of symptoms is a gradual onset of fever, malaise, and weight loss

    C. A history of pharyngitis within the preceding three months occurs in about 20% of the children diagnosed with ARF

    D. Criteria for the diagnosis of rheumatic fever have been revised (see table that follows)

CHARACTERISTICS OF ACUTE RHEUMATIC FEVER (JONES CRITERIA, UPDATED 1992)	
Two major manifestations or one major and 2 minor manifestations are required to make the diagnosis:	
Major manifestations	*Minor manifestations*
Carditis	Clinical
Polyarthritis	Fever
Chorea	Arthralgias
Erythema marginatum	Previous acute rheumatic fever or evidence of preexisting rheumatic heart disease
Subcutaneous nodules	
	Laboratory
	Acute phase reaction
	Leukocytosis
	Elevated erythrocyte sedimentation rate
	Abnormal C-reactive protein
	Prolonged PR interval or other electrocardiographic changes
Plus Evidence of a preceding streptococcal infection such as elevated or increasing antistreptolysin-O or other streptococcal antibodies, positive throat culture for group A streptococcus, recent scarlet fever	

Adapted from Dajani, A.S., et al. (1993). Guidelines for the diagnosis of rheumatic fever: Jones criteria, updated 1992. Circulation, 87, 302-307.

    E. Carditis, a major manifestation, is defined as a new or changed murmur, a pericardial friction rub or effusion, and a recent or worsening heart enlargement with or without heart failure

    F. Polyarthritis, the most common major manifestation, is a benign condition
        1. The arthritis is migratory and usually involves the larger joints such as the knees, ankles, elbows and wrists
        2. If untreated, the arthritis lasts for about 4 weeks and almost never results in permanent joint deformity

    G. Sydenham's chorea is a benign sign which presents as purposeless, involuntary, rapid movements of the trunk and/or extremities; often accompanied with muscle weakness and emotional lability

    H. Erythema marginatum is a rare manifestation
        1. Presents as red, nonpruritic, macular lesions with rounded or serpiginous margins and pale centers
        2. The exanthem is transient and migratory and occurs mainly on trunk and proximal extremities; rash may be brought out by application of heat

    I. Subcutaneous nodules are painless and freely movable nodules under the skin which are found over the extensor surfaces of certain joints, particularly the elbows, knees, and wrists

    J. Arthralgias and fever are nonspecific, minor manifestations which support the diagnosis of ARF when only a single major manifestation is present

K. Other common symptoms not included in the Jones criteria are weight loss, fatigue, irritability, abdominal pain, and epistaxis

L. Diagnostic test abnormalities are often present
1. Prolonged P-R interval on the electrocardiogram and elevated erythrocyte sedimentation rate (ESR) and C-reactive protein are nonspecific findings but provide supporting data that ARF is present
2. Patients may have positive throat cultures or rapid antigen tests for group A streptococci; patients may have elevated or rising streptococcal antibody titers

M. ARF lasts an average of less than 3 months; fewer than 5% of the cases persist for more than 6 months

N. The major complications are chronic cardiac valve disease and mitral regurgitation; aortic and mitral stenosis murmurs are not heard acutely, but may be present in adults who had ARF as children

IV. Diagnosis/Evaluation:

A. History
1. Specifically, inquire about onset, duration, and severity of any sore throat within preceding 3 months
2. Ask about duration and presence of all major and manifestations of ARF as well as nonspecific complaints such as weight loss, fatigue, and abdominal pain
3. Question about history of heart murmur or previous cardiac diseases
4. Determine family history of ARF
5. Ask about medication use; use of aspirin can mask signs of inflammation and tends to prolong the course of ARF

B. Physical Examination
1. Measure vital signs, noting elevated temperature
2. Inspect skin for exanthems, lesions, and nodules
3. Perform a complete exam of the ears, nose, and throat
4. Palpate for lymph nodes
5. Perform a complete cardiac exam
6. Auscultate the lungs
7. Assess all joints for tenderness, erythema, warmth and swelling
8. Perform a complete, neuromuscular exam

C. Differential Diagnosis: Diagnosis of ARF must be differentiated from other immunologic and infectious diseases such as the following:
1. Juvenile rheumatoid arthritis
2. Kawasaki syndrome
3. Reiter's syndrome
4. Rheumatoid arthritis
5. Systemic lupus erythematosus
6. Lyme disease

D. Diagnostic Tests
1. Obtain specimens for rapid antigen test and throat culture on all patients with sore throats who are at high risk for ARF (children between 4 to 17 years old, individuals with previous ARF, and close contacts of patients with a history of ARF); if rapid test is negative, send throat culture
2. To document a recent streptococcal infection, obtain acute and convalescent serum samples at 2-4 week intervals; all samples should be tested simultaneously
    a. A rise in titer of two or more dilution increments between the acute-phase and convalescent-phase specimens is significant
    b. The most commonly used antibody assays are antistreptolysin O, antistreptokinase, and anti-deoxyribonuclease B
3. Order C-reactive protein and erythrocyte sedimentation rate

V.   Plan/Management

A.   Treatment of acute rheumatic fever varies depending on severity of attack; consultation with a specialist is recommended
1.   Because anti-inflammatory therapy such as aspirin may mask inflammation and prolong the duration of attacks, codeine is the analgesic of choice for mild attacks
2.   Corticosteroid therapy is reserved for patients with severe carditis; Dose is 1 mg/kg/day; once the disease is controlled, taper drug over 2-3 weeks
3.   Bed rest should be maintained until the C-reactive protein level has been normal for 2 weeks
4.   Carditis is treated with inotropic agents, diuretics, vasodilators and possibly corticosteroids
5.   Chorea is treated with sedatives and minor tranquilizers

B.   Prevention of initial attacks or primary prevention of ARF involves adequate treatment of group A beta-hemolytic streptococcal infections of the upper respiratory tract
1.   Treatment of choice is penicillin oral or intramuscular:
a.   Adolescents: Penicillin V (Pen-Vee-K) 500 mg BID or TID for at least 10 days
b.   Children: Penicillin V (Pen-Vee-K) 250 mg BID or TID for 10 days. Available 125 mg/5 mL and 250 mg/5 mL liquid
c.   Benzathine penicillin 600,000 units for children <60 pounds;1,200,000 units (1.2 million units) for larger children and adolescents
(1)   Be familiar with signs, symptoms and treatment of anaphylaxis and observe patient for 30 minutes after injection.
(2)   Bring medication to room temperature before injecting to reduce discomfort
2.   Alternative antibiotics:
a.   Erythromycin: For adolescents prescribe erythromycin estolate (E-mycin): 20-40 mg/kg/day BID or TID for 10 days; for children prescribe erythromycin ethyl succinate (Eryped) 40mg/kg/day BID or TID for 10 days; available 200mg/5mL and 400mg/5mL susp
b.   Cefadroxil monohydrate (Duricef): For adolescents prescribe 500 mg capsules BID for 10 days; for children prescribe 30 mg/kg once a day or in 2 divided doses. Available formulations include 125 mg/5mL, 250 mg/5 mL, and 500 mg/5mL suspensions for 10 days; do not use in patients with allergies to penicillin

C.   Prevention of recurrent attacks of ARF or secondary prevention
1.   Patients with history of ARF are at a high risk for recurrence of ARF if they develop a streptococcal group A upper respiratory tract infection
2.   Because both asymptomatic and symptomatic infections can trigger a recurrence, continuous prophylaxis is recommended for patients with a well-documented history of ARF
3.   Begin prophylaxis, after full course or antibiotics to eradicate residual Group A Beta-hemolytic streptococcus even if throat culture is negative; promptly treat family members who have current or previous rheumatic fever
4.   Prescribe one of the following medication regimens (see following table)

SECONDARY PROPHYLAXIS OF ACUTE RHEUMATIC FEVER		
Drug	**Dose**	**Frequency**
Benzathine penicillin G IM	>60 pound: 1,200,000 units. ≤60 pound: 600,000 units.	Every 3-4 weeks
Penicillin V PO	250 mg	BID
Sulfadiazine PO	>60 pound (27 kg): 1 gm ≤60 pound (27 kg): 500mg	QD QD
Erythromycin PO*	250 mg	BID

*For patients allergic to penicillin and sulfadiazine

*Adapted from Dajani, A., et al., 1995. Treatment of acute streptococcal pharyngitis and prevention of rheumatic fever: A statement for health professionals. Pediatrics, 96, 758-764.

5. The duration of continuous prophylaxis is controversial. Duration of treatment is dependent on risk of recurrence. Risk increases with multiple, previous attacks and in persons who have increased risk of exposure to streptococcal infections such as school teachers, health professionals, or military recruits; recommendations for therapy duration are as follows:

    a. Patients who have had rheumatic carditis need long-term antibiotic prophylaxis into adulthood or possibly for life

        (1) Patients with persistent valvular disease need prophylaxis for at least 10 years after the last episode of ARF and at least until age 40 (continue prophylaxis even after valve surgery)

        (2) Patients with carditis but no residual heart disease such as persistent valvular disease need prophylaxis for 10 years or well into adulthood whichever is longer

    b. Patients who have had ARF without carditis should be carefully assessed, but providers can consider discontinuing prophylaxis in 5 years or until age 21 whichever is longer

D. Prophylaxis for bacterial endocarditis prior to medical or surgical procedures is important; antibiotic regimens used to prevent the recurrence of ARF are inadequate for prevention of bacterial endocarditis (see two tables on RECOMMENDED STANDARD PROPHYLACTIC REGIMEN on the following page)

    1. Endocarditis prophylaxis is recommended for high and medium-risk patients:

        a. High risk patients: prosthetic cardiac valves, previous bacterial endocarditis, complex, cyanotic congenital heart disease, surgically constructed systemic pulmonary shunts or conduits

        b. Medium risk patients: ARF patients who have acquired valvular dysfunction but NOT for patients with previous ARF without valvular dysfunction; other moderate risk patients include those with uncorrected cardiac congenital defects, hypertrophic cardiomyopathy, mitral regurgitation, mitral valve prolapse with murmur, and possibly men >45 years with mitral valve prolapse without murmur

    2. Prophylaxis is recommended for procedures likely to cause bacteremia (see table that follows)

PROCEDURES IN WHICH ENDOCARDITIS PROPHYLAXIS IS RECOMMENDED			
Dental	**Respiratory Tract**	**Gastrointestinal Tract**	**Genitourinary Tract**
Periodontal surgery Scaling Professional teeth cleaning	Tonsillectomy Adenoidectomy Surgery - resp. mucosa Bronchoscopy with bronchoscope	Sclerotherapy for esophageal varices Esophageal stricture dilation Endoscopic retrograde cholangiography Biliary tract surgery Surgery assoc. with intestinal mucosa	Prostatic surgery Cystoscopy Urethral dilation

Adapted from Dajani, A.S. et al. (1997). Prevention of bacterial endocarditis: Recommendations by the American Heart Association. JAMA, 277, 1794-1801.

	RECOMMENDED STANDARD PROPHYLACTIC REGIMEN FOR DENTAL, ORAL, RESPIRATORY TRACT, AND ESOPHAGEAL PROCEDURES		
Situation	**Drug**	**Timing**
Standard general prophylaxis	Amoxicillin Adolescent: 2 g Child: 50 mg per kg	One hour before procedure and not continued more than 6-8 hours
Patients unable to take PO medications	Ampicillin Adolescent: 2 g Child: 50 mg per kg	Given IM or IV 30 minutes before procedure
Patients allergic to penicillin	Clindamycin (Cleocin) Adolescent: 600 mg Child: 20 mg per kg -or-	One hour before procedure and not continued more than 6-8 hours
	Cefadroxil (Duricef) or Cephalexin (Keflex) Adolescent: 2 g Child: 50 mg per kg -or-	One hour before procedure and not continued more than 6-8 hours
	Azithromycin (Zithromax) or Clarithromycin (Biaxin) Adolescent: 500 mg Child: 15 mg per kg	One hour before procedure and not continued more than 6-8 hours
Patients allergic to penicillin and unable to take oral medication	Clindamycin (Cleocin) Adolescent: 600 mg Child: 20 mg per kg -or-	Given IM or IV within 30 minutes of procedure
	Cefazolin (Kefzol) Adolescent: 1 g Child: 25 mg per kg	Given IM or IV within 30 minutes of procedure

Adapted from Dajani, A.S. et al. (1997). Prevention of bacterial endocarditis: Recommendations by the American Heart Association. JAMA, 277, 1794-1801.

	RECOMMENDED STANDARD PROPHYLACTIC REGIMEN FOR GENITOURINARY AND GASTROINTESTINAL PROCEDURES		
Situation	**Drug**	**Adolescents' Dose**	**Children's Dose**
Standard general prophylaxis for patient with ARF and valvular dysfunction	Amoxicillin -or- Ampicillin	2 g PO one hour before procedure -or- 2 g IM or IV within 30 minutes of procedure	50 mg per kg PO one hour before procedure -or- 50 mg per kg IM or IV within 30 minutes of procedure
Patients with ARF and valvular dysfunction who are allergic to penicillin	Vancomycin	1 g IV over one to two hours; infusion should be completed within 30 minutes of procedure	20 mg per kg IV over one to two hours; infusion should be completed within 30 minutes of procedure

Adapted from Dajani, A.S. et al. (1997). Prevention of bacterial endocarditis: Recommendations by the American Heart Association. JAMA, 277, 1794-1801.

3. Patient Education for preventing bacterial endocarditis
    a. Teach patient to maintain good oral health with regular brushing, flossing, and visits to dentist to reduce sources of bacterial seeding
    b. Teach about the risks and sequella of bacterial endocarditis; emphasize that patients must take responsibility in communicating to health care providers about their cardiac condition and possible need for prophylaxis before procedures

E.   Follow Up
1.   For primary prevention or prevention of ARF with penicillin for Group A beta-hemolytic streptococcal pharyngitis no "test of cure" throat culture is needed unless the patient is at unusually high risk for developing ARF
2.   For patients with ARF, return visits depend on their clinical condition
a.   Typically, patients can be reevaluated when they return for prophylaxis every 3-4 weeks if they receiving an intramuscular antibiotic, otherwise schedule visits for every 4-6 weeks
b.   C-reactive protein needs to be closely monitored until it returns to normal levels; after C-reactive protein is normalized, monitor periodically for 6-8 additional weeks

ROCKY MOUNTAIN SPOTTED FEVER

I.   Definition: Systemic, febrile illness with characteristic rash that results from bite of infected tick

II.   Pathogenesis

A.   Infectious agent is *Rickettsia rickettsii*

B.   Mode of transmission
1.   Tick must attach and feed on blood for approximately 4-6 hours to become infectious in humans
2.   No person-to-person transmission

C.   Incubation period ranges from 2-14 days

III.   Clinical Presentation

A.   Most common arthropod-borne disease

B.   Most cases are in south Atlantic, southeastern, and south central states; other areas include the upper Rocky Mountain states, Canada, Mexico and South and Central America

C.   Patient typically presents with sudden onset of moderate to high fever (which persists if untreated for 2-3 weeks), severe headache, myalgia, conjunctival injection, nausea and vomiting

D.   Characteristic maculopapular rash usually appears before the sixth day of illness
1.   Rash spreads from wrists and ankles to trunk, neck and face
2.   In untreated patients, the lesions become petechial in about 4 days, then purpuric and coalesced

E.   Thrombocytopenia develops in most patients; anemia is present in about 30% of cases

F.   Disease can persist for 3 weeks and can be severe with central nervous system, cardiac, pulmonary, gastrointestinal, and renal involvement as well as disseminated intravascular coagulation which can lead to shock and ultimately to death; case fatality rate is 15-20% in untreated individuals but death is uncommon when diagnosis and treatment are prompt

IV.   Diagnosis/Evaluation

A.   History
1.   Inquire about onset, duration, and characteristics of all symptoms
2.   Ask patient to describe characteristics and progression of any rashes or skin lesions
3.   Inquire about possible exposure to tick bites such as recent camping trip or frequent yard work
4.   May need to do a complete review of systems to detect complications from the infection

B. Physical Examination
1. Measure vital signs, noting fever
2. Observe general appearance for signs of distress and lethargy
3. Carefully inspect skin for rashes and lesions
4. Inspect eyes for conjunctival injection
5. Palpate for lymphadenopathy
6. Perform complete heart, lung, and neurological examinations to rule out complications

C. Differential Diagnosis
1. In early stage, disease resembles systemic viral infections
2. In advanced disease, bacterial sepsis, meningitis, and meningococcemia are part of differential diagnosis

D. Diagnostic Tests
1. Consider ordering acute and convalescent sera, group-specific serologic tests (a fourfold rise in antibody titer is diagnostic of the disease)
   a. Titers can be determined by indirect fluorescent antibody, complement fixation, latex agglutination, indirect hemagglutination, or microagglutination
   b. Never delay initiation of antimicrobial treatment to confirm clinical suspicion of the disease
2. Consider ordering a CBC with differential, BUN, serum albumin, serum electrolytes, and liver function studies

V. Plan/Management (consult specialist)

A. Important to treat patients with antimicrobial therapy early in the course of disease; mortality sharply increases when therapy is delayed until the sixth day of illness
1. For children older than 8 years and adolescents, oral doxycycline (Vibramycin) is the drug of choice. Dose is 100 mg BID after a loading dose of 200 mg; therapy is continued until patient is afebrile for at least 2-3 days; usual course is 7-10 days
2. In children less than 8 years and patients with severe disease in whom meningococcemia is also in the differential diagnosis, chloramphenicol should be considered for use
   a. Some authorities, however, recommend using doxycycline in young children because of its superior benefits and less serious side effects when compared with chloramphenicol; prescribe oral doxycycline (Vibramycin) 3 mg/kg/day in two divided doses. Available in 50mg/5ml syrup
   b. For children older than 2 weeks and adolescents prescribe chloramphenicol (Chloromycetin) 50-100 mg/kg/day orally or intravenously in 4 divided doses. Therapy is continued until patient is afebrile for at least 2-3 days; usual course is 7-10 days

B. Patients who have any signs of complications should have a specialist consult and probably be admitted to the hospital because of the dangers of vascular collapse

C. Prevention: Teach patient about measures to avoid tick bites (see section on LYME DISEASE)

D. Follow Up
1. Because of the possible dangerous complications of the disease, close monitoring is needed
   a. Teach patients to return to clinic if any danger signs such as alterations in mental status, stiff neck, severe headache, prolonged nausea and vomiting, shortness of breath, decreased urine output, high fever, severe weakness and dizziness occur
   b. Patients should return to clinic within 24-48 hours of initial visit; then patient should be reevaluated at the end of the antimicrobial therapy
2. Patients using chloramphenicol need frequent serum platelet counts and CBCs

ROSEOLA (EXANTHEM SUBITUM)

I. Definition: Acute viral infection occurring primarily in children under 3 years of age

II. Pathogenesis

   A. Causal agent is human herpesvirus-6 (HHV-6) or a virus closely related to HHV-6

   B. Mode of transmission is unknown

   C. Incubation period ranges from 5-15 days

   D. Period of communicability is unknown, but is most likely greatest during the febrile phase, before the appearance of the exanthem

III. Clinical Presentation

   A. Occurs in children between the ages of 6 months and 3 years; 90% of the cases involve 2 year-olds

   B. Most common exanthem of children younger than 3 years of age; recent research suggests that most children are infected with the virus early in life but have no symptoms and the condition usually goes unrecognized

   C. Children with symptoms present with acute onset of prodromal fever, lasting 3-4 days, which can be as high as 105°F (40.6°C)

   D. Abrupt resolution of fever and eruption of a rash occur together
      1. Rash begins on trunk and spreads to face and extremities
      2. Discrete, pinkish maculopapular rash which lasts only one or two days

   E. Usually, child has no accompanying symptoms, but may have mild adenopathy

   F. Only complication is the possible onset of febrile seizures due to high fever

IV. Diagnosis/Evaluation

   A. History
      1. Question about degree, onset and duration of fever
      2. Question about self-treatment of fever
      3. Ask parents to describe progression of rash
      4. Determine whether there are other symptoms such as coryza, cough, sore throat, watery eyes (accompanying symptoms suggests a diagnosis other than roseola)
      5. Determine whether other family or household members have similar symptoms (infection of close contacts suggests a diagnosis other than roseola)
      6. Determine medication use (side effects of several medications present with rash)
      7. Ask about history of febrile seizures

   B. Physical Examination
      1. Measure vital signs, carefully assessing temperature
      2. Assess general appearance, noting lethargy and respiratory distress
      3. Carefully inspect skin
      4. To rule out other viral exanthems perform a complete head, eyes, ears, nose, throat and mouth exam
      5. Assess neck for nuchal rigidity and adenopathy (adenopathy may be present with roseola)
      6. Auscultate heart and lungs (normal findings are present with roseola)

C. Differential Diagnosis: The rash accompanying roseola may be confused with other viral exanthematous diseases; the following characteristics help differentiate roseola from other conditions
   1. Roseola occurs in children 6 months to 3 years (children younger than 6 months who have exanthem do not have roseola)
   2. Children with roseola are often playful without change in appetite even with the high fever (typically, with other viral exanthems, children are uncomfortable or lethargic)
   3. Abrupt onset of fever followed by rash with rapid resolution of both is characteristic of roseola

D. Diagnostic Tests: No tests are needed unless diagnosis is uncertain

V. Plan/Management

A. Treatment is symptomatic
   1. Administer acetaminophen to control temperature (see section on FEVER for dosage)
   2. Encourage fluids to prevent dehydration from high fever

B. Patient Education
   1. Parents need reassurance that the high fever does not mean a serious disease
   2. Teach parents to be alert for other symptoms such as lethargy, decreased fluid intake, cough, and irritability which suggest a diagnosis other than roseola and the need for a further evaluation

C. Follow Up: No follow up is needed if there are no further problems

RUBELLA (GERMAN MEASLES)

I. Definition: Febrile viral disease with diffuse maculopapular rash; postnatal rubella is usually mild and congenital rubella is associated with high incidence of congenital anomalies

II. Pathogenesis

A. Causal agent is rubella virus which is a RNA virus

B. Spread by direct contact with secretions of nose and throat

C. Incubation period ranges from 14-21 days

D. Period of communicability
   1. One week before and 5-7 days after onset of rash
   2. Infants with congenital rubella may shed virus for months after birth

III. Clinical Presentation

A. Importance of this viral illness is not the morbidity of the disease itself, but rather the consequences that can occur to a fetus during a maternal infection

B. Before the use of vaccines, rubella was a wide-spread disease; today the incidence of disease has declined by more than 99% from the prevaccine era

C. Most cases today occur in young, unvaccinated adults and outbreaks in colleges and occupational settings; approximately 10% of young adults are susceptible to rubella

D. Postnatal rubella
   1. Prodrome may or may not be present; typically lasts 1-5 days; younger children present with a mild coryza and diarrhea; older children and adolescents may have headache and sore throat
   2. Exanthem is typically a pink, maculopapular eruption which begins on the face and spreads downward to the trunk and extremities
      a. Facial rash clears as extremity rash erupts; rash usually completely cleared by third or fifth day after initial presentation
      b. Lesions remain discrete and pink which contrasts with the rash of rubeola which is deep red and becomes confluent
   3. Lymphadenopathy is impressive with enlarged posterior auricular and suboccipital nodes
   4. Transient polyarthralgia and polyarthritis are common in adolescents and may occur in children
   5. Disease is usually self-limited and patient does not usually manifest any complications

E. Congenital Rubella
   1. Most common anomalies: eye (cataracts,retinopathy), heart (patent ductus arteriosus, pulmonary artery stenosis), sensorineural deafness and neurologic disorders (meningoencephalitis, mental retardation)
   2. Also, infants may have growth retardation, hepatosplenomegaly, thrombocytopenia and purple skin lesions

IV. Diagnosis/Evaluation

A. History
   1. Inquire about duration and occurrence of rash, fever, and enlarged lymph nodes which indicate rubella as well as other symptoms such as cough, coryza, conjunctivitis, pharyngitis which are associated with other exanthematous diseases
   2. Ask about recent exposure to persons with a rash
   3. Ask about medication and drug use
   4. Inquire about history of rubella illness and/or illnesses with exanthems (history of rubella illness is not a reliable indicator of immunity; identification of immune status is based on the presence of demonstrable antibody)

B. Physical Examination
   1. Measure vital signs
   2. Inspect skin, noting characteristics of exanthem
   3. To eliminate other exanthematous diseases as the diagnosis, examination of the following areas is often needed
      a. Eyes, noting signs of conjunctivitis
      b. Head, ears, nose, and throat
      c. Mouth for signs of Koplik's spots which indicate measles, not rubella
      d. Neck, noting nuchal rigidity and adenopathy
      e. Heart, noting murmurs associated with Kawasaki syndrome

C. Differential Diagnosis
   1. Rubeola
   2. Roseola
   3. Rocky Mountain spotted fever
   4. Scarlet fever
   5. Kawasaki syndrome
   6. Infectious mononucleosis
   7. Enterovirus
   8. Drug reaction

D. Diagnostic Tests
   1. Order acute (within 7-10 days after onset of disease) and convalescent sera (2-3 weeks later); a fourfold or greater rise in titer or seroconversion is indicative of infection
   2. Many virology laboratories can detect specific rubella IgM antibody (presence of this antibody indicates a recent postnatal infection or congenital infection in a neonate)

3. To determine immune status and presence of antibodies, order latex agglutination, fluorescence immunoassay, passive hemagglutination, hemolysis-in-gel or enzyme immunossay; the hemagglutination inhibition antibody test is not as sensitive and is no longer recommended
4. The virus may be isolated from the pharynx one week before until 2 weeks after exanthem; blood, urine, and cerebrospinal fluid can also yield virus

V. Plan/Management

A. Treatment: Patient's condition is usually mild and only symptomatic treatment is needed such as rest and increased fluid intake

B. Primary prevention of rubella
1. Rubella vaccine is recommended to be administered in combination with measles and mumps vaccine when child is 12-15 months of age and then a second dose at 4-6 years; persons who do not have dose at school entry should be given second dose at 11-12 years
2. Efforts should be made to vaccinate all postpubertal adolescent and adult males and females who have not been immunized or who have not been proven serologically to be immune to rubella
   a. Females should be counseled to avoid pregnancy for 3 months after vaccination
   b. Do not give vaccine in the 2 weeks before or 3 months after administration of immunoglobulin or blood
   c. Serious illness is a contraindication for vaccine, but minor illness with or without fever should not preclude vaccination

C. Treatment of exposed persons
1. Pregnant females need blood specimens tested for rubella antibody; consult specialist for further treatment of exposed pregnant females; routine use of immune globulin is not recommended and only considered if termination of pregnancy is not an option
2. Live rubella vaccine given after exposure does not prevent the disease, but may be indicated in nonpregnant persons for protection against developing rubella in the future

D. Control procedures
1. All cases of rubella and congenital rubella should be reported to the local health unit
2. In institutions such as hospitals, patients suspected of having rubella should be isolated
3. Patients should not go to work or school for 7 days after onset of rash; patients with congenital rubella should be considered contagious until they are one year old, unless nasopharyngeal and urine cultures after 3 months of age are repeatedly negative
4. Efforts should be made to identify and counsel all pregnant females who had contact with patient with infection

E. Follow up is usually not needed unless the patient must return for convalescent titers after 2-3 weeks of initial illness

RUBEOLA (MEASLES)

I. Definition: Acute, highly communicable viral disease consisting of fever, rash, and presence of cough, coryza or conjunctivitis

II. Pathogenesis

A. Causal agent is the measles virus which is an RNA virus

B. Transmitted between individuals by direct contact with infectious droplets, or less frequently, by air-borne spread

C. Incubation period is 8-12 days from exposure to onset of symptoms

D. Period of communicability: Patient is infectious 1-2 days before onset of symptoms and 3-5 days prior to rash to approximately 4 days after rash

III. Clinical Presentation

A. One of most serious exanthematous diseases

B. Prior to widespread immunization, measles were common in childhood; effective immunization programs have reduced rate by 99%

C. About 5% of all measles cases are due to vaccine failure

D. Center for Disease Control's clinical case definition is as follows:
1. Generalized rash lasting 3 or more days
2. Fever greater than 38.3°C (100.9°F)
3. At least one of the following symptoms: cough, coryza and conjunctivitis (sometimes referred to as the 3 "C"s)

E. Typically, patients have a prodrome with fever and the 3 "C"s which lasts between 1-4 days; patients are usually very ill during this time

F. As prodromal symptoms reach a peak, the exanthem appears and is characterized by the following:
1. Deep, red macular rash which begins on face and neck and spreads down trunk and extremities
2. Rash begins as discrete lesions but then becomes confluent and salmon-colored (referred to as a morbilliform rash)
3. When fever subsides, around the sixth day, a faint brown stain on the skin remains and desquamation of the skin often begins

G. Koplik's spots are pathognomonic for measles; this enanthem presents as tiny, bluish white spots on an erythematous base which cluster adjacent to the molars on the buccal mucosa

H. Most patients recover rapidly after the first 3-4 days

I. Complications are common occurring in approximately 1/3 of infected children <5 years old and include otitis media, pneumonia, croup, and encephalitis

IV. Diagnosis/Evaluation

A. History
1. Inquire about duration and occurrence of rash, cough, conjunctivitis, coryza and Koplik's spots
2. Explore the presence of other symptoms which denote complications of measles such as chest pain, ear pain and confusion
3. Ask about immunization status
4. Ask about recent exposure to persons with a rash
5. Inquire about medical history (immunosuppressed patients may need different treatment regimens; patients who are chronically ill often develop life-threatening symptoms)
6. Ask about medication use

B. Physical Examination
1. Measure vital signs
2. Inspect skin, noting characteristics of exanthem
3. Examine eyes, noting signs of conjunctivitis
4. Examine head, ears, nose, and throat because complications of measles often involve these parts of the body

5. Examine mouth for signs of Koplik's spots
6. Examine neck for adenopathy and nuchal rigidity
7. Auscultate heart
8. Patients need daily examination of chest to rule out complications such as pneumonia
9. Perform a mental status examination and a neurological exam to rule out complications such as encephalitis

C. Differential Diagnosis
1. Rubella
2. Roseola
3. Rocky Mountain spotted fever
4. Scarlet fever
5. Infectious mononucleosis
6. Secondary syphilis
7. Enterovirus
8. Drug reaction
9. Kawasaki syndrome

D. Diagnostic Tests: Order one of the following:
1. Antibody titers when rash first appears and then at convalescence or 2-4 weeks later (significant rise in antibody concentrations between acute and convalescent sera is characteristic of measles)
2. Serum IgM antibody levels (presence of measles-specific IgM antibodies is characteristic; IgM antibody peaks ten days after rash onset and disappears after 20 to 60 days)
3. Measles virus can be detected by viral isolation in cell culture from nasopharyngeal secretions, conjunctiva, blood or urine during the febrile period of illness

V. Plan/Management

A. The following patients should be considered for Vitamin A supplementation:
1. Patients with measles who live in communities where Vitamin A deficiency is a problem and where mortality related to measles is ≥1%
2. Children 6 months to 2 years of age who are hospitalized with measles and its complications
3. Patients > 6 months with measles who have one of the following risk factors:
   a. Immunodeficiency
   b. Ophthalmologic evidence of vitamin A deficiency including night blindness, Bitot's spots, or evidence of xerophthalmia
   c. Impaired intestinal absorption
   d. Moderate to severe malnutrition, including that associated with eating disorders
   e. Recent immigrants from areas where high mortality rates from measles have occurred
4. Recommended dose: Available in 50 000 IU/mL solution
   a. Single dose of 100 000 IU orally for children 6 months to 1 year of age
   b. Single dose of 200 000 IU orally for children 1 year of age and older
   c. Dose needs to be repeated the next day and at 4 weeks for children who have ophthalmologic evidence of vitamin A deficiency

B. Symptomatic Treatment
1. Provide rest and fluids
2. Instruct patient to avoid bright lights due to problems with photosensitivity
3. Frequently monitor for signs and symptoms of complications of measles

C. Treatment of exposed persons
1. Give live measles vaccine if exposure was within 72 hours (may give to infants as young as 6 months). Recommended dose is 0.5 mL, given subcutaneously
2. Give immune globulin to induce passive immunity and to prevent or modify symptoms within 6 days of exposure. Do not give immune globulin with the live measles vaccine
   a. Recommended dose of immune globulin is 0.25 mL/kg/dose IM (immunocompromised patients should receive 0.5 mL/kg). Maximum dose is 15 mL

173

     b.   Immune globulin is especially indicated for susceptible household contacts of measles, particularly immunocompromised contacts, and contacts younger than 1 year of age, and pregnant females

     c.   Live measles virus vaccine should be given approximately 5-6 months after immune globulin administration, provided patient is >12 months

D.   Primary prevention of measles:
1.   By 12 years of age all children should have had 2 doses of live measles immunization [doses on or after first birthday (12-15 months) and at school entry (4-6 years)]
2.   Anyone born after 1956 needs serological evidence of immunity or 2 documented measles immunizations

E.   Control Procedures
1.   Infected patients should be isolated for at least 4 days after appearance of rash
2.   Persons exposed to measles who are susceptible to developing the infection should be isolated from 5th day post-exposure up to and including the 21st day
3.   All reports of measles cases should be reported to the local health unit and investigated promptly
4.   All patients who cannot provide documentation of measles immunity should be vaccinated or excluded from school, work, or other public places
5.   Investigate immune status of family members and other immediate contacts; prescribe vaccine if appropriate

F.   Patient Education
1.   Teach patient to take daily temperature readings; fever lasting more than 4 days suggests presence of complications
2.   Teach patient and/or parents to monitor for signs of complications of measles such as how to count respirations and how to assess for changes in respiratory status and changes in level of consciousness

G.   Follow Up
1.   Patient with measles should be examined by health care provider (can be a nurse) every day during acute phase to rule out development of complications
2.   Patient should be seen in the clinic office about 3-4 days after onset of exanthem

SCARLET FEVER (SCARLATINA)

I.   Definition: Acute, infectious disease with vascular response to bacterial exotoxin and usually associated with streptococcal pharyngitis

II.   Pathogenesis

A.   Caused by circulating erythrogenic toxin that is produced by group A hemolytic *Streptococcus* and to a lesser extent, certain strains of staphylococci
1.   If streptococcus is the source of the toxin, it usually has a pharyngeal focus
2.   May rarely follow infection of wounds, burns or streptococcal or staphylococcal skin infections

B.   Mode of transmission is usually via direct projection of large droplets or physical transfer of respiratory secretions
1.   Rarely may be due to contaminated articles or ingestion of contaminated milk or other food
2.   Prolonged carriage of streptococci may occur in the throat or upper respiratory tract for weeks to months

C.   Incubation period usually ranges from 3-5 days

D.   Period of communicability: During incubation period and clinical illness or approximately 10 days; person is no longer infectious after 24 hours of antibiotic therapy

III.   Clinical Presentation

A.   In the past, disease had a high morbidity and mortality from systemic toxicity and the sequella of rheumatic fever and glomerulonephritis; complications less common today due to use of antibiotics

B.   Streptococcal infections are uncommon in children under 2 years of age; incidence highest in children 6-12 years of age but can occur in adulthood

C.   Usually an abrupt onset of fever, pharyngitis, and headache; less common is abdominal pain

D.   Exanthem appears 24-48 hours after infection and lasts 4-10 days
1.   Presents as fine, pin-head sized eruptions, often confluent, on an erythematous base which blanches on pressure
2.   Rash has the texture of sandpaper
3.   Rash rapidly becomes generalized but is typically absent on the face which usually has a flushed appearance with circumoral pallor
4.   Petechia may be present in a linear pattern along the major skin folds in the axillae and antecubital fossa (Pastia's sign)
5.   Rash fades 3-4 days after onset
6.   Desquamation of the skin usually occurs at the end of first week and usually disappears by end of 3 weeks

E.   Patient may have enanthem of a "strawberry" tongue which presents as a thick white coat with hypertrophied red papillae

F.   Staphylococcal scarlet fever can be differentiated from streptococcal scarlet fever in the following ways:
1.   There is no circumoral pallor or strawberry tongue
2.   The erythematous skin is often painful or tender
3.   Desquamation of the superficial epidermis occurs as with the streptococcal illness; if the superficial skin separates and sloughs after only a few days, the patient should be classified as having scalded skin syndrome

G.   Generalized lymphadenopathy is common in both streptococcal and staphylococcal scarlet fever

H.   Complications include otitis media, sinusitis, bacteremia, rheumatic fever, glomerulonephritis; rarely occur with prompt diagnosis and treatment

IV.   Diagnosis/Evaluation

A.   History
1.   Inquire about onset and duration of symptoms, particularly pharyngitis, rash, headache, fever, and abdominal pain
2.   Ask about any associated symptoms such as ear pain, chest pain, edema which may be related to complications of scarlet fever
3.   Inquire about the possibility of infected skin wounds
4.   Question whether other members of the household, classmates, or work colleagues have been ill with streptococcal pharyngitis or other communicable diseases
5.   Ask about medication history
6.   Ask about previous medical history
7.   Determine whether patient is allergic to penicillin

B. Physical Examination
   1. Measure vital signs
   2. Observe general appearance for signs of toxicity and respiratory distress
   3. Inspect skin; noting exanthem, Pastia's lines, facial flushing with circumoral pallor
   4. Palpate skin, noting any rough texture
   5. Perform a complete eyes, ears, nose, and mouth exam
   6. Perform a thorough examination of the pharynx, noting exudate, color, and swelling
   7. Perform a complete cardiovascular and chest exam
   8. Palpate abdomen for organomegaly

C. Differential Diagnosis
   1. Kawasaki disease is the eruption that needs to be most carefully differentiated from scarlet fever; Kawasaki has additional signs of conjunctivitis, cracking lips, and diarrhea
   2. Rubeola
   3. Rubella
   4. Infectious mononucleosis
   5. Toxic shock syndrome
   6. Drug reactions (sulfonamides, penicillin, streptomycin, quinine, and atropine)

D. Diagnostic Tests
   1. Obtain throat swab for rapid antigen test and a duplicate swab for a throat culture; if rapid test is positive, treat for streptococcal infection; if rapid test is negative, process throat culture
   2. Household contacts of index patient who have symptoms should be cultured, but do not culture asymptomatic household contacts unless there is an outbreak

V. Plan/Management: Treatment of scarlet fever is no different from that of streptococcal pharyngitis (see section on PHARYNGITIS)

A. Treatment of choice is penicillin oral or intramuscular:
   1. Adolescents: Penicillin V (Pen-Vee-K) 250 mg TID or QID for 10 days
   2. Children: Penicillin V (Pen-Vee-K) 40-60 mg/kg/day in 4 divided doses for 10 days. Available 125 mg/5 mL and 250 mg/5 mL liquids
   3. Benzathine penicillin 600,000 units for children <60 pounds, 900,000 units for children between 60-90 pounds, and 1.2 million units for children >90 pounds and adolescents. Be familiar with signs, symptoms and treatment of anaphylaxis and observe patient for 30 minutes after injection

B. Alternative antibiotics:
   1. Erythromycin: Adolescents prescribe (E-mycin): 250 mg q 6 hours for 10 days; Children prescribe (Eryped) 30-50 mg/kg/day in 4 divided doses
   2. Cefadroxil monohydrate (Duricef): Adolescents prescribe 500 mg capsules BID for 10 days; Children prescribe 30 mg/kg once a day or in 2 divided doses for 10 days. Available formulations include 125 mg/5mL, 250 mg/5 mL, and 500 mg/5mL suspensions

C. If staphylococcal scarlet fever is suspected, prescribe dicloxacillin (Dynapen) 15-20 mg/kg/day in divided doses every 6 hours for 10 days

D. Patient Education
   1. Discuss communicability of disease; patient should not return to work or school until at least 24 hours after beginning antimicrobial therapy
   2. Warn patient that skin desquamation may occur
   3. Assure family that rheumatic fever does not occur with appropriate antimicrobial therapy

E. Follow Up
   1. Posttreatment throat cultures are indicated only for patients who have a high risk for rheumatic fever or who are still symptomatic after treatment
   2. No follow up is needed for patients with uncomplicated illnesses

VARICELLA (CHICKENPOX)

I.   Definition: Viral disease with a pruritic, vesicular exanthem that appears in crops

II.   Pathogenesis

    A.   Causal agent is varicella-zoster virus (VZV) which is a member of the herpesvirus family

    B.   Transmission (highly contagious disease)
        1.   Primarily, spread by respiratory secretions which become airborne
        2.   Contact with fluid from vesicles can spread disease
        3.   Direct contact with patient with shingles may also spread the virus and cause chickenpox in the susceptible host

    C.   Incubation period is 10-21 days with an average of 14-16 days

    D.   Patient is communicable one to two days before the rash is apparent until all the vesicles have crusted, typically 5 days after onset of rash

III. Clinical Presentation

    A.   Commonly occurs in children between 5 and 10 years old, but is becoming more common in adolescents and young adults

    B.   In children, usually there is no prodrome or a mild prodrome with slight malaise and a low-grade fever

    C.   In adolescents the prodrome and illness are more severe and the course is prolonged; there also is a 25-fold increased risk of mortality

    D.   In both children and adolescents, a few hours to days after the prodrome a macular rash, typically on the scalp, neck or upper trunk emerges:
        1.   Exanthem occurs in stages: begins as macules, then turns to papules, and then to vesicles all within 12-24 hours
        2.   When vesicles begin to resolve, crusts develop
        3.   Rash spreads centrifugally (away from center) and lesions may occur on mucous membranes of mouth, conjunctivae, esophagus, trachea, rectum and vagina
        4.   Usually patient has little scarring unless infection of skin occurs

    E.   Certain groups of patients have more severe cases
        1.   Neonates and patients with leukemia may suffer severe, prolonged or fatal chickenpox
        2.   Older children and adolescents often have prolonged and severe illness
        3.   Immunocompromised children often have eruption of lesions and high fever for 2 weeks
        4.   AIDS patients may develop chronic chickenpox

    F.   Complications are uncommon but may include the following:
        1.   Secondary bacterial skin infection (*Group A Streptococcus* or *Staphylococcus aureus*), acute cerebellar ataxia, meningoencephalitis, thrombocytopenia, glomerulonephritis, and varicella pneumonia (which is rare in normal children, but the most common complication in older patients)
        2.   Reye syndrome was more common in the past due salicylate therapy

    G.   The virus remains in a latent form after the primary infection; zoster or shingles results with reactivation

IV.   Diagnosis/Evaluation

    A.   History
        1.   Ask patient to specifically describe when and where the first lesion occurred
        2.   Ask about the spread and changes that have occurred in the characteristics of the lesions
        3.   Ask about prodromal symptoms
        4.   Question about associated symptoms or potential complications such as pulmonary and nervous problems
        5.   Inquire about recent exposure to chickenpox
        6.   Ask about any self-treatments
        7.   Determine whether patient is immunocompromised or has any other risk factors
        8.   Ask whether any household contacts lack immunity to varicella and if there are immunocompromised individuals who were exposed to infected patient

    B.   Physical Examination
        1.   Observe skin and describe types of lesions, location of lesions, arrangement of lesions
        2.   Palpate for adenopathy
        3.   Auscultate heart and lungs
        4.   Perform a focused neurological examination

    C.   Differential Diagnosis
        1.   Scabies
        2.   Herpes simplex
        3.   Folliculitis
        4.   Viral exanthems such as coxsackievirus and echovirus have vesicles, but these vesicles do not usually crust as occurs in chickenpox
        5.   Contact dermatitis
        6.   Insect bites
        7.   Drug eruptions
        8.   Impetigo
        9.   Hand-foot-and-mouth disease
      10.   Secondary syphilis

    D.   Diagnostic Tests
        1.   Usually none needed
        2.   Immunofluorescent staining of vesicular scrapings from skin lesion with monoclonal antibodies can detect virus
        3.   To demonstrate a recent infection, can order acute and convalescent titers
        4.   Serologic tests include enzyme immuno-assay, latex agglutination, indirect fluorescent antibody, and fluorescent antibody-to-membrane antigen

V.   Plan/Management

    A.   Consider oral acyclovir therapy. Acyclovir (Zorvirax) therapy can reduce the rate of acute complications, pruritus, spread of infection, and duration of absence from school or work with no significant adverse effects if given within 24 hours of illness
        1.   Acyclovir therapy is <u>not</u> recommended routinely for treatment of uncomplicated varicella in otherwise healthy children but is used in healthy adolescents
        2.   Acyclovir is recommended, if it can be initiated within the first 24 hours after the onset or rash, in the following groups:
            a.   Otherwise healthy, nonpregnant individuals 13 years of age or older
            b.   Children older than 12 months with a chronic cutaneous or pulmonary disorder and those receiving long-term salicylate therapy
            c.   Children receiving short, intermittent or aerosolized course of corticosteroids (if possible, corticosteroids should be discontinued)
            d.   Some experts also suggest oral acyclovir for secondary household cases who typically have most severe infection
        3.   If therapy can be initiated within the first 24 hours of rash onset, prescribe oral acyclovir 20 mg/kg/dose in 4 divided doses for 5 days; maximum dose is 800 mg per dose QID. Patient should be maintained in a well-hydrated state

4. Intravenously administered acyclovir is recommended for treatment of immunocompromised patients
5. In the pregnant adolescent with uncomplicated varicella, oral acyclovir therapy is not advised, because of unknown risks to fetus. Intravenous therapy should be considered for pregnant females with serious viral mediated complications of varicella
6. Because of limited research, no recommendations for using oral acyclovir in infants less than 12 months can be made

B. Measures to control pruritus:
1. Can apply calamine or cetaphil lotion to lesions
2. Prescribe hydroxyzine (Atarax). Adolescent dosage is 25 mg TID/QID; in children prescribe 2 mg/kg/day in 3-4 divided doses (available in syrup 10 mg/5 mL)
3. Alternatively, can prescribe diphenhydramine HCl (Benadryl). Adolescent dosage is 25-50 mg TID/QID; in children, prescribe 5 mg/kg/day in 3-4 divided doses (Available as 12.5 mg/5 mL elixir)
4. Daily baths with baking soda or Aveeno may relieve pruritus and prevent bacterial superinfection
5. Cut patient's nails

C. Symptomatic treatment to reduce fever and discomfort: Use acetaminophen (Tylenol) (see section on FEVER for dosage); NEVER USE ASPIRIN IN CHILDREN AND ADOLESCENTS

D. Control Measures: Patients may return to school/work on the sixth day after the onset of the rash or in mild cases, after all the lesions are crusted

E. Care of Exposed Persons: Administration of varicella-zoster immune globulin (VZIG) within 72-96 hours after exposure to varicella may prevent or modify the disease (obtain VZIG from American Red Cross Blood Services)
1. VZIG should be given to the following persons if they have had signficant exposure such as residing in same household, indoor face-to-face contact, hospital contact:
   a. Immunocompromised persons known to be susceptible
   b. Susceptible, pregnant females
   c. Newborns whose mothers have had onset of varicella within 5 days before or within 2 days after delivery
   d. Hospitalized premature infant
      (1) ≥28 weeks gestation whose mother has no history of varicella or seronegativity
      (2) <28 weeks of gestation or ≤1000 g regardless of maternal history
   e. Dosage: One vial VZIG containing 125 units is given for each 10 kg of body weight. The maximum dose is 625 units or 5 vials
   f. Because of the availability of acyclovir, it is no longer recommended that normal adults who have close contact with infected patient use VZIG
2. Postexposure prophylactic administration of varicella vaccine is not FDA-approved but it may be effective in preventing or reducing clinical symptoms of the contact and carries little risk

F. Active or primary immunization is recommended for the following patients:
1. Children 12 months to 13th birthday
   a. 12-19 months: one dose for children who lack history of varicella
   b. 19 months to 13th birthday: one dose any time before 13th birthday who lack history of varicella or lack proof of vaccination
2. Healthy adolescents and adults: prescribe two doses of vaccine 4 to 8 weeks apart
3. Adults: vaccination of susceptible adults is encouraged (two doses 4-8 weeks apart); priority given to persons at high risk for complications such as health care personnel and family contacts of immunocompromised individuals, those at high risk for exposure, and non-pregnant females of child-bearing age

4. Vaccination is contraindicated in individuals with moderate to serious illness, immunocompromised persons, children receiving corticosteroids, persons with acute lymphocytic leukemia, and persons with allergies to vaccine component
   a. Salicylates should not be administered for 6 weeks and VZIG should not be given for 3 weeks after vaccine
   b. Vaccine should not be given for at least 5 months after patient has taken VZIG

G. Follow Up
   1. Teach patients to identify potential complications such as secondary skin infections, central nervous system problems, and pneumonia
   2. In uncomplicated cases, no follow up is needed

REFERENCES

American Academy of Pediatrics. (1997). Summaries of infectious diseases. In Peter, G. (Ed.). 1997 Red Book: Report of the committee on infectious diseases (24th ed.). Elk Grove Village, IL: Author.

American College of Physicians. (1997). Clinical guideline, part 1: Guideline for laboratory evaluation in the diagnosis of Lyme disease. Annals of Internal Medicine, 127, 1106-1108.

American College of Rheumatology and the Council of the Infectious Diseases Society of America (1993). Appropriateness of parenteral antibiotic treatment for patients with presumed Lyme disease. Annals of Internal Medicine, 119, 518.

Baraff, L.J, Bass, J.W., Fleisher, G.R., et al. (1993). Practice guidelines for the management of infants and children 0 to 36 months of age with fever without source. Pediatrics, 92, 1-12.

Castiglia, P.T. (1996). Kawasaki Disease. Journal of Pediatric Health Care, 10, 124-126.

Centers for Disease Control and Prevention. (1996). Prevention of varicella: Recommendations of the Advisory Committee on Immunization Practices. MMWR,45(No. RR-11), 1-27.

Centers for Disease Control and Prevention. (1997). Prevention and control of influenza: Recommendations of the Advisory Committee on Immunization Practices. MMWR, 46(No. RR-9), 1-25.

Committee on Infectious Diseases. American Academy of Pediatrics. (1993). Vitamin A treatment of measles. Pediatrics, 91(5), 1014-1015.

Cozad, J. (1996). Infectious mononucleosis. Nurse Practitioner, 21 (3), 14-28.

Daaleman, T.P. (1996). Fever without source in infants and young children. American Family Physician, 54, 2503-2512.

Dajani, A.S., Ayoub, E., Bierman, F.Z., Bisno, A.L., Denny, F.W., Durack, D.T., Ferrieri, P., Freed, M., Gerber, M., Kaplan, E.L., Karchmer, A.W., Markowitz, M., Rahimtoola, S.H., Shulman, S.T., Stollerman, G., Takahashi, M., Taranto, A., Taubert, K.A., & Wilson, W. (1993). Guidelines for the diagnosis of rheumatic fever: Jones criteria, updated 1992. Circulation, 87, 302-307.

Dajani, A., Taubert, K., Ferrieri, P., Peter, G., Shulman, S. and other committee members. (1995). Treatment of acute streptococcal pharyngitis and prevention of rheumatic fever: A statement for health professionals. Pediatrics, 96, 758-764.

Dajani, A.S., Taubert, K.A., Gerber, M.A., Shulman, S.T., Ferrieri, P., Freed, M., Takahashi, M., Bierman, F.Z., Karchmer, A.W., Wilson, W., Rahimtoola, S.H., Durack, D.T., & Peter, G. (1993). Diagnosis and therapy of Kawasaki disease in children. Circulation, 87, 1776-1780.

Dajani, A.S.,Taubert, K.A., Takahashi, M., Bierman, F.Z., Freed, M.D., Ferrieri, P., Gerber, M., Shulman, S.T., Karchmer, A.W., Wilson, W., Peter, G., Durack, D.T., & Rahimtoola, S.H. (1997). Guidelines for long-term management of patients with Kawasaki Disease: Report from the Committee on Rheumatic Fever, Endocarditis, and Kawasaki Disease, Council on Cardiovascular Disease in the Young, American Heart Association. Circulation, 89, 916-922.

Dajani, A.S.,Taubert, K.A., Wilson, W., Bolger, A.F., Bayer, A., Ferrieri, P., Gewitz, M., Shulman, S.T., Nouri, S., Newburger, J.W., Hutto, C. Pallasch, T.J., Gage, T.W. Levison, M.E., Peter, G., & Zuccaro, G. Jr. (1997). Prevention of bacterial endocarditis: Recommendations by the American Heart Association. JAMA, 277, 1794-1801.

Dattwyler, R.J., Luft, B.J., Kunkel, M.J., et al. (1997). Ceftriaxone compared with doxycycline for the treatment of acute disseminated Lyme disease. New England Journal of Medicine, 337, 289-294.

Habif, T.P. (1996). Clinical dermatology: A color guide to diagnosis and therapy (3rd ed.). St. Louis: Mosby.

Joffe, A., Kabani, A., & Jadavji, T. (1995). Atypical and complicated Kawasaki Disease in infants: Do we need criteria? Western Journal of Medicine, 162, 322-327.

Lopez, J.A., McMillin, K.J., Tobias-Merrill, E.A., & Chop, W.M., Jr. (1997). Managing fever in infants and toddlers: Toward a standard of care. Postgraduate Medicine, 101, 241-251.

McCarthy, P.L., Sharpe, M.R., Spiesel, Z., et al. (1982). Observation scales to identify serious illness in febrile children. Pediatrics, 70, 802-809.

Nightingale, S.L. (1997). Public health advisory: Limitations, use, and interpretation of assays for supporting clinical diagnosis of Lyme disease. JAMA, 278, 805.

Rubin, B., & Cotton, D.M. (1998). Kawasaki disease: A dangerous actue childhood illness. Nurse Practitioner, 23(2), 34-48.

Smith, D.L. (1997). Cat scratch disease and related clinical syndromes. American Family Physician, 55, 1783-1789.

Spach, D.H., Liles, W.C., Campbell, G.L., Quick, R.E., Anderson, D.E. & Fritsche, T.R. (1993). Tick-borne diseases in the United States. The New England Journal of Medicine, 329(13), 936-945.

Still, M.M., & Ryan, M.E. (1997). Pitfalls in diagnosis of Lyme disease. Postgraduate Medicine, 102, 65-72.

Straus, S.E., Cohen, J.E., Tosato, G., & Meier, J. (1993). Epstein-Barr virus infections: Biology, pathogenesis, and management. Annals of Internal Medicine, 118, 45-55.

Tugwell, P., Dennis, D.T., Weinstein, A., Wells, G., Shea, B., Nichol, G., Hayward, R., Lightfoot, R., Baker, P., & Steere, A.C. (1997). Clinical guideline, part 2: Laboratory evaluation in the diagnosis of Lyme disease. Annals of Internal Medicine, 127, 1109-1121.

Vernon, M.E., & Igal, L.H. (1997). Recognition and management of Lyme disease. American Family Physician, 56, 427-436.

Wilson, D. (1995). Assessing and managing the febrile child. Nurse Practitioner, 20,(11), 59-74.

Zangwill, K.M., Hamilton, D.H., Perkins, B.A. (1993). Cat scratch disease in Connecticut: Epidemiology, risk factors, and evaluation of a new diagnostic test. New England Journal of Medicine, 329, 8-13.

Skin Problems in Children

Fungal and Yeast Infections
Candidiasis
Tinea Versicolor
Dermatophyte Infections

Infestations and Bites
Scabies
Pediculosis (Lice Infestation)
Cutaneous Larva Migrans (Creeping Eruption)

Papulosquamous Disorders
Pityriasis Rosea

Disorders of Pigmentation
Pityriasis Alba
Café au Lait Spots

Viral Infections
Herpes Simplex
Molluscum Contagiosum
Warts

CARE OF DRY AND OILY SKIN

I.   Definition: Care aimed at preserving or restoring the normal physiologic state of the skin

II.   Pathogenesis

    A.   Dry skin results from reduced water content of the stratum corneum and may result from exposure to irritating substances (household/industrial chemicals), decreased humidity, and frequent or prolonged exposure to water

    B.   Oily skin is a result of excess sebum production by sebaceous glands which are largest and most numerous on face, chest, and upper back

III.   Clinical Presentation

    A.   Dry skin presents as scaly, dry appearing skin which feels dry to touch, and is most often located on extensor surfaces of legs and arms

    B.   Dry skin is sensitive (that is, easily irritated) and usually pruritic

    C.   Oily skin presents as moist appearing, shiny skin which feels oily to touch and is most often located on face, chest, and upper back

    D.   Oily skin may occur at any age, but is most common among adolescents

IV.   Diagnosis/Evaluation

    A.   History
        1.   Inquire about distribution, onset, duration
        2.   Ask about skin cleansing practices, occupational, and household exposures
        3.   Ask about treatments tried and results

    B.   Physical Examination
        1.   Examine entire skin surface
        2.   For patients complaining of dry skin, focus on legs, extensor surfaces, and hands, where drying is likely to be worse
        3.   For oily skin, focus on face, upper back, and chest

    C.   Differential Diagnosis
        1.   Atopic dermatitis
        2.   Contact dermatitis
        3.   Ichthyosis
        4.   Dyshidrotic eczema

    D.   Diagnostic Tests: None indicated

V.   Plan/Management

A.   For dry skin, the following recommendations should be provided to patients

---

ADVICE FOR PATIENTS WITH DRY SKIN

➡ Soak, rather than shower, immersed in water no warmer than 90° for 10 minutes (**Note:** Experts in previous years discouraged frequent bathing–daily soaking is now recommended for dry skin)

➡ Use a mild, non-drying synthetic detergent (syndet) bar such as Dove, Caress or Eucerin and rinse well

➡ A waterless liquid cleanser such as Cetaphil or Aquanil may also be used, especially for washing face

➡ Omit use of bubble baths and bath oils which pose hazard (falls)

➡ Pat skin dry–brush away excess water with hands, then pat or blot skin with towel

➡ Apply moisturizers from the following list after bathing and while skin is somewhat moist to seal moisture into skin

➡ **Note:** Lotions are the least moisturizing but the most acceptable to patients; ointments are the most moisturizing but patients dislike the greasy feel of ointments

Moisturizing Lotions	**Moisturizing Creams**	**Moisturizing Ointments**
Petrolatum-based	Petrolatum-based	Petrolatum-based
Dermasil	Purpose Dry Skin Cream	Vaseline Pure Petroleum Jelly
SML Lotion	Cetaphil Cream	(Fragrance, preservative, and
Moisturel Lotion	Keri Cream	lanolin free)
Replenaderm		
Mixtures of lanolin and petrolatum	Mixtures of lanolin and petrolatum	Mixtures of lanolin and petrolatum
Eucerin Lotion	Eucerin Creme	Aquaphor Natural Healing Ointment
Lubriderm Lotion		(Fragrance and preservative free)
Nivea Moisturizing	Without lanolin or petrolatum	
Without lanolin or petrolatum	Neutrogena Norwegian	
Corn Huskers Lotion	Formula Hand Cream	
Cetaphil Lotion		

B.   For patients with extremely dry skin, products containing urea may be helpful (**Note:** Urea removes excess adherent scales and make skin more pliable but use cautiously, as erythema and peeling may occur)

UREA CREAMS AND LOTIONS

Cream 10% (Aquacare, Nutraplus)
Cream 20% (Carmol 20)
Lotion 10% (Aquacare, Carmol 10)
Lotion 5% (Eucerin Plus)

C.   For oily skin, the following recommendations should be provided to patients

---

ADVICE FOR PATIENTS WITH OILY SKIN

➡ Use a deodorant soap such as Dial or Safeguard containing an antibacterial or a mildly drying soap (Ivory)

➡ Avoid using preparations containing oils

➡ Use an astringent or toner on face

➡ For adolescent girls, use cosmetics such as those listed here

---

Allercreme
  Matte-Finish Makeup
  (Waterbase, oil free)
Charles of the Ritz
  T-Zone Controller
Clinique
  Pore Minimizer Makeup
  (Fragrance and oil free)
  Stay True Oil-Free
  (For sensitive skin, SPF 15)
Covergirl
  Fresh Complexion, 100% Oil-Free
Estee Lauder
  Tender Matte Makeup
  (Fragrance and oil free)
  Simply Sheer
  Fresh Air Makeup Base, Oil-free

Lancome
  Maquicontrol, Oil-Free Liquid Makeup
Mary Kay cosmetics
  Oil-Free Foundation
  (Fragrance and oil-free)
Max Factor
  Shine-Free Makeup
Revlon
  Spring Water Matte Makeup
Shisheido
  Pureness Oil-Control Makeup

D.   Follow up: None indicated

BENIGN SKIN LESIONS OF INFANTS AND CHILDREN

I.   Definition: Cutaneous disorders commonly present in infants and children that are of no consequence in terms of the child's physical health

II.   Pathogenesis

   A.   Milia: Superficial epithelial cysts in the papillary dermis; the cyst cavity is filled with keratin

   B.   Mongolian spots: Spindle-shaped pigment cells located deep in dermis

   C.   Erythema toxicum: Associated with obstruction of the pilosebaceous orifice; unknown etiology

   D.   Raised hemangiomas (capillary and cavernous): Dilated proliferating capillaries and dilated venous channels

   E.   Flat hemangiomas (port-wine stains and nevus flammeus): Permanent dilation of mature capillaries

   F.   Freckles: Areas with increased pigment within epidermal cells without an increase in number of melanocytes

   G.   Lentigines: Increased numbers of melanocytes along the basal layer of the epidermis

III.   Clinical Presentation

BENIGN SKIN LESIONS IN INFANTS AND CHILDREN: CLINICAL PRESENTATION	
Milia	Multiple, white, 1-2 mm papules occurring on forehead, cheeks, and nose of infant Called Epstein's pearls when in oral cavity Up to 40% of newborns have on skin and 64% on palate Exfoliate and disappear a few weeks after birth
Mongolian spots	Blue-black macule found in lumbosacral area in up to 90% of African-American, Asian, Hispanic, and Native American infants Tend to fade with time and usually disappear by age 3 years
Erythema toxicum	Multiple 2-3 cm lesions with erythema and a tiny central papule or pustule resembling a flea bite (called flea-bite dermatitis) Occur on face, back, chest, and extremities of infants, sparing the face Fade spontaneously within 5-7 days
Raised hemangiomas	Capillary hemangiomas also called "strawberry hemangiomas," are characterized by marked vascular overgrowth that produces bright red elevated lesions ranging from 0.5-4.0 cm Cavernous hemangiomas are located deep beneath the surface of the skin and appear bluish in color Natural history of both types of raised hemangiomas is the same Usually not present at birth Emerge during early months of life Slowly involute so that 90% disappear by age 9 years
Flat hemangiomas	Port-wine stains are purplish-red discolorations of the skin present at birth A permanent discoloration that does not fade Does not enlarge but tends to remain stable and flat Most commonly located on face in unilateral distribution May be associated with Sturge-Weber syndrome Nevus flammeus, also called "salmon patch" are light red splotchy areas seen in 40% of newborns and considered a normal variant Usually located on nape of neck, the glabella, forehead, or upper eyelids Usually more apparent with episodes of crying Tend to fade by age 1 year
Freckles	Small, 1-5 mm light brown pigmented macules that occur in UVL exposed skin Most frequent in light-haired, blue-eyed children and adults Autosomal dominant and first appear at ages 3-5 years
Lentigines	Small 1-2 mm brown to brown-black macules found sparsely scattered over body including mucous membranes Do not appear with sun exposure First appear during school age and number about 30 in any one individual

IV.   Diagnosis/Evaluation

 A.   History
  1.   Ask about onset, location, and a description of the lesion
  2.   Ask if there are any associated symptoms
  3.   Inquire about treatments tried and results

 B.   Physical Examination
  1.   Examine the entire skin surface
  2.   Use good lighting and magnification if needed

 C.   Differential Diagnosis
  1.   Milia: Molluscum contagiosum (does not appear in immediate neonatal period)
  2.   Mongolian spots: Bruising secondary to trauma
  3.   Erythema toxicum: Herpes simplex and bacterial folliculitis (exclude with Gram's stain, cultures, and Tzanck smear)

 D.   Diagnostic Tests: None indicated

V. Plan/Management

    A.   Milia: No treatment needed; reassure parents that normal variation which disappears in weeks

    B.   Mongolian spots: No treatment needed; reassure parents that normal variation which disappears over months

    C.   Erythema toxicum: No treatment necessary as eruption fades spontaneously within 5-7 days

    D.   Raised hemangiomas
        1.   No treatment necessary given the natural history of involution
        2.   If obstruction of vital orifice, refer for treatment

    E.   Flat hemangiomas
        1.   Port wine stains: Refer for treatment with pulsed dye laser which can begin in infancy
        2.   Nevus flammeus: No treatment necessary as fades by 1 year of age

    F.   Freckles and lentigines: No treatment necessary

    G.   Follow Up: None indicated for these benign conditions

ACNE VULGARIS

I.   Definition: A disease of the pilosebaceous unit that is most intense in areas where sebaceous glands are numerous

II.   Pathogenesis

    A.   A number of factors and events work in concert to make the pathogenesis of acne multifactorial in nature

    B.   Excessive sebum produced by the androgen-dependent sebaceous glands, combined with excessive numbers of desquamated cells from the walls of the sebaceous follicles cause obstruction of the follicles (which are located primarily on the face and trunk)

    C.   As a consequence of this obstruction, a microcomedo is formed that may eventually evolve into either a comedo or an inflammatory lesion

    D.   A resident anaerobic organism, Propionibacterium acnes (found in very low numbers on normal skin) finds the environment created by the excessive sebum and desquamated follicular cells very conducive to growth and produces chemotactic factors and proinflammatory mediators that may lead to inflammation

III.   Clinical Presentation

    A.   Acne is the most common skin disorder, affecting almost 80% of persons at some point in their lives, most often between the ages of 11 and 30
        1.   Acne begins in the pre-pubertal period when the adrenal glands begin secreting increased amounts of adrenal androgens which leads to increased production of sebum
        2.   Androgen production and sebaceous gland activity are further stimulated with gonad development during puberty

B. Most patients with acne are probably hyperresponsive to androgens rather than overproducers of androgens; androgen excess, however, has been implicated in the development of acne

C. **Comedonal acne** represents the **earliest** clinical expression of acne, occurring in the pre-teen and early teenage years
   1. Characteristic lesions are noninflammatory comedones located on central forehead, chin, nose, paranasal area
   2. Comedones are open (blackheads) or closed (whiteheads)
   3. Colonization with *P. acnes* has not yet occurred; thus, no inflammatory lesions are present

D. **Mild inflammatory acne** usually develops in teenagers **after the first phase** of non-inflammatory comedonal acne; also occurs in adult women in their 20s
   1. Characterized by scattered small papules or pustules with a minimum of comedones
   2. Arises from microcomedones in which two factors are present
      a. Abnormal desquamation of epithelial cells in the follicles
      b. Proliferation of *P. acnes*

E. **Inflammatory acne** represents the **final** phase in the evolution of acne from noninflammatory comedonal acne, to small numbers of inflammatory lesions on the face, to a more generalized eruption, first on the face, and then on the trunk
   1. Most patients with acne have inflammatory acne, with comedones, papules, and pustules on the face and trunk
   2. In a minority of patients, large, deep inflammatory nodules (called cysts) develop reflecting the presence of a very destructive type of inflammation
   3. Cystic acne requires prompt attention since ruptured cysts may result in scar formation

IV. Evaluation/Diagnosis

A. History
   1. Question regarding onset, type of lesions, distribution
   2. In females, question about history of cyclic menstrual flares, use of oral contraceptives
   3. Inquire about types of cleansers and lubricants used on face
   4. Document previous treatments and results

B. Physical Examination
   1. Examine skin to determine form of acne:
      a. Comedonal acne--noninflammatory comedones
      b. Mild inflammatory acne--scattered small papules or pustules with a minimum of comedones
      c. Inflammatory acne -- comedones, papules, and pustules on the face and trunk
      d. Inflammatory acne with large, deep inflammatory nodules
   2. Determine areas of involvement
   3. Use chart such as the one below to document location, type, and number of lesions during initial and follow up visits:

CHART OF ACNE LESIONS BY TYPE, NUMBER, AND VISIT			
Location		Date of Visit	
1:_____ 2:_____		3:_____ 4:_____	
R Cheek			
L Cheek			
Forehead			
Nose			
Chin			
Other (Back/Chest)			

C. Differential Diagnosis
1. Rosacea
2. Steroid Rosacea
3. Molluscum contagiosum
4. Folliculitis

D. Diagnostic Tests: None indicated

V. Plan/Management

A. Explain the mechanism of acne and treatment plan to the patient
1. Emphasize that little improvement may be evident for 2-3 months
2. Use written patient education materials to reinforce teaching

B. Counsel patient regarding the following general measures:
1. Wash affected area gently with mild soap (Purpose, Basis) no more than 2-3 x day (emphasize that use of topical agents such as soaps and astringents have no effect on sebum production but only remove sebum from the surface of the skin which has little value therapeutically)
2. Avoid picking at lesions to prevent scarring
3. Avoid oil-based cosmetics, hair styling mousse, and face creams which have no effect sebum production but do increase the amount of oil on the face
4. Use cleansers such as Cetaphil lotion, nonacnegenic moisturizers such as Moisturel, and cosmetics from the table that follows

---

NONACNEGENIC COSMETICS FOR ADOLESCENT GIRLS

Allercreme
    Matte-Finish Makeup
    (Waterbase, oil free)
Charles of the Ritz
    T-Zone Controller
Clinique
    Pore Minimizer Makeup
    (Fragrance and oil free)
    Stay True Oil-Free
    (For sensitive skin, SPF 15)
Covergirl
    Fresh Complexion, 100% Oil-Free
Estee Lauder
    Tender Matte Makeup
    (Fragrance and oil free)
    Simply Sheer
    Fresh Air Makeup Base, Oil-free
	Lancome
	    Maquicontrol, Oil-Free Liquid Makeup
	Mary Kay cosmetics
	    Oil-Free Foundation
	    (Fragrance and oil-free)
	Max Factor
	    Shine-Free Makeup
	Revlon
	    Spring Water Matte Makeup
	Shisheido
	    Pureness Oil-Control Makeup

5. Dietary factors have no effect on sebum production; thus patient should be counseled to eat a normal, well-balanced diet

C. Treatment of acne is outlined in the following table

TREATMENT OF ACNE

Treatment Aims	Treatment	Comments

Reduce or counteract abnormal desquamation of follicular epithelium	**Comedonal Acne**
	
	Topical comedolytic agents are the treatment of choice
	Select a comedolytic agent from the following list
	
	Comedolytic agents
	
	Topical tretinoin (Retin-A) available as cream, gel, or liquid
	  Cream: 0.025, 0.05, and 0.1% concentrations, supplied as 20 g, 45 g
	  Gel: 0.01, 0.025% concentrations, supplied as 15 g, 45 g
	  Liquid: 0.05% concentration, supplied as 28 mL
	
	Apply QD, at bedtime, beginning with a lower concentration of the cream, gel, or liquid and increasing if local irritation does not occur
	(Note: Considered the standard against which all other comedolytics are judged)
	
	Adapalene (Differin), [a naphthoic derivative with retinoid activity] available as gel or solution
	  Gel: 0.1%, supplied as 15g, 45g
	  Solution: 0.1%, supplied as 30 mL
	
	Apply QD at bedtime, beginning with a lower concentration of the solution or gel, and increasing if local irritation does not occur
	(Note: Causes less irritation than topical tretinoin and is often effective in patients who cannot tolerate topical tretinoin)
	
	Azelaic acid (Azelex) [has both comedolytic and antibacterial effects], available as cream (one concentration only); supplied as 30 g
	Apply BID, in the morning and evening to clean dry skin
	(Note: Also causes less irritation than tretinoin; may cause hypopigmentation which may be desirable for some patients)
		Advise patient to apply thin layer of the topical agent to the entire face, not just the individual lesions
		Warn about increased photosensitivity--patient must apply sunscreen daily for any sun exposure
		Gels are usually preferred in hot/humid climates and creams in cold/dry climates
		Several months may be necessary to achieve good results
		Treatment should be continued until no new lesions are developing

(continued)

Treatment Aims	Treatment	Comments
	Mild Inflammatory Acne	
Reduce or counteract abnormal desquamation of follicular epithelium	Topical therapy with a combination of a comedolytic **and** an antibiotic is the treatment of choice	Most patients respond to treatment after 2-4 weeks
Prevent proliferation of *P. acnes*	Select a comedolytic agent from the list above	Treatment should be continued until no new lesions develop, then slowly discontinued
	Select an antibiotic agent from the list below	
	(**Note:** When used in combination, **once** daily dosing for the comedolytic and the antibiotic is acceptable; each product should be used at separate time of day: Use comedolytic in AM and antibiotic in the PM. **The BID dosing schedule for both comedolytic and antibiotic agents in the lists given here are the dosing recommendations when the agents are used alone!**)	
	Topical Antibiotics	
	Benzoyl peroxide, (Benzac) available as a gel with alcohol-base in 5, 10% concentrations; also available as aqueous-base gel (Benzac-W) in 2.5, 5, 10% concentrations	
	Both products supplied as 60 g	
	Apply QD to clean, dry skin	
	(**Note:** Very effective anti-P. acnes agent; major disadvantage is irritation which can be minimized by using lower concentrations and water-base form)	
	Erythromycin, 2% solution (A/T/S) and gel (A/T/S GEL) [alcohol base]	
	Supplied as solution--60 mL and gel--30g	
	Apply BID to clean, dry skin	
	Clindamycin, 1% (Cleocin-T) available as solution, pads, lotion, and alcohol-base gel	
	Supplied as solution--30, 60 mL; pads--boxes of 60; lotion--60 mL; gel--30 g, 60 g	
	Apply BID to clean, dry skin	
	Benzoyl peroxide plus erythromycin (Benzamycin), contains 3% erythromycin and 5% benzoyl peroxide in gel form (alcohol base)	
	Supplied as gel--23.3 g, 46.6 g	
	Apply BID to clean, dry skin	
	(**Note:** Considered by experts to be the **most effective** topical antibiotic therapy against *P. acnes*)	

(continued)

193

TREATMENT OF ACNE (CONTINUED)

Treatment Aims	Treatment	Comments
Reduce or counteract abnormal desquamation of follicular epithelium Prevent proliferation of *P. acnes* and the resultant inflammation produced by the organism	**Inflammatory Acne** Topical therapy with comedolytic and systemic antibiotic therapy Select a comedolytic agent from list above Select an antibiotic from the following list **Oral antibiotics** Doxycycline (Vibramycin), available as 50, 100 mg caps 100 mg BID x 1 day, then 50 mg BID; dose can be reduced to 50 mg QD after improvement Minocycline (Minocin), available as 50, 100 mg caps 50 mg BID; dose can be reduced to 50 mg QD after improvement (**Note:** Above two agents are more lipid-soluble than tetracycline and erythromycin and are generally considered to be more effective than tetracycline and erythromycin) Tetracycline (Achromycin V), available as 250, 500 mg caps 1 gram/day in 2 divided doses, then 125-500 mg/day with further reduction after improvement Erythromycin (E-Mycin), available as 250, 333 mg tabs 500 mg BID or 333 mg BID, with reduction after improvement	Deciding between topical and systemic antibiotics should be guided by two factors: Extent of skin involvement and severity of inflammation **Do not use tetracycline derivatives** in pregnant women, nursing mothers, or children under the age of 12 Patients treated with oral antibiotics may also be given topical antibiotics once the oral dose is reduced to a maintenance level

194

D. Refer patients with widespread, nodular cystic lesions to a dermatologist for treatment aimed at therapy to suppress sebum production

E. Follow Up: Three follow up visits (over 8-10 weeks) are generally needed to establish a successful treatment program
    1. For patients with comedonal and mild inflammatory acne on topical agents:
        a. Use chart to document location, type, and number of lesions to determine treatment response on each visit
        b. Adjust strength and frequency of topical agents depending on irritation and effectiveness
        c. If skin dryness is a problem that interferes with compliance, suggest use of a nonacnegenic moisturizer such as Moisturel, Purpose lotion, or Neutrogena Moisture after application of gel, or switch to a cream preparation
    2. For patients with inflammatory acne using topical comedolytics as well as **oral** antibiotics:
        a. Do a., b., and c. in E.1. above
        b. Begin tapering oral antibiotic dose by 4-6 weeks into treatment (depending upon when development of new inflammatory lesions ceases); once the oral dose is reduced to a maintenance level, can add topical antibiotics to provide control
        c. Most patients require prolonged courses (months) or frequent, intermittent courses before complete and final remission occurs. **Consult PDR regarding need to monitor blood, renal, and hepatic function in patients on long-term antibiotic use!**
    3. For patients who are not on a successful treatment program after a total of 10-12 weeks of therapy, referral to a dermatologist is indicated

ATOPIC DERMATITIS

I. Definition: Extremely pruritic inflammatory skin disorder involving cutaneous hypersensitivity that is chronic or chronically relapsing

II. Pathogenesis

A. Exact pathogenesis is unknown, but abnormalities of the immune system have been documented with contributions of IgG-medicated inflammation, other pro-inflammatory mechanisms, and immunoregulatory dysfunction

B. Epidermal barrier dysfunction and increased genetic susceptibility are also believed to be causative factors

III. Clinical Presentation

A. Approximately 90% of affected persons have age of onset between 6 weeks and 5 years of age; occasionally, age of onset is in later childhood or less often, in adulthood

B. Abnormally dry skin and lowered threshold for itching are significant factors

C. Itching occurs in paroxysms and may be severe, especially in evenings; once itch-scratch cycle is established, characteristic lesions are created

D. Some children are chronically affected while others have disease-free periods between exacerbations

E. Patterns of inflammation begin with severe pruritus and erythema. As skin changes are produced by scratching, skin becomes dry and scaly (xerosis)

F. Several patterns of lesions may be produced: erythematous papular lesions that become confluent; diffuse erythema and scaling; lichenification (thickening of dermis with accentuation of skin lines)

G. A personal or family history of atopy (asthma or allergic rhinitis) is usually present

H. Atopic dermatitis is divided into 3 phases which are outlined in the following table

ATOPIC DERMATITIS	
Infant phase (birth to 2 years)	Usually appears at about 3 months of age especially during cold, dry weather Erythema and scaling of cheeks, chin with sparing of perioral and paranasal areas is frequently seen and there is sparing of the diaper area as well. May have generalized eruption of papules that are erythematous and scaly Exudative lesions (oozing, weeping) are typical in infancy
Childhood phase (2-12 years)	Characteristic appearance at this age is flexural area involvement; perspiration produced by act of flexing and extending stimulates itching and itch-scratch cycle Erythematous papules coalesce into plaques and scratching produces lichenification Exudative lesions are seen less frequently
Adult phase (12 years to adult)	New onset as adult is rare Onset of puberty may be associated with exacerbation Localized inflammation of flexural areas with lichenification is most common pattern Hand dermatitis occurs much more frequently in the adult phase

IV. Diagnosis/Evaluation

A. History
   1. Inquire about personal or family history of atopy -- allergic rhinitis, asthma, atopic dermatitis -- and age of onset
   2. Question about itching, appearance and distribution of lesions, if dermatitis is chronic or chronically relapsing
   3. Question regarding hand dermatitis
   4. Ask about routine skin care at home including frequency of bathing and products used

B. Physical Examination
   1. Have patient disrobe completely
   2. Examine the skin methodically and determine the extent of the eruption and its distribution
   3. Determine the primary lesion and the nature of the secondary lesions
   4. Examine flexural areas for erythema and scaling but also look for lichenification in these areas
      a. Examine the hands. Look for erythema and scaling on dorsal aspects of hands
      b. Look for dry, fissured fingertip pads

C. Differential Diagnosis
   1. Contact dermatitis, irritant or allergic
   2. Seborrheic dermatitis
   3. Nummular dermatitis
   4. Scabies
   5. Tinea

D. Diagnostic Tests: None indicated

V. Plan/Management

A. Emphasize to patient that this is a chronic condition and exacerbating factors must be controlled for successful management

B. Counsel patient how to control exacerbating factors using guidelines in the following table

---

KEYS TO REDUCING OR ELIMINATING FACTORS THAT PROMOTE DRYNESS AND INCREASE DESIRE TO SCRATCH

- Keep environment slightly cool and well humidified (home or office humidifiers)
- Avoid frequent hand washing
- Daily soaks in tepid water using syndet bars such as Dove or soap substitutes such as Cetaphil or Aquanil is acceptable
- Wear 100% cotton clothing; avoid wool and synthetics
- Use fragrance-free laundry products such as Ivory Snow Flakes, Cheer-Free
- Recognize that emotional stress can worsen but not cause the disorder

---

C. Systematic lubrication of the skin must be done daily
1. Bathing should always be followed by immediate application of emollients applied after patting the skin dry
2. Remind patient to lubricate skin more frequently during winter months
3. Recommend moisturizers from the table below
4. Lotions are the least moisturizing but the most acceptable to patients; ointments are the most moisturizing but patients dislike the greasy feel of ointments

---

RECOMMENDED MOISTURIZERS

Moisturizing Lotions
Petrolatum-based
  Dermasil
  Moisturel Lotion
  Replenaderm Lotion

Mixtures of lanolin and petrolatum
  Eucerin Lotion
  Lubriderm Lotion
  Nivea Moisturizing Lotion

Without lanolin or petrolatum
  Corn Huskers Lotion
  Cetaphil Lotion

Moisturizing Creams
Petrolatum-based
  Purpose Dry Skin Cream
  Cetaphil Cream
  Keri Cream

Mixtures of lanolin and petrolatum
  Eucerin Creme

Without lanolin or petrolatum
  Neutrogena Norwegian Formula Hand Cream

Moisturizing Ointments
Petrolatum-based
  Vaseline Pure Petroleum Jelly
  (Frangrance, preservative, and lanolin free)

Mixtures of lanolin and petrolatum
  Aquaphor Natural Healing Ointment
  (Fragrance and preservative free)

D. To reduce inflammation, may use topical corticosteroids applied thinly 2x/day until controlled (up to 7 days); creams are the preferred formulation
1. Hydrocortisone cream 2.5% (use 1% on face and intertriginous areas) [**Note:** Systemic absorption of topical corticosteroids in infants and children can cause growth retardation and hypothalamic-pituitary-adrenal axis suppression!]
2. Apply lubricant to inflamed area 3-4x/day also
3. Once inflammation is controlled, continue frequent daily use of emollients only
4. Use the topical corticosteroid of the lowest potency that will control the condition

E. Pruritus control is important for all patients (see following table)

PRURITUS CONTROL USING PHARMACOLOGIC INTERVENTIONS
Oral Antihistamines
Hydroxyzine (Atarax), supplied as 10 mg/5mL syrup and 10, 25, 50, 100 mg tablets
Infants and children, 0.5 mg/kg/dose TID PRN
Adolescents, 25-50 mg/dose TID PRN
A single dose at bedtime is frequently all that is necessary
Oral Antihistamines for Use in the Daytime (Nonsedating)
Loratidine (Claritin) may be used in children ≥6 years of age
Begin with 10 mg every other day; then 10 mg/day
Supplied as Claritin Reditabs, 10mg, which are dissolved on tongue and swallowed with or without water
Supplied also as Claritin syrup, 1mg/1mL (alcohol free, dye free)
Important to prescribe nonsedating antihistamines for patients who attend school or who have other daytime responsibilities that require alertness
Topical Antipruritic Agents
Sarna lotion, Prax lotion and Itch-X gel are all OTC products
Cetaphil with menthol 0.25% and phenol 0.25% is an Rx product
Topical agents may be used in addition to or instead of oral antihistamines

F.   Counsel patient to avoid exposure to chemicals, and to use gloves for protection when engaging in "wet work"

G.   Consider referral to a specialist for patients who have severe skin eruptions or for those who do not respond to conservative treatment after a 2 week trial

H.   Follow up visit should be monthly, then every 3 months until using lubricants only, then every 6 months
      1.   Patient should understand that this is a chronic, recurrent disorder and should be offered practical counseling on each visit regarding ways to deal with the disorder
      2.   Reliable patients should be given ample refills of topical corticosteroids so that they can control the condition themselves (if there is not a concern about overuse/inappropriate use)

DYSHIDROSIS (POMPHOLYX)

I.   Definition: A disease of unknown etiology that disrupts the skin of the palms and soles

II.   Pathogenesis

    A.   The name dyshidrosis implies, incorrectly, an abnormality of sweating

    B.   The cause of dyshidrosis is unknown, but there may be some relationship to stress

III.   Clinical Presentation

    A.   Condition is characterized by itchy vesicles on the palms, side of fingers, and soles (acute phase)

    B.   After 3-4 weeks vesicles slowly resolve, and are replaced by scaling, redness, and lichenification (chronic phase)

    C.   Waves of vesiculation may occur

    D.   Moderate to severe itching usually precedes the emergence of the vesicles

IV.   Diagnosis/Evaluation

    A.   History
        1.   Question about location of lesions, onset, duration, and changes in lesions over time
        2.   Ask about associated symptoms
        3.   Inquire about skin allergies
        4.   Ask about treatments tried and results

    B.   Physical Examination
        1.   Examine lesions looking for vesicles, or if the acute process has ended, exfoliation of skin revealing a red, cracked base
        2.   Examine all skin areas to determine if vesicles are located in areas other than palms and soles

    C.   Differential Diagnosis
        1.   Contact dermatitis
        2.   Tinea
        3.   Atopic dermatitis
        4.   Pustular psoriasis of palms and soles (with this disease, vesicles are cloudy with purulent fluid and pain is the chief complaint); referral is needed

    D.   Diagnostic Tests: Skin patch testing for cell mediated allergy may be arranged if problem perseveres or if allergy is suspected

V.   Plan/Management

    A.   Topical corticosteroids: Triamcinolone acetonide cream, 0.025% (Aristocort cream, 0.025%) TID x 14 days **AND**

    B.   Oral antibiotics:
        1.   Adolescents: Erythromycin (as base) [E-Mycin] 250 mg QID x 10 days
        2.   Children: Erythromycin (as ethylsuccinate) suspension [Eryped], 200 mg/5 mL, 400 mg/5 mL; give 30 mg/kg/day, divided into 4 doses x 10 days. Also available in 200 mg chewable tablets **AND**

    C.   Cold wet compresses: Apply cold, sopping wet compresses (consisting of 4-8 layers) to affected area; leave in place at least 30 minutes; repeat 3-4 x day

    D.   Follow up: None indicated

CONTACT DERMATITIS

I.   Definition: Skin inflammation due to irritants (irritant contact dermatitis) or allergens (allergic contact dermatitis)

II.   Pathogenesis

    A.   Irritant contact dermatitis
        1.   Damage to one of the components of the water-protein-lipid matrix of the outer layer of the epidermis of the skin caused by irritants including chemicals, dry, cold air, and friction
        2.   An eczematous response in the skin is produced that is nonallergic in origin

B. Allergic contact dermatitis
1. A form of cell mediated immunity that occurs in 2 phases
2. The sensitization phase which occurs when allergens penetrate the epidermis and produce proliferation of T lymphocytes (sensitization phase; can take days or months)
3. In the elicitation phase, the antigen-specific T lymphocytes present in the skin combine with the subsequent exposures to the allergen to produce inflammation

III. Clinical Presentation

A. Irritant contact dermatitis
1. Intensity of inflammation is related to the concentration of the irritant and the exposure time
2. Everyone is at risk for the dermatitis, but people vary in their response to the irritant
3. Frequent hand washing with harsh detergents is a very common cause
4. Mild irritants cause erythema, dryness, and fissuring
5. Chronic exposure can cause oozing, weeping lesions
6. Irritant diaper dermatitis is a common dermatitis in infants

B. Allergic contact dermatitis
1. A genetically predisposed hypersensitivity reaction
2. May correspond exactly to contactant (e.g., fabric treatments, clothing, nickel in jewelry)
3. Poison ivy, oak, and sumac produce more cases of allergic contact dermatitis than all other contactants combined
   a. Observe for highly characteristic sharply demarcated linear lesions caused from leaves brushing skin or from streaking oleoresin when scratching
   b. Classic lesions are vesicles and blisters on erythematous base
   c. Diffuse patterns may occur when oleoresin is contacted from contaminated pets or smoke from burning plants

C. Distribution often provides clues to diagnosis
1. Scalp and ears: Hair care products, jewelry
2. Eyelids: Cosmetics, contact lens solution
3. Face/neck: Cosmetics, cleansers, medications, jewelry
4. Trunk/axilla: Clothing, deodorants
5. Arms/hands: Poison oak, ivy, sumac, soaps, detergents, frequent hand washing chemicals, jewelry, rubber gloves
6. Legs/feet: Clothing, shoes
7. Preservatives in OTC and prescriptive topical products may produce dermatitis at area of application

IV. Diagnosis/Evaluation

A. History
1. Question regarding location of eruption, time and rate of onset (abrupt or insidious), and associated symptoms such as pruritus
2. Ask about occupation and recreational pursuits
3. Question regarding exposures to such substances as chemicals, detergents, medications, poison plants, lubricants, cleansers, and rubber gloves, both at home and at work or in recreational pursuits
4. Obtain family history, personal history of allergies, treatments tried and results

B. Physical Examination
1. Examine skin to determine the location of the inflammation
2. Determine the primary lesion
3. Determine the distribution of the eruption as a clue to diagnosis

C. Differential Diagnosis
    1. Atopic dermatitis (usually more chronic, occurs in flexural distribution, onset in childhood)
    2. Scabies (usually begins in fingerwebs, wrists, spreading to groin, axilla; other household contacts are symptomatic)
    3. Nummular dermatitis (discrete, coin-shaped, erythematous, scaling plaques)
    4. Dermatitis herpetiformis (usually localized to elbows, knees, buttocks, posterior scalp)

D. Diagnostic Tests: None indicated

V. Plan/Management

A. For both types of contact dermatitis, the first step in management is to identify the offending agent and limit or eliminate further exposure

B. Pruritus control is important for all patients

PRURITUS CONTROL USING PHARMACOLOGIC AND NONPHARMACOLOGIC INTERVENTIONS

Oral Antihistamines

Hydroxyzine (Atarax), supplied as 10 mg/5mL syrup and 10, 25, 50, 100 mg tablets
Infants and children, 0.5 mg/kg/dose TID PRN
Adolescents, 25-50 mg/dose TID PRN
A single dose at bedtime is frequently all that is necessary

Oral Antihistamines for Use in the Daytime (Nonsedating)

Loratidine (Claritin) may be used in children ≥6 years of age
Begin with 10 mg every other day; then 10 mg/day
Supplied as Claritin Reditabs, 10 mg, which are dissolved on tongue and swallowed with or without water
Supplied also as Claritin syrup, 1 mg/1mL (alcohol free, dye free)

Important to prescribe nonsedating antihistamines for patients who attend school or who have other daytime responsibilities that require alertness

Topical Antipruritic Agents

Sarna lotion, Prax lotion and Itch-X gel are all OTC products
Cetaphil with menthol 0.25% and phenol 0.25% is an Rx product
Topical agents may be used in addition to or instead of oral antihistamines

Nonpharmacologic Treatment Modalities to Soothe Itchy Skin

Cool tub baths with or without colloidal oatmeal can provide relief
Topical compresses (washcloths wet with plain water and kept in freezer) can be applied to affected skin for 15-20 minutes, 3-4 x day

---

C. When skin involvement is limited but the dermatitis is moderate, not mild, treatment with topical corticosteriods is indicated
    1. Children ≥6 years of age: Prescribe intermediate potency preparation such as Triamcinolone 0.1% cream
        a. Apply thin layer of cream 2 x daily; do not occlude
        b. Maximum 7 days of treatment
        c. Do not use on face, groin, or axillary area; use hydrocortisone 1% cream on these areas
        d. Always exclude viral disease before use of a topical steroid
    2. When skin involvement is generalized, the face and groin areas are involved, and pruritus is poorly controlled with topical therapies, use of an oral corticosteroid may be indicated in adolescents
        a. Prednisone: 50 mg/day x 2 days, 45 mg/day x 2 days, 40 mg/day x 2 days, 30 mg/day x 2 days, 20 mg/day x 2 days, 10 mg/day for 2 days, and 5 mg/day x 2 days (for a total of 14 days of treatment)
        b. Avoid dose packs as dosage is usually inadequate
    3. Infants and children with generalized dermatitis should be referred to a specialist for management

D. Follow Up
    1. None indicated if dermatitis is mild
    2. Follow up in 2-3 days for moderate dermatitis requiring topical or oral corticosteroid treatment

KERATOSIS PILARIS

I.   Definition: An eruption consisting of sterile pustules on the posterolateral aspects of the upper arms, anterior thighs, and the buttocks that is common in person with atopic dermatitis

II. Pathogenesis

     A. Unknown

     B. One theory is that the condition is caused by a disorder in keratinization so that follicular plugging with keratin debris occurs

     C. A second theory is that it represents a response to drying of the skin surface; the scaling produced is trapped in follicular opening

III. Clinical Presentation

     A. Commonly occurs in individuals with atopic dermatitis with children, adolescents, and young adults most often affected

     B. Appears as small, pinpoint, follicular papules and pustules on the extensor aspects of the extremities, and the buttocks–a "gooseflesh" appearance

     C. The affected skin surface feels rough and dry; hair in the center of the papule/pustule confirms a follicular location

     D. Condition is aggravated by cold, dry climates, and is usually associated with extremely dry skin

IV. Diagnosis/Evaluation

     A. History
         1. Ask about location of eruption, onset, duration, and appearance of lesions
         2. Determine if there is a history of atopic dermatitis
         3. Ask if condition gets better or worse at any time of the year
         4. Question about associated symptoms (there should be none)

     B. Physical Examination
         1. Examine skin, focusing on areas typically affected -- extensor aspects of arms, legs, and the buttocks
         2. Feel affected areas for rough skin; examine all skin surfaces for signs of dryness

     C. Differential Diagnosis
         1. Microcomedones of acne (distribution of acne is face, chest, upper back)
         2. Molluscum contagiosum (lesions are waxy-appearing with central umbilication)
         3. Drug eruption (drug eruption usually has acute onset and keratosis pilaris is chronic)

     D. Diagnostic Tests: None indicated

V. Plan/Management

    A. Mild forms: Lubricants applied to moist skin immediately after bathing are usually effective (see CARE OF DRY AND OILY SKIN for table of moisturizers)

    B. Moderate to severe forms
       1. Lubricants and keratolytics (to remove keratin debris from the follicles) are effective
       2. Use of a urea-containing lotion such as Eucerin Plus lotion usually controls the condition

    C. Advise patient to soak daily for 10 minutes in tepid water, to use bars such as Dove, Purpose, or Basis, and to apply moisturizers after bathing while skin is still damp after having been patted dry (**Note:** Persons who shower typically use hotter water than those who take tub baths–experts now recommend daily soaks in tepid water to keep skin hydrated)

    D. Follow up: None indicated

SEBORRHEIC DERMATITIS

I. Definition: A common, chronic, inflammatory disease with a characteristic pattern for different age groups

II. Pathogenesis

    A. The yeast Pityrosporum ovale is believed to play a role in the etiology

    B. Both genetic and environmental factors seem to influence onset and course of disease

III. Clinical Presentation

    A. Affects all age groups, including infants and children, but is most common in adults age 20-50 or older

    B. An extremely common condition which waxes and wanes and may be aggravated by stress

    C. Mild seborrheic dermatitis presents as fine, dry, white or yellow scale, on an inflamed base

    D. More severe eruptions appear as dull, red plaques with thick, white or yellow scale in a diffuse distribution

    E. Occurs in seborrheic areas
       1. Infants: Scalp ("cradle cap") and diaper area
       2. Adolescents: Scalp, eyebrows, paranasal, nasolabial fold, external ear canals, posterior auricular fold, and presternal areas

    F. Seborrheic dermatitis is one of the most common early cutaneous manifestations of HIV infection

IV. Diagnosis/Evaluation

    A. History
       1. Question regarding onset, duration, and location of lesions
       2. Inquire about personal or family history of seborrheic dermatitis
       3. Question regarding immunosuppressed status
       4. Ask about treatments tried and results

B. Physical Examination
   1. Examine skin for characteristic lesions: fine, dry, white or yellow scale on inflamed base or dull, red plaques with thick white or yellow greasy appearing scale
   2. Determine distribution

C. Differential Diagnosis
   1. Psoriasis (lesions are usually on elbows/knees and consist of thick, silvery scales; facial involvement is less common; psoriasis of scalp may be difficult to differentiate from seborrheic dermatitis)
   2. Tinea capitis/faciale (fungal culture/KOH prep can help differentiate; tinea faciale is usually unilateral)

D. Diagnostic Tests: None indicated if typical lesions, distribution

V. Plan/Management

   A. Infants with seborrheic dermatitis should be treated as follows

TREATMENT OF INFANTS AND SMALL CHILDREN	
Cradle cap	* Use bland shampoos such as Johnson's baby shampoo left on 5-10 minutes and then rinsed off * Repeat 2-3x/week * Apply topical steroid lotions of low potency such as hydrocortisone lotion 1% BID for 2 weeks
On the face	* Use low potency topical steroid cream such as Hytone cream 1% once a day or every other day * Use no longer than 2 weeks
In diaper area	* Use low potency topical steroid cream as above * May use once daily for 2 weeks * Leave diaper area open to air as much as possible

   B. Adolescents with seborrheic dermatitis should be treated as follows

TREATMENT OF ADOLESCENTS
For scalp involvement, medicated shampoos may be prescribed * Selenium sulfide: Exsel, Selsun blue (OTC) * Coal tar: Denorex, T/Gel, Tegrin (OTC) * Above shampoos must be left on a minimum of 5-10 minutes before rinsing * Ketoconazole: Nizoral (Rx): Use 2-3x/week x 1 month; may need to use once a week for maintenance **For scalp involvement**, topical corticosteroid lotions/solutions may also be used on the scalp if shampoo fails to control the condition after 2-3 weeks, or for initial treatment of moderate to severe scalp involvement * Intermediate potency drug such as betamethasone valerate 0.1% lotion, available in 20, 60 mL bottles may be used BID for 2 weeks; after 2 weeks, use hydrocortisone lotion, 1% or 2.5% QD for control, tapering to every other day and then discontinuing over the next 2 weeks * Should be used only on scalp and not on face and should not be used for maintenance therapy **For face/groin involvement**, low-potency agents such as hydrocortisone 1% cream or lotion, QD or BID to control erythema and scale; lotion works best in eyebrows For facial involvement that is unresponsive to topical steroids, may use Ketoconazole 2% cream QD to address a possible yeast component (Note: May be used as a combination treatment with topical steroids, applied at different times during the day) **For chest involvement**, medicated shampoos may be used on chest skin; may also use triamcinolone 0.1% lotion BID OR Ketoconazole (Nizoral) 2% cream BID until clear; then use once or twice weekly

   C. Recalcitrant cases should be referred to a specialist for management

   D. Follow up: Not indicated except in treatment failures

IMPETIGO AND ECTHYMA

I.   Definition: Bacterial skin infection caused by invasion of the epidermis by pathogenic Staphylococcus aureus or Streptococcus pyogenes, or a combination of these organisms

II.   Pathogenesis

   A.   Microscopic breaks in the epidermal barrier allows penetration by two major pathogens S. aureus and/or S. pyogenes

   B.   The depth of invasion in impetigo is superficial; the entire epidermis is involved in ecthyma

   C.   Poststreptococcal glomerulonephritis may follow skin infections involving strains of nephritogenic streptococci; rheumatic heart disease is not a sequelae of this infection

III. Clinical Presentation

   A.   Impetigo begins as small (1-2 mm) superficial vesicles with fragile roofs that are quickly lost; vesicles rupture leaving erosions covered by moist, honey-colored crusts

   B.   Multiple lesions are usually present, and face and extremities are the most common sites of involvement

   C.   The terms bullous and nonbullous impetigo have been used to describe two patterns of infection with bullous impetigo suggesting staphylococcal origin and nonbullous, streptococcal origin. The preferred term presently is simply, "impetigo," since differentiation is difficult based on appearance, and many infections are caused by both organisms

   D.   In ecthyma, ulcers form with a dry, dark crust, and surrounding erythema; lesions are usually found on legs

   E.   Both ecthyma and impetigo may occur simultaneously

   F.   Both infections occur most frequently in children but also occur in adults

   G.   Enhanced by poor hygiene and warm, moist climates; disease is self-limiting

IV.   Diagnosis/Evaluation

   A.   History
        1.   Question about location of lesions, onset, duration, and any associated symptoms
        2.   Ask if other family members are affected; treatments tried and results

   B.   Physical Examination
        1.   Examine skin (focus on areas of typical involvement--face, arms, legs) looking for erosions covered by moist, honey-colored crusts that characterize impetigo, and firm, dry, dark crusts with surrounding erythema that characterize ecthyma
        2.   Check for regional lymphadenopathy

   C.   Differential Diagnosis
        1.   Tinea (with tinea, there is central clearing, and KOH test is positive)
        2.   Herpes simplex infections (HSV is characterized by clusters of lesions, prodromal illness, and a positive Tzank smear)
        3.   Second-degree burn may be confused with ecthyma (careful history is important; Gram's stain for bacteria should be negative unless burn site contaminated with bacteria)
        4.   Allergic contact dermatitis (itching is prominent symptom in allergic contact dermatitis)

D. Diagnostic Tests: None required as clinical features are so characteristic; if uncertain about diagnosis, perform Gram's stain of fluid from intact vesicle/pustule looking for gram-positive cocci in clusters (*S. aureus*) or chains (*S. pyogenes*)

V. Plan/Management

A. For multiple lesions, oral antibiotics are the preferred therapy

B. Treatment of choice is dicloxacillin supplied as suspension, 62.5 mg/5 mL, and caps, 250, 500 mg
1. 12.5-25 mg/kg/day divided into 4 doses
2. Treat for 10 days OR

C. Erythromycin (as ethylsuccinate) [Eryped] supplied as suspension, 200 mg/5 mL, 400 mg/5 mL, and chewable tabs, 200 mg
1. 30-50 mg/kg/day divided into 4 doses
2. Treat for 10 days OR

D. Cephalexin (Keflex) supplied as suspension (250 mg/5 mL), caps, 250 mg, 500 mg, and tabs, 250, 500 mg
1. 25-40 mg/kg/day divided into 2 doses
2. Better compliance with this drug than with either dicloxacillin or erythromycin

E. Please note that strains of staphylococci resistant to erythromycin have been encountered in US; thus dicloxacillin is the drug of choice

F. If only a few lesions are present, consider use of topical mupirocin ointment (Bactroban) applied TID x 7-10 days or until all lesions have cleared (Note: Reevaluate if no response in 3-5 days)

G. Gentle washing of lesions to remove loose crusts may be helpful and must be done if mupirocin is used; scrubbing of lesions with antibacterial soaps has not been shown to be effective and is not routinely recommended

H. Good hand washing and personal hygiene are recommended to reduce likelihood of spread; use of a mild antibacterial soap such as Lever 2000 for bathing may be helpful

I. Follow up is not routinely recommended but is indicated for resistant or recurrent cases

CELLULITIS

I. Definition: An acute, diffuse, inflammation of the skin and subcutaneous structures characterized by hyperemia, edema, and leukocytic infiltration

II. Pathogenesis

A. Invasion of bacteria (usually pathogenic streptococci) into the dermis and subcutaneous fat with subsequent spread through the lymphatic

B. Haemophilus influenzae and Staphylococcus aureus are also frequent causative organisms May develop in apparently normal skin, but more often trauma to the skin provides a portal of entry for invading organisms

III.   Clinical Presentation

    A.   Erythema, warmth, edema, and pain are usual clinical features

    B.   Fever, chills, malaise, and lymphadenopathy are also frequently present

    C.   Typically, there is a preceding wound or trauma to the skin which compromises lymphatic drainage

    D.   Findings that signal an emergent condition are listed in the following table

INDICES OF AN EMERGENT CONDITION
✔ Extensive cellulitis
✔ Fever, or other signs and symptoms of septicemia
✔ Diminished arterial pulse in a cool, swollen, infected extremity
✔ Presence of cutaneous necrosis
✔ Closed space infections of the hand
✔ Periorbital cellulitis because of proximity to brain
✔ Immunosuppressed or diabetic host

    E.   Erysipelas, a distinctive type of superficial cellulitis is virtually always caused by group A streptococci

    F.   In erysipelas, infection is more superficial, with margins that are more clearly demarcated from normal skin than in cellulitis

    G.   Lower legs, face, and ears are most frequently involved in erysipelas

    H.   Lymphatic involvement ("streaking") is prominent in erysipelas which also differentiates it from other types of cellulitis

IV.   Diagnosis/Evaluation

    A.   History
        1.   Question about location, onset, duration, degree of spread, and presence of pain
        2.   Ask if there was a preexisting wound or trauma to involved area
        3.   Determine if systemic symptoms are present (fever, chills, malaise)

    B.   Physical Examination
        1.   Vital signs and BP to determine if febrile, and to evaluate cardiovascular status
        2.   Examine involved area of skin to determine how extensive infection is, degree of erythema, presence of purulent discharge, presence of necrotic tissue
        3.   Examine adjacent skin/lymph nodes to determine presence of "streaking," degree of lymphadenopathy

    C.   Differential Diagnosis
        1.   Pressure erythema
        2.   Contact dermatitis
        3.   Swelling over septic joint

    D.   Diagnostic Tests
        1.   Obtain Gram's stain and culture and sensitivity of wound before treatment is instituted
        2.   Obtain CBC and blood cultures if cellulitis is extensive or associated with marked systemic toxicity

V. Plan/Treatment

    A. Treatment of erysipelas and cellulitis depends on the patient's condition and underlying risk factors

    B. Refer for hospitalization any patient with emergent conditions described in section III.D.

    C. Most patients with erysipelas and localized cellulitis can be treated with oral antibiotics

    D. For uncomplicated cases, choose ONE of the following antibiotics, and **treat for 10-14 days** (except for Zithromax):
        1. Oxacillin
            a. Children < 20 kg: 50-100 mg/kg/day divided into 4 doses
            b. Children >20 kg: 1-2 g/day divided into 4 doses, OR
        2. Cephalexin (Keflex) supplied as suspension, 250 mg/5 mL; caps, 250, 500 mg; tabs, 250, 500 mg: 25-40 mg/kg/day divided into 4 doses OR
        3. Erythromycin (Eryped) supplied as suspension, 200 mg/5 mL, 400 mg/5 mL; chewable tabs, 200 mg: 30-50 mg/kg/day divided into 4 doses, or
        4. Azithromycin (Zithromax) supplied as suspension, 100 mg/5 mL, 200 mg/5 mL; 10 mg/kg (maximum 500 mg/day) once daily x 1 day, then 5 mg/kg (maximum 250 mg/day) once daily for next 4 days

    E. In all cases, antibiotic therapy may require changing based on culture results and clinical response

    F. Local measures such as immobilization, elevation, application of moist heat (3-4 x day for 15-20 minutes) should be used with all patients to provide symptomatic relief and speed resolution of the infection

    G. Follow up in 48 hours to determine response to therapy

FOLLICULITIS, FURUNCULOSIS, AND CARBUNCULOSIS

I. Definition: Bacterial invasion of the follicular wall

II. Pathogenesis

    A. Most commonly due to Staphylococcus aureus

    B. Other organisms may be involved, and, in general, the microbiology of cutaneous infection reflects the microflora of the part of body involved

III. Clinical Presentation

    A. Folliculitis is inflammation of the hair follicle caused by infection, chemical irritation, or injury

    B. Furuncle (abscess or boil) is a deep folliculitis, consisting of a walled-off, pus filled mass that is painful, firm, or fluctuant

    C. Furuncle may appear at any site, but most often occurs in areas of friction (waistline, groin, buttocks, axilla)

D.   Carbuncles are aggregates of infected follicles located deep in dermis; it points and drains through multiple openings

E.   Carbuncles are painful and systemic signs such as chills, fever may be present. Occur in areas with thick dermis (back of neck, lateral aspect of thigh)

IV.   Diagnosis/Evaluation

A.   History
1.   Ask about location, appearance of lesion, onset, duration, and if purulent drainage is exuding from surface
2.   Inquire about associated symptoms of pain and systemic symptoms of fever and chills
3.   Inquire about frequency of occurrence

B.   Physical Examination
1.   Take temperature to determine if systemic involvement
2.   Inspect lesion(s) for signs of local inflammation (erythema, swelling, and pustular surface)
3.   Palpate surface of lesion for fluctuance, indicating accumulation of purulent matter; palpate adjacent lymph nodes

C.   Differential Diagnosis
1.   Acne pustules
2.   Keratosis pilaris
3.   Epidermal cyst
4.   Hidradenitis suppurative

D.   Diagnostic Tests: Wound culture should be done to verify antibiotic choice

V.   Plan/Management

A.   For folliculitis, application of 5% benzoyl peroxide gel (Desquam-X) BID x 10 days is usually sufficient
1.   Alternative: Erythromycin 2% solution (A/T/S) BID x 10 days
2.   Clindamycin solution (Cleocin T) BID x 10 days may also be used

B.   For carbuncles and furuncles, frequent warm, moist compresses provide relief and promote localization and spontaneous draining

C.   Incision and drainage is commonly required for carbuncles and furuncles

D.   Systemic antistaphylococcal antibiotics should be used to treat furuncles and carbuncles
1.   Treatment of choice is dicloxacillin supplied as suspension, 62.5 mg/5 mL, and caps, 250, 500 mg: 12.5-25 mg/kg/day divided into 4 doses x 10 days
2.   Alternative treatment is cephalexin (Keflex) supplied as suspension, 250 mg/5 mL; caps, 250, 500 mg; tabs, 250, 500 mg: 25-40 mg/kg/day divided into 4 doses

E.   Refer patients with cutaneous abscesses located on face, scalp, and neck

F.   Culture recurrent abscesses and refer patients for evaluation for diseases that may underlie recurrent furunculosis: Immunodeficiency, diabetes mellitus, alcoholism, malnutrition, and severe anemia

G.   To prevent recurrence, stress role of good hygiene to patient and family. **Most useful: Frequent hand washing and daily skin cleansing** with an antibacterial soap such as Dial or Hibiclens antimicrobial skin cleanser

H.   Follow Up: None indicated

CANDIDIASIS

I. Definition: Skin and mucous membrane infections caused by the yeast-like fungus, *Candida albicans*

II. Pathogenesis: *C. albicans* is part of the normal flora of skin and mucous membranes; invasion of the epidermis occurs when moisture, warmth, and breaks in epidermal barrier allows overgrowth

III. Clinical Presentation

    A. **Oral** cavity: In infants, appears as white plaque on erythematous base (thrush). In immunocompromised patients, acute process is similar to the infection in infants. Tongue is almost always involved; may spread into trachea, esophagus, and angles of mouth, and become a chronic process

    B. **Diaper** area: Beefy red, well-demarcated lesions with elevated margins and satellite lesions; may also present as erosions, pustules, and erythematous papules; scrotum may be involved

    C. **Intertriginous** areas: Occurs most often in obese individuals (inframammary, axillary, neck, and inguinal body folds). Presents as red, moist, glistening plaque or moist red papules and pustules

    D. **Vagina**: Appears as a cheesy discharge with white plaques on erythematous base. External genitalia becomes red, swollen, with some skin erosions (see GYNECOLOGY section for discussion of vulvovaginal candidiasis)

    E. **Male genitalia**: Occurs mainly in uncircumcised but also occurs in circumcised. Multiple, round red erosions on glans and shaft (candida balanitis); usually painful. Often involves scrotum whereas tinea spares scrotum

    F. **Nails**: A common result of thumb/finger sucking. Non-tender erythema and swelling at nail margin

    G. Pain, discomfort usually symptoms regardless of site. Itching usually occurs with vulvovaginitis

IV. Diagnosis/Evaluation

    A. History
        1. For infants/children, inquire about location of lesions (remember that with thrush, there is frequently co-existing diaper dermatitis and vice versa). If nail involvement, ask if child sucks involved thumb/finger
        2. In older children, inquire about location of lesions, medications used (e.g., inhaled steroids or oral corticosteroids) and underlying chronic conditions (diabetes, HIV+).
        3. If vagina, penis involved, ask about associated symptoms of discharge, itching, and pain

    B. Physical Examination
        1. Examine skin, mucous membranes, and nails for characteristic lesions
            a. White plaques on erythematous base (oral); red moist plaques with satellite lesions (diaper/intertriginous)
            b. Red erosions on glans, shaft (penis); non-tender erythema of nail margins (nail)
            c. For vulvovaginal candidiasis, see under GYNECOLOGY
        2. Palpate adjacent lymph nodes

    C. Differential Diagnosis
        1. Oral
            a. Geographic tongue
            b. Aphthous stomatitis
            c. Leukoplakia

2. Diaper
   a. Bacterial infection
   b. Linea IgA dermatosis
   c. Irritant contact dermatitis
3. Intertriginous areas
   a. Miliaria
   b. Bacterial
4. Vaginal: See GYNECOLOGY section
5. Male genitalia
   a. Bacterial
   b. Psoriasis
   c. Tinea
6. Nails
   a. Bacterial
   b. Tinea

D. Diagnostic Tests
   1. None indicated when typical lesions present
   2. Potassium hydroxide (KOH) wet mount that is positive for pseudohyphae and budding spores confirms the diagnosis

V. Plan/Management
   A. Oral candidiasis: For the majority of patients, topical treatments are effective

---

TREATMENT FOR ORAL CANDIDIASIS

Topical treatment is preferred for limited disease in normal hosts
➡ Nystatin (Mycostatin) oral suspension (100,000 U/mL) QID x 10 days
  • Infants: 2 mL (1/2 dose in each side of mouth)
  • Older children and adolescents: 4-6 mL (1/2 dose in each side of mouth)
  • Medication should be retained in mouth as long as possible before swallowing
➡ Alternative for adolescents: 10 mg clotrimazole (Lotrimin) buccal troches,dissolve 1 PO 5x day for 2 weeks
Systemic therapy is necessary for moderate to severe disease that occurs in immunocompromised persons (see HIV/AIDS section for treatment recommendations)

B. Treatment of diaper candidiasis is outlined below

TREATMENT FOR DIAPER CANDIDIASIS

➡ Wash skin with plain water with each diaper change
➡ Dry completely; allow to air dry 15 minutes, 4x day
➡ Discontinue all powder, creams
➡ Nystatin cream, 3-4x day x 7-10 days

C. For candidal vaginitis, see GYNECOLOGY section

D. Candida balanitis: For limited disease, select one of the topical agents from the table

---

TREATMENT FOR CANDIDA BALANTITIS

➡ Nystatin cream, 2-3x day for 10 days
➡ Miconozole (Monistat-Derm) or clotrimazole (Lotrimin) cream 2x day for 10 days
➡ Econazole (Spectazole) cream, BID x 10 days
➡ Relief occurs quickly once treatment begins; remind patient to use for 10 days even though pain is gone

---

E.   Candida intertrigo: Select one of the topical agents from the table

TREATMENT FOR CANDIDA INTERTRIGO
➡ Nystatin cream applied 2-3x day after thorough drying of the skin x 10 days
➡ Econazole (Spectazole) cream; apply BID x 10 days
➡ Clotrimazole (Lotrimin) cream, solution, lotion; apply BID x 10 days
➡ Counsel regarding weight reduction and elimination of conditions leading to maceration of skin
➡ If there is maceration, use wet Burrow's compress 3-4x day for 15-20 minutes to promote drying
➡ Advise patient to expose areas to light and air several times a day to promote drying

F.   Candida paronychia (chronic): The following treatment is recommended

TREATMENT FOR CANDIDA PARONYCHIA
➡ 3% thymol in 95% ethanol (must be compounded by pharmacist) TID
➡ **In addition, select one** of the following to be used BID 2-4 weeks
• Clotrimazole (Lotrimin) solution
• Ciclopirox (Loprox) lotion
➡ Advise patient to avoid excess exposure to water
➡ For refractory cases, refer to specialist

G.   Treat predisposing factors. Rule out HIV+ and diabetes mellitus in patients with recurring infection

H.   Follow up is not indicated; patient should return if no improvement after 2 weeks and drug from another class should be prescribed

TINEA VERSICOLOR

I.   Definition: Common non-inflammatory fungal infection of the skin caused by lipophilic yeast

II.   Pathogenesis

    A.   Fungal infection of skin caused by *Pityrosporum orbiculare*

    B.   *P. orbiculare* is part of normal flora; overgrowth occurs for unknown reasons

III.   Clinical Presentation

    A.   Occurs at any age, but most likely to occur in adolescence and young adulthood

    B.   Presents as multiple small, circular macules of various colors -- white, pink, or brown -- thus the name "versicolor"

    C.   Infection is limited to the outermost layers of the skin; lesions enlarge rapidly and have mild scaling

    D.   Upper trunk most commonly affected, rarely located on face; may itch, but usually asymptomatic; not contagious

    E.   Proliferation exacerbated by heat, humidity, pregnancy, corticosteroid therapy, oral contraceptives, and immunosuppression

    F.   Infection is most evident in summer because the organism produces azelaic acid, a substance that inhibits pigment transfer to keratinocytes

IV. Diagnosis/Evaluation

    A. History
        1. Ask about location, onset, duration, and appearance of lesions
        2. Inquire if associated symptoms present
        3. Ask if any medications, including oral contraceptives are being taken
        4. Determine if patient is immunocompromised

    B. Physical Examination
        1. Examine skin for characteristic lesions
        2. Use Wood's light to look at skin. While not useful as a diagnostic aid (because fluorescence is not predictably present) can demonstrate extent of the infection better than ordinary light

    C. Differential Diagnosis
        1. Vitiligo
        2. Tinea corporis
        3. Seborrheic dermatitis
        4. Pityriasis alba

    D. Diagnostic Tests
        1. Microscopy of KOH-cleared scrapings
        2. Short, curved hyphae and clusters of round yeast cells "spaghetti and meatballs" are diagnostic

V. Plan/Management

    A. For limited disease, **topical** therapies are usually effective. Select **one** from the following from the table below

TREATMENT FOR TINEA VERSICOLOR USING TOPICAL THERAPIES

Selenium sulfide 2.5% lotion (Selsun), supplied as 4 oz
  ❖ Applied and then washed off **after** 24 hours; repeat once each week for a total of 4 weeks **OR**
  ❖ Applied daily x 7 days, rinsing off after 10 minutes
  ❖ Advise patient to apply Selsun from neck down
  ❖ Allow skin to repigment for one month; if not cleared in one month, have patient repeat above treatment
  ❖ Repeat the treatment monthly until satisfactory result obtained; treatment is cheap and usually effective

Sulconazole (Exelderm) supplied as cream, 15, 30 g and solution, 30 mL
  ❖ Apply once or twice daily for 3 weeks
  ❖ Not recommended for use in children <12

Ketoconzaole (Nizoral) supplied as shampoo, 4 oz
  ❖ Apply to damp skin in affected area with wide margins
  ❖ Lather, and leave in place for 5 minutes
  ❖ One application should be sufficient (No need to repeat)
  ❖ Repeat treatment if necessary
  ❖ Not recommended for use in children <12

Ketoconazole (Nizoral) cream, supplied as 25, 30 g
  ❖ Apply QD x 2 weeks
  ❖ Not recommended for use in children <12

    B. Tell patients that clearing may be temporary; since infection is caused by an inhabitant of normal skin, it often recurs

    C. Recommend prophylactic monthly use of selenium sulfide lotion (especially during summer) to prevent recurrences

    D. Advise that treatment does not repigment the skin; once the infection is cleared up, the skin with normally repigment itself, but it will take 2 months or longer

    E. Follow Up: None indicated

DERMATOPHYTE INFECTIONS

I.   Definition: Infections by a group of fungi that have the ability to infect and survive only on keratin

II.   Pathogenesis

    A.   Causative organisms belong to 3 genera:
        1.   Microsporum
        2.   Trichophyton
        3.   Epidermophyton

    B.   Predisposing factors include debilitating diseases, poor nutrition, poor hygiene, tropical climates, and contact with infected persons or animals

III. Clinical Presentation

    A.   Tinea capitis, or ringworm of the scalp
        1.   Occurs mainly in prepubertal children (ages 2-10); rarely occurs in adults
        2.   Erythema and scaling of the scalp with patchy hair loss are characteristic
        3.   Usually asymptomatic unless kerion, a tender, boggy, lesion representing a hypersensitivity reaction to the fungal infection is present
    B.   Tinea corporis, or ringworm of the body and face (excluding beard area in men)
        1.   Occurs in all age groups; more common in warm climates
        2.   Lesion is generally circular, erythematous, well-demarcated with a raised, scaly, vesicular border
        3.   The central area becomes hypopigmented, and less scaly as the active border progresses outward
        4.   Pruritus is common

    C.   Tinea cruris, or ringworm of the groin and upper thighs
        1.   Frequent in males, usually obese ones; rare in females
        2.   Eruption is sharply demarcated, scaling patches; usually extremely pruritic
        3.   Involvement of the scrotum is uncommon (unlike candidal infections in which scrotal involvement is common)

    D.   Tinea pedis, or ringworm of the foot
        1.   Common infection in adolescents and adults (uncommon in prepubertal children)
        2.   Lesions are fine, vesiculopustular or scaly and usually itch
        3.   Any area of the foot may be involved, but likely to occur on the instep or between the toes

    E.   Tinea unguium, or ringworm of the nails (onychomycosis)
        1.   Occurs in adolescents and adults; rare in children
        2.   May occur simultaneously with hand or foot tinea or present independently
        3.   Usually involves only 1 or 2 nails; toenails more often than fingernails
        4.   Distal thickening and yellowing of the nail plate are characteristic features

IV.   Evaluation/Diagnosis

    A.   History
        1.   Question regarding onset, duration, distribution, morphology of lesions, and presence of symptoms
        2.   Question regarding contact with others (or infected dogs, cats) with similar lesions, symptoms
        3.   Ask about predisposing conditions -- sweaty feet, occlusive footwear
        4.   Inquire about treatments used and outcomes

B. Physical Examination
    1. Examine skin to determine type, distribution of lesions
    2. Use of Wood's light may aid in exam as some species cause tinea to fluoresce (pale or brilliant green). The most common fungus infecting the scalp, *T. tonsurans* does not fluoresce. Also, lint, scales, serum exudate, and hair preparations containing petrolatum fluoresce a bluish or purplish color which may be misleading

C. Differential Diagnosis
    1. Seborrheic dermatitis
    2. Psoriasis
    3. Alopecia areata
    4. Atopic dermatitis
    5. Contact dermatitis

D. Diagnostic Tests

DIAGNOSTIC TESTS FOR DERMATOPHYE INFECTIONS
Microscopic examination for fungus
❖ Scrape the border of lesion with a sterile scalpel blade (No. 15) moistened with tap water to contain scales; can also "pluck" 2 or 3 hairs using a hemostat. Transfer specimen to slide with a small droplet of plain water
❖ Add 1 or 2 drops of KOH solution, put on coverslip and warm the slide carefully for 15-30 seconds with a flame
❖ Examine the specimen under low power with minimal illumination
❖ Identify hyphae -- thin, often branching strands of uniform diameter; switch to high dry (43X) objective to confirm finding
❖ While a positive exam establishes the diagnosis, a negative test does not rule out the disease
Dermatophyte test medium (DTM)
❖ Using a hemostat, remove 5-10 hairs from a scaling area or rub a moistened 2 x 2 gauze vigorously over an area of scaling and alopecia
❖ Inoculate the plucked hair/scrapings from the gauze directly onto the culture medium and incubate at room temperature (with cap on loosely)
❖ After 1-2 weeks, phenol red indicator in agar will turn from yellow to red in area surrounding dermatophte colony

V. Plan/Management

    A. Treatment for tinea capitis is contained in the table below

TREATMENT FOR TINEA CAPITIS
Tinea capitis requires systemic antifungal therapy
Griseofulvin microsize (Grifulvin V), supplied as 250, 500 mg tabs; 125 mg/5 mL suspension
❖ Dosing: 10 to 20 mg/kg/day x 4-8 weeks. May be given as a single daily dose (maximun 1g in a single dose) or divided into 2 doses per day
❖ Take with high fat food such as whole milk, peanut butter, ice cream to enhance absorption
❖ 4-6 weeks of therapy are needed; some patients require longer
❖ Continue medication for 2 weeks after clinical resolution
Selenium sulfide, 2.5% shampoo, used 2x week for 2 weeks may reduce fungal shedding
❖ If kerion present, a short course of oral steroid therapy to reduce inflammation and prevent scarring of scalp may be needed
❖ Prednisone, 1-2 mg/kg/day for 7-10 days is recommended
❖ Taper dose over last half of therapy
❖ Children receiving treatment may attend school
❖ Cutting hair, shaving head, wearing cap unnecessary
❖ Advise parent/child that hair regrowth is slow

B.   Treatment for tinea corporis, pedis, and cruris is outlined in the table below

TREATMENT FOR TINEA CORPORIS, PEDIS, AND CRURIS				
Topical Antifungal Agents	**Supplied As**	**Dosing**	**Duration of Treatment**	**Use in Children**
Miconazole (Monistat-Derm)	Cream, 15 g, 1 oz, 3 oz	BID	Tinea corporis, cruris--2 wks Tinea pedis--1 month	Yes
Econazole (Spectazole)	Cream, 15, 30 g	QD	Tinea corporis, cruris--2 weeks Tinea pedis--1 month	Yes
Ciclopirox (Loprox)	Cream, 15, 30 g Lotion, 30, 60 mL	BID	Up to 4 weeks	< 10--not recommended
Oxiconazole (Oxistat)	Cream, 15, 30 g Lotion, 30 mL	QD or BID	Tinea corporis, cruris--2 wks Tinea pedis--4 wks	Yes

C.   Treatment for onychomycosis in children should be by a specialist since there are no oral therapies approved for use in children

D.   Follow Up: Every 2-4 weeks for patients receiving long-term (more than 2 week) oral antifungal treatment to monitor LFTs and CBC

SCABIES

I.   Definition: Skin infestation of the mite, *Sarcoptes scabies*

II.   Pathogenesis

A.   A fertilized female mite excavates a burrow in the stratum corneum and deposits eggs and fecal pellets

B.   The larvae hatch and reach maturity in about 14 days, mate, and repeat the cycle

C.   Humans are the source of infection with transmission occurring most often by close personal contact

D.   A hypersensitivity reaction rather than a foreign-body response is responsible for the intense pruritus

E.   Incubation period in persons without previous exposure is 4-6 weeks

III. Clinical Presentation

A.   Occurs mainly in children, young adults; also among institutionalized persons of all ages (e.g., elderly in nursing homes)

B.   Primary lesions are burrows, vesicles, and papules
1.   Burrows appear as gray or skin-colored ridges up to a few centimeters in length; scratching destroys burrows, so they may be difficult to find
2.   Vesicles are isolated, pinpoint and filled with serous fluid; may contain mites
3.   Papules are small, isolated, represent a hypersensitivity reaction and rarely contain mites

C.   Secondary lesions with erythema and scaling caused by scratching are present in more chronic cases

D. A generalized urticarial rash may occur, especially in infants and the elderly. This condition, called Norwegian scabies, is the result of penetration of the underlying epidermis by hundreds of mites

E. In infants <2 years of age, lesions are often vesicular and are likely to occur on the head, neck, palms and soles, areas that are largely spared in older children and adults

F. In older children and adolescents, common sites are hands (90%), especially fingerwebs, flexor aspects of the wrists, belt line, thighs, navel, intergluteal cleft, penis, areola, and axillae

G. Main symptom is intense itching which is usually more intense at night and the diagnosis should be considered with widespread pruritus presenting primarily with skin excoriation

IV. Diagnosis/Evaluation

A. History
1. Question regarding onset, duration, morphology and location of lesions
2. Ask if itching is present, and if it is worse at night
3. Ask about exposures to friends or family members with similar symptoms
4. Inquire what treatments have been tried and their effectiveness

B. Physical Examination
1. Examine the skin for typical burrows
2. Pay particular attention to the hands, especially the fingerwebs and wrists (flexor aspect), axillary folds, belt line, navel, penis, areas surrounding the areolae
3. A magnifying glass and good lighting are essential

C. Differential Diagnosis
1. Atopic dermatitis
2. Allergic and irritant contact dermatitis
3. Papular urticaria
4. Pediculosis

D. Diagnostic Tests
1. Microscopic identification of mite, ova, or feces proves the diagnosis. Two ways to do this:
   a. Locate tiny black dot at end of burrow; insert a 25 gauge hypodermic needle at dot. Mite, ova, or feces (dot) will stick to it and can be transferred to immersion oil on slide; cover with slip and examine under low power
   b. Slice off whole burrow with sterile scalpel blade (No. 15) held parallel to skin; put slice on slide, add immersion oil, cover with slip and examine under low power
2. If no burrows are found, no diagnostic test indicated

V. Plan/Management

A. Use a scabicide from the following table

TREATMENT OF SCABIES
Drug of choice is 5% permethrin (Elimite) cream
→ Children: Apply cream over the entire body below the head
→ Infants and toddlers: Apply cream over the head, neck, and body (avoid the eyes)
→ Remove by bathing in 8-14 hours
→ Of drugs available to treat scabies, this drug is safest for use in infants, young children, pregnant and lactating women
Alternatives: Lindane (Kwell, Scabine) and crotamiton (Eurax) cream or lotion
→ Apply as for permethrin cream above
→ Lindane, remove in 8-12 hours
→ Crotamiton, remove in 48 hours; repeat application for 2 to 5 days
→ **Caution: Lindane should not be used in infants and toddlers and pregnant women**

B. Control Measures/Patient Education
   1. Prophylactic therapy recommended for household members; therefore all household members should be treated simultaneously to prevent reinfection
   2. Launder all clothing and bedding in hot water and hot drying cycle
   3. Clothing that cannot be laundered should be placed in plastic storage bags for at least a week. (Parasites cannot survive off the skin for longer than 3-4 days)
   4. Children in day care or school can return the day after treatment completed
   5. Advise patient that pruritus may continue a week after cure due to local irritation (see CONTROL OF PRURITUS table below)

PRURITUS CONTROL USING PHARMACOLOGIC AND NONPHARMACOLOGIC INTERVENTIONS

Oral Antihistamines

Hydroxyzine (Atarax), supplied as 10 mg/5 mL syrup and 10, 25, 50, 100 mg tablets
Infants and children, 0.5 mg/kg/dose TID PRN
Adolescens, 25-50 mg/dose TID PRN
A single dose at bedtime is frequently all that is necessary

Oral Antihistamines for Use in the Daytime (Nonsedating)

Loratidine (Claritin) may be used in children ≥6 years of age
Begin with 10 mg every other day; then 10 mg/day
Supplied as Claritin Reditabs, 10 mg, which are dissolved on tongue and swallowed with or without water
Supplied also as Claritin syrup, 1 mg/1 mL (alcohol free, dye free)

Important to prescribe nonsedating antihistamines for patients who attend school or who have other daytime responsibilities that require alertness

Topical Antipruritic Agents

Sarna lotion, Prax lotion and Itch-X gel are all OTC products
Cetaphil with menthol 0.25% and phenol 0.25% is an Rx product
Topical agents may be used in addition to or instead of oral antihistamines

Nonpharmacologic Treatment Modalities to Soothe Itchy Skin

Cool tub baths with or without colloidal oatmeal can provide relief
Topical compresses (washcloths wet with plain water and kept in freezer) can be applied to affected skin for 15-20 minutes, 3-4 x day

---

C. Follow up: None indicated unless patient fails to respond to treatment

PEDICULOSIS (LICE)

I. Definition: Infestation with one of the three species of lice that infest humans

   A. *Pediculus humanus* var. *capitis* (head louse)

   B. *Pediculus humanus* var. *corporis* (body louse)

   C. *Pthirus pubis* (pubic or crab louse)

II. Pathogenesis

   A. Transmission of head lice occurs by direct contact with infested persons or through hats, brushes, and combs

   B. Fomites play a major role in transmission of body lice, but almost no role in transmission of pubic lice, which are transmitted through sexual contact

C. Ova hatch in a week; lice feed on human blood

D. Incubation period from laying of eggs to hatching of first nymph is 6-10 days; mature lice (capable of reproducing) do not appear until 2-3 weeks later

III. Clinical Presentation

CLINICAL PRESENTATION OF LICE

Pediculosis capitis (head lice)
- ➡ Most common in children with all socioeconomic groups affected; African Americans are less likely than other races to become infested
- ➡ Head lice are not responsible for the spread of any disease
- ➡ Most commonly seen in hair on back of the head near nape of neck
- ➡ Nits (ova) are cemented to hair shaft and may be seen; few adult lice are seen
- ➡ Head lice can survive only 1-2 days away from the scalp
- ➡ Excoriation from scratching, secondary bacterial infections, and cervical adenopathy are common

Pediculosis corporis (body lice)
- ➡ Generally found on persons with poor hygiene; lice cannot survive away from blood source for longer than 10 days
- ➡ Body lice are vectors of disease including typhus, trench fever, and relapsing fever
- ➡ Excoriation and secondary bacterial infection are common
- ➡ Body lice and nits may be found in seams of clothing

Pediculosis pubis (pubic lice)
- ➡ Highly contagious; chance of acquiring from one exposure is about 90%
- ➡ Common in adolescents and young adults; African-Americans and other racial groups are affected with same frequency
- ➡ Pubic hair is most common site of infestation, but can also infest hair on chest, abdomen, and thighs
- ➡ Infested adults may spread pubic lice to eyelashes of children
- ➡ Eyelash infestation is seen almost exclusively in children
  - ✦ Acquired from other children or adult infested with pubic lice
  - ✦ May be a sign of sexual abuse in children
- ➡ Frequently coexists with other sexually transmitted diseases

---

IV. Diagnosis/Evaluation

A. History
1. Determine if nits, lice have been visualized and when they were first noticed
2. Ask if itching present, especially nocturnal; determine if itching is generalized or localized
3. Question if nits, lice present in close contacts
4. If lice in eyelashes of child, explore with parent/care giver how this might have occurred

B. Physical Examination
1. Examine appropriate body part for lice, nits; a magnifying glass is helpful
2. Check eyelashes closely
3. Examine skin of infested site for excoriation secondary to scratching
4. If body lice suspected, examine seams of clothing for lice

C. Differential Diagnosis
1. Scabies
2. Neurotic excoriation

D. Diagnostic Tests
1. Identification of eggs, nymphs, and lice with naked eye or magnifying glass
2. Microscopic exam usually unnecessary

V.   Plan/Management

   A.   The following products are recommended for the treatment of head lice

---

TREATMENT OF HEAD LICE

Permethrin 1% cream rinse (Nix) OTC
- ➡ Children over 2 months of age
- ➡ Apply cream rinse to shampooed, rinsed, and towel dried hair (and scalp)
- ➡ Leave on for 10 minute; rinse
- ➡ A single treatment is usually adequate, but some experts recommend retreatment 7-10 days after the initial treatment

Lindane 1% shampoo (Kwell shampoo)
- ➡ Do not use in infants and pregnant women
- ➡ Apply to dry hair until thoroughly wet.; allow to remain for 4 minutes
- ➡ Add water to lather, rinse thoroughly
- ➡ Repeat application in 7-10 days is often recommended

Pyrethrins 0.33% shampoo, gel (A-200) (RID) OTC
- ➡ Apply to area until thoroughly wet, massage in, wait 10 minutes, rinse
- ➡ Use gel for body lice, shampoo for head or pubic lice

   B.   To remove nits for aesthetic reasons (not necessary to prevent spread)
      1.   Soak hair with white vinegar for 30-60 minutes, or use a commercial formic acid rinse (Step 2) made for this purpose
      2.   Use fine-tooth comb to mechanically remove nits
      3.   With heavy involvement, a haircut may be preferable to tedious nit removal (child should not be forced to have hair cut, however, if he/she would find it humiliating)

   C.   Children can return to daycare/school the next day after their first treatment for head lice; provide a note for school

   D.   Combs and brushes should be soaked in hot water with pediculicide shampoo for 15 minutes

   E.   Treatment of pubic lice is described below

TREATMENT OF PUBIC LICE

For the treatment of pubic lice, any of the pediculocides listed above for treatment of head lice are effective
- ➡ Retreatment is recommended in 7-10 days following initial treatment
- ➡ All sexual contacts of persons with pubic lice should be treated

For infestation of eyelashes, use petrolatum ointment, applied BID x 8-10 days; nits should be removed mechanically from the eyelashes

---

   F.   Treatment of body lice is described below

TREATMENT OF BODY LICE

For the treatment of body lice, pediculocides are not necessary
- ➡ Treatment consists of improving hygiene and laundering clothing
- ➡ Infested clothing should be washed and dried at very hot temperatures to kill lice

---

   G.   Household and other close contacts should be examined and treated if they have head or body lice; bed mates should be treated prophylactically

   H.   Clothing, bedding should be laundered in hot soapy water and dried on hot cycle or dry cleaned

   I.   Follow Up: Unnecessary

CUTANEOUS LARVAE MIGRANS

I. Definition: A skin disease caused by infected larvae of cat and dog hookworms with *Ancylostoma braziliense* and *Ancylostoma caninum* the usual causes; often referred to as creeping eruption

II. Pathogenesis

   A. Ova of *A. braziliense* or *A. caninum* are deposited in cat or dog feces

   B. Larvae in soil or sand penetrate human skin that contacts soil

III. Clinical Presentation

   A. A disease of persons likely to come into contact with sandy soil contaminated with cat/dog feces (i.e., children, gardeners, sunbathers, outdoor workers)

   B. Disease is most prevalent in the southeastern part of the US

   C. Classically presents as pruritic, erythematous, thread-like (or serpiginous) lesions that advance about 1 cm/day

   D. Lesions are usually located on feet, hands, buttocks, or upper thighs; excoriation may obscure the otherwise typical serpiginous lesion

IV. Diagnosis/Evaluation

   A. History
       1. Inquire about location, onset, duration, and if pruritus is present
       2. Ask if sitting or playing in soil/sand has occurred recently

   B. Physical Examination: Examine skin for typical serpiginous, thread-like lesions; look for signs of scratching

   C. Differential Diagnosis
       1. Tinea
       2. Urticaria
       3. Erythema chronicum migrans
       4. Scabies

   D. Diagnostic Tests: None indicated

V. Plan/Treatment

   A. Treatment of choice is topical application of oral thiabendazole suspension (Mintezol); apply suspension to affected areas QID x 7-10 days

   B. Patient Education: Should be advised not to sit, lie, or walk barefoot on wet soil or sand in areas where cats or dogs are likely to deposit feces

   C. Follow Up: None indicated

PITYRIASIS ROSEA

I. Definition: A common, benign, often asymptomatic, self-limiting skin eruption of unknown etiology

II. Pathogenesis: Unknown, but some evidence suggests it is viral in origin

III. Clinical Presentation

    A. More than 75% of cases are in persons 10-35 years of age

    B. Incidence is higher during cold months

    C. In its typical form, a 2-10 cm round-to-oval lesion (the herald patch) appears on the trunk
        1. Precedes the appearance of the generalized eruption by 7-14 days
        2. Herald patch usually has central clearing

    D. The herald patch is followed by a generalized eruption consisting of multiple, erythematous (appears as hyperpigmentation in dark-skinned patients) macules progressing to papules which enlarge and become oval; a fine scale is present

    E. Long axes of oval lesions tend to run parallel to each other, creating a "Christmas tree" distribution on trunk

    F. Lesions usually last 4-8 weeks and mild itching is common

IV. Diagnosis/Evaluation

    A. History
        1. Question regarding recent occurrence of herald patch and location and presence of other lesions
        2. Question regarding medications currently taking
        3. Question if symptoms such as pruritus are present

    B. Physical Examination
        1. Examine skin for characteristic lesions; look specifically for herald patch which is usually on trunk
        2. Determine distribution of lesions, looking to see if long axes of oval-shaped lesions are parallel to each other
        3. Check the mucous surfaces, palms, and soles which are spared by pityriasis rosea

    C. Differential Diagnosis
        1. Tinea corporis
        2. Tinea versicolor
        3. Viral exanthems
        4. Drug eruptions
        5. Syphilis

    D. Diagnostic Tests: **Always** order VDRL or RPR as syphilis can mimic this disorder

V. Plan/Management

    A. No therapy is required, but symptomatic management of pruritus may be indicated

Oral Antihistamines

Hydroxyzine (Atarax), supplied as 10 mg/5mL syrup and 10, 25, 50, 100 mg tablets
Infants and children, 0.5 mg/kg/dose TID PRN
Adolescents, 25-50 mg/dose TID PRN
A single dose at bedtime is frequently all that is necessary

Oral Antihistamines for Use in the Daytime (Nonsedating)

Loratidine (Claritin) may be used in children ≥6 years of age
Begin with 10 mg every other day; then 10 mg/day
Supplied as Claritin Reditabs, 10 mg, which are dissolved on tongue and swallowed with or without water
Supplied also as Claritin syrup, 1 mg/1 mL (alcohol free, dye free)

Important to prescribe nonsedating antihistamines for patients who must work or attend school, or who have other daytime responsibilities that require alertness

Topical Antipruritic Agents

Sarna lotion, Prax lotion and Itch-X gel are all OTC products
Cetaphil with menthol 0.25% and phenol 0.25% is an Rx product
Topical agents may be used in addition to or instead of oral antihistamines

Nonpharmacologic Treatment Modalities to Soothe Itchy Skin

Cool tub baths with or without colloidal oatmeal can provide relief
Topical compresses (washcloths wet with plain water and kept in freezer) can be applied to affected skin for 15-20 minutes, 3-4 x day

B. Sunlight exposure to the point of minimal erythema will hasten disappearance of lesions and decrease itching; caution against sunburn

C. Follow Up: None required

PITYRIASIS ALBA

I. Definition: A disorder of pigmentation of unknown etiology which may be a form of atopic dermatitis

II. Pathogenesis

A. A thickening in the stratum corneum with subsequent edema

B. The thickened stratum corneum reduces UVL penetration

C. The edema interferes with pigment transfer from melanocytes to keratinocytes

III. Clinical Presentation

A. Occurs primarily in children before puberty

B. Presents as multiple, oval, scaly, hypopigmented patches on the face, extensor surfaces of upper arms, and on neck

C. Lesions range in size from 5-20 mm in diameter with 10-20 lesions commonly seen

D. Lesions are asymptomatic but are cosmetically bothersome

E. A chronic dermatitis that may persist for several years

IV.   Diagnosis/Evaluation

    A.   History
        1.   Inquire about location, onset, duration, and any symptoms of lesions
        2.   Ask about treatments tried and results

    B.   Physical Examination: Examine skin for characteristic lesions

    C.   Differential Diagnosis
        1.   Tinea versicolor
        2.   Vitiligo (dead white appearing; does not scale)

    D.   Diagnostic Tests: Do KOH exam to exclude tinea versicolor

V.   Plan/Treatment

    A.   Triamcinolone acetonide, 0.025% (Aristocort) cream applied BID x 14 days

    B.   After 2 week course of topical steroids, apply moisturizers such as Moisturel at bedtime to control scaling

    C.   Treatment does not affect pigmentation

    D.   Condition gradually improves after puberty

    E.   Follow Up: None indicated

CAFÉ AU LAIT SPOTS

I.   Definition: Uniformly brown macules found on any cutaneous surface

II.   Pathogenesis

    A.   Increased levels of melanin in melanocytes and in keratinocytes of the basal cell layer occurs for unknown reasons

    B.   There is no increase in the actual number of melanocytes

    C.   Benign lesion in most cases, but also a cutaneous marker of neurofibromatosis, an autosomal dominant disease

III.   Clinical Presentation

    A.   Hyperpigmented (pale brown) macules with distinct borders ranging in size from 0.5-2.0 cm

    B.   May be present at birth; occurs in 10-20% of normal children and are usually of little significance in the vast majority of children

    C.   Increase in number and size with age

    D.   Five or more lesions >0.5 cm in children <5 years of age suggests the diagnosis of neurofibromatosis; six or more lesions >1.5 cm in children >5 years of age strongly suggests the diagnosis

IV. Diagnosis/Evaluation

   A. History
      1. Question about location, onset, and duration of lesions; ask if lesions were present at birth
      2. Inquire if lesions have increased in number or size
      3. Ask about family history of neurofibromatosis, an autosomal dominant disease

   B. Physical Examination
      1. Examine skin surface for characteristic lesions
      2. Carefully count and measure lesions, mapping location and size in chart

```
Lesion Measurement Tool
To order MediRules, which are disposable plastic sheets
for measuring the size of lesions or wounds:
Briggs Corp.
7887 University Bend
DesMoines, IA 50306
1-800-247-2343
```

   C. Differential Diagnosis
      1. Freckles
      2. Lentigo

   D. Diagnosis Tests: None indicated

V. Plan/Treatment

   A. Children <5 years with fewer than 5 lesions that are ≥ 0.5 cm (but <1.5 cm) in size and with a negative family history should be observed at yearly health maintenance visit for changes

   B. Parent of child should be instructed to bring child to clinic if number or size of lesions increases

   C. Child of any age with >5 lesions that are ≥ 0.5 cm should be referred for evaluation of neurofibromatosis

   D. Café au lait spots cannot be lightened by hydroquinone bleaching agents

   E. Follow Up: Yearly to evaluate for change

HERPES SIMPLEX

I. Definition: Cutaneous infections with herpes simplex viruses which are large, enveloped DNA viruses of two types that have major genomic and antigenic differences

   A. HSV-1 is usually associated with oral/labial infections

   B. HSV-2 is usually associated with genital infections (Genital herpes is considered under SEXUALLY TRANSMITTED DISEASES)

II.   Pathogenesis

    A.   HSV-1 and HSV-2 are epidermotropic viruses with infection occurring within keratinocytes

    B.   Transmission is only by direct contact with active lesions, or by virus-containing fluid such as saliva or cervical secretions in persons with no evidence of active disease

    C.   Inoculation of the virus into skin or mucosal surfaces produces infection, with an incubation period of 2-12 days

    D.   About 48 hours after entering the host, the virus transverses afferent nerves to find host ganglion
        1.   The trigeminal ganglia are the target of the oral virus -- primarily HSV-1
        2.   The sacral ganglia are the target of the genital virus -- most often HSV-2

    E.   Upon reactivation, the virus retraces its route, causing recurrence in the cutaneous area affected by the same nerve root, but not necessarily in the original site

    F.   Generally HSV-1 is associated with infection of the lips, face, buccal mucosae, and throat; HSV-2, with the genitalia (see SEXUALLY TRANSMITTED DISEASES section for a full discussion of this topic)

    G.   An increasing number of genital herpes cases are attributable to HSV-1

    H.   In neonates, Type 2 (HSV-2) is the most common cause of infection

III.   Clinical Presentation

    A.   Three clinical stages define the course of herpes viruses: primary infection, latency, and recurrent infection

    B.   During primary infection with HSV-1 virus, the following usually occurs:
        1.   Lesions may appear 2-14 days following inoculation; lesions are typically grouped vesicles on an erythematous base, usually located on the lips, facial area, buccal mucosa, and throat
        2.   Vesicles rupture, leaving erosions that slowly form crusts; crusting signals the end of viral shedding; lesions are intraepidermal and usually heal without leaving a scar
        3.   There may be tenderness, pain, mild paresthesia, or burning prior to eruption of lesions; some persons have no prodrome
        4.   Almost 60% of HSV-1 infections in infants and children appear as a gingivostomatitis (extensive erosions in oral cavity) with symptoms of pain in mouth and throat, accompanied by fever and irritability
        5.   Persons may be asymptomatic during the primary infection stage, or may have fever, myalgia, malaise, or cervical lymphadenopathy

    C.   During the second clinical stage called latency, the virus remains dormant in the ganglia

    D.   During the recurrent or third clinical stage, the virus is reactivated and travels down the peripheral nerves to the site of the initial infection, causing the characteristic focal infection; recurrent infection is not inevitable and may be triggered by one or more of the following:
        1.   Local skin trauma
        2.   Sunlight exposure
        3.   Systemic changes such as menses, fatigue, or fever

    E.   The severity of the disease increases with age

IV. Diagnosis/Evaluation

    A. History
        1. Question regarding location, onset, duration, and appearance of lesions; ask if pain, burning, or paresthesia present prior to eruption
        2. Ask about associated symptoms of fever, myalgia, malaise
        3. Ask regarding previous occurrence of similar lesions, symptoms
        4. Inquire about exposures to infected persons

    B. Physical Examination
        1. Examine lesions for characteristic location, distribution, and appearance
        2. Check for cervical lymphadenopathy

    C. Differential Diagnosis
        1. Erythema multiform
        2. Pemphigus

    D. Diagnostic Tests
        1. Tzanck preparation
        2. Use of a commercially available rapid office test such as Kodak SureCell Herpes (uses enzyme immunoassay for HSV)
        3. Most definitive test: Viral culture
           a. Unroof vesicle and scrape the material with Dacron-tipped swab
           b. Place swab in viral transport media
           c. Viral detection usually requires 1-3 days after inoculation

V. Plan/Management

    A. Treatment of primary episode of mild to moderate HSV that is localized
        1. For symptomatic management of lesions of the mouth
           a. Apply Orabase, a dental protective paste QID to prevent irritation of lesion by teeth
           b. Diphenhydramine (Benadryl) elixir mixed 1:1 with aluminum hydroxide/magnesium hydroxide (Maalox) may also be used QID as an oral rinse
           c. Sucking on frozen juice bars, drinking ice water can also be helpful
        2. For symptomatic management of lesions of the lip
           a. Apply ice to reduce swelling
           b. Use Blistex to prevent drying and reduce pain
           c. Use sun-screen containing lip protectants prior to sun exposure
        3. Use acetaminophen (Tylenol) PO for pain relief

    B. Follow Up: None indicated

MOLLUSCUM CONTAGIOSUM

I. Definition: A benign, viral disease of the skin characterized by discrete, white to flesh-colored, dome-shaped papules

II. Pathogenesis

    A. Caused by a poxvirus that induces epidermal cell proliferation

    B. Humans are the only known source of the virus and infectivity is relatively low

C.   Spreads by direct contact, including sexual contact, or by fomites

D.   Incubation period varies between 2-7 weeks and may be as long a 6 months

III.   Clinical Presentation

A.   More common in children and adolescents, but may affect any age group

B.   Tiny (2-5 mm), early lesions are shiny, white to flesh-colored, dome-shaped discrete papules with a firm, waxy appearance
1.   As lesions mature, the center becomes soft and umbilicate
2.   Usually number of lesions ranges from 2-20

C.   Lesions occur in groups; usually on genital area in adults

D.   Erythema may surround the lesions as a result of inflammation from scratching, or may be a hypersensitivity reaction

E.   Self-limiting; usually spontaneously clears in 6-9 months

F.   A common, cutaneous manifestation of HIV+ infection

IV.   Diagnosis/Evaluation

A.   History
1.   Inquire about location, appearance of lesions, onset and duration
2.   Ask about past medical history, HIV+ infection

B.   Physical Examination
1.   Examine skin looking for lesions in groups, 3-5 mm in size, with a waxy appearance
2.   Magnification may assist in seeing central umbilication in more mature lesions
3.   Palpate the lesions to reveal their solid versus fluid-filled nature (wear gloves)

C.   Differential Diagnosis
1.   Basal cell carcinoma
2.   Epidermal cyst
3.   Wart
4.   Herpes simplex

D.   Diagnostic Tests: None indicated

V.   Diagnosis/Treatment

A.   For small number of asymptomatic lesions that are stable (not spreading), observe for spontaneous resolution over next few months

B.   If patient prefers, removal via curettage of the central core or via liquid nitrogen therapy is also an option

C.   Another option is to use one of the following topical agents for removal
1.   Duofilm (available as 15 mL) OR
2.   Viranol solution (available as 10 mL) OR
3.   Duoplant (available as 7.5 mL gel), OR
4.   Tretinoin 0.01% or 0.025% gel (available as 15 g)
a.   Products should be used sparingly at bedtime
b.   Dead skin should be removed nightly with washcloth before reapplying preparation
c.   Use petroleum jelly to protect the surrounding skin

D.   Follow Up: None required

WARTS

I. Definition: Virus-induced epidermal tumors

II. Pathogenesis

    A. Wart virus is located within epidermal cell nucleus

    B. Cells proliferate to form a mass which remains confined to the epidermis

III. Clinical Presentation

    A. May appear at any age but commonly occur in young adults

    B. Warts are transmitted by touch and commonly appear at sites of trauma on the hands, periungual regions from biting, and on plantar surfaces from weight bearing

    C. Most warts resolve in 12-24 months without treatment

    D. Generally, warts are asymptomatic except for plantar warts which may be painful

    E. Presentation is variable depending on type:
        1. Common wart (verruca vulgaris) may arise anywhere on body and appears as solitary flesh-colored papule with a scaly, irregular surface
        2. Filiform warts are usually seen on face (lips, nose, eyelids) and appear as thin projections on a narrow stalk
        3. Flat warts (verruca plana) are usually located on face and extremities and appear in groups as flat-topped, skin-colored papules
        4. Plantar warts occur on weight-bearing areas of the feet; papule is pushed into skin and verrucous surface appears level with skin surface
        5. Venereal warts are considered under SEXUALLY TRANSMITTED DISEASES section

IV. Diagnosis/Evaluation

    A. History
        1. Question about location, onset, duration, and if any symptoms are present
        2. Ask about treatments tried and results

    B. Physical Examination
        1. Examine lesion looking for characteristic appearance
        2. Use hand lens to aid in visualizing surface characteristics

    C. Differential Diagnosis
        1. Calluses (have smooth rather than rough irregular surface)
        2. Lichen planus (look for Wickham's striae)
        3. Seborrheic keratosis (have stuck on appearance with horn cysts visible on close inspection)

    D. Diagnostic Tests: None indicated

V. Plan/Management

    A. Common wart: Topical salicylic acid preparations applied at bedtime for 6-8 weeks; may use liquid nitrogen in cooperative patients (can be quite uncomfortable for young children)
        1. Examples of 17% concentrations are Occlusal HP, Duoplant, Compound W, Duofilm, Wart-Off; all are OTC and in liquid form

2. An example of a 15% solution in karaya gum base patches for use on isolated thicker lesions is Trans Ver Sal (40 patches of varying size with securing tapes and emery file)

B. Filiform wart: Refer for removal by snip excision

C. Flat wart: Refer for removal; these warts are resistant to treatment and are usually located in cosmetically important areas

D. Plantar wart: Use 40% salicylic acid plasters; examples are Mediplast and Duofilm Patch
   1. Plaster is cut to size of wart and applied over wart
   2. Plaster is removed in 24-48 hours and pliable dead white keratin is removed with pumice stone
   3. Process is repeated every 24-48 hours until wart is removed (usually 6-8 weeks)
   4. Pain relief occurs early because a large part of wart is removed in first few days of treatment

E. Follow Up: None indicated

REFERENCES

Abramowicz, M. (1998). Drugs for parasitic infections. The Medical Letter, 40(1017), 1-11.

American Academy of Pediatrics, Committee on Infectious Diseases. (1997). Red book: Report of the committee on infectious diseases (24th ed.). Elk Grove Village, IL: Author.

Bernhard, J.D. (1994). Itch: Mechanisms and management of puritus. New York: McGraw-Hill.

Bisno, A.L., & Stevens, D.L. (1996). Streptococcal infections of skin and soft tissues. New England Journal of Medicine, 334, 240-245.

Chapel, K.L., & Rasmussen, J.E. (1997). Pediatric dermatology: Advances in therapy. Journal of the American Academy of Dermatology, 36(3), 513-523.

Goldstein, B.G., & Goldstein, A.O. (1997). Practical dermatology. St. Louis: Mosby.

Habif, T.P. (1996). Clinical dermatology. St. Louis: Mosby.

Kligman, A.M. (1997). The treatment of acne with topical retinoids: One man's opinions. Journal of the American Academy of Dermatology, 36, S-92-95.

Leyden, J.J. (1997). Therapy for acne vulgaris. New England Journal of Medicine, 336, 1156-1162.

Leyden, J.J. (1998). Emerging topical retinoid therapies. Journal of the American Academy of Dermatology, 38, S1-4.

Rosen, T., & Ablon, G. (1997, Sept). Cutaneous herpes virus infection update. Consultant, 2443-2455.

Sadick, N.S. (1997). Current aspects of bacterial infections of the skin. Dermatologic Clinics of North America, 15(2), 341-346.

Weston, W.L., Lane, A.T., & Movelli, J.C. (1996). Color textbook of pediatric dermatology. St. Louis: Mosby.

Woodmanse, D., & Christiansen, S. (1998). Atopic dermatitis. Pediatric Annals, 27, 710-716.

Problems of the Eyes

AMBLYOPIA

I. Definition: Marked decrease in visual acuity in one eye due to an interruption of normal visual development during a critical period in the first few years of life (before age 7)

II. Pathogenesis

  A. Exact mechanism is unknown, but there appears to be a microscopic defect in wiring of the retina-to-brain connections that results from disuse of one eye

  B. There are three main causes of amblyopia: physical occlusion (e.g., cataract, ptosis), refractive errors, and strabismus

  C. A marked difference in visual acuity between 2 eyes (anisometropia) is especially amblyopiogenic

III. Clinical Presentation

  A. Amblyopia affects up to 5% of population

  B. Condition is potentially reversible when identified before visual development is complete (no later than age 7)

  C. Typical presentation is a young child with an acuity difference between the eyes or with bilateral vision less than expected for the age of the child

  D. Child with amblyopia usually tests poorly on standard visual acuity charts using rows of letters or symbols because of difficulty in separating out individual letters/symbols (crowding phenomenon); vision testing is more accurate using single, isolated, letters or symbols

IV. Diagnosis/Evaluation

  A. History
    1. Ask parents when symptoms were first noticed and what in particular was observed
    2. In infant, ask parent if child can fixate on and follow objects
    3. In infant, ask parent if fine motor coordination is at appropriate level based on age
    4. Ask parent if child has abnormal face or head position (head turn or chin tilt may improve acuity or correct diplopia)
    5. In older child, ask parent if developmental tasks were achieved at appropriate age
    6. Inquire about other eye problems and their treatment

  B. Physical Examination
    1. Test for visual acuity (testing both eyes separately) using the Tumbling E (also called Illiterate E) or the Allen picture cards (see VISUAL IMPAIRMENT for details on how to test visual acuity in children)
    2. Inspect eyelids, conjunctiva, cornea, height and equality of the level of upper eyelids
    3. Assess pupils for shape, size, equality, reaction to light
    4. Assess extraocular movement using an interesting target
    5. Perform cover test (see STRABISMUS for technique and interpretation of cover testing)
    6. Perform corneal light reflex test (shine light directly in eyes from a distance of about 24 inches; observe the position of the reflection of the light on each cornea with respect to the location of the pupil)
    7. Assess for presence of red reflex

  C. Differential Diagnosis
    1. Optic nerve hypoplasia
    2. Abnormalities of the retina

3. Cortical blindness
4. Cataract
5. Anisometropia (Unequal refractive error between the eyes)
6. Strabismus

D. Diagnostic Tests: Additional testing will be done by pediatric ophthalmologist

V. Plan/Management

A. Referral to an ophthalmologist is necessary

B. Recognition and treatment of underlying cause is the first step in treatment (e.g., if a cataract is interfering with vision, it needs to be removed)

C. The second component of treatment by the ophthalmologist is use of occlusive therapy

D. Follow Up: Make certain the parent keeps appointment with the ophthalmologist

BLEPHARITIS

I. Definition: Inflammation of the eyelid margins

II. Pathogenesis:

A. Often due to infection (usually Staphylococcal)

B. May also be caused by hypersecretory or inflammation of sebaceous glands (often associated with seborrhea of face/scalp)

C. May be associated with conjunctivitis

III. Clinical Presentation

A. A common, chronic problem which usually begins in early childhood and continues throughout adulthood

B. Characterized by hypertrophy and desquamation of the epidermis near the lid margin which results in erythema and scaling of the lid border

C. Main complaint is redness of the eyelid margin but burning and discomfort of the eyes may be additional symptoms

D. Severe cases may produce purulent discharge and over time permanent changes in the eyelid structure can occur (lost lashes and distortion of lid contour)

E. Patient usually has a history of recurrent chalazia and hordeola

IV. Diagnosis/Evaluation

A. History
1. Determine onset and duration of symptoms
2. Ask about presence of flaking, crusting at lid margins
3. Inquire about eye pain, visual disturbances, dry eyes and tearing
4. Ask about past episodes and previous treatments
5. Inquire about previous and present skin problems, particularly of the face and scalp

233

6. Ask about chronic exposure to irritants such as smoke, cosmetics, and chemicals
7. Inquire about frequency of eye rubbing

B. Physical Examination
1. Determine visual acuity
2. Perform a complete eye examination, paying particular attention to the following components:
   a. Inspect eyelid margins with magnifying glass for crusting, scaling, erythema, and ulcers
   b. Examine sclera and conjunctiva for abnormalities
   c. Palpate lid margins and lid for masses
3. Palpate for preauricular adenopathy

C. Differential Diagnosis
1. Chalazion, stye, conjunctivitis, and keratitis may result from blepharitis
2. Sebaceous cell carcinoma is a rare condition, but should be suspected if blepharitis persists despite extensive treatment

D. Diagnostic Tests: None are usually indicated

V. Plan/Management:

A. If an underlying source of the lid irritation can be identified, it is important to treat the source as the first step in management
1. If seborrheic dermatitis of the scalp and face is present, institute appropriate treatment (see section on SEBORRHEIC DERMATITIS for treatment recommendations)
2. If dry eyes are present, advise patient to use agents such as Cellufresh or Lacrisert

B. For patients with **acute** phase of blepharitis, the following treatment should be instituted
1. Instruct patient in eye hygiene
   a. Patient should be directed to scrub eyelids with wet washcloth (or cotton-tipped applicator) and baby shampoo (or commercial cleansing pads such as Eye Scrub or Lid Wipes SPF) in order to remove crusts and scale
   b. Scrubs should be repeated up to four times a day depending on symptoms
   c. May also apply warm, moist compresses for 15 minutes throughout the day
2. If condition is moderate to severe, prescribe erythromycin, 5 mg/g (Ilotycin) ophthalmic ointment BID x 7 days OR sulfacetamide sodium 10% (Bleph-10) available as ophthalmic solution or ointment (solution: 1-2 drops Q3H during day; ointment: QID and at HS) x 7 days

C. For patients with chronic blepharitis, the following treatment is recommended
1. Instruct patient to continue daily eye hygiene of the lid margins
2. For flares, also use warm moist compresses throughout day and apply ophthalmic antibiotics intermittently when needed

D. For severe blepharitis, referral to an ophthalmologist is indicated

E. Follow Up
1. None needed for mild cases
2. Reevaluate moderate cases in 10-14 days

CHALAZION

I.   Definition: Focal chronic inflammation of a meibomian gland

II. Pathogenesis

   A.   Chronic granuloma from obstructed meibomian gland

   B.   May occur as a result of a chronic hordeolum

   C.   Secondary infection of the surrounding tissues may develop

III. Clinical Presentation

   A.   Usually hard, non-tender nodule is found on midportion of the tarsus, away from the lid border; may develop on lid margin if the opening of the duct is involved and can present with lid tenderness, pain, and swelling

   B.   Chalazia which become infected result in painful swelling of the entire lid

   C.   Small chalazia may resolve spontaneously without treatment

   D.   History of chronic blepharitis and prior excision of chalazia is often present

IV. Diagnosis/Evaluation

   A.   History
        1.   Determine onset and duration of symptoms
        2.   Inquire about pain or tenderness of the lid
        3.   Inquire about any changes in visual acuity level
        4.   Ask about past episodes and previous treatments

   B.   Physical Examination
        1.   Assess visual acuity
        2.   Perform a complete eye examination, paying particular attention to the following components
             a.   Inspect eyelids for inflammation and masses
             b.   Palpate eyelids for masses and tenderness
             c.   Evert the eyelid and examine inner surface for pointing
             d.   Inspect sclera and conjunctiva for abnormalities
        3.   Palpate for preauricular adenopathy

   C.   Differential Diagnosis
        1.   May be associated with a hordeolum and blepharitis
        2.   Sebaceous cell carcinoma is a rare condition which should be considered

   D.   Diagnostic Tests: None indicated

V.   Plan/Management

   A.   Small, asymptomatic chronic chalazia do not require treatment and usually disappear spontaneously within a few months

B. If chalazia are large or if there is secondary infection, treatment is needed
   1. Apply warm, moist compresses for 15 minutes throughout the day
   2. Prescribe erythromycin, 5 mg/g (Ilotycin) ophthalmic ointment BID x 7 days OR polymyxin B-trimethoprim drops (Polytrim) BID x 7 days

C. If the chalazion does not respond to conservative therapy, patient should be referred to an expert for injection of the lesion or incision and curettage

D. Follow Up
   1. Small chalazia do not require follow up
   2. Follow up for chalazia that do not respond to conservative therapy should be with ophthalmologist

CONGENITAL NASOLACRIMAL DUCT OBSTRUCTION

I. Definition: A defect of the lacrimal drainage system in which a lack of patency affects drainage function

II. Pathogenesis: An imperforate membrane at the distal end of the nasolacrimal duct is the usual cause of occlusion

III. Clinical Presentation

   A. The most common abnormality of the infant's lacrimal apparatus

   B. Incidence of this condition in newborn infants is approximately 6%

   C. Usually presents within the first few weeks of life with persistent tearing, crusting of the lashes, and mucopurulent discharge

   D. Tears spill over the lower lid and there is a persistent "wet look" in the involved eye or eyes

   E. Reflux of mucopurulent material from either punctum can be elicited by gently pressing over the nasolacrimal sac of the involved eye(s)

   F. Discharge is most evident after the infant awakens and parent must use a moistened cloth to loosen dried mucus on the lashes

   G. There are no systemic manifestations

   H. Most (almost 90%) congenital obstructions of the nasolacrimal duct clear spontaneously within one year

IV. Diagnosis/Evaluation

   A. History
      1. Ask parent when condition was first noticed, and if one or both eyes are affected
      2. Inquire regarding appearance of discharge, and if matting of lashes occurs
      3. Ask if condition is worse in mornings and after naps when child first awakens
      4. Ask about treatments tried and results
      5. Ask parent if child's vision seems normal

B. Physical Examination
1. Assess visual acuity (ability to fix and follow an interesting object)
2. Examine the lids and adnexa for symmetry, swelling, abnormal discharge, erythema; examine sclera, cornea, and conjunctiva for signs of inflammation
3. Palpate the soft tissue of the orbit, lids, and zygoma
4. Inspect and palpate the lacrimal apparatus, including the lacrimal gland, superior and inferior puncta, canaliculi, and lacrimal sac
5. Gently press over the nasolacrimal sac on the affected side to elicit material from the puncta
6. Note appearance of discharge (if present) from affected eye(s)

C. Differential Diagnosis
1. Conjunctivitis
2. Blepharitis
3. Dacryocystitis

D. Diagnostic Tests: None indicated

V. Plan/Treatment

A. Conservative treatment is the recommended approach to management of nasolacrimal duct obstruction in children less than 12 months of age

B. Instruct parent to massage the lacrimal sac several times a day in an effort to rupture the membrane at the lower end of the duct
1. As illustrated, instruct parent to place index finger over the nasolacrimal sac and exert downward pressure
2. Then slide finger downward toward the mouth
3. Theoretically, fluid is trapped in the lacrimal sac, and then the downward motion breaks the obstruction in the lacrimal duct with hydrostatic pressure

C. The technique is shown in Figure 8.1

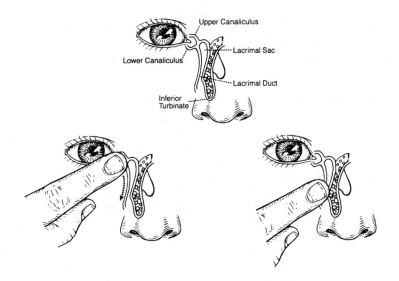

Figure 8.1. Nasolacrimal Duct Massage.

D. If there is evidence of secondary conjunctivitis (conjunctiva is inflamed) or significant discharge that is purulent or mucopurulent, administration of topical antibiotics is indicated
1. Sodium sulfacetamide, 10% (Sulamyd) 1-2 drops TID x 7 days
2. Erythromycin ointment (Ilotycin) 0.5 cm strip of ointment in lower conjunctival sac QID x 7 days

3. Advise parent that antibiotic drops or ointment reduce the infectious component of the discharge, but do not cure the blockage
4. Aim of antibiotic therapy is to alter the character of the discharge so that it is mucoid
5. Prolonged use of antibiotics for tearing without purulent or mucopurulent discharge is not indicated

E. Controversy exists regarding when to surgically treat the condition
1. Some authorities recommend conservative treatment for a short time and then referral of the child for surgery at less than 6 months of age (early probing may be more successful and may obviate need for general anesthesia)
2. Other experts recommend that conservative therapy be continued for almost the first year of life, and then referral for surgery at that time if the condition has not spontaneously resolved (late probing [at 12-13 months of age] may reduce the number of unnecessary probings)

F. Follow Up: In 2 weeks if child placed on topical antibiotics to determine efficacy of treatment

CONJUNCTIVITIS

I. Definition: Inflammation of the conjunctiva characterized by vascular dilation, cellular infiltration, and exudation

II. Pathogenesis

A. Conjunctivitis can be caused by bacterial or viral agents, by allergic reaction, or by toxic factors
1. Acute bacterial conjunctivitis
   a. *Staphylococcus aureus* (probably the most common cause of bacterial conjunctivitis and the most common causative organism in adults)
   b. *Streptococcus pneumoniae* (more commonly a causative organism in children rather than adults)
   c. *Haemophilus influenzae* (more commonly a causative organism in children rather than adults)
2. Hyperacute bacterial conjunctivitis
   a. Most commonly caused by *Neisseria gonorrhoeae* and less often by *Neisseria meningitidis;* occurs in adults via autoinoculation from infected genitalia
   b. Conjunctivitis in the newborn caused by *Neisseria gonorrhoeae* represents the most serious type of ophthalmia neonatorum, defined as conjunctivitis that occurs during the first month of life
3. Ocular chlamydial infections are of two types
   a. Trachoma is associated with serotypes A through C and causes a chronic keratoconjunctivitis which frequently results in blindness; this condition is rare in the US but occurs in rural areas of developing countries, particularly Africa, Asia, and the Middle East
   b. Inclusion conjunctivitis is associated with serotypes D through K and is a common, primarily sexually transmitted disease that occurs in both newborns and adults in the US; it is the most frequent cause of conjunctivitis in neonates
4. Viral conjunctivitis
   a. Usually caused by adenovirus
   b. *Herpes simplex* virus is a less common cause
5. Noninfectious conjunctivitis
   a. Allergic conjunctivitis (hay fever conjunctivitis)
   b. Contact lens associated
   c. Toxic (often occurs as a chemical reaction in patients using ocular medications)

B. Systemic infections such as rubella, rubeola, and Kawasaki disease may present with conjunctivitis

III. Clinical presentation

A. Acute bacterial conjunctivitis
1. Characterized by acute onset of mucopurulent or purulent discharge with burning, irritation, and tearing
2. Eyelids are often edematous with matting of the eyelashes upon awakening
3. Inflammation is more prominent in the palpebral conjunctiva than in the bulbar conjunctiva with mild injection of the conjunctival vessels
4. Typically, the infection begins in one eye and then becomes bilateral in 2 to 5 days
5. Usually the condition is self-limited but antibiotics can shorten the time course of infection

B. Hyperacute bacterial conjunctivitis
1. A severe, sight-threatening ocular infection most often affecting sexually active adolescents and newborn infants
   a. In adolescents, organism is transmitted from genitalia to hands, and then to eyes
   b. In newborns, transmission is via vaginal delivery from an infected woman and symptoms usually present at 3-5 days of age
2. Characterized by marked yellow-green purulent discharge that is bilateral, lid edema, erythema, and chemosis
3. Preauricular lymphadenopathy often present

C. Chlamydial conjunctivitis in adolescents
1. Usually presents in young sexually active persons between the ages of 18 and 30
2. Transmission occurs most often via autoinoculation from infected genital secretions
3. Typically, an indolent infection which is characterized by a thin, mucoid discharge
4. Patient may have photophobia and enlarged, tender preauricular nodes
5. Subacute or chronic in nature, with patients presenting with symptoms that have been present for as long as 6 months

D. Chlamydial conjunctivitis in newborns
1. By far the most common cause of conjunctivitis in newborn
2. Usually presents 5 to 12 days after birth in infants exposed during vaginal delivery
3. Presents with more mucopurulent discharge and inflammation than in adolescents

E. Viral conjunctivitis due to adenoviruses
1. Often occurs in community epidemics and is highly contagious
2. Usual modes of transmission are contaminated fingers and swimming pool water
3. Onset is usually acute and discharge is usually watery
4. A mild injection of the conjunctiva lasting 3-4 days is often present
5. Always self-limited and rarely results in sequelae

F. Viral conjunctivitis due to herpes simplex
1. Type 1 herpes simplex virus is the type that is usually involved in ocular disease
2. Occurs very infrequently especially in view of the fact that by age 60, approximately 97% of all persons have been infected with type 1 HSV, and less than 1% of these infections present as ocular disease
3. May be accompanied by fever blister on lip or face
4. Preauricular nodes are usually enlarged
5. Occurs most frequently in immunosuppressed persons

G. Noninfectious conjunctivitis
1. **Allergic**: Itching is the hallmark of this condition; systemic manifestations of hay fever such as rhinorrhea and sneezing which is usually seasonal may also be present
   a. Characterized by itchy, red eyes, with discharge that is watery and bilateral
   b. Eyelids may be edematous and have a cobblestone appearance

c. **Note**: Vernal catarrh is a serious form of allergic conjunctivitis and is seen most often in children and adolescents (more common in male African Americans); may result in severe corneal ulceration and loss of vision

2. **Contact lens associated**: Soft contact lenses are most often involved
   a. Ocular irritation with erythema, pruritus, and mucoid discharge is common
   b. Characteristic papillae are present on the upper tarsal conjunctiva

3. **Toxic**: Presents most commonly in patients using ocular medication
   a. Discharge is usually watery or mucoid
   b. Chemosis may be present but no preauricular nodes are palpable
   c. Examination will reveal a follicular and papillary response

IV. Diagnosis/Evaluation

A. History
   1. Inquire regarding onset and duration of symptoms (Is the condition acute, subacute, chronic, or recurrent?)
   2. Determine if condition is unilateral or bilateral; ask about the type and amount of discharge
   3. Determine if ocular pain, photophobia, or blurred vision (that fails to clear with a blink) are present
   4. Ask if itching and other symptoms of seasonal allergic rhinitis are present
   5. Ask about contact with a person with "pink-eye"
   6. Inquire about personal and family history of hay fever, allergic rhinitis
   7. Obtain past medical and medication history, specifically asking about use of any ocular medications (including OTCs)

B. Physical Examination
   1. Determine visual acuity, visual fields, pupillary function and extraocular movements
   2. Examine eyelids for inflammation or tenderness
   3. Examine sclera and conjunctiva for hyperemia and edema; check cornea for clarity
   4. Determine type of discharge
   5. Examine face for presence of herpes labialis or a dermatomal vesicular eruption suggesting shingles
   6. Palpate for regional lymphadenopathy

C. Differential Diagnosis: Patients typically present with the main complaint of red eye; there is need to distinguish conjunctivitis from other conditions causing red eye
   1. In conjunctivitis, redness of the conjunctiva is diffuse, pain is minimal, and vision, pupil size, and reactivity are normal
   2. Acute angle-closure glaucoma presents with severe ocular pain, headache, and blurred vision
   3. Iritis presents with pain, moderately decreased vision, dull and swollen iris, and sluggishly reacting pupil; injection is usually bulbar near limbus
   4. Lacrimal duct obstruction presents with pain, redness, and edema around lacrimal sac; pressure over lacrimal sac will express mucopurulent material from the upper and lower canaliculi
   5. Blepharitis may have similar presentation as conjunctivitis with burning and itching of the conjunctiva, but with blepharitis there also is inflammation of lid margins
   6. Corneal abrasions usually have a history of trauma with mild to moderate bulbar injection and a foreign-body sensation

D. Diagnostic Tests
   1. Culture and smears of discharge are usually not recommended for mild conjunctivitis with a suspected viral, bacterial, allergic, or toxic origin
   2. If there is severe inflammation as occurs with hyperacute conjunctivitis, or if the condition is chronic or recurrent, a culture is indicated
   3. If testing for chlamydia is indicated based on history, enzyme immunoassays for Chlamydia organisms or DNA assays may be used

V.   Plan/Management

   A.   Acute bacterial conjunctivitis: If treatment is based on clinical diagnosis alone, select a broad spectrum topical antibiotics such as ONE of the following
   1.   Erythromycin ointment (Ilotycin): Apply small amount 2-3x/day for 7-10 days
   2.   Polymyxin B-trimethoprim solution (Polytrim) Children >2 months: 1 gtt Q 3-4 hours (maximum 6 doses/day) x 7-10 days
   3.   Sodium sulfacetamide 10% solution (Bleph-10) Children >2 months: 1-2 gtts Q 2-3 hours during day for 7-10 days (**Note**: About 50% of staphylococci are now resistant to the sulfonamides)

   B.   Hyperacute bacterial conjunctivitis: Systemic antibiotics are required and most patients with this condition should be admitted to the hospital for IV therapy

   C.   Chlamydial conjunctivitis in adolescents: Prescribe systemic antibiotics Doxycycline (Vibramycin) 100 mg BID for 7 days
   1.   Once a diagnosis has been established, a genital work-up of the patient and sexual partner is indicated
   2.   Pregnant and lactating females: Use erythromycin, 250 mg QID x 21 days
   3.   Diagnosis of chlamydial disease in an infant, child, or adolescent should prompt investigation for other sexually diseases, including syphilis, gonorrhea, hepatitis B and HIV infection

   D.   Chlamydial conjunctivitis in newborns: Systemic erythromycin is the treatment of choice
   1.   Oral erythromycin 50 mg/kg/day in 4 divided doses for 14 days
   2.   Topical treatment of chlamydial conjunctivitis is ineffective and unnecessary
   3.   See V.C.3 above

   E.   Viral infections primarily due to adenoviruses
   1.   Usually self-limiting and treatment is supportive (application of cold compresses and use of topical vasoconstrictor)
   2.   Antiviral agents have not proven to be effective
   3.   Topical antibiotics are not necessary as secondary bacterial infection is uncommon

   F.   Viral infection due to herpes simplex
   1.   Refer to ophthalmologist
   2.   Never prescribe steroid medication if herpes simplex virus is a possibility as steroid preparations can enhance proliferation of virus and result in permanent eye damage

   G.   Allergic conjunctivitis
   1.   Prescribe cromolyn sodium (Crolom) ophthalmic solution: Children >4 years, 1-2 gtts 4 times a day OR
   2.   Patanol solution, an antihistamine/mast cell stabilizer: Children >3 years, 1-2 gtts BID at 6-8 hour intervals
   3.   Systemic antihistamines are also often recommended
       a.   Loratadine (Claritin), supplied as 10 mg tabs and I mg/mL syrup
       b.   Children >6 years: 10 mg QD

   H.   Toxic conjunctivitis
   1.   Eliminate the suspected medication
   2.   Prescribe mild ocular lubricants such as Tears Naturale or Naturale Free to promote comfort
   3.   Suggest frequent cold compresses

   I.   Contact lens associated conjunctivitis
   1.   Discontinuation of contact lens use is curative, but is not often acceptable to patient
   2.   Trials of stopping the use of various agents and substituting others (example, change the contact lens solution) or changing the type of contact lens may be helpful

J. Refer the patient for expert management if any of the following occur
1. There is no improvement in 24-48 hours
2. Patient has moderate to severe ocular pain, decreased visual acuity, abnormal eye exam
3. Infection from herpes simplex virus

K. Patient Education
1. Instruct patients to instill medication in the inner aspect of the lower eyelid
2. Teach patients that infection is easily spread to unaffected eye and to other household members
3. The role of frequent handwashing in limiting the spread of ocular infections cannot be overemphasized
4. Discuss with patient that eye secretions are contagious for 24 to 48 hours after therapy begins
5. Patients with viral infections should be instructed that the ocular infection is contagious for at least seven days after the onset

L. Follow Up
1. If no improvement in 24-48, or if condition worsens, patient should return for referral for expert care
2. No follow up is indicated for mild cases which resolve without problems

HORDEOLUM (STYE)

I. Definition: Acute inflammation of the follicle of an eyelash or the associated gland of Zeis (sebaceous) or Moll (apocrine sweat gland)

II. Pathogenesis: An acute infectious process involving the sebaceous, sweat or meibomian glands of the eyelid usually caused by *Staphylococcus aureus*

III. Clinical Presentation

A. More common in children and adolescents than adults

B. Patient often presents with sudden onset of localized tenderness, redness, and swelling of the eyelid

C. May occur in crops because the infecting pathogen may spread from one hair follicle to another

D. May point to the conjunctival side of the lid (internal hordeolum involving the meibomian glands) or may involve the lid margin (external hordeolum involving the sebaceous or sweat glands)

IV. Diagnosis/Evaluation

A. History
1. Determine onset and duration of symptoms
2. Inquire about pain and visual disturbances
3. Ask about past episodes and previous treatments

B. Physical Examination
1. Assess visual acuity
2. Inspect eyelids for inflammation, swelling, and discharge
3. Palpate eyelids for induration and masses
4. Evert the eyelid and examine inner surface for pointing
5. Examine sclera and conjunctiva for abnormalities
6. Palpate for preauricular adenopathy

C. Differential Diagnosis: The main differential diagnosis is chalazia; chalazia point on the conjunctival side of the eyelid and do not usually affect the margin of the eyelid

D. Diagnostic Tests: None indicated

V. Plan/Management

A. Apply warm, moist compresses for 15 minutes throughout the day

B. Prescribe erythromycin, 5 mg/g (Ilotycin) ophthalmic ointment BID x 7 days OR polymyxin B-trimethoprim drops (Polytrim) BID x 7 days

C. Cleanse eyelids daily with a neutral soap such as Neutrogena

D. If not responsive to medical therapy, refer to expert for incision and drainage

E. If crops of styes occur, diabetes mellitus must be excluded and patient should be told not to rub eyes; some authorities recommend a course of tetracycline to stop recurrences

F. Patient Education
1. Advise patient that good periorbital hygiene will help prevent recurrence
2. Advise against wearing eye makeup until clear and disposing of all old make up as it may be contaminated.

G. Follow Up: None indicated

STRABISMUS

I. Definition: Abnormal ocular alignment

II. Pathogenesis

A. Strabismus may be divided into two general types according to underlying pathophysiology:
1. Nonparalytic strabismus: a condition due to muscle weakness, focusing difficulties, unilateral refractive error, nonfusion, or anatomical differences in the eyes
2. Paralytic strabismus: a motor imbalance caused by paresis or paralysis of an extraocular muscle

B. Because visual axes are not parallel, the brain receives two images thereby interfering with binocular vision

C. Familial tendencies toward strabismus have been well documented, but no clear-cut genetic mode of inheritance has been identified

III. Clinical Presentation

A. Whereas the eyes of the newborn infant are rarely aligned during the first few weeks of life, by the age of three months, normal oculomotor behavior is usually established and an experienced examiner may be able to document the existence of abnormal alignment by that time

B. Strabismus involves a number of complex clinical entities and only the common patterns are listed here. This discussion is limited to Nonparalytic strabismus
1. Convergent deviation: a crossing or turning in of the eyes is designated by the prefix eso-
2. Divergent deviation: a turning outward of the eyes is designated by the prefix exo-
3. Vertical deviations are designated by the prefixes hyper- (upward) and hypo- (downward)

C. Pseudostrabismus is one of the most common reasons a pediatric ophthalmologist is asked to evaluate an infant
   1. A false appearance of strabismus when visual axes are in reality aligned accurately
   2. Appearance may be due to flat, broad nasal bridge, prominent epicanthal folds, or narrow interpupillary distance
   3. Observer may see less white sclera nasally than expected due to above factors

D. Esotropia (nonparalytic strabismus) is the condition of inward or convergent deviation of the eyes
   1. Most common ocular misalignment representing more than half of all ocular deviations in the pediatric population
   2. Infantile esotropia occurs in infancy and whether it is congenital or has onset soon after birth is undetermined
   3. Accommodative esotropia occurs between 6 months and 7 years with an average age of 2.5 years and may be intermittent or constant

E. Exotropia (nonparalytic strabismus) is characterized by divergent misalignment of the eyes that may be intermittent or constant
   1. Intermittent exotropia is the most common type of exotropic strabismus and is characterized by an outward drift of one eye most often occurring when child is fixating at distance
      a. Deviation more frequent with fatigue or illness
      b. Photophobia in the exotropic eye is common
      c. Visual acuity tends to be good in both eyes with normal binocular vision
      d. Age of onset is usually between infancy and age 4 years
   2. Constant exotropia (nonparalytic strabismus) may be congenital but most often results from the following:
      a. Deterioration of intermittent exotropia
      b. Significant loss of vision in one eye (usually after age 5 years)
      c. Overcorrection following surgery for esotropia

IV. Diagnosis/Evaluation

   A. History
      1. Ask when were symptoms first noticed (age of onset) and what in particular was observed (description of deviation)
      2. Ask about frequency and duration of deviation, symptoms, and previous treatment
      3. Request that parents bring in unposed photos of the child at various ages to help evaluate deviation over time
      4. In infants, ask does child fix and follow objects
      5. In infants, ask if fine motor coordination is at appropriate level based on age
      6. Ask if child has abnormal face or head position (head turn or chin tilt may improve acuity or correct diplopia)
      7. Ask if child spontaneously closes one eye (squint)
      8. Ask about presence of eye deviations in blood relatives
      9. In older children, ask if developmental tasks have been achieved at appropriate age

   B. Physical Examination
      1. Test for visual acuity (testing both eyes separately using the Tumbling E (also called Illiterate E) or the Allen picture cards for preschoolers and school-aged children and fixation and following testing for infants (See VISUAL IMPAIRMENT for details on how to test visual acuity in children and infants)
      2. Inspect eyelids, conjunctiva, cornea, height and equality of the level of upper eyelids
      3. Assess pupils for shape, size, equality, reaction to light
      4. Perform corneal light reflex test (shine light directly in eyes from a distance of about 24 inches; observe the position of the reflection of the light on each cornea with respect to the location of the pupil)
      5. Assess extraocular movement using an interesting target
      6. Assess for presence of red reflex
      7. Perform cover test which depends on the fixation reflex

TECHNIQUE AND INTERPRETATION FOR COVER TESTING

Overview

▲ A prerequisite to cover testing is the ability of each eye to focus when the fellow eye is covered; if organic disease (such as cataract) or functional conditions (for example, eccentric fixation) prevent central fixation, the test is invalid. Because the child begins the test with both eyes viewing, the cover test examines a binocular circumstance

Technique

▲ Have child look at fixation target with both eyes viewing (use interesting toy or picture at about a 24" distance)

▲ Place an occluder over one eye while watching the fellow eye for shift in fixation

▲ If no shift occurs, the occluder may have been placed in front of the deviating eye in which case the fellow eye would already be fixed on the target

▲ Allow the child to return to binocular vision for several seconds, so that fusion (if it exists) can take place

▲ The second eye is then covered and the first eye is observed for movement

Interpretation

▲ If a shift occurs, the shift is evidence that the uncovered eye was not regarding the target with its fovea when both eyes were viewing

▲ This deviation is called a heterotropia, or a manifest deviation (i.e., it exists under normal seeing circumstances, both eyes viewing)

Summary: Sequence of Cover Test

▲ Child's attention is drawn to fixation target

▲ Cover one eye, observing the fellow eye

▲ Uncover that eye and wait for a few seconds to allow fusion (if it exists) to take place

▲ Cover the second eye while observing the first eye

    C.   Differential Diagnosis: Pseudostrabismus

    D.   Diagnostic Tests: Additional diagnostic testing should be done by the ophthalmologist

V.   Plan/Management

    A.   All children in whom strabismus is suspected must be evaluated by a pediatric ophthalmologist

    B.   When poor fixation is present, the preferred eye must be patched to allow vision to develop in the other eye

    C.   The decision to perform muscle surgery is based on the degree and frequency of deviation

    D.   Follow up is by an ophthalmologist

VISUAL IMPAIRMENT IN CHILDREN

I.   Definition: A decline in vision in one or both eyes

II.   Pathogenesis

    A.   Etiology of impaired vision can be divided into two general categories

        1.   Refractive errors or those problems that can be improved by glasses (common causes: myopia, hyperopia, presbyopia, anisometropia, and astigmatism)

        2.   Non-refractive errors (retinal abnormalities, glaucoma, cataract, retinoblastoma, eye muscle imbalance, and systemic disease with ocular manifestations) that cannot be corrected by glasses alone

B.   For clear vision, light must focus precisely on the retina
1.   In nearsightedness, or myopia, light is focused in front of the retina and the person sees near objects best
2.   In farsightedness, or hyperopia, light is focused behind the retina and the person sees far objects best

C.   Myopia is a condition in which objects can be seen clearly if held close enough to the eye (the person is "nearsighted"); person typically has no problem with reading or close work

D.   Hyperopia is called farsightedness, and means that the individual cannot see near objects; because children have strong focusing or accommodative mechanisms that enable them to overcome moderate amounts of hyperopia and still maintain clear vision, this condition is relatively uncommon in children

E.   Anisometropia is a state in which there is a difference in the refractive error of the two eyes; condition may be congenital or acquired (due to asymmetric age changes or disease)

F.   Astigmatism is a condition in which curvature variations of the optical system result in unequal light refraction and impaired vision

G.   Pathophysiology of conditions causing non-refractive errors is dependent on the condition

III.   Clinical Presentation

A.   Refractive errors requiring the use of corrective lenses exist in almost 20% of the pediatric population

B.   Children with refractive errors most often have difficulty with far vision. Typically, the child is unable to read the blackboard from back of the room, or see movie from back of the theater

C.   Myopia is the most common clinically significant refractive error seen in childhood
1.   Condition is rarely present at birth
2.   Often begins to develop as the child grows and is usually detected by age 9 or 10 in school vision testing
3.   Usually stabilizes in mid-teens, at about 5 diopters or less

D.   Hyperopia usually does not necessitate correction in children unless it causes the eyes to cross, or causes reduced vision

E.   In anisometropia, the visual acuity differences between the two eyes may result in suppression strabismus or amblyopia

F.   Astigmatism can begin in either childhood or adulthood and can be easily corrected if it causes blurred vision or eye discomfort

G.   Children with non-refractive errors have impaired vision at both near and far distances
1.   Children with open-angle glaucoma are usually asymptomatic until neural damage has occurred; visual dysfunction in glaucoma is first expressed in the mid-peripheral field of vision (central vision functions such as acuity remain relatively intact until late in the disease process)
2.   Children with cataract may be observed to have nystagmus of the wandering or searching type (nystagmus of the blind)
3.   Young children with impaired vision from both refractive and non-refractive causes rarely complain but may rub the eye (if pain present) or may squint
4.   See STRABISMUS and AMBLYOPIA for more information on impaired vision due to these causes

H.   Visual acuity correctable by glasses or contact lenses to 20/200 or worse in both eyes, or visual fields <10° centrally, constitutes legal blindness in the US

IV. Diagnosis/Evaluation

  A. History
      1. Determine if vision in one or both eyes is impaired and if both near and far vision are affected
      2. Ask if there are associated symptoms of eye discomfort, increased tearing, cloudy vision, or flashing lights
      3. In infants and toddlers, ask parent if vision seems normal
          a. Ask if there are any behaviors present that suggest vision is a problem
          b. Ask regarding achievement of developmental tasks particularly in the area of eye-hand (fine motor) coordination
      4. In school-age child, ask about school performance, reading ability, and parent's observations about child's visual acuity
      5. Ask about chronic or past eye problems, previous treatments and response
      6. Ask if there is a family history of eye disease

  B. Physical Examination
      1. Examine external eye for swelling, ptosis, injection of the conjunctiva, and corneal clarity
      2. Determine extraocular movement: In small children, have them fixate on and follow a brightly colored or interesting object
      3. Measure peripheral vision (recognizing that this is only a very gross assessment of visual fields)
          a. Children can be tested by using a threatening gesture from the periphery and observing response
          b. Older children can be tested by direct confrontation
      4. Perform the cover test (described in detail under STRABISMUS)
      5. Perform corneal light reflex test (shine light directly in eyes from a distance of about 24 inches; observe the position of the reflection of the light on each cornea with respect to the location of the pupil)
      6. Elicit red reflex and perform fundoscopic exam
      7. Determine visual acuity

KEY POINTS TO KEEP IN MIND IN THE ASSESSMENT OF VISUAL ACUITY IN CHILDREN

General Principles for Testing Children
It is essential to test each eye independently, with the other eye occluded
For older children, use of a hand held occluder is usually satisfactory
For young children, eye occlusion with an adhesive patch is preferred to avoid intentional/unintentional peeping
Subjects who wear corrective glasses should be tested with and without glasses

Older Children: Measure far vision using Snellen chart (read at 20 feet away) and near vision using hand-held Rosenbaum Pocket Vision Screening Card [Use the Tumbling E chart for children or adults who cannot read--patient identifies the direction that E is open by pointing in that direction]

Pinhole vision is tested if the patient is unable to read the 20/30 line
Place a pinhole aperture in front of the eye to ascertain any improvement in acuity (the pinhole will correct for any uncorrected refractive error due to nearsightedness, farsightedness, and astigmatism)
Through the pinhole, a patient with refractive error should read close to 20/20
If the pinhole fails to improve the patient's visual acuity, another cause for reduced vision such as opacities in the ocular media, or macular or optic nerve disease should be suspected

Preschool Children (3, 4, 5): Use the Tumbling E test or the Allen cards which are pictures of well-known objects (telephone, tree, house) [AAP recommends testing children at 10-feet testing distance which may result in better compliance due to closer interaction with the examiner]

Note the position of the child's head as he/she tries to read vision chart
*Head position is described in 3 parameters: Chin up or down; face turned right or left; head tilted right or left
*Any one or a combination of 2 or 3 is possible

Infants and Toddlers: The very earliest that vision testing is possible with picture cards is at approximately 2 years of age

(continued)

For toddlers younger than 2, testing vision using a picture book and asking the child to point to familiar objects such as dog, baby, flower can provide a gross measure of visual acuity (testing eyes independently may not be possible at this age as child usually refuses to have one eye covered)

In infants over 3 months, evaluate ability to fixate and follow interesting object over a wide range (90-180°); evaluate for social response to mother's face

In infants ages 4-6 weeks, assess ability to follow a light or large object over a short range (45-90°)
*Move a brightly colored object or own face across the visual field of a quiet but alert infant at a distance of one foot
*Observe infant's fixation and following behavior (over short range -- 4-6 weeks; over long range --≥3 months)

In newborns, assess for pupillary response to light and assess for blinking response to bright light

     C.   Differential Diagnosis
          1.   Refractive errors
          2.   Non-refractive errors (common causes: glaucoma, cataract, retinal detachment, uveitis, macular degeneration, strabismus, and amblyopia)

     D.   Diagnostic Tests: None indicated

V.   Plan/Management

     A.   Indicators requiring further evaluation are outlined in the table below

PATIENTS REQUIRING FURTHER EVALUATION

- Children ≥5 years of age with visual acuity of 20/30 or worse
- Children 3 years of age with visual acuity of 20/50 or worse
- Infants who fail gross visual acuity testing as outlined in the table above
- All age groups who demonstrate more than a **one-line** difference between eyes

     B.   If the cause of the impaired vision is not believed to be a refractive error, refer to ophthalmologist for further evaluation

     C.   Children with acute onset of impaired vision need immediate referral for emergency care

     D.   Patients requiring visual acuity determination for purposes of legal blindness or disability determination or for any medicolegal cases should be referred to an ophthalmologist

     E.   Follow Up: By ophthalmologist or optometrist

REFERENCES

American Academy of Pediatrics, Committee on Practice and Ambulatory Medicine. (1996). Eye examination and vision screening in infants, children, and young adults. Pediatrics, 98(1), 153-1577.

Beauchamp, G.R. & Meisler, D.M. (1991). Disorders of the conjunctiva. L.B. Nelson, J.H. Calhoun, & R.D. Harley (Eds.), Pediatric ophthalmology. Philadelphia: Saunders.

Bedrossian, E.H. (1997, March). Treatment of hordeolums: Styes and chalazia. Hospital Medicine, 59-64.

Boyer, W.P., & Peterson, R.A. (1996). Pediatric ophthalmology. In D. Pavan-Langston (Ed.), Manual of ocular diagnosis and therapy. Boston: Little-Brown.

Carter, S.R. (1998). Eyelid disorders: Diagnosis and management. American Family Physician, 57, 2695-2702.

Catalano, R.A., & Nelson, L.B. (1999). Conjunctivitis. In R.A. Dershewitz (Ed.), Ambulatory pediatric care. Philadelphia: Lippincott.

Centers for Disease Control and Prevention. (1998). 1998 Sexually transmitted diseases treatment guidelines. MMWR, 47, (No. RR-1).

Garcia, G.E., & Pavan-Langston, D. (1996). Refractive errors and clinical optics. In D. Pavan-Langston (Ed.), Manual of ocular diagnosis and therapy. Boston: Little-Brown.

Grove, A.S. (1996). Eyelids and lacrimal system. In D. Pavan-Langston (Ed.), Manual of ocular diagnosis and therapy. Boston: Little-Brown.

Kushner, B.J. (1991). Amblyopia. In L.B. Nelson, J.H. Calhoun, & R.D. Harley (Eds.), Pediatric ophthalmology. Philadelphia: Saunders.

Metz, H.S. (1999). Visual testing. In R.A. Dershewitz (Ed.), Ambulatory pediatric care. Philadelphia: Lippincott.

Metz, H.S. (1999). Visual disturbances. In R.A. Dershewitz (Ed.), Ambulatory pediatric care. Philadelphia: Lippincott.

Morrow, G.L, & Abbott, R.L. (1998). Conjunctivitis. American Family Physician, 57, 735-745.

Nelson, L.B. (1991). Strabismus disorders. In L.B. Nelson, J.H. Calhoun, & R.D. Harley (Eds.), Pediatric ophthalmology. Philadelphia: Saunders.

Pavan-Langston, D. (1996). Ocular examination: Techniques and diagnostic tests. In. D. Pavan-Langston (Ed.), Manual of ocular diagnosis and therapy. Boston: Little-Brown.

Ragge, N.K. & Easty, D.L. (1990). Immediate Eye care. St. Louis: Mosby.

Repka, M.X. (1991). Refraction in infants and children. In L.B. Nelson, J.H. Calhoun, & R.D. Harley (Eds.), Pediatric ophthalmology. Philadelphia: Saunders.

Schachat, A.P. (1995). The red eye. In L.R. Barker, J.R. Burton, & P.D. Zieve (Eds.), Principles of ambulatory medicine. Baltimore: Williams & Wilkins.

Sutherland, J.E., & Mauer, R.C. (1997). Conjunctivitis and other causes or red eye. In R.B. Taylor, D. Haxby, & C. Blem (Eds.), Manual of family practice. Boston: Little, Brown.

US Department of Health and Human Services, Office of Disease Prevention and Health Promotion. (1994). Put prevention into practice. Washington, DC: Author.

Varma, R. (1997). Essentials of eye care. Philadelphia: Lippincott-Raven.

Weber, C.M., & Eichenbaum, J.W. (1997). Acute red eye. Postgraduate Medicine, 101(5), 185-196.

Zwaan, J. (1999). Amblyopia. In R.A. Dershewitz (Ed.), Ambulatory pediatric care. Philadelphia: Lippincott.

Zwaan, J. (1999). Strabismus. In R.A. Dershewitz (Ed.), Ambulatory pediatric care. Philadelphia: Lippincott.

Zwaan, J. (1999). Styes and chalazia. In R.A. Dershewitz (Ed.), Ambulatory pediatric care. Philadelphia: Lippincott.

CHAPTER 9

Problems of the Ears, Nose, Sinuses, Throat, Mouth and Neck

HEARING LOSS

I.   Definitions: Reduction in a person's ability to perceive sound

   A.   Hearing loss is measured according to hearing thresholds (the softest tone heard by patient at a given frequency) during pure tone audiometric testing
      1.   Normal hearing: 0-15 decibels (dB)
      2.   Mild impairment: 15-30 dB
      3.   Moderate impairment: 30-50 dB
      4.   Severe: 50-70 dB
      5.   Profound: 70 dB or greater

   B.   Conductive hearing loss occurs when sound is inadequately conducted through the external or middle ear to the sensorineural apparatus of the inner ear
      1.   Normally, bone conduction thresholds are the same or better than air conduction thresholds
      2.   An air-bone gap (difference between air conduction thresholds and bone conduction thresholds) of 10 dB at two or more frequencies with bone conduction thresholds within normal limits indicates conductive hearing loss

   C.   Sensorineural hearing loss occurs when sound is normally carried through the external and middle ear but there is a defect within the inner ear which results in sound distortion

II.   Pathogenesis

   A.   Common causes of conductive hearing loss
      1.   Impacted cerumen
      2.   Foreign bodies
      3.   Otitis externa
      4.   Benign tumors of middle ear
      5.   Carcinoma of external auditory canal and/or middle ear
      6.   Eustachian tube dysfunction
      7.   Otitis media
      8.   Serous otitis media with effusion
      9.   Cholesteatoma
      10. Otosclerosis
      11. Tuberculosis of the temporal bone

   B.   Common causes of sensorineural hearing loss
      1.   Congenital and neonatal hearing loss may be hereditary (albinism, Alport's syndrome, User's syndrome, or Waardenburg's syndrome) or caused by maternal rubella, prematurity, traumatic delivery, or other infections during the perinatal period
      2.   Presbycusis which occurs because of atrophy of the basal end of the organ of Corti, a loss in number of auditory receptors, vascular changes, and stiffening of the basilar membranes
      3.   Noise exposure
      4.   Meniere's disease (see VERTIGO section)
      5.   Acoustic tumors (see VERTIGO section)
      6.   Trauma
      7.   Other diseases
         a.   Syphilis
         b.   Paget disease
         c.   Collagen diseases
         d.   Endocrine disease such as diabetes mellitus or hypothyroidism
         e.   Bacterial meningitis
         f.   Tuberculosis of the temporal bone

g. Basilar migraines

h. Viral illnesses such as mumps, cytomegalovirus, and herpes zoster

i. Demyelinating processes such as multiple sclerosis

8. Drug ototoxicities

a. Antibiotics such as streptomycin, neomycin, gentamicin, and vancomycin

b. Diuretics such as ethacrynic acid and furosemide

c. Salicylates

d. Antineoplastic agents such as cisplatin

III. Clinical presentation of common causes of hearing loss

A. Congenital hearing loss may be either conductive or sensorineural

1. Approximately 1 of every 1000 infants is born deaf; incidence of congenital hearing loss is approximately 1 per 600 live births

2. Typically diagnosed around 30 months of age when language and developmental skills may already be delayed

3. In infants, hearing loss of 30 dB and greater in the frequency region is important for speech recognition (about 500 through 4000 Hz) and will impede normal language and speech development

4. Infants with one or more of the following factors are at risk for hearing loss and should be referred for comprehensive auditory testing:

a. Birthweight <1500 g

b. Apgar score of 5 or less at 5 minutes

c. Delayed growth and development

d. More than 24 hours in neonatal intensive care unit

e. Hyperbilirubinemia requiring prolonged phototherapy or exchange transfusion

f. Seizures or other neurologic abnormalities

g. Known physical abnormalities of skull, ear, nose, or throat at birth

h. History of maternal or neonatal infection or sepsis

i. History of head injury at birth

j. Family history of hereditary hearing loss

B. In acquired conductive hearing loss, sensitivity to sound is diminished, but clarity is unchanged; if volume is increased to compensate for loss, the hearing is normal

1. Serous otitis media

a. Most frequent cause of hearing loss in children

b. Patient usually has fullness and decreased hearing in one or both ears

2. Otosclerosis is associated with slow, progressive hearing loss (usually bilateral)

a. Hereditary condition of unknown etiology in which there is an irregular ossification in the bony labyrinth of the inner ear, particularly of the stapes

b. Patients have tinnitus and hearing loss which may progress to deafness

c. On physical examination, the tympanic membrane (TM) is normal

3. Osteogenesis imperfecta is associated with multiple fractures of the long bone and blue sclera; results in delayed hearing loss

C. Acquired sensorineural hearing loss

1. Infections such as otitis media, bacterial meningitis, measles, mumps, and syphilis should be considered

2. Noise-induced hearing loss

a. Early in condition there is isolated pure tone loss at 4000 Hz unilaterally or bilaterally

b. Pure tone loss progresses to other frequencies with increased exposure

3. Acoustic neuroma presents with tinnitus and unilateral, unexplained hearing loss

4. Meniere's disease is characterized by episodic vertigo, fluctuating sensorineural hearing loss, and roaring tinnitus (see VERTIGO section)

IV.   Diagnosis/Evaluation

A.   History
1.   Question about nature of onset of hearing loss (unilateral, bilateral, progressive, acute versus chronic, fluctuating)
2.   Inquire about associated symptoms such as fever, ear pain, discharge from ear, vertigo, tinnitus, and neurologic disturbances
3.   Explore predisposing factors such as exposure to noise, trauma, barotrauma (airplane travel or diving), antecedent viral infection, and medication use
4.   Obtain a thorough past medical history
5.   Ask about family history of hearing loss and neoplastic diseases
6.   Question patient about the impact of the hearing loss on activities of daily living
7.   Infants:
a.   Ask parents if child has inappropriate response to sound such as lack of eye blinking, startling, head turning or eye widening
b.   Ask parents if there was any birth trauma, anoxia, and prenatal or perinatal infections such as rubella or cytomegalovirus
8.   Children:
a.   Ask parents if child must watch television with increased volume
b.   Question about school performance and development

B.   Physical Examination
1.   Examine eyes including funduscopy to detect congenital abnormalities
2.   Perform visual examination of TM and external auditory canal
3.   Perform pneumatic otoscopy to determine mobility of TM
4.   Perform clinical hearing test in older children and adolescents: whispered voice should be done with the patient using a finger to occlude the opposite ear to prevent crossover
5.   In infants and toddlers, assess communication skills:
a.   Birth to 3 months: Infant should blink eye or turn head to clap of hands
b.   Infants orient to familiar voice by 3-6 months
c.   By 9 months, infant responds to simple phrases such as "no" or "bye-bye."
d.   Around 12-15 months, infants speak first words
e.   By 24-36 months, toddler should follow simple commands and have vocabulary of 100 words
6.   Perform Weber and Rinne tests (see table that follows)

TUNING FORK TESTS		
	Weber Test	Rinne Test
Procedure	Strike fork and hold in middle of forehead or apex of skull and ask patient to localize sound	Strike fork, then place firmly on mastoid tip [(measure of bone conduction (BC)], and ask patient to raise hand when sound is no longer present; then move fork so that it resonates beside ear [measure of air conduction (AC)]
Conductive Loss	Sound louder in ear in which patient perceives the hearing loss	In affected ear, sound is louder when on mastoid tip than beside ear (BC>AC)
Sensorineural Loss	Sound louder in unaffected ear	In normal ear or ear with sensorineural hearing loss, the sound is louder beside the ear than on the mastoid tip (AC>BC)

7.   Complete head, neck and cranial nerve examination are often indicated; craniofacial abnormalities are often present in children with congenital or hereditary hearing loss disorders
8.   Assess developmental level

C. Differential Diagnosis: See common causes of hearing loss under pathogenesis; important to determine the following:
1. Is hearing loss acute versus chronic? (acute hearing loss almost always requires immediate intervention such as removal or cerumen or treatment with antibiotics with otitis media)
2. Is hearing loss conductive versus sensorineural?

D. Diagnostic Tests
1. Joint Committee for Infant Hearing recommends that newborns should ideally be evaluated for hearing loss before discharge from the hospital with one physiologic measure (either auditory brainstem response or otoacoustic emissions)
2. Behavioral tests can be performed in infants > 6 months: common form uses sound generators and observation of the auropalpebral reflex, the startle reflex, and arousal
3. 70% of children at 2 years of age can be evaluated by play audiometry
4. Puretone audiometry should be used in children >5 years; it characterizes the extent of impairment; air-conduction and bone-conduction measurements are made for sounds of varying intensity (decibels) and frequency (Hertz or cps): Indicated for all cases of chronic hearing loss and in cases of acute hearing loss when the etiology is uncertain
   a. Presbycusis: higher frequency loss at 8000 than at 4000 cycles (smooth, ski slope curve)
   b. Noise-induced hearing loss: high frequency loss, greatest at 4000 cycles and improvement at 8000 cycles
   c. Conductive hearing loss: Low frequency hearing loss (125-500 cycles)
5. Vestibular testing should be considered if there are tinnitus and vertigo: electronystagmometry, rotational tests, and posturography are useful adjuncts
6. Computerized tomography should be considered if tumors and bony lesions are suspected
7. Magnetic resonance imaging should be considered if acoustic neuromas are diagnostic possibilities
8. Fluorescent treponemal-antibody-absorption test should be ordered if there is a possibility of late latent syphilis
9. Tympanometry should be considered to assess TM stiffness
10. Impedance audiometry evaluates middle ear function by testing tympanic membrane compliance and acoustic reflex thresholds; particularly useful for children
11. Based on history and physical, consider CBC, chemistry panel, thyroid function tests, and urinalysis

V. Plan/Management

A. Referral to otolaryngologist is needed for patients with acute hearing loss who do not have an apparent diagnosis or for patients with apparent treatable acute or chronic causes for hearing loss who do not improve with appropriate treatments

B. Referral to audiologist is needed for patients with chronic deficits who may benefit from a hearing device

C. Most patients with otosclerosis and congenital or acquired causes of conductive hearing loss can be helped by surgical procedures

D. Aural rehabilitation is often beneficial for patients with sensorineural hearing loss
1. Hearing aids are the mainstay of therapy
2. Inexpensive auditory amplifiers are available and include telephone receiver amplifiers and radio and television earphones
3. Cochlear implants stimulate the eighth cranial nerve directly and can provide sound awareness for patients with severe hearing loss
4. Lip reading and sign language may be helpful

E. Patient Education
    1. Discuss with the patient's family ways to enhance communication
        a. Face patient, obtain patient's attention before speaking, speak slowly, use gestures, and only speak louder or move closer if the patient states that it is helpful
        b. Take time to carefully enunciate all words to patient
    2. Because many patients are embarrassed about wearing a hearing aid, emphasize that today's hearing aids are small and less noticeable; inform patient that due to advanced technology, today's hearing aids are more efficient
    3. Discuss prices of hearing aids: older analog models range from $500 to $2000 whereas digital hearing aids with better sound quality may cost $3000; medicare does not cover cost
    4. Discuss prevention of hearing loss
        a. Ear plugs or ear muffs with tight seal may reduce noise by 10-30 dB
        b. People vary in their susceptibility to noise-induced trauma, but typically if sound causes pain, tinnitus, or temporary blocking of ear, extended exposure to this noise will cause permanent hearing loss
        c. Limit exposure to loud noise; prolonged or repeated exposure to any noise above 85 dB can cause hearing loss; most lawn mowers, motorcycles, chainsaws, and powerboats produce noise > 85 dB; personal stereos, rock concerts, and firecrackers may produce noise at 140 dB or more

F. Follow up is dependent on the type and cause of the hearing loss

IMPACTED CERUMEN

I. Definition: Obstruction of the ear canal by cerumen (earwax)

II. Pathogenesis

    A. Cerumen is produced by the ceruminous glands in the outer portion of the canal and is a naturally occurring lubricant and protectant of the external ear canal

    B. While cerumen is normally cleared from the ears through the body's natural mechanisms, excessive accumulation may occur and partially or totally occlude the canal

III. Clinical Presentation

    A. Removal of cerumen may be necessary in the following situations
        1. Accumulation is causing the patient to have a problem with decreased hearing, tinnitus, feeling of fullness, vertigo, or ear discomfort
        2. Accumulation is causing the patient no problem, but is obstructing the examiner's view of the tympanic membrane

    B. Symptoms may include pain, itching, and sensation of fullness on the affected side; conductive hearing loss may also be present with total occlusion of the canal

    C. Ear pain may be present if cerumen hardens and touches the tympanic membrane, or if the external canal is irritated by build up of hardened cerumen

IV. Diagnosis/Evaluation

    A. History
        1. Ask about onset, and if ear discomfort or a feeling of fullness is present
        2. Ask patient/parent how ears are usually cleaned (Are cotton-tipped swabs used?)

3. Ask if wax removal has been required in the past
4. Determine if patient has history of previous ear surgery with resultant scarring and increased risk of perforation (Procedure using either curette or irrigation technique is **contraindicated** if patient responds positively)

B. Physical Examination
1. Examine both ear canals
2. Attempt to visualize the tympanic membranes around the wax to ascertain intactness
3. Test hearing to determine if the affected ear is the only hearing ear (if so, referral to a specialist is indicated)

C. Differential Diagnosis
1. Foreign body
2. Otitis media
3. Otitis externa

D. Diagnostic Tests: None indicated

V. Plan/Management

A. Removal of cerumen using either the curette or irrigation technique is usually successful and both techniques are described in tables that follow

B. The irrigation technique takes longer than the curette technique and is usually implemented when the curette technique fails or is poorly tolerated by patient; irrigation technique rarely fails

REMOVAL USING CURETTE TECHNIQUE	
Equipment needed/types of curette	Metal and plastic Metal curettes are either rigid or flexible Plastic are either the flex-loop ear curette or infant ear scoop
Positioning patient	For infant/young child, place in supine position and restrain head carefully
	For older children and adolescents, seat comfortably on exam table and explain procedure and the importance of remaining still
Visualize cerumen	Using otoscope, look into the canal using posterior traction on helix
Select the appropriate curette	Gently remove the impacted cerumen, working through the otoscope or by direct vision (after having identified where the impaction is and keeping in mind the anatomy of the external auditory canal)
If hard wax is encountered	Stop the procedure and instill a few drops of mineral oil into the canal to soften for 10 minutes and then resume removal
If wax appears to be adherent to the tympanic membrane itself	Removal must be via gentle irrigation
Immobilization	Absolutely necessary to avoid risk of perforation and trauma to the ear canal!
If removal is via direct vision	Use the otoscope to assess progress during procedure

Removal Using Irrigation Technique

Equipment needed	Use a soft-tipped syringe such as a 22-gauge butterfly intravenous catheter tubing with needle and butterfly removed and a 20 to 50 cc syringe, or A bulb syringe, or A water jet device such as Water-Pik
Irrigate with lukewarm water	**Caution**: Use of cold or hot water may lead to dizziness and nausea! Squirt water on your wrist to verify that temperature is correct
Positioning patient	Place in supine postion, or seat comfortably on exam table Cover the patient's shoulder with towel Instruct the patient to tilt head toward side being irrigated and place a small kidney-shaped basin under the ear to catch water (patient can hold basin)
Visualize cerumen	Use otoscope to determine location
Place the tip of the tubing or syringe just inside the canal	Infuse the water with a moderately strong and steady force If the water jet irrigator is used, set at **lowest** setting to reduce risk of perforation
Direct the jet of water superiorly toward the occiput	Allow for space in the canal for the return of water and cerumen **Do not** direct the stream of water onto the tympanic membrane Try to direct the stream of water past the plug of cerumen so as to create outward pressure on it
Evaluate the effluent	Sometimes an intact plug of cerumen is expelled and at other times the effluent will be tinted yellow but no obvious plug will be seen
Reassess progress using the otoscope	It will be necessary to dry the external canal with gauze for good visualization
If pain or bleeding occur	STOP!
If the irrigation is not successful after a few minutes	Terminate the procedure
Instruct the patient to	Instill 1-2 drops of baby oil in the affected ear twice a week to soften wax, or Use 3 drops of hydrogen peroxide and water solution (1:1 solution) in affected ear 2-3 times a week
Ask the patient to return	In one week for evaluation and removal of cerumen

C.   Cerumen solvents that are commercially available are not recommended because they frequently make the condition worse

D.   To prevent recurrences, direct patient to apply 1 or 2 drops of baby oil in each ear once or twice weekly to help soften wax; patient may also use a squeeze bulb syringe filled with lukewarm water to gently irrigate canals every month or so (best to do about 10 minutes after oil has been instilled into canals)

E.   Follow Up: None indicated unless cerumen removal fails

OTITIS EXTERNA

I. Definition: Inflammation of the external auditory canal

II. Pathogenesis

    A. Predisposing factors
        1. Frequent exposure to moisture (e.g., swimming; humid, warm climates), aggressive cleaning of the canal, or trauma
        2. Allergies or skin conditions such as psoriasis or seborrhea

    B. Pathogens
        1. Bacterial: *Pseudomonas* species, staphylococci coliform, *Proteus* species and anaerobes
        2. Fungal (account for 9% of cases): *Candida* and *Aspergillus*

III. Clinical Presentation

    A. Ear pain (occurs approximately 85% of cases) may begin gradually or suddenly; increases when pressure is placed on the tragus or when the pinna is moved; pain may increase with movement

    B. Sensation of fullness or obstruction of the ear occurs early in the process

    C. Itching may occur and it is the predominant symptom with fungal infections

    D. Purulent discharge and conductive hearing loss may occur

    E. Systemic symptomatology such as fever or chills is uncommon

    F. An uncommon, serious complication is malignant or necrotizing external otitis which can lead to cranial neuropathies and infection of the temporal bone
        1. Characterized by deep-seated nocturnal pain and granulation tissue at the bony-cartilaginous junction
        2. Foul-smelling, purulent drainage and facial nerve paralysis and cranial neuropathies may be present
        3. Most common in immunocompromised persons

IV. Diagnosis/Evaluation

    A. History
        1. Ask about the location of pain/discomfort and time of onset
        2. Ask about the occurrence of itching, and bleeding/purulent exudate
        3. Question about hearing loss
        4. Ask about location and frequency of swimming
        5. Obtain history of recent ear trauma; ask type of ear cleaning method
        6. Ask if there is a history of previous episodes and risk factors such as diabetes and immunosuppression

    B. Physical Examination
        1. Determine if febrile
        2. Assuming the ear is extremely tender, carefully examine the external canal with the otoscope; the following are signs of otitis externa:
            a. Erythema and edema of the canal
            b. Weeping secretions, purulent otorrhea, and exudate or crusting of the skin
        3. Apply pressure to the tragus and move the pinna, noting degree of tenderness
        4. If possible, observe the tympanic membrane which is usually normal; edema may impede observation
        5. Palpate the infra-auricular cervical lymph nodes for signs of lymphadenitis

C. Differential Diagnosis
    1. Cyst, furuncle or abscess
    2. Carcinoma
    3. Herpes zoster oticus (characterized by tiny vesicles which may be difficult to visualize; pain usually precedes eruption of vesicles)
    4. Otitis media
    5. Mastoiditis
    6. Foreign body

D. Diagnostic Tests: Culture should be performed if resistance to initial management occurs

V. Plan/Management: Objectives are to decrease edema and pain and restore the acidic pH, flora, cerumen and canal epithelium to normal

A. Referral is recommended whenever malignant otitis externa cannot be ruled-out or for severe, recalcitrant infections and recurrent otitis externa

B. Before treatment, remove all exudative and epidermal debris
    1. Best approach is to use a Frazier suction tip (5F or 7F) or a cotton-tipped metal applicator
    2. Otherwise, use gentle irrigation with isotonic saline; irrigation of the canal should be done cautiously until perforation is ruled out

C. If swelling prevents the passage of topical medications, insert cotton wick
    1. Insert by gently twisting the wick into the canal
    2. Patient or parent should place drops on wick for first two days, then remove wick and place drops directly in ear

D. Ear drops containing combinations of antibiotics, hydrocortisone, and propylene glycol are effective in treating bacterial infections: Use polymyxin B sulfate, neomycin, hydrocortisone (Cortisporin Otic suspension): 3 drops in canal, QID x 7 days

E. If cortisporin suspension causes localized reaction due to neomycin, switch to tobramycin, dexamethasone (TobraDex) 4 gtts. TID or QID x 7 days; Ciprofloxacin hydrochloride and hydrocortisone otic suspension (Cipro HC Otic) and ofloxacin otic solution 0.3% (Fioxin Otic), both 3 drops BID for 7 days are other effective topical agents (to minimize dizziness, warm suspension by holding bottle in hand 1-2 minutes before use; not recommended in children <1 year)

F. For fungal infections prescribe one of the following for 7 days:
    1. Acetic acid, aluminum acetate solution (Otic Domeboro) 5 drops QID
    2. Propylene glycol solution of acetic acid (Vosol) 5 drops QID
    3. Clotrimazole (Lotrimin) solution 3 gtts. BID for 5-7 days

G. Severe cases require systemic antibiotics; consider consultation with ENT specialist; prescribe broad spectrum antimicrobial such as cefaclor (Ceclor) or amoxicillin-clavulante (Augmentin)

H. Advise patient to keep moisture out of ear for 4-6 weeks; may bathe or shower but plug ear with cotton impregnated with petroleum jelly; swimming is not permitted

I. Teach patients to prevent recurrence
    1. Advise to instill 2-3 drops of 1:1:1 solution of vinegar/isopropyl alcohol/water after each contact with water
    2. Use ear plugs while swimming, showering or shampooing
    3. Parent/patient should be instructed in proper way to clean ears
    4. Remind of importance of avoiding strong jets of water from shower heads or dental water jet systems
    5. Instruct in proper way to clean ears (see section on IMPACTED CERUMEN)

J. Follow Up
1. If properly treated, otitis externa should resolve in 7 days; mild cases do not require follow-up
2. Moderate and severe case should return to office in 3 days and 24 hours, respectively

ACUTE OTITIS MEDIA

I. Definition: Presence of fluid in the middle ear in association with signs and symptoms of acute local or systemic illness; other terms synonymous with acute otitis media (OM) include suppurative otitis media, acute bacterial otitis media, and purulent otitis media

II. Pathogenesis

A. Single most important factor is eustachian tube dysfunction which prevents effective drainage of middle ear fluid
1. Typically, patient has an antecedent event such as an infection or allergy which results in edema and congestion of the mucosa of the nasopharynx, eustachian tube, and middle ear
2. The congestion of the eustachian tube impedes the flow of middle ear secretions
3. Negative pressure often increases which further pulls fluid into the middle ear
4. As middle ear secretions increase microbial pathogens grow resulting in otitis media; common pathogens are as follows:
    a. *Streptococcus pneumoniae*
    b. *Haemophilus influenzae*
    c. *Moraxella catarrhalis*
    d. Viruses; most common is respiratory syncytial virus (RSV) in children
    e. Other bacteria such as *Streptococcus pyogenes* and *Staphylococcus aureus*
5. Recently, there has been an increase in infections due to beta-lactamase producing organisms *(M. catarrhalis* and *H. influenzae)* and drug-resistant *S. pneumoniae*

B. Recurrent episodes of otitis media may be related to anatomical or physiological eustachian tube abnormality

C. Predisposing factors to developing otitis media include the following:
1. Active or passive smoking
2. Caucasian or Native American race
3. Male gender
4. Congenital disorders such as cleft palate and trisomy 21
5. Family history of otitis media

III. Clinical Presentation

A. Occurs most frequently in winter months in children <7 years old, with highest incidence in children between 6 months and 3 years of age

B. Commonly seen following a viral upper respiratory infection

C. Symptoms include the following:
1. Ear pain, otorrhea, hearing loss and/or vertigo
2. Fever is a common but not a universal symptom
3. Patients, particularly children, may be asymptomatic or just have behaviors perceived as irritability
4. Other symptoms include nausea, vomiting, and diarrhea (these occur primarily in children)

D. Complications include hearing loss, perforation of eardrum, cholesteatoma, acute mastoiditis, meningitis, and epidural abscess

E. Diagnosis is based on the appearance of the tympanic membrane (TM), the following are characteristic:
1. Full or bulging TM
2. Absent or obscured bony landmarks
3. Distorted light reflex
4. Decreased of absent mobility of TM by pneumatic otoscopy
5. Erythema of TM is an inconsistent finding; TM may be red due to crying or vascular engorgement due to fever rather than infection
6. Bullae may form between layers of TM; often associated with *Mycoplasma pneumoniae*

IV. Diagnosis/Evaluation

A. History
1. Determine onset and duration of symptoms
2. Ask about ear pain, fever, irritability
3. Inquire about hearing loss, tinnitus and dizziness
4. Ask about drainage from ear
5. Inquire about associated symptoms such as nasal congestion, headache, sore throat, mouth pain, cough, hearing loss
6. Carefully document the number and if possible dates of previous occurrences; ask about successes and failures of previous treatments
7. Determine whether an upper respiratory infection preceded the fever or ear pain
8. Inquire about history of allergies and other risk factors such as active or passive smoking and congenital disorders such as cleft palate
9. In infants, inquire about manner of bottle feeding

B. Physical Examination
1. Measure vital signs
2. Inspect conjunctivae, pharynx, and nasal mucosa
3. Palpate sinuses
4. Palpate for auricular and cervical adenopathy
5. Examine auricle and external auditory canal
6. Carefully examine tympanic membranes bilaterally for position, color, degree of translucency and mobility (may require removal of cerumen)
   a. Position: Process of the malleus should be visible but not prominent through the membrane; retraction and bulging indicate effusion
   b. Color: Normal TM is gray; an amber color often indicates an effusion; erythema may indicate infection but also may be due to crying, severe coughing, or vascular engorgement
   c. Translucency: Middle ear landmarks should be visible through the TM; air fluid level, bubbles, and inability to visualize middle ear landmarks suggest effusion
   d. Mobility: Normal ear will move with pneumatic otoscopy; **to be diagnosed with acute otitis media there must be presence of fluid in middle ear; this can only be detected with pneumatic otoscopy**
7. Perform a lung examination

C. Differential Diagnosis [Health care providers can generally detect OM 90% of time when it is present, but over diagnosis frequently occurs (as high as 40%)]
1. External otitis media
2. Transient middle ear effusion may result with flying or traveling in high altitudes (barotrauma)
3. Mastoiditis
4. Furuncle
5. Temporomandibular joint dysfunction
6. Mumps
7. Dental abscess
8. Tonsillitis
9. Foreign body
10. Trauma

D. Diagnostic Tests
1. Usually no diagnostic tests are ordered
2. Rarely, may perform tympanocentesis for culture and sensitivity of middle ear effusion in toxic patients, patients with complications such as mastoiditis, immuno-compromised patients, patients in whom treatment is unsatisfactory or who have recurrent infections
3. Tympanometry may be indicated in recurrent cases and when there is suspicion of fluid behind the TM without clinical signs
4. Acoustic reflectometry helps diagnose OM by analyzing sound pressure and reflected sound in the eardrum
5. Consider ordering sinus films in patients with recurrent otitis media or otitis media with effusion
6. Order CBC with differential and blood cultures in children who appear toxic, have a high fever, are not drinking and voiding, or are immunocompromised
7. Consider audiometry post treatment

V. Plan/Management

A. General management concepts (see following table)

GENERAL CONCEPTS OF MANAGEMENT	
1. Be cautious	Remember favorable natural history of OM (80% of cases resolve spontaneously)
2. Prescribe antibiotics sparingly	-Antibiotics improve resolution by only about 15% -Antibiotics increase risk of bacterial resistance
3. Modify risk factors	Improve odds of resolution: -Avoid passive smoking -Control food and inhalant allergies -Treat sinusitis -Limit pacifier use in day -Consider alternatives for group day care
4. Practice prevention	-Encourage breast feeding -Advise parents not to prop infant's bottle and to elevate infant's head when feeding -Consider pneumococcal vaccine (age 2 or more) -Consider influenza vaccine (day care)
5. Avoid unproven therapies	-Antihistamines/decongestants -Homeopathy and naturopathy -Folk remedies such as "sweet oil"

B. Some experts only recommend antibiotics for patients with pus drainage, recurrent infections, and history of serous otitis media or ear tubes; most experts, however, recommend antibiotics to reduce the development of delayed suppurative complications such as mastoiditis
1. Use first-line antibiotics for initial empiric treatment (see following table)

RECOMMENDED FIRST-LINE ANTIBIOTICS FOR MEDICAL MANAGEMENT		
Generic (Trade) Name *Duration of treatment*	Dosing	Comment
Amoxicillin (Amoxil) *10 day treatment**	40 mg/kg/day - TID (Available 125 mg/5 mL and 250 mg/5 mL liquid) **Adolescents**: 250-500 mg tabs TID	-Inexpensive, few adverse effects -In 1998 still recommended as **drug of choice** for initial therapy -Disadvantage: Not effective against beta-lactamase producing organisms
Trimethoprim- sulfamethoxazole (Bactrim, Septra) *10 day treatment**	8 mg/kg/day trimeth. and 40 mg/kg/day sulf. - BID (available 200 mg sulfa. component/5 mL liquid) **Adolescents**: One DS tab BID	-Effective against beta-lactamase producing organisms -**Drug of choice** - pts. allergic to penicillin -Disadvantage:Less effective than amoxil against common pathogen, *S. pneumonia*

* Duration of treatment may be 5-7 days for patients >2 years of age, who have mild, uncomplicated AOM, and no underlying medical condition and no history of chronic or recurrent otitis media

2. Use second-line antibiotics for following cases (see following table)
   a. Initial treatment failures
   b. Complicated infections
   c. Patients with ipsilateral conjunctivitis suggesting *H. Influenzae* infection

RECOMMENDED SECOND-LINE ANTIBIOTICS FOR MEDICAL MANAGEMENT		
Generic (Trade) Name *Duration of treatment*	**Dosing**	**Comment**
Amoxicillin-clavulanate (Augmentin) *10 day treatment**	40 mg/kg/day - TID (available 125 mg/5 mL and 250 mg/5 mL liquid) **Adolescents:** 250-500 mg tabs TID	-Broad spectrum -15-20% patients have gastrointestinal upset
Azithromycin (Zithromax) *5 day treatment*	Over 6 months: 10 mg/kg QD Day 1; 5 mg/kg QD Days 2-5 (available 100 mg/5 mL & 200mg/5mL); **Adolescents:** 500 mg tab QD Day 1; 250 mg Days 2-5	-Broad spectrum -Oral suspension: Take 1 hour before or 2 hours after meals
Cefprozil (Cefzil) *10 day treatment**	Over 6 months: 30 mg/kg/day - BID (available 125 mg/5 mL & 250 mg/5 mL liquid) **Adolescents:** 500 mg tab BID	-Broad spectrum
Cefpodoxime (Vantin) *10 day treatment**	Over 5 months: 10 mg/kg QD (available 50 mg/5 mL & 100 mg/5 mL liquid) **Adolescents:** 200 mg tab BID	-Broad spectrum -Convenient dosing for children -For adolescents, take tabs with food
Cefibuten (Cedax) *10 day treatment**	Over 6 months: ≤45 kg: 9 mg/kg QD; (available 90 mg/5 mL) **Adolescents & children >45 kg:** 400 mg cap QD	-Broad spectrum -Convenient dosing -Take suspension on empty stomach; caps may be taken without regard for meals
Cefuroxime (Ceftin) *10 day treatment**	Over 3 months: 30 mg/kg/day - BID (available 125 mg/5 mL) **Adolescents:** 250-500 mg cap BID	-Broad spectrum -Bitter taste -Take with food
Clarithromycin (Biaxin) *10 day treatment**	Over 6 months: 15 mg/kg/day - BID (available 125 mg/5 mL & 250 mg/5 mL liquid) **Adolescents:** 250-500 mg cap BID	-Broad spectrum -Well tolerated
Loracarbef (Lorabid) *10 day treatment**	Over 6 months: 30 mg/kg/day - BID (Available 100 mg/5 mL & 200 mg/5 mL liquid) **Adolescents:** 200-400 mg caps BID	-Broad spectrum -Must take on an empty stomach

* Duration of treatment may be 5-7 days for patients >2 years of age, who have mild, uncomplicated AOM, and no underlying medical condition and no history of chronic or recurrent otitis media

3. Use third-line antibiotics for special cases; for example, infections with resistant *S. pneumoniae* or patients who have difficulty taking a course of oral medications

RECOMMENDED THIRD-LINE ANTIBIOTICS FOR MEDICAL MANAGEMENT		
Generic (Trade) Name *Duration of treatment*	**Dosing**	**Comment**
Clindamycin (Cleocin) *10 day treatment*	8-12 mg/kg/day -TID (available 75mg/5mL oral solution) **Adolescents:** 150-300 mg caps QID	-Excellent choice for resistant S. pneumoniae -Take with full glass of water
Ceftriaxone (Rocephin) *1-5 day treatment*	50-75mg/kg/day IM injection - QD	-Useful for refractory cases -Inconsistent findings of efficacy of drug -Reserve as third-line drug and for cases with intra-cranial complications

C. Cases involving penicillin-resistant *S. pneumoniae* (suspect when patient has persistent AOM)
   1. Drug of choice: clindamycin (see previous table)
   2. Alternatives:
      a. High dose amoxicillin (60-80 mg/kg/day)
      b. Ceftriaxone IM (5 day treatment)

D. Management of pain
   1. Usually, an analgesic such as acetaminophen (5-15 mg/kg/dose every 4 hours PRN or in adolescents 300-600 mg every 4 hours) is all that is needed; codeine may be prescribed
   2. Topical pain relievers such as Americaine Otic solution, 4 to 5 gtts q 1-2 hours or Auralgan Otic solution every 1-2 hours may be prescribed

E. Nasal and oral decongestants are usually not effective in preventing otitis media, but may provide symptomatic relief of associated symptoms which often accompany otitis media

F. Antihistamines are not recommended unless the predisposing factor for developing otitis media is an allergy; antihistamines may thicken the secretions and aggravate the problem

G. Treatment of persistent, recalcitrant, or subacute otitis media
   1. If no response in 2-3 days and patient is not toxic switch to a second-line antibiotic (see previous table); consider the possibility of infection with penicillin-resistant *S. pneumoniae* (see V.C. for treatment)
   2. Consider consultation with specialist if 2-3 courses of recommended treatments fail

H. Treatment of recurrent infections is controversial; recurrent infections are those in which the middle ear effusion clears between episodes.
   1. Always try preventive measures such as limiting passive smoking, administering vaccines, etc. before prescribing prophylactic antibiotics (see table - General Concepts)
   2. Roark & Berman (1997) found only a marginal benefit of antibiotic prophylaxis; they recommend treating individual episodes of AOM rather than using antibiotics preventively and to refer to a specialist when child has frequent infections
   3. Others recommend prophylaxis therapy for selected patients who have recurrent infections after an acute episode with a normal exam and normal tympanogram
      a. Previously, the rule of thumb was to begin prophylaxis treatment when the patient had 3 or more episodes in 6 months or 2 episodes before 6 months old; today, because of antibiotic resistance, clinicians must individually weigh the benefits and risks of prophylactic antibiotics
      b. For prophylaxis, prescribe: Sulfisoxazole (Gantrisin) 50 mg/kg as single dose at bedtime or erythromycin-sulfisoxazole (Pediazole) 75 mg/kg/day BID.
      c. Prophylactic treatment should be continued for approximately 3-6 months or until regimen fails.
      d. Evaluate children every 4 weeks to ensure that acute otitis media is not overlooked.
      e. If acute infection occurs, treat with full dose of a different antimicrobial (second-line)
      f. When prophylaxis fails and there are signs and symptoms of eustachian tube dysfunction, consider alternatives after consulting specialist:
         (1) Placement of tympanotomy tubes
         (2) Myringotomy
         (3) Adenoidectomy or tonsillectomy or both

I. Treatment of tympanic membrane perforation involves prescription of oral antibiotic supplemented with topical antibiotic such as a combination of neomycin sulfate, polymyxin-ß and hydrocortisone (Cortisporin otic suspension) 4 drops in each ear, 3-4 times a day for maximum of 10 days

J. Consult specialist and consider surgery for following:
   1. Hearing loss bilaterally of 20 dB or more
   2. Chronic or persistent infection with evidence of mastoid involvement
   3. Cholesteatoma formation or chronic perforation
   4. Children with febrile seizures, antibiotic intolerance, speech problems, or chronic otitis media with effusion

K. Follow Up
1. Return to clinic in 2-3 days if condition is not significantly improved.
2. Typically, return visits are scheduled several days after completion of drug therapy or recheck in 2-3 weeks from initial visit; recently some authorities recommend delaying follow-up for 4-6 weeks if the patient is older than 15 months, asymptomatic, and parents/patient report that the infection has resolved
3. For patients treated with prophylactic antibiotics, evaluate every 4 weeks

OTITIS MEDIA WITH EFFUSION

I. Definition: Accumulation of serous fluid in the middle ear longer than 2 or 3 months without signs and symptoms of acute infection (sometimes referred to as serous otitis media)

II. Pathogenesis

   A. Loss of patency of the eustachian tube with subsequent negative pressure and effusion behind the tympanic membrane

   B. Common causative factors:
      1. Adenoidal hypertrophy
      2. Recent upper respiratory infection
      3. Allergies
      4. Deviated nasal septum
      5. Post purulent otitis media
      6. Rarely due to nasopharyngeal neoplasm

III. Clinical Presentation

   A. Often asymptomatic or may have mild pain

   B. Common symptoms include sensation of stuffiness or fullness in ear or popping and crackling sounds in ear with chewing, yawning or blowing nose

   C. A small number of patients may experience vertigo or ataxia

   D. Tympanic membrane is often retracted with diffuse light reflex
      1. Bubbles or a fluid level may be present behind the tympanic membrane
      2. Decreased tympanic membrane movement with insufflation (pneumatic otoscopy)

   E. Chronic effusion may result in the following:
      1. Hearing loss which, in children, may lead to a delay in language development
      2. Delay of gross motor skills in children

   F. Complications are rare, but may include chronic drainage and perforation, cholesteatoma, and facial nerve paralysis

IV. Diagnosis/Evaluation

   A. History
      1. Determine onset, duration, character of symptoms
      2. Inquire about rhinitis, cough, and fever
      3. Question about pain and decreased hearing acuity level
      4. Inquire about recent upper respiratory infection and allergies
      5. Inquire about past episodes of otitis media and treatments received
      6. Ask about family history of allergies

B. Physical Examination
   1. Measure vital signs
   2. Examine nasal passages and pharynx
   3. Examine tympanic membranes for fluid level, retraction, diffuse light reflex and/or bubbles
   4. Assess TM mobility with pneumatic otoscopy
      a. Recommended for primary diagnosis
      b. Accuracy of diagnosis with pneumatic otoscopy is 70-79%
   5. Perform Rinne and Weber tests
   6. Palpate neck and jaw for adenopathy
   7. Examine neck and head for anatomical abnormalities
   8. Assess language development

C. Differential Diagnosis
   1. Nasopharyngeal carcinoma
   2. Anatomic abnormalities

D. Diagnostic Tests
   1. Tympanometry (Indirect measure of tympanic membrane compliance and estimate of middle ear pressure)
      a. Tympanometry is reliable for detecting otitis media with effusion (OME) in children older than 4-6 months
      b. Often falsely positive due to impacted cerumen, foreign body, TM perforation, or improper placement of instrument tip on the ear canal wall
      c. Pneumatic otoscopy recommended for primary diagnosis, followed by tympanometry as confirmatory test
      d. Tympanogram is flat with an effusion
   2. Audiometry
      a. Patients with fluid in both ears for three months should undergo hearing evaluation; prior to three months, audiometry is an option
      b. Hearing impairment is defined as equal to or worse than 20 decibels (dB) hearing threshold level in the better-hearing ear
   3. Acoustic reflectometry; experts disagree about the value of this test but probably best viewed as complement to tympanometry
      a. Accurate testing method after age 3 months
      b. Analyzes sound pressure and reflected sound on eardrum
   4. Otoacoustic emissions are responses emitted by the cochlea in the form of acoustic energy; in the future this test may be used as a supplement to tympanometry in assessing auditory recovery from OME

V. Plan/Management

A. For asymptomatic children (normal hearing, speech, school performance) choose either watchful waiting with vigilant monitoring **OR** antibiotic therapy
   1. Watchful waiting is becoming the preferred approach due to accumulating evidence that antibiotic use increases the risk for both colonization and invasive disease with penicillin-resistant *Streptococcus pneumoniae*; additional rationale for this recommendation:
      a. Most cases spontaneously resolve without antibiotic treatment (about 90%)
      b. Effect of antibiotics is marginal and often short-lived; antibiotics increase short-term resolution by approximately 15%
      c. Incidence of delayed suppurative complications from effusion is small
   2. If antibiotic therapy is chosen, prescribe a beta-lactamase stable antibiotic such as the following:
      a. Amoxicillin-clavulanate (Augmentin) 40 mg/kg/day in three divided doses for 2-3 weeks. Available in 125 mg/5 mL and 250 mg/5 mL liquids
      b. Clarithromycin (Biaxin) 15 mg/kg/day in two divided doses for 2-3 weeks. Available in 125 mg/5 mL and 250 mg/5 mL liquids

B. Assess hearing status and structural integrity of TM with audiometry and pneumatic otoscopy every 3-4 months

C. Children with bilateral OME for greater than 3 months and hearing loss, defined as 20 dB hearing threshold level or worse in the better-hearing ear, should be referred to an ENT specialist for possible placement of tympanostomy tubes; tympanostomy tubes are recommended after total of 4-6 months of bilateral effusion with bilateral hearing deficit

D. Oral corticosteroids are sometimes recommended for children **>3 years old** as a last-resort alternative to surgery:
   1. Dangers of this approach: chickenpox exacerbation, immunosupression and adverse effects such as insomnia, changes in behavior, weight gain
   2. Prescribe prednisolone (Pediapred) 1 mg/kg/day QD for 5 days, Available 5 mg/5 mL liquid (Do not prescribe steroids if child has NOT had chickenpox or is not immunized for chickenpox and if there has been exposure to chickenpox in last 4 weeks)

E. For older children and adolescents, consider autoinflation of eustachian tube with plastic nasal cannula attached to balloon

F. Patient education, modification of risk factors, and controlling concurrent illness are important
   1. Limit passive smoke exposure, and, if possible, group day-care attendance, and bottle-feeding in infants
   2. Consider milk-free diet for several weeks as a diagnostic trial in children <2 years as allergy to milk proteins may cause middle ear inflammation
   3. Treat concurrent illnesses such as sinusitis and allergic rhinitis
   4. Emphasize importance of follow up
   5. Discuss with family the possibility of hearing loss due to this condition
   6. Children should be seated in front of the class until hearing is normal

G. Most studies indicate that decongestants and antihistamines are ineffective; the role of allergies in patients with effusions is still uncertain

H. Referral to speech therapist may be needed for language delay or a speech problem.

I. Adenoidectomy combined with tympanostomy tubes may be beneficial for children >3 years

J. Follow Up
   1. Assess every 4-6 weeks or sooner if ear pain or other bothersome symptoms occur
   2. If effusion still persists at 6-week follow-up visit, watchful waiting or antibiotic therapy are acceptable approaches
   3. If effusion persists at 3-month follow-up visit, hearing evaluation is indicated

CARE OF PATIENT WITH TYMPANOSTOMY TUBES

I. Definition: Middle ear ventilation tubes placed in tympanic membrane (TM) after myringotomy

II. Procedure

A. Tubes restore hearing to pre-effusion threshold, permit normal vibration of TM and middle ear bones, permit ventilation of middle ear tissues, equalize middle ear and atmospheric pressures, and prevent accumulation of fluid or mucus in middle ear

B. Tubes are placed in pars tensa of the tympanic membrane, in any location except the posterosuperior quadrant, overlying the incus and stapes

C. Generally, tubes are made of plastic, metal or Teflon and are designed for short-term placement (8-15 months) or long-term placement (>15 months)

D. Possible candidates for tube placement:
   1. Patients with bilateral middle ear effusion and hearing deficiency for more than 3 months; recommended if condition existed for 4-6 months
   2. Patient with middle ear effusion and structural changes of tympanic membrane
   3. Experts consider earlier tube placement for patients with recurrent painful ear infections, language delay, and craniofacial anomalies

III. Clinical Presentation

A. Potential benefits in children include improvements in behaviors, sleep, communication and hearing

B. Potential Risks
   1. Auditory canal wall laceration, persistent otorrhea, granuloma formation, cholesteatoma and permanent TM perforation
   2. Structural changes in TM such as flaccidity, retraction and/or tympanosclerosis have occurred; long-term effects on hearing are unknown but estimated as small
   3. Risks associated with general anesthesia
   4. Intrusion of tube into middle ear cleft rather than normal extrusion through external ear canal
   5. Approximately 30 percent of children have repeat tympanostomy tube insertion within 5 years of initial surgery

IV. Diagnosis/Evaluation

A. History
   1. Question about pain and ear discharge
   2. Inquire about noticeable changes in hearing, speech, and/or development

B. Physical Examination
   1. Inspect ear canal for possible tube extrusion and signs of ear discharge
   2. Inspect TM for placement of tube and color and degree of translucency (TM should be gray and translucent if tube is properly functioning)
   3. Assess for mobility with pneumatic otoscopy (TM should be immobile if tube is properly functioning)

C. Diagnostic tests
   1. If tube functioning is questionable, order tympanometry which should be flat if tube is properly functioning
   2. Audiometry helps to confirm status of tube functioning

V. Plan/Management

A. In past, an otolaryngologist was responsible for complete care and follow-up of patients with tympanostomy tubes; today, experienced, health care providers in primary care are caring for minor problems with tubes in collaboration with an otolaryngologist

B. For tubes clogged with dried middle ear effusion, consider consultation with specialist and prescribe topical antibiotic such as Cortisporin otic suspension for 5-7 days; hydrogen peroxide and cerumolytics are **contraindicated**

C. Posttube otorrhea occurs in 10-30% of patients
   1. Prescribe amoxicillin (Amoxil) 40 mg/kg/day PO in three divided doses. Available 125 mg/5mL and 250 mg/5mL liquid or a beta-lactamase stable antibiotic in areas with prevalence of resistant organisms (see second-line antibiotics under OTITIS MEDIA)
   2. If unresponsive to first course of antibiotics, consider the possibility of water contamination with *Pseudomonas aeruginosa* and *Staphylococcus aureus* and prescribe Cortisporin otic suspension for 5-7 days

D. Refer the following cases to an otolaryngologist
   1. Recurrent or chronic tube otorrhea
   2. Recurrent episodes of acute otitis media
   3. Occluded tube with middle ear effusion which does not readily clear
   4. Bloody otorrhea
   5. Decreased hearing acuity
   6. Suspicion of cholesteatoma
   7. TM perforation surrounding tube
   8. Retention of tube for more than 2 years

E. Patient Education
   1. Teach patient and family to watch for tube extrusion and possible complications such as discharge from ear and fever
   2. Emphasize importance of follow-up visits with otolaryngologist
   3. Wear fitted ear plugs when swimming or bathing especially during diving and head dunking in lakes, ponds, rivers and bath water which may have higher bacterial counts

F. Follow Up
   1. Typically patients have routine postoperative visits with otolaryngologist at the following times: 2-4 weeks after tube placement; 4-6 months after tube placement; 6-12 months after tube extrusion
   2. Patients should return to primary care provider after treatment for clogged tube or posttube otorrhea

ALLERGIC AND NONALLERGIC RHINITIS

I. Definition of rhinitis: Inflammation of mucous membranes of the nose, usually accompanied by edema of mucosa and a nasal discharge. Rhinitis may be allergic or nonallergic

II. Pathogenesis

A. Allergic rhinitis: An IgE-mediated inflammatory disease involving the nasal mucosa membranes
   1. When a person with a genetic predisposition to allergy is exposed to a strong allergic stimulus, antigen IgE-antibody molecules are produced and bind to mast cells in the respiratory epithelium
   2. Reexposure to offending allergen causes a hypersensitivity to offending allergen and triggers the release of histamines and other mediators
   3. Histamine release results in immediate local vasodilation, mucosal edema, and increased mucous production
   4. A late-phase reaction sometimes occurs 4-8 hours after the original reaction in persons with severe disease; results in hyperresponsiveness to antigenic and nonantigenic stimuli and is linked to development of chronic disease
   5. Most common form is the seasonal pattern due to inhalant pollen allergens
   6. Year-round perennial type which is difficult to diagnose and treat is usually related to house dust mites, mold, cockroaches, and animal dander; in adults, food allergies are a rare cause of rhinitis

B. Nonallergic Rhinitis
   1. Vasomotor rhinitis: Perennial nonallergic rhinitis which represents a hyperreactive state of the nasal mucosa
   2. Rhinitis medicamentosis or rebound rhinitis is due to overuse of topical decongestant
   3. Rhinitis of pregnancy is due to hormonal increase (will not be discussed further)

III.	Clinical Presentation

A.	Allergic rhinitis
1.	Onset of symptoms is most common between ages 10-20; rarely begins before age 4 or after age 40
2.	Usually involves the triad of nasal congestion, sneezing and clear rhinorrhea
3.	Coughing, sore throat, and itching and puffiness of eyes may occur
4.	Signs include the following:
a.	Pale, boggy nasal mucosa with clear thin secretions
b.	Enlarged nasal turbinates which may obstruct airway flow
c.	"Allergic shiners" or a dark discoloration beneath both eyes
d.	Cobblestone appearance of the conjunctiva
e.	"Dennie's lines" or extra wrinkles below the lower eyelids
f.	Transverse nasal crease due to chronic upward wiping of the nose
g.	Nasal salute
h.	Mouth-breathing
i.	Short, upper lip
j.	Enlarged tonsils and adenoids
5.	Predisposing factors include serous otitis media, chronic sinusitis, asthma, nasal polyposis, respiratory infections, nasal speech, and abnormal facial development

B.	Vasomotor rhinitis
1.	May be due to abnormal autonomic responsiveness and vascular dilatation of submucosal vessels
2.	Vasomotor rhinitis or persistent nasal congestion does not have a correlation to specific allergen exposures
3.	May begin in early childhood, but onset is usually in adulthood
4.	Patients have a rapid onset of nasal congestion and a pronounced and noticeable postnasal drip
5.	Triggers of attacks are the following: abrupt changes in temperature and barometric pressure, odors, and emotional stress
6.	Negative family history of allergy
7.	Nasal smear and skin tests are negative
8.	Patients are usually unresponsive to environmental controls and medications

C.	Rhinitis medicamentosa
1.	When the beneficial effects of topical nasal decongestants subside, a secondary vasodilation occurs, resulting in increased nasal congestion
2.	Addiction may develop as the patient's relief becomes shorter and the rebound more severe within a short time

IV.	Diagnosis/Evaluation

A.	History
1.	Question about onset, duration, and progression of symptoms
2.	Explore relationship of symptoms to season, place, time of day, and activity
3.	Ask about environmental factors such as pets, cigarette smoking in house, and type of heating system
4.	Question about triggers such as exposure to cold air, ingestion of spicy foods, odors, and changes in temperature and barometric pressure
5.	Question about nasal stuffiness or obstruction, sensation of pressure over and under the eyes, itching of the eyes, nose and pharynx, sneezing, color, consistency, and amount of nasal and postnasal discharges, and sensation of needing to constantly clear throat
6.	Ask about mouth breathing, changes in hearing and smell acuity, snoring during sleep, and fatigue
7.	Inquire about self-treatment, particularly duration and use of nasal sprays
8.	Inquire about family history and past history of allergies

B. Physical Examination
1. Check pulse and blood pressure as sympathomimetic decongestants may increase both
2. Measure temperature which should be normal
3. Inspect eyes for allergic "shiners," tearing, conjunctival injection, lid swelling, and periorbital edema
4. Palpate for sinus tenderness.
5. Examine ears to rule out otitis media and to check for serous otitis media
6. Assess for nasal obstruction and polyps
7. Inspect nasal mucosa noting color, edema, and type and color of nasal discharge
8. Assess pharynx for tonsillar enlargement and inflammation
9. Palpate lymph nodes
10. Always check breath sounds to rule out concurrent asthma

C. Differential Diagnosis
1. Upper respiratory infections typically have a history of contagion, presence of fever, purulent nasal discharge, inflamed nasal mucosa, and absence of eosinophils on nasal smear
2. Sinusitis
3. Otitis media
4. Foreign body, if blockage is unilateral
5. Deviated septum, if blockage is unilateral
6. Nasal polyps
7. Endocrine conditions such as hypothyroidism
8. Pregnancy and oral contraceptives

D. Diagnostic tests (most of the time the diagnosis is made from the history and physical and no tests are required)
1. Skin testing for allergies is often recommended and the results must be compared with clinical history
    a. Gold standard test
    b. No age limit to testing but less relevant in children <18 months
    c. In preschool children, limit testing to allergens that relate to the history of exposure or symptoms
2. Nasal smear for eosinophils is often helpful and eosinophils are elevated with allergic rhinitis; peripheral eosinophil count is not useful
3. Serum IgE levels are elevated in 30-40% of patients with allergic rhinitis and increased levels occur in nonallergies. Thus, the test has limited value
4. In vitro serum allergy tests (radioallergosorbent tests: RAST, FAST, MAST) are expensive and not as specific nor sensitive as skin testing; use in patients with severe skin problems such as extensive eczema
5. If there is any question of an infectious process obtain a CBC

V. Plan/Management

A. Allergic rhinitis
1. Patient Education: Allergen avoidance is the most effective form of treatment.
    a. The bedroom is considered the room that must be the most allergen-free
    b. Try to eliminate dust and allergen exposure in the household (see table that follows)

MEASURES OF ENVIRONMENTAL CONTROL IN THE HOME

➡ Vacuum weekly (some vacuums spread dust and mites, so the vacuum should be cleaned regularly) or perform damp mopping

➡ Dust furniture and all horizontal surfaces weekly with a damp cloth

➡ Encase mattress and pillow in allergen-impermeable cover; wash sheets and blankets in hot water weekly

➡ Remove carpets from bedroom; avoid lying on upholstered furniture; remove carpets laid on concrete

➡ Avoid rubber mattress

➡ Recommend keeping windows and doors closed to decrease influx of mold and pollen; may necessitate air conditioning in the summer (have AC unit professionally cleaned to clear mold/mildew off coils)

➡ Reduce indoor humidity to less than 50%

➡ Eliminate or restrict exposure to pets

➡ To control cockroaches, use poison traps or bait; do not leave food or garbage exposed

➡ Use clothes dryer rather than hanging clothes outside to air dry

➡ Wear high-efficiency mask and long-sleeved shirt when gardening; bathe and change clothes immediately after coming inside

2. Drug therapy is indicated when allergen avoidance is ineffective or impractical

3. There is no recommended first-line drug of choice; Choice of medication depends on symptoms patient is experiencing as well as adverse reactions of drugs, adherence factors, risk of drug interactions, and cost (See table on the EFFICACY OF PHARMACOTHERAPEUTIC AGENTS)

EFFICACY OF PHARMACOTHERAPEUTIC AGENTS

Therapeutic Agents	Itching/ Sneezing	Runny Nose	Nasal Blockage	Eye Symptoms
Oral Antihistamines	+++	++	---	+++
Intranasal corticosteroids	+++	+++	+++	+
Oral decongestants	---	+	+++	---
Antihistamine/decongestant combinations	+++	++	++	+++
Nasal decongestants	---	+	+++	---
Cromolyn sodium	++	++	---	---
Intranasal ipratropium	---	+++	---	---

Adapted from Kaiser, H.B., Kay, G.G., & Palakanis, K. (1998). Contemporary issues in the management of allergic disorders: A focus on respiratory and dermatologic manifestations. Clinical Courier, 16 (46), 1-7.

4. First generation antihistamines (see table that follows)

    a. Advantage: Inexpensive; anticholinergic properties may be beneficial for patient who is bothered by rhinorrhea; early onset of action which is useful for intermittent symptoms

    b. Disadvantage: Numerous adverse effects: drowsiness, impaired performance, anticholinergic effects such as dry mouth, urinary retention and constipation; do not relieve nasal congestion; do not control underlying inflammatory response

    c. Hydroxyzine is the most potent

    d. Rule of thumb is to use the smallest dose that is effective

    e. Slowly titrate drugs beginning with one dose at bedtime for several days, then adding a small morning dose and so on (base titration on symptom control and adverse effects); tolerance to sedative effects usually occurs after 1-2 weeks of continued dosing

    f. May be necessary to try several antihistamines from different classes before effective one is found; administer 2-3 weeks before switching to an agent of another class; may need to switch occasionally to prevent increased tolerance

5. Azelastine HCl 0.1% nasal spray (Astelin) is the first topical antihistamine
   a. Advantage: Effective in reducing allergic symptoms, has good safely profile, and is more beneficial in relieving nasal obstruction than oral antihistamines
   b. Disadvantage: Few studies to determine long-term effectiveness
   c. Prescribe 2 sprays per nostril BID
   d. Not recommended for children <12 years old

FIRST GENERATION ANTIHISTAMINES		
	Older Adolescent Dose (mg)	Child's Dose (liquid forms)
Ethanolamine		
Diphenhydramine (Benadryl)	25-50 TID/QID	5 mg/kg/day (12.5 mg/5 mL)
Clemastine (Tavist)	1-2 BID	---
Ethylenediamine		
Tripelennamine (Pyribenzamine)	25-50 TID/QID	---
Alkylamine		
Chlorpheniramine (Chlor-Trimeton)	4 QID	>6 yrs, 2 mg QID (2 mg/5 mL)
Brompheniramine (Dimetane)	4 QID	2-6 yrs, 1 mg QID; >6 yrs, 2 mg QID (2 mg/5 mL)
Piperazine		
Hydroxyzine (Atarax, Vistaril)	10-25 TID/QID	<6 yrs, 50 mg daily; >6 yrs, 50-100 mg daily (10 mg/5 mL)
Phenothiazine		
Trimeprazine (Temaril)	2.5 QID	6 mos-3 yrs, 1.25 mg hs/TID; >3 yrs, 2.5 mg hs/TID (2.5 mg/5 mL)
Piperidine		
Azatadine (Optimine)	1-2 BID/TID	---
Cyproheptadine (Periactin)	4 TID	2-6 yrs, 2 mg BID/TID; 7-14 yrs, 4 mg BID/TID (2 mg/5 mL)

6. Second generation antihistamines (see table that follows)
   a. Advantage: Fewer adverse drug effects and simpler dosing schedule than first-generation antihistamines
   b. Disadvantage: Expensive; less effective than first-generation antihistamines and other medications in reducing rhinorrhea; no relief for nasal congestion; do not control underlying inflammatory response

COMPARISON OF SECOND GENERATION ANTIHISTAMINES				
	Astemizole (Hismanal)	**Loratadine (Claritin)**	**Fexofenadine (Allegra)**	**Certirizine (Zyrtec)**
Dosage Person >18 years	10 mg tab QD (Take on empty stomach)	10 mg tab QD (Initially 10 mg EOD)	60 mg cap BID (Initially 60 mg QD)	10 mg tab QD
Children	Not recommended	<6 years not recommended; ≥6 years 10 mg QD; available 1 mg/mL syrup	Not recommended	<2 years not recommended; 2-5 years 2.5-5 mg QD; ≥6 years 5-10 mg QD; available 1 mg/mL syrup
Risk of Torsades de Pointes (Cardiotoxicity)	Yes	No	No	No
Sedation	No	No	No	Yes
Dry mouth & urinary retention	No	No	No	Yes
Weight gain	Yes	<astemizole	Not reported	Yes
Interactions	Avoid erythromycin, clarithromycin, keto-conazole, itracon-azole, quinine	None known	None known	Potentiates CNS depres-sion with alcohol & other CNS depressants

7. Oral decongestants are often combined with antihistamines to enhance effectiveness and counterbalance sedative side effects (see table that follows)

COMMON COMBINATION ANTIHISTAMINE/DECONGESTANT PRODUCTS			
Antihistamine/-Decongestant	**Brand Name**	**Older Adolescent Dose (mg)**	**Child Dose**
Brompheniramine/-phenylpropanolamine	Dimetapp	1 tab q 4 hours	1-6 mos, 1.25 mL po TID/QID; 7 mos-2 yrs, 2.5 mL po TID/QID; 2-4 yrs, 3.75 mL po TID/QID, >5 yrs, 5 mL po TID/QID
Chlorpheniramine/-pseudoephedrine	Deconamine	1 tab TID/QID	2-6 yrs, 2.5 mL TID/QID; >6 yrs, 2.5-5.0 mL TID/QID
Chlorpheniramine/-pyrilamine/phenylephrine	Rynatan	1-2 tabs BID	2-6 yrs, 2.5-5.0 mL; >6 yrs, 5-10 mL
Chlorpheniramine/-phenylpropanolamine	Triaminic-12	1 tab q 12 hours	3-12 mos, 0.75 mL; 12-24 mos, 1.25 mL; 2-6 yrs, 2.5 mL; 6-12 yrs, 5 mL; q 4 hrs
Fexofenadine/pseudoephedrine	Allegra-D	1 tab BID	Not recommended
Loratadine/pseudoephedrine	Claritin-D 12 hr Claritin-D 24 hr	1 tab BID/QD 1 tab QD	Not recommended

8. For patients with significant congestion of mucous membranes, a topical decongestant may be needed first. Topical pharmacotherapy provides direct delivery of drug to nasal mucosa and has minimal side effects but will be ineffective for pulmonary and ocular allergic symptoms. Prescribe phenylephrine HCl (Neo-Synephrine spray or drops) 1-2 sprays or 2-3 drops of 0.25% or 0.5% in each nostril every 3-4 hours; use no longer than 3-4 days (not recommended for children <6 years)
9. Steroid sprays are often drug of choice, particularly for patients who have moderate or severe symptoms (see table that follows for dosing and prescribing information)

INTRANASAL CORTICOSTEROID SPRAYS			
Medications	Dose per Actuation	Formulation (Aq/MDI)	Adolescent Dosage
Beclomethasone dipropionate (Vancenase, Beconase)	42 mcg 84 mcg	+/+ +/0	1-2 sprays each nostril BID-QID 2 sprays each nostril QD
Budesonide (Rhinocort)	32 mcg	0/+	2 sprays each nostril BID or 4 sprays each nostril QD
Dexamethasone (Dexacort)	100 mcg	0/+	2 sprays each nostril BID-TID
Flunisolide (Nasarel)	25 mcg	+/0	2 sprays each nostril BID-TID
Fluticasone propionate (Flonase)	50 mcg	+/0	2 sprays each nostril QD
Mometasone furoate (Nasonex)	50 mcg	+/0	2 sprays each nostril QD
Triamcinolone acetonide (Nasacort)	55 mcg	+/+	2-4 sprays each nostril QD

Aq = Aqueous, MDI = Metered-dose inhaler, + = Available, 0 = Not available

Adapted from Kaiser, H.B., Kay, G.G., & Palakanis, K. (1998). Contemporary issues in the management of allergic disorders: A focus on respiratory and dermatologic manifestations. Clinical Courier, 16 (46), 1-7.

      a.   Advantages: Control nasal congestion as well as rhinorrhea; few adverse effects; most effective and potent agents available for treatment; controls underlying anti-inflammatory response

      b.   Disadvantages: Expensive; slow onset of activity; do not relieve ocular symptoms

      c.   May be combined with antihistamines for enhanced effectiveness

      d.   Steroid sprays have a slow onset of activity; warn patients they might not see effects for 2 weeks after initiating therapy

      e.   Medication must be used on a regular basis to be effective

10.   Oral corticosteroids are reserved for short-term therapy for patients with severe, debilitating disease

11.   Mast cell stabilizers are usually reserved for patients with chronic or severe symptoms

      a.   Advantages: Good safety profile, control underlying inflammatory response

      b.   Disadvantages: Less effective than other therapies in relieving nasal obstruction; frequent dosing makes it difficult for patients to adhere; more expensive than other therapies

      c.   These medications prevent symptoms from starting and are generally not beneficial once an attack has started; relief of symptoms may be delayed 3-4 weeks after initiation of therapy

          (1)   Recommend over-the-counter, intranasal cromolyn sodium (Nasalcrom) 1-2 sprays in each nostril 3-6x daily at regular intervals; use prophylactically before known or suspected allergen contact (not recommended <6 years)

          (2)   Nedocromil is considered ten times more potent than cromolyn

          (3)   Concomitant use of decongestants may be useful to relieve congestion

12.   Application of saline to nasal mucosa acts as a mild decongestant and can liquify mucus and prevent crusting; administer 2-4 times a day

13.   Intranasal ipratropium may be used for relief of rhinorrhea with allergic and nonallergic rhinitis

      a.   Advantage: excellent safety profile and few adverse reactions

      b.   Disadvantage: effective for only rhinorrhea; minimal effect on other symptoms

      c.   Prescribe ipratropium bromide 0.03% aqueous solution (Atrovent nasal spray) 2 sprays in each nostril 2-3 times daily (not recommended <6 years)

14.   Allergic conjunctivitis which often accompanies allergic rhinitis may require flushing eyes with artificial liquid tears; may use naphazoline HCl 0.025% and pheniramine maleate (0.3%) (Naphcon A) ophthalmic solution 1-2 drops every 3-4 hours prn (not recommended <6 years). May also use cromolyn sodium 4% ophthalmic solution (Crolom) 1-2 drops 4-6 times daily (not recommended <4 years)

15.   For patients with nasal polyps, refer to specialist

16. Patient Education
    a. Remind patients with perennial allergic rhinitis to take medications regularly rather than sporadically when symptoms occur
    b. Teach patients to read drug labels before taking over-the-counter medication as many cold products and sleep aids contain antihistamines
    c. Teach patient proper administration of intranasal medications (see following table)

INSTRUCTIONS FOR USE OF INTRANASAL MEDICATION
➡ Clear nasal passages or blow nose before administering medication
➡ Keep head upright and spray medication quickly and firmly into each nostril
➡ Spray medication away from nasal septum
➡ Spray each nostril separately and wait at least 1 minute before second spray
➡ If possible, avoid sneezing or blowing nose for 5-10 minutes after spraying
➡ Cleanse medicine canister device after each use

17. Referral to a specialist for allergen immunotherapy is recommended when patients cannot eliminate environmental allergens or have severe symptoms, poor response to medications, long-term need for medications, or presence of secondary complications

B. Vasomotor rhinitis
    1. Difficult to relieve symptoms; best medication is a nasal spray of physiological saline solution
    2. More thorough cleansing of nose may be accomplished by powered irrigators such as the Grossan irrigator
    3. Topical ipratropium often relieves symptoms
    4. Oral anti-histamines/decongestants and steroid sprays are usually less efficacious than the above recommendations, but for some patients are helpful

C. Follow up of all types of rhinitis
    1. Schedule follow up visit in 2-3 weeks to review patient education topics and check results of therapies
    2. Schedule quarterly or biannual rechecks depending on patient's level of comfort and health

EPISTAXIS

I. Definition: Nasal bleeding from any cause

II. Pathogenesis

A. The nose acts as a conduit to allow air into the lungs and has a very well vascularized mucosa with a complex interior surface composed of folds and irregularities

B. The blood supply of the nose comes from both the internal and external carotid systems

C. The anterior portion of the septum contains a plexus of vessels known as Kisselbach's plexus which is particularly vulnerable to digital as well as direct blunt trauma

D. Bleeding occurs as a result of disruption of the nasal mucosa, whether due to trauma, inflammation, or neoplasm

E. More than 90% of bleeds are related to local irritation and most occur in the absence of a specific underlying anatomic lesion

F. Epistaxis is rarely associated with systemic diseases, such as liver disease, hypertension (hypertension does not cause nasal bleeding but may exacerbate the problem), clotting abnormalities, thrombocytopenia, or platelet dysfunction

III. Clinical Presentation

A. Approximately 10% of the population experiences at least one significant nosebleed

B. Commonly seen in children and episodes are typically infrequent, mild, and self-limiting

C. Over 90% of nosebleeds are anterior, and usually involve the Kisselbach's triangle of the anterior portion of the septum

D. Anterior nosebleeds are generally less severe and easier to control than nosebleeds originating in posterior area of nose

E. Epistaxis is rare in hemophiliacs without trauma, but is characteristic of von Willebrand's disease (a heritable coagulation disorder)

IV. Diagnosis/Evaluation

A. History
   1. Question about onset and duration of nasal bleeding; ask how frequently does it occur and how much bleeding is there (quantity)
   2. Ask if there has been an increase in nasal mucus production; if yes, determine color, character, and quantity
   3. Ask if nasal obstruction is present, and if so, is it an acute or chronic occurrence
   4. Ask about occupational exposure to irritating chemicals or dust; ask about cocaine use if appropriate
   5. Inquire about previous episodes and treatments
   6. Determine if patient has any clotting abnormalities, thrombocytopenia, or platelet dysfunction; is the patient hypertensive? (A **rare** hypertensive patient with severe pressure elevation may experience epistaxis)

B. Physical Examination
   1. Assess blood pressure and pulse
   2. Use gentle suction with a bulb syringe to remove blood and secretions and make visualization of the involved vessels possible
   3. Locate bleeding site if possible; 90% are in the anterior septum (Kisselbach's plexus). Posterior site is indicated by persistent drainage of blood down the pharynx

C. Differential Diagnosis
   1. Coagulation disorders
   2. Intranasal foreign bodies
   3. Familial hereditary telangiectasia

D. Diagnostic Tests
   1. Extensive evaluation should be reserved for those cases that are recurrent or particularly severe
   2. Hemoglobin or hematocrit if significant blood loss suspected
   3. CBC with differential, platelets, PT and PTT if bleeding disorders suspected

V.   Plan/Management

A.   Use the approaches outlined in the table below

MANAGEMENT OF NOSE BLEEDS
✓ First, apply pressure to anterior nasal septum while head tilted forward; continue pressure for 10-15 minutes
✓ Then, if clot formation and bleeding cessation do not occur, do the following
✱ Place a small piece of cotton soaked in 1:1000 epinephrine or a vasoconstricting nosedrop such as phenylephrine (Neo-Synephrine) into the vestibule of the nose
✱ Press against the bleeding site for 5 to 10 minutes to promote vasoconstriction
✱ Remove to observe for bleeding (almost all venous types of anterior nosebleeds are stopped with this treatment)
✓ If bleeding continues, but has slowed considerably,
✱ Repeat treatment
✱ Apply ice pack over the nose as an additional therapy
✓ Finally, if these remedies fail,
✱ Anesthetize the mucous membrane with 4% lidocaine (apply to cotton ball and hold in place for several minutes)
✱ Apply a silver nitrate stick to the bleeding site

B.   If still not responsive, refer to local emergency department

C.   Instruct parent/patient regarding management of simple nose bleeds at home

D.   Advise increasing humidity in home through use of humidifier, especially during winter months

E.   Advise liberal use of lubricant such a petrolatum in nares to promote hydration

F.   All cases that are recurrent or are particularly severe should be referred to a specialist

G.   Follow Up: None indicated for cases due to local trauma or inflammation

FOREIGN BODY IN THE NOSE

I.   Definition: Presence of object(s) in the nasal cavity

II.   Pathogenesis: Intentional placement of an object in nose, or occasionally accidental placement of a foreign body while child is attempting to sniff or smell the object

III. Clinical Presentation

A.   Boredom or curiosity may lead a child to place an object in his/her nose

B.   Typically, these objects are soft materials such as tissues, erasers, clay, or part of a toy

C.   Research has shown that the most common underlying factor in children placing objects in their nose is a history of chronic rhinitis

D.   Symptoms include unilateral obstruction, mild discomfort, sneezing; unilateral purulent nasal discharge can also occur over time

E.   A key feature is that it is unilateral

F. Unilateral nasal discharge in a young child should be considered evidence of a foreign body until proven otherwise

IV. Diagnosis/Evaluation

A. History
1. Inquire about onset and duration of symptoms
2. Ask parent/child if this has occurred in the past
3. Ask child if object has been placed in nose (child will usually not confess that he/she has done this)

B. Physical Examination
1. Test both nares for patency
2. Examine both nares with nasal speculum to visualize the object

C. Differential Diagnosis
1. Rhinitis
2. Sinusitis

D. Diagnostic Tests: None indicated

V. Plan/Management

A. Remove secretions with a small suction tip and use topical decongestant such as Neosynephrine to reduce mucosal edema

B. Occlude the uninvolved nostril and have the child blow forcefully out

C. In infants, briskly force air through the oropharynx (as in mouth-to-mouth resuscitation) and object may be dislodged out the nose

D. If the above intervention is not successful, use alligator forceps if child is cooperative; instruments introduced into the nasal passage require a steady hand resting on the child's head

E. For uncooperative child, or when the nasal passage is completely occluded by an expanding foreign object such as plant materials, beans, or other seeds, or when there is marked edema and inflammation, referral to a specialist is indicated

F. Follow Up: Instruct patient/parent to use saline irrigation 2-3 times/day for 2-3 days, and follow up in 2 days to evaluate healing of mucosa

SINUSITIS

I. Definition: Acute, subacute, or chronic inflammation of the mucous membranes that line the paranasal sinuses

A. Acute sinusitis is the abrupt onset of infection of one or more of paranasal sinuses with resolution of symptoms with therapy

B. Subacute sinusitis is the persistent occurrence of purulent nasal discharge despite therapy; epithelial damage is usually reversible, symptoms last <3 months

C. Chronic sinusitis occurs with episodes of prolonged inflammation and/or repeated or inadequately treated acute infection; irreversible damage to the mucosa is present, symptoms last >3 months

II.   Pathogenesis

    A.   Etiological factors

        1.   Main factor is obstruction of ostiomeatal unit which leads to lower levels of oxygen within sinuses, decreased clearance of foreign material, and mucus stasis which creates a good environment for pathogens to grow; any factor or condition which blocks flow of secretions can lead to sinusitis:

            a.   Recent upper respiratory infection

            b.   Allergic response to airborne allergens

            c.   Anatomical abnormalities such as deviated septum

            d.   Adenoidal hypertrophy

            e.   Diving and swimming

            f.   Extension of dental abscess

            g.   Neoplasms

            h.   Trauma

            i.   Foreign body

        2.   Other patients have problems with mucus stasis due to immune deficiency, immotile cilia syndrome, or cystic fibrosis

    B.   Pathogens in acute sinusitis

        1.   Common

            a.   *Streptococcus pneumoniae*

            b.   *Haemophilus influenzae* (may be ß-lactamase producing)

            c.   *Moraxella catarrhalis* [(may be ß-lactamase producing); prevalence greater among children than adults]

        2.   Less common

            a.   *Chlamydia pneumoniae*

            b.   *Streptococcus pyogenes*

            c.   Viruses

            d.   Fungi (e.g., *Aspergillus fumigatus*) (more common in patients who are immunosuppressed or have diabetes mellitus)

        3.   Penicillin-resistant *Streptococcus pneumoniae* is becoming more common

    C.   Pathogens in chronic or subacute sinusitis are usually polymicrobial

        1.   Anaerobic bacteria

        2.   *Staphylococcus aureus*

    D.   Anaerobes are common in sinusitis resulting from dental infections

III.   Clinical Presentation

    A.   Most sinus disease in adults and children involves the maxillary and anterior ethmoidal sinuses

        1.   After age 10 the frontal sinus becomes a more common site of infection and may be focus of serious albeit rare intracranial infection

        2.   Sphenoid sinuses are rarely site of isolated infection but may be involved in cases of pansinusitis

    B.   Once believed an adult disease, today acute sinusitis is considered a common, pediatric problem, complicating 5-10% of upper respiratory infections and affecting all age groups even infants

        1.   Younger children are at greater risk due to their small anatomic structures, frequency of viral infections, increased exposure to pathogens, allergens, and irritants, as well as their "immature" immune systems

        2.   Children usually have more nonspecific complaints than adults

            a.   Typically children <5 years do not complain of headaches and facial pain

            b.   Purulent nasal discharge is almost always present in children with sinusitis, which is not characteristic of adults

C.   Acute sinusitis has the following characteristics:
1.   Yellow or green nasal discharge with fever
2.   Nasal congestion with an intermittent sore or raw sensation in throat
3.   Complaint of facial pain, toothache, or headache over the affected sinus.
4.   Increased pain with coughing, bending over or sudden head movement
5.   Cough which may worsen with lying down
6.   Early morning periorbital swelling
7.   Fetid breath is often reported by parents
8.   Fever and malaise are common systemic symptoms
9.   Classic study by Williams & Simel (1993) found that three symptoms (maxillary toothache, poor response to nasal decongestants, and history of colored nasal discharge) and two signs (purulent nasal secretion and abnormal transillumination) were the best predictors of acute sinusitis
    a.   According to the Canadian Sinusitis Symposium Panel, acute sinusitis can be ruled out when there are fewer than 2 of the preceding signs and symptoms
    b.   When 4 or more of the preceding signs and symptoms are present the likelihood of acute sinusitis is very high
10.   According to O'Brien et al. (1998) the clinical diagnosis of sinusitis requires one of the following:
    a.   Prolonged nonspecific upper respiratory signs and symptoms without improvement for >10-14 days
    b.   More severe upper respiratory tract signs and symptoms such as facial swelling, facial pain , and fever $\geq 39.0^{\circ}C$

D.   Thick, tenacious, brown secretions are characteristic of fungal sinusitis

E.   Subacute or chronic sinusitis has the following characteristics:
1.   Nasal discharge, nasal congestion, or cough lasting >30 days
2.   Hallmark is dull ache or pressure across midface or headache
3.   Other symptoms include thick postnatal drip, "popping" ears, eye pain, halitosis, chronic cough, and fatigue

F.   Chronic sinusitis is less common in children than adults

G.   All types of sinusitis may exacerbate asthma

H.   Diabetics and immunosuppressed patients often experience severe, invasive sinus disease

I.   Complications of sinusitis include contiguous spread or hematogenous dissemination of infection and can result in life-threatening intraorbital or intracranial suppuration; patients with frontal headaches and associated frontal sinusitis are at greatest risk for intracranial complications

IV.   Diagnosis/Evaluation

A.   History
1.   Question regarding onset, duration, and seasonality of symptoms
2.   Inquire about the laterality and quality (mucoid, purulent, serous) of nasal discharge
3.   Ask about fever and systemic symptoms such as fatigue
4.   Question about character (dry, productive) and timing (day, night, continual) of cough
5.   Ask patient to describe pain and what aggravates it
6.   Ask about timing and quality of headaches and morning puffiness about the eyes
7.   Ask about history of allergies
8.   Ask about past episodes and treatments
9.   Inquire about past medical history such as diabetes mellitus, immunodeficiency, asthma
10.   Question about smoking, recent trauma to the nose, recent upper respiratory infections
11.   Inquire about family history of allergies, immunodeficiency, chronic respiratory complaints

B. Physical Examination
1. Determine vital signs
2. Examine eyes, noting peri-orbital swelling and presence of allergic shiners
3. Examine nasal mucosa for erythema, edema, and discharge
4. Determine patency of both nasal nares
5. Inspect nose for septal deviation and polyps
6. Examine ears, throat, and mouth for signs of inflammation
7. Transilluminate and percuss frontal and maxillary sinuses (not reliable in young children)
8. Examine teeth and gingivae for caries and inflammation; tap maxillary teeth with tongue blade because 5% to 10% of maxillary sinusitis is due to dental root infection
9. Palpate neck and jaw for lymphadenopathy
10. Auscultate heart and lungs.
11. Perform a neurological examination to rule-out complications

C. Differential Diagnosis:
1. Dental abscess
2. Cluster and migraine headaches
3. Allergic rhinitis
4. Vasomotor rhinitis
5. Nasal polyp
6. Tumor
7. Uncomplicated upper respiratory infection

D. Diagnostic Tests
1. None indicated for typical presentation and for first episodes of acute sinusitis
2. Radiologic studies are not routinely ordered and must be intrepreted cautiously
    a. The common cold often includes radiologic evidence of sinus involvement (abnormal images only reflect inflammation; they do not pinpoint whether the inflammation is viral, bacterial or allergic in origin)
    b. Order radiographs to confirm clinical impression and in following: patients with frontal headaches, refractory cases, when complications are suspected, and when diagnosis is unclear
        (1) Sinus x-rays
            (a) Need antero-posterior, lateral and occipitomental (Waters view) views
            (b) An air-fluid level or complete opacification of the sinuses and thickening of the mucosal lining are most diagnostic
            (c) Accuracy of diagnosing ethmoid disease is questionable with x-rays
        (2) Computerized tomography (CT scan) is gold standard of radiographic study, but is reserved for recalcitrant cases and patients in need of surgery
3. To confirm diagnosis of maxillary and frontal sinusitis and to identify causative pathogen, obtain sinus aspirates by antral puncture (impractical in most primary care settings)
4. Flexible fiber optic rhinoscopy, after the topical application of a vasoconstrictor and anesthetic may be indicated
5. CBC with differential indicated for severely, ill patients
6. Allergy testing when the history suggests an allergic disease

V. Plan/Management

A. Treatment of acute sinusitis and acute episodes in patients who have subacute and chronic sinusitis includes antibiotics and drugs to reduce obstruction of the ostiomeatal unit
1. Antibiotics for acute sinusitis are similar to those recommended for otitis media (see tables on pages 263 and 264 of recommended antibiotics in OTITIS MEDIA section)
    a. For adolescents: Amoxicillin (Amoxil) 500 mg TID is the first-line drug. Prescribe trimethoprim sulfamethoxazole (Bactrim) 1 double strength tab q 12 hours for patients allergic to penicillin; duration of antibiotic therapy is 10-14 days or 7 days beyond the point of resolution of signs and symptoms

b. For children <12 years of age with acute sinusitis, use amoxicillin (Amoxil) 40 mg/kg/day PO in 3 divided doses for 10-14 days (available in 125 mg/5 mL and 250 mg/5 mL strengths) or 7 days beyond the point of resolution of signs and symptoms. If allergic to penicillin, use trimethoprim sulfamethoxazole (Bactrim) suspension 1 mL/kg/day PO q 12 hours

2. Patients with chronic sinusitis are likely to have acute exacerbations; for these acute episodes prescribe a beta-lactamase stable antibiotic and extend therapy for a total of 2-4 weeks; prescribe one of following:

    a. Amoxicillin/clavulanate (Augmentin) 500 mg TID; in children: 40 mg/kg/day in 3 divided doses

    b. Clarithromycin (Biaxin) 500 mg tab every 12 hours; in children: 7.5mg/kg every 12 hours. Available 125mg/5mL and 250mg/5mL suspensions

    c. See table for other recommended second-line antibiotics in OTITIS MEDIA section

3. Decongestants or saline nasal spray at the time of diagnosis of acute sinusitis and in acute episodes of subacute and chronic sinusitis can improve patency of ostiomeatal unit

    a. Topical decongestants should be used no longer than 3-4 days. For patients over 6 years of age use phenylephrine (Neo-Synephrine spray or drops) 1-2 sprays or 2-3 drops of 0.25% or 0.5% in each nostril every 3-4 hours

    b. In children under 6 years of age, use saline nasal drops, 2-3 drops in each nostril BID-QID (1/4 tsp of salt in 8 oz of boiled water)

    c. Oral decongestants are not as effective as topical agents but can be used for a longer time period

        (1) Use cautiously in patients with hypertension

        (2) Adolescents: suggest pseudoephedrine hydrochloride (Sudafed) 60 mg, 1 tablet every 4-6 hours or Pseudoephedrine sulfate (Afrin) 120 mg, 1 tablet every 12 hours

        (3) In children 2-6 years, use pseudoephedrine hydrochloride (Sudafed) 2.5 mL every 4-6 hours. Available 30 mg/5 mL liquid. Over 6 years old, 30 mg tablets or 5 mL liquid every 4-6 hours

        (4) In infants less than 6 months of age, oral decongestants are not recommended. For older infants, can cautiously prescribe pseudoephedrine hydrochloride (Pediacare Infants' Oral Decongestant): 12-17 lbs, 1 dropper; 18-23 lbs, 1-1/2 droppers; 24-35 lbs, 2 droppers every 4-6 hours

B. For recurrent acute infections or for persons with acute sinusitis or acute exacerbations who do not have a clinical response to first antibiotic in 48 to 72 hours, prescribe a beta-lactamase-stable agent or second-line drug (see OTITIS MEDIA section)

C. Acute sinusitis due to dental infection: Prescribe amoxicillin clavulanate (Augmentin)

D. Unresponsive cases may be due to infection with *Chlamydia pneumoniae*; trial with doxycycline (Vibramycin) 100 mg caps every 12 hours for 10-14 days (not recommended in children <8 years) or clarithromycin (dosage-see preceding V.A.2.b.) may be beneficial

E. Treatment of fungal infections involves surgery and broad-spectrum antibiotics for intercurrent bacterial infections

F. Treatment of chronic sinusitis

1. Prescribe: Nasal steroids sprays such as beclomethasone dipropionate (Beconase, Vancenase) 1-2 sprays in each nostril BID; triamcinolone acetonide (Nasacort AQ) or mometasone furoate (Nasonex) both prescribed 2 sprays in each nostril QD and then may decrease as symptoms improve; use cautiously in children

2. Do not use topical steroids when patient has an acute episode of sinusitis

3. Some experts do not recommend that children be treated with intranasal steroids

G. Oral antihistamines should not be used unless patient has allergies. Antihistamines tend to slow the movement of secretions out of the sinuses

H. Referral to a specialist is needed for the following:
   1. Exquisite pain with palpation or percussion of the face
   2. Possibility of cellulitis
   3. Periorbital swelling

I. Functional endoscopic sinus surgery which removes only affected tissue has revolutionized surgical treatment of sinus disease

J. Patient Education
   1. Instruct patient to return for further evaluation if symptoms are not improved within 48 hours
   2. Teach patient about the complications of sinusitis, particularly the need to return if there is swelling in the periorbital area
   3. Humidify the air
   4. Increase fluid intake
   5. Steam inhalation and warm compresses often help relieve pressure
   6. Avoid allergens and excessively dry heat
   7. Avoid swimming/diving and air travel during acute period
   8. Avoid use of antihistamines unless there is an allergic basis to disease
   9. Encourage cessation of smoking
   10. Teach proper application of nasal sprays (see table on instructions for use of intranasal medications in ALLERGIC RHINITIS section)
   11. Patients who have recurrent sinusitis should be instructed to begin decongestants at the first sign of sinusitis to facilitate sinus drainage and decrease development of infection

K. Follow Up
   1. If no decrease in symptoms in 48-72 hours, patient should be reevaluated; refer to specialist if symptoms are actually worsening.
   2. Schedule return visit for 10-14 days.
   3. Patients with chronic sinusitis who do not have marked improvement in four weeks with continuous medical therapy may be candidates for needle aspiration of a maxillary sinus or sinus surgery

PHARYNGITIS

I. Definition: Inflammation of the pharynx, and surrounding lymph tissue (tonsils)

II. Pathogenesis

A. Viruses are the most common pathogens; the following are viral infections
   1. Infections due to rhinovirus, adenovirus, parainfluenza, coronavirus, and echovirus
   2. Herpangina due to Coxsackie virus and echovirus
   3. Hand-Foot-and-Mouth disease due to Coxsackie virus
   4. Infectious mononucleosis caused by Epstein-Barr virus
   5. Human Immunodeficiency Virus (HIV)

B. Bacteria (listed common to rare)
   1. Group A β-hemolytic *streptococcus*
   2. *Neisseria gonorrhoea*
   3. *Corynebacterium diphtheriae*
   4. *Streptococci of Lancefield Groups C* and *G* (often associated with contaminated food)

C. Other atypical agents usually in adults or adolescents include *Mycoplasma pneumoniae* and *Chlamydia trachomatis* (rare)

D. Fungus: *Candida albicans*

E.   Peritonsillar abscess: Often due to anaerobic bacteria, but can be due to Group A *streptococci*, *Haemophilus influenzae*, or *Staphylococcus aureus*

F.   Noninfectious causes
1.   Allergic rhinitis or post-nasal drip
2.   Mouth breathing
3.   Trauma from heat, alcohol, irritants such as marijuana or sharp objects
4.   Subacute thyroiditis in females

III.   Clinical Presentation

A.   Herpangina
1.   Small oral vesicles or ulcers may be on tonsils, pharynx, or posterior buccal mucus
2.   Fever, headache, and malaise often accompany sore throat

B.   Hand-Foot-and-Mouth syndrome: usually oral lesions and sore throat accompanied by lesions on hands and feet; may have lesions on arms, legs, buttocks as well

C.   Infectious mononucleosis: May have exudative tonsillitis with fever, fatigue, lymphadenopathy, and palatal petechiae (see section on INFECTIOUS MONONUCLEOSIS)

D.   Primary HIV infection resembles signs and symptoms of mononucleosis with sorethroat, fever, malaise, myalgia, photophobia, lymphadenopathy, and rash; duration is few days to 2 weeks

E.   Pharyngitis due to *Group A ß-hemolytic streptococcus*
1.   Commonly seen in 15-40% of school age children with pharyngitis but uncommon in children <3 years old
2.   Symptoms include fever >101°F, headaches and sore throat with dysphagia
3.   Erythema of tonsils and pharynx with white or yellow exudate
4.   Tender and enlarged anterior cervical lymph nodes are often present
5.   Erythematous "sand paper" rash and Pastia's lines (petechiae in flexor skin creases of joints) occur with scarlet fever
6.   Abdominal pain, vomiting, and headache may occur whereas upper respiratory symptoms suggest other causes of pharyngitis
7.   Without proper antimicrobial treatment, streptococcal pharyngitis can lead to serious suppurative (direct extension from pharyngeal infection) and nonsuppurative complications (arise from immune responses to acute infection)
     a.   Suppurative adenitis involving tender, enlarged nodes (see section on CERVICAL ADENITIS)
     b.   Scarlet fever (suppurative) (see section on SCARLET FEVER)
     c.   Peritonsillar abscess (suppurative) (discussed later)
     d.   Glomerulonephritis (nonsuppurative) which appears 1-3 weeks after pharyngeal infection (proper treatment with antimicrobials does not prevent)
     e.   Rheumatic fever (nonsuppurative) (see section on RHEUMATIC FEVER)

F.   Pharyngitis due to *Corynebacterium diphtheriae*
1.   Gray adherent membrane on the nasal mucosa, tonsils, uvula or pharynx
2.   Bleeding occurs when membrane is removed

G.   Pharyngitis due to *Neisseria gonorrhoea* and *Chlamydia trachomatis*
1.   Seen in those patients who practice orogenital sex and sexually abused children
2.   Commonly presents as a chronic sore throat

H.   Pharyngitis due to *Mycoplasma pneumoniae*
1.   Uncommon in children <5 years of age, but seen in adolescents and adults
2.   Signs and symptoms indistinguishable from streptococcal disease

I.   *Candida albicans*
1.   Thin diffuse or patchy exudate on mucous membranes
2.   Patients have history of antibiotic use or are immunosuppressed

J. Peritonsillar abscess
1. Most common in older children and adolescents following an episode of tonsillitis
2. Often presents with gradually increasing unilateral ear and throat pain
3. Dysphagia, dysphonia, drooling, and trismus are common
4. The affected tonsil is usually grossly swollen medially and erythematous and may displace uvula and soft palate to contralateral side
5. Swelling and erythema of the soft palate is noted
6. Fluctuance may be felt with palpation of affected side
7. Enlarged and very tender lymph nodes are usually present

IV. Diagnosis/Evaluation

A. History
1. Determine onset and duration of symptoms
2. Question about rhinorrhea and coughing (suggestive of viral agent)
3. Inquire regarding trismus, excessive drooling and dysphagia (suggestive of peritonsillar abscess)
4. Ask about lesions in the mouth (suggestive of herpangina, hand-foot-mouth syndrome, and thrush)
5. Inquire about skin changes and exanthems (rash with scarlet fever)
6. Determine other associated symptoms such as abdominal pain, headache, and fatigue
7. Ascertain that sore throat is not significantly reducing intake of fluids
8. Inquire about possible streptococcal exposure
9. Inquire about immunization status
10. If applicable, inquire about sexual practices

B. Physical Examination
1. Do not attempt to examine the pharynx of a patient (particularly if the patient is between 3-7 years old) who has drooling, stridor or trouble breathing (may have epiglottitis)
2. Measure vital signs
3. Inspect skin for color and exanthems
4. Palpate skin for texture and turgor, noting whether the skin has a "sand paper" rash
5. Inspect mouth for lesions and thrush
6. Examine ears for concurrent otitis media or effusion
7. Visualize throat and pharynx for exudate and swelling (unilateral swelling occurs with peritonsillar abscess)
8. Palpate neck and jaw for adenopathy
9. Completely examine pharynx
10. Assess for nuchal rigidity
11. Auscultate chest
12. Depending on history of sexual activity, may need to perform genitourinary examination
13. Palpate abdomen

C. Differential Diagnosis
1. Stomatitis
2. Rhinitis or sinusitis with post nasal drip
3. Epiglottitis
4. Thyroiditis

D. Diagnostic Tests
1. Perform rapid strep test (sensitivity may be as low as 60%)
2. Perform throat culture: It is advisable to collect the rapid antigen strep and the throat culture at the same time; if rapid test is negative and suspicion is high, send throat culture
3. Consider heterophil agglutination, or mono spot test
4. Consider CBC with differential; expect WBC elevation with bacterial infection and WBC decrease with viral agent
5. Consider culture for gonorrhoea
6. Consider viral cultures of throat and mouth lesions

V. Plan/Management

A. For viral pharyngitis (i.e., herpangina, hand-foot-and-mouth disease, and infectious mononucleosis), treatment is symptomatic

B. Antibiotic treatment for possible and probable strep throat: According to Schwartz et al. (1998), never prescribe antibiotic without a positive throat culture or positive antigen-detection test
   1. Therapy is aimed at preventing complications such as rheumatic fever
   2. Begin therapy on all patients suspected of strep throat and who have a history of rheumatic fever, appear toxic, have clinical scarlet fever, have symptoms suggesting peritonsillar abscess
   3. Treatment of choice is oral or intramuscular penicillin
      a. Adolescents: Penicillin V (Pen-Vee-K) 500 mg BID or TID for at least 10 days
      b. Children: Penicillin V (Pen-Vee-K) 250 mg BID or TID for 10 days. Available 125 mg/5 mL and 250 mg/5 mL liquid
      c. Benzathine penicillin 600,000 units for children <60 pounds; 1,200,000 units for larger children and adolescents
         (1) Be familiar with signs, symptoms and treatment of anaphylaxis and observe patient for 30 minutes after injection.
         (2) Bring medication to room temperature before injecting to reduce discomfort
   4. Alternative antibiotics:
      a. Erythromycin: Adolescents prescribe erythromycin estolate (E-mycin): 250 mg TID/QID for 10 days; Children prescribe erythromycin ethyl succinate (Eryped) 40mg/kg/day BID or TID for 10 days; available 200mg/5mL and 400mg/5mL susp.
      b. Cefadroxil monohydrate (Duricef): Adolescents prescribe 500 mg capsules BID for 10 days; Children prescribe 30 mg/kg once a day or in 2 divided doses. Available formulations include 125 mg/5mL, 250 mg/5 mL, and 500 mg/5mL suspensions for 10 days. Do not use in patients with allergies to penicillin
   5. Treatment of patient who has recurrence of streptococcal pharyngitis shortly after completing recommended antibiotic therapy includes one of following:
      a. Retreat with same antibiotic
      b. Prescribe an alternative oral antibiotic
      c. Administer IM dose of benzathine penicillin G
   6. Treatment of streptococcal pharyngeal carriers
      a. Antibiotics are not indicated except for the following:
         (1) During outbreaks of acute rheumatic fever or poststreptococcal glomerulonephritis
         (2) During an outbreak of strep. pharyngitis in a closed or semi-closed community
         (3) Family history of rheumatic fever exists
         (4) Multiple episodes of documented, symptomatic strep. pharyngitis continue to occur within a family over weeks despite appropriate antibiotic therapy
         (5) Family with excessive anxiety of strep. pharyngitis
         (6) When tonsillectomy is considered due to chronic strep carriage
      b. To eliminate carriage, prescribe clindamycin (Cleocin) 20 mg/kg/day (maximum 1.8 g/day) in three divided doses for 10 days

C. Pharyngeal gonorrhea is usually treated with ceftriaxone (Rocephin) 250 mg IM

D. Diphtheria needs immediate specialist consult and is usually treated with equine antitoxin and penicillin or erythromycin; notify public health department

E. For pharyngitis due to mycoplasma pneumoniae and *Chlamydia trachomatis*, treat with erythromycin (E-mycin) 250 mg TID/QID for 10 days

F. *Candida albicans* (see section on CANDIDIASIS)

G. Peritonsillar abscess needs an immediate referral to a specialist
   1. Initially, in outpatient setting, prescribe drug of choice, penicillin, and a pain medication
   2. Needle aspiration, incision and drainage, or abscess tonsillectomy are current surgical approaches to management

H. Patient Education
   1. Teach parents and patients to immediately call office if the pain becomes more severe or if dyspnea, drooling, difficulty swallowing, and inability to fully open mouth develop
   2. Advise increased fluid intake
   3. May use hard candy, lozenges or warm saline gargles to soothe throat
   4. Patients with streptococcal pharyngitis should not return to school or work until they have been on antibiotic therapy for a full 24 hours
   5. Reinforce that patients will usually feel well in 24-48 hours, but that it is important to take full 10-day course of antibiotic to prevent complications, particularly rheumatic fever

I. Follow Up
   1. If no significant improvement in 3-4 days patient should return to health care provider
   2. Patients with streptococcal pharyngitis: Posttreatment throat cultures are indicated only for patients who have high risk for rheumatic fever or who are still symptomatic after treatment

APHTHOUS STOMATITIS

I. Definition: Chronic Inflammation of the oral mucosal tissue with ulcers often called canker sores

II. Pathogenesis: Etiology is uncertain, but the following factors play an important role:

   A. Immunopathologic processes
      1. Common in persons with leukemia, neutropenia, and human immunodeficiency virus infection
      2. Increased prevalence in patients with autoimmune diseases such as Crohn's disease, Behcet's syndrome, Reiter's syndrome, and ulcerative colitis

   B. Allergies; coffee, chocolate, potatoes, cheese, figs, nuts, citrus fruits, and gluten are predisposing factors

   C. Stress

   D. Viral and bacterial pathogens

   E. Trauma

   F. Nutritional deficiencies such as vitamin B_{12}, folate, and iron

   G. Hormones

   H. Medications such as antihypertensives, antineoplastics, gold salts, and nonsteroidal anti-inflammatory drugs

III. Clinical Presentation

   A. Peak onset is between 10 and 19 years of age

   B. Less prevalent in males and in chronic smokers

   C. In approximately 1/3 of patients, reoccurrences continue for numerous years

D. Lesions divided into 3 classifications: minor, clusterform ulcers, and major
1. Minor: Lesions appear on vestibular and buccal mucosa, tongue, soft palate, fauces, and floor of mouth; rarely do lesions appear on attached gingiva and hard palate as occurs with herpetic ulcers
   a. Most common type
   b. Occasionally, patient may have a burning prodrome
   c. Lesions usually occur singly
   d. Lesions start as indurated papules that progress to ulcers (1 cm) which are covered by a yellow fibrinous membrane and surrounded with an erythematous halo; lesions are never vesicular as occurs in herpetic stomatitis
   e. No fever or lymphadenopathy is noted
   f. Typically lesions heal in 7-14 days and tend to recur
2. Clusterform:
   a. Typically present as crops of small (1-5 mm) painful ulcers from 3 to over 12
   b. Lesions are intially round or oval and later coalesce to form large ulcers with irregular margins
3. Major:
   a. This severe form presents with lesions that are large (>0.5 cm), and take 6 weeks or longer to heal with possible scarring
   b. Severe pain, tender lymphadenopathy and facial edema are sometimes present

IV. Diagnosis/Evaluation

A. History
1. Ask about onset and duration of symptoms
2. Inquire about fever and systemic symptoms
3. Question regarding nutritional deficiencies and stressors
4. Ask about past episodes and treatments received
5. Inquire about systemic diseases
6. Inquire regarding contact with irritants or allergens

B. Physical Examination
1. Determine vital signs
2. Assess hydration status; patients may not be drinking fluids due to mouth pain
3. Perform complete head, ears, eyes, nose, mouth, and throat exam; note location, number and distribution of lesions
4. Palpate neck and jaw for adenopathy
5. Auscultate chest

C. Differential Diagnosis
1. Oral cancer (consider if lesions are present for more than 6 weeks, are unresponsive to therapy, and have unusual presentations such as indurated or rolled borders)
2. Oral candidiasis (white patches in mouth) (see CANDIDIASIS section)
3. Hand-foot-and-mouth disease (lesions on hands and feet as well as mouth)
4. Herpes simplex virus (vesicles form before ulcers develop) (see HERPES SIMPLEX section)
   a. In primary herpes simplex, lesions are confined to pharynx, tonsils and soft palate
   b. In secondary herpex simplex, lesions are at the vermillion border of lips
5. Vincent's stomatitis (uclers appear on gingivae and are covered by purulent, gray exudate)
6. Herpangina
   a. More common in children than adults
   b. Distinctive papular, vesicular, and ulcerative, multiple lesions on anterior tonsillar pillars, soft palate, tonsils, pharynx, and posterior buccal mucosa
7. Acute necrotizing ulcerative gingivitis
8. Trauma due to dental appliances or rough surfaced teeth
9. Varicella (chicken pox)
10. Pemphigus (presence of bullous lesions in mouth and other parts of body)

D.   Diagnostic Tests
1.   Usually none indicated
2.   Vitamin B_{12}, folate and iron levels if nutritional deficiencies are suspected
3.   CBC with differential to assist in ruling out anemias
4.   Consider Tzanck smear for distinguishing herpetic stomatitis from other causes
5.   Biopsy is needed if cancer is suspected

V.   Plan/Management

A.   Pharmacologic treatment of minor lesions include one of following:
1.   Liquid antacids or 3% hydrogen peroxide/water solution, 1:1 as a gargle
2.   Ulcer Ease is a sodium bicarbonate based mouth rinse which acts as a soothing, cleansing, and buffering agent
3.   Xylocaine (Lidocaine 2%) viscous solution. Adolescents: May apply to lesions every 3 hours or use 15 mL as a gargle or mouthwash and swallow every 3 hours (maximum 8 doses/day). Children <3 years: apply 1.25 mL to affected area with applicator every 3 hours (maximum 8 doses/day). Adjust dosage for older children
4.   Diphenhydramine (Benadryl) elixir mixed 1:1 with attapulgite (Kaopectate) or aluminum hydroxide, magnesium hydroxide (Maalox). May be used as mouth rinse QID
5.   Corticosteroid creams can provide pain relief and promote healing, but be cautious as they worsen viral infections; apply thin layer of triamcinolone acetonide 0.1% (Kenalog) in paste vehicle, Orabase, after meals and HS (moderate potency); not recommended for young children

B.   For acute clusterform lesions, treat simulteneously with the following two syrups:
1.   Tetracycline syrup (Sumycin) 250mg/10mL syrup QID for 7-14 days; rinse for 2 minutes and swallow; contraindicated in pregnant females and children <8 years old
2.   Dexamthasone elixir (Decadron); rinse for 2 minutes QID and then expectorate
3.   Remind patient not to eat or drink for 20 minutes after this treatment

C.   Treat severe recurrent aphthous ulcers with one of following:
1.   May require oral corticosteroids
2.   Ask pharmacist to mix clobetasol propionate 0.05% (Temovate) ointment with an equal amount of Orabase; dry ulcer site lightly and apply sufficient paste to cover lesion three to six times daily

D.   Patient Education
1.   Stress the importance of good oral hygiene, even for infants
2.   Encourage good nutrition and increased fluid intake
3.   Avoid spicy, salty, and acidic foods and drinks
4.   Use soft-bristled toothbrush and avoid foods with sharp surfaces and talking while chewing
5.   Aphthous ulcers are not contagious, so no danger in spreading

E.   Follow Up
1.   Immediately in infants not taking fluids
2.   In severe cases, reschedule in 2-3 days
3.   Consult specialist if not healed in 2-3 weeks

TOOTHACHE (PULPITIS)

I.   Definition: A suppurative process that usually results from pulpal infection

II.   Pathogenesis

A.   Inflammation involving pulp tissue, the central portion of the tooth containing vital soft tissue, occurs due to injury of some type

B.   Dental caries, a disease of the calcified tissues of the teeth, is the most frequent type of injury that causes pulpitis

C.   Diverse flora, including gram-positive anaerobes and Bacteroides are the organisms most often involved in the infectious process

III.   Clinical Presentation

    A.   Constant, throbbing pain is the most frequent presenting complaint

    B.   Affected tooth is extremely sensitive to touch and pain is intensified with the application of heat or cold (thermal sensitivity)

    C.   Tooth may be slightly extruded so that occlusal contact gives rise to exquisite pain

    D.   The affected area of the jaw is tender to palpation

    E.   Systemic manifestations may or may not be present and are usually limited to regional lymphadenopathy, malaise, and fever

IV.   Diagnosis/Evaluation

    A.   History
        1.   Inquire about recent toothache
        2.   Inquire about occurrence of fever and chills
        3.   Inquire about heart murmur or defect
        4.   Determine type of medication taken for pain relief and when it was last taken

    B.   Physical Examination
        1.   Determine if febrile
        2.   Inspect and gently percuss teeth to determine location of affected tooth
        3.   Examine adjacent tissue for signs of inflammation
        4.   Observe for facial symmetry and examine jaw in area for signs of cellulitis
        5.   Auscultate heart (risk of sepsis and complications increase with valvular disease)
        6.   Examine for regional lymphadenopathy

    C.   Differential Diagnosis
        1.   Mumps
        2.   Cellulitis
        3.   Pericoronitis (painful wisdom teeth)

    D.   Diagnostic Tests: Should be done by dentist who will see patient

V.   Plan/Management

    A.   Patients with toothaches generally fall into one of three categories ranging from least to most serious and should be managed as follows

TREATMENT OF TOOTHACHE

Category 1: Patients who are afebrile, with no extraoral swelling (no facial asymmetry present) or intraoral swelling
  ✓ Prescribe analgesics: **Adolescents:** Prescribe acetaminophen (300 mg) with codeine (30 mg) (Tylenol #3), 1-2 tabs, every 4 hours. **Children:** Prescribe acetaminophen or ibuprofen. See PAIN MANAGEMENT section for dosing
  ✓ Recommend warm salt water rinses (swish and spit) every 3-4 hours
  ✓ Refer to dentist within 24 hours

Category 2: Patients who have either slight extraoral or intraoral swelling, or who have a low-grade fever
  ✓ Prescribe analgesics (as above) and
  ✓ Prescribe antibiotics: Treatment of choice is Penicillin V (Pen-Vee-K). **Adolescents:** 250-500 mg Q 6 hours x 5-7 days. **Children:** 40-60 mg/kg/day in 4 divided doses x 5-7 days
  ✓ Patients allergic to penicillin should be treated with erythromycin; consult PDR for dosing recommendations
  ✓ Recommend warm salt water rinses (swish and spit) every 3-4 hours
  ✓ Refer to dentist within 12-24 hours

Category 3: Patients who have fever ≥101F (38.5°) with intraoral and/or extraoral swelling (causing facial asymmetry)
  ✓ Emergency consultation and treatment by dentist is needed
  ✓ Management must be immediate because the consequences of delayed treatment can be serious and occasionally life threatening!

B. Treatment by the dentist for these three categories of toothache varies from extraction to root canal to incision and drainage, and to hospitalization for IV antibiotic therapy for patients with cellulitis

C. Follow up should be done by dentist

PERIODONTAL DISEASE

I. Definition: General term used to describe diseases that destroy the gingival and bony structures that support the teeth

A. Usually divided into two types, gingivitis and periodontitis

B. Major difference in the two types is that in periodontitis, there is loss of supporting bony structure of the teeth

II. Pathogenesis

A. Poor dental hygiene which allows plaque to accumulate on the teeth is the major causative factor

B. Initiating factors in the development of periodontal disease include bacterial plaque and calculus
  1. The initial changes in healthy gingiva after only a few days of plaque accumulation include an acute inflammation of the junctional epithelium (attachment of the gingiva to the enamel surface of the tooth)
  2. Within 2-4 weeks after the beginning of plaque formation, the gingivitis becomes established
  3. At some point, chronic gingivitis may progress to periodontitis, which is characterized by suppuration, bone loss, loss of attachment, pocket formation, tooth mobility, and loss of teeth

C. Systemic factors that alter inflammatory and immune responses so that the host's defenses against bacteria or their metabolites are compromised include the following:
  1. Hormonal--pregnancy gingivitis is an exaggerated inflammatory response that may be caused by hormonal changes, especially in the third trimester
  2. Nutritional--Vitamin C deficiency in the development of periodontal disease is well established

3. Drug Therapy--hyperplasia is associated with the use of phenytoin (Dilantin), cyclosporine, and calcium channel blockers

D. Local factors that modify the immunoinflammatory response and contribute of the progress of plaque-induced periodontal disease include the following:
   1. Trauma from occlusion (bruxism) which tends to accelerate pocket formation and bone loss
   2. Food impaction which occurs most frequently due to an impinging overbite
   3. Mouth breathing and continued exposure and drying of the facial gingiva of the maxillary anterior teeth

III. Clinical Presentation

A. Approximately two-thirds of young adults and 80% of middle-aged and older adults suffer from periodontal disease; also seen in up to 50% of children

B. Most common cause of tooth loss in adults; occurs at all ages, but increases in prevalence and severity with age

C. Whereas dental caries damages the tooth itself, the supporting structures for the tooth, the gingiva, cementum, alveolar bone, and periodontal membrane are damaged by periodontal disease

D. Gingivitis presents in one of four forms: acute, subacute, recurrent, and chronic
   1. Acute form, is characterized by rapid onset, short duration, and pain
   2. Subacute form is less severe than acute
   3. Recurrent form reappears after treatment or spontaneous remission
   4. Chronic (most common form) is characterized by slow onset, long duration, and most often painless

E. Early signs of gingivitis include the following:
   1. Inflammation of the gingiva (the normally coral-pink gingiva becomes bright red due to increased vascularity and decrease in keratinization)
   2. Increased gingival fluid secretion
   3. Bleeding from the gingival sulcus (usually with brushing)

F. Both acute and chronic forms produce changes in the gingiva which normally has a firm, resilient consistency
   1. In acute forms (acute, subacute), gingiva appears diffusely edematous
   2. In chronic forms (recurrent, chronic), gingiva has a fibrous appearance that pits with pressure

G. Major complication of untreated gingivitis is periodontitis
   1. Patients with periodontitis present with red, bleeding gums, unpleasant taste in mouth, but usually has no pain (unless acute infection superimposed on chronic process)
   2. Signs of gingivitis as described above are present and there is also periodontal pockets around the teeth containing purulent matter
   3. As periodontitis progresses, teeth loosen, spread apart, causing difficulty chewing and pain
   4. Eventually, destruction of the alveolar bone occurs and teeth are deprived of support and lost

IV. Diagnosis/Evaluation

A. History
   1. Ask about onset and duration of symptoms
   2. Ask about bleeding from gums after brushing
   3. Inquire regarding dental hygiene habits
   4. Question about bruxism, mouth breathing, and problems with occlusion
   5. Obtain medication history

B. Physical Examination
1. Examine teeth and gingiva for presence of plaque, and for hyperplasia or recession of gums
2. Examine gums for areas of erosion
3. Determine if gingival hyperplasia is generalized or localized

C. Differential Diagnosis
1. Dental abscess
2. Stomatitis

D. Diagnostic Tests: None indicated.

V. Plan/Management

A. Treatment of the four forms of gingivitis described above usually require 1-3 dental visits and is aimed at elimination of local etiologic factors (plaque and calculus) which will result in a reversal of the gingival inflammation
1. Plaque and calculus are removed using appropriate instruments
2. Patients are instructed in proper plaque control measures (use of soft-bristled toothbrush that facilitates cleaning of teeth and gingiva; use of dental floss)
3. Patients are scheduled for return visits for professional cleaning every 6 months
4. Mouthwashes such as Peridex are helpful in the treatment of gingivitis
5. Colgate Total is the first toothpaste FDA approved to prevent gingivitis (as well as cavities); it reduces plaque up to 50% and contains the antibacterial triclosan)

B. Patients with phenytoin-induced gingival hyperplasia usually require periodontal surgery

C. Mouth-breathing associated gingivitis usually is difficult to correct, but good plaque control can control the process in most cases

D. Most patients with periodontitis can be effectively treated although early diagnosis and referral are important
1. The first phase of treatment is similar to that for gingivitis described above
2. Phase 2 of treatment involves surgery to improve the gingival architecture that remains

E. Follow up should be by the dentist to whom patient was referred

CERVICAL ADENITIS

I. Definition: Acute pyogenic infection of a cervical lymph node

II. Pathogenesis

A. Usually reactive or secondary to an upper respiratory tract infection or dental infection; less frequently due to trauma

B. Pathogens:
1. *Staphylococcus aureus* and *Streptococcus pyogenes* account for 80% of unilateral cervical adenitis
2. Increasingly, anaerobic pathogens are being identified
3. Less common pathogens: viruses and group B streptococci

III. Clinical Presentation

    A. More common in children than adults

    B. Typically, patient has a low-grade or no fever, malaise, and an upper respiratory infection or dental infection

    C. Usually presents as tender, soft, warm, rapidly enlarging lymph node with erythema of the overlying skin; node ranges from 2-6 cm.

    D. Most common site is the submandibular and anterior cervical areas

IV. Diagnosis/Evaluation

    A. History
        1. Ascertain duration and onset of node enlargement
        2. Ask if node is increasing in size and whether overlying skin has changed in color
        3. Ask about pain during eating which suggests parotid gland involvement
        4. Question about dysphagia, odynophagia, strider, speech disorders, or a sensation of a lump in the throat
        5. Inquire about associated constitutional symptoms
        6. Question about recent infections, trauma, insect bites, pet scratches, TB contact, drug usage, and foreign travel

    B. Physical Examination
        1. Measure vital signs
        2. Observe for general state of health
        3. Thoroughly examine head, ears, eyes, nose, throat and mouth
        4. Carefully examine neck for other masses and nuchal rigidity
        5. Carefully palpate cervical mass to determine exact anatomic location, presence of tenderness, mobility, and consistency; examine skin overlying node for color
        6. Thoroughly examine areas of lymph nodes
        7. Inspect skin for lesions and rashes
        8. Assess respiratory status
        9. Palpate abdomen for organomegaly

    C. Differential Diagnosis (see Figure 9.1 for common location of masses of the neck); vast majority of neck masses in children are cervical adenitis
        1. Congenital cysts (these conditions need referral and usually surgery)
            a. Thyroglossal duct cyst (located at midline and typically moves with swallowing or tongue protrusion)
            b. Branchial cleft cysts (small dimple or opening anterior to middle portion of the sternocleidomastoid muscle)
            c. Cystic hygromas (fluid-filled, compressible mass in the posterior triangle just behind the sternocleidomastoid muscle and the supraclavicular fossa)
        2. Salivary gland disorders; salivary glands are located in area of lymph nodes and enlarged glands may be confused as cervical adenitis; care must be taken to distinguish glands from nodes; for example, enlargement of the parotid gland obliterates the angle of the mandible

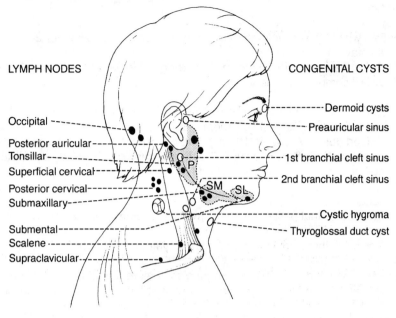

LYMPH NODES   CONGENITAL CYSTS

Occipital ------   -----Dermoid cysts
                                                     ---- Preauricular sinus
Posterior auricular----
Tonsillar----   ----1st branchial cleft sinus
Superficial cervical----
Posterior cervical----   ----2nd branchial cleft sinus
Submaxillary----
                                                     ----- Cystic hygroma
Submental----   ------- Thyroglossal duct cyst
Scalene----
Supraclavicular----

P = Parotid gland, S = Submandibular gland, SL = Sublingual gland

Figure 9.1. Common Location of Masses of the Face and Neck.

3. Cervical lymphadenopathy (see section on LYMPHADENOPATHY)
    a. Viral infections (most common)
        (1) Often due to herpesviruses, adenoviruses, enteroviruses, and Ebstein-Barr virus
        (2) Nodes are typically bilateral, discrete, oval, soft, and minimally tender
    b. Bacterial infections of the upper respiratory tract and mouth
    c. Cat Scratch Disease (see CAT SCRATCH DISEASE section)
    d. Kawasaki Disease (see KAWASAKI DISEASE section)
    e. Atypical mycobacterium
    f. Toxoplasmosis
    g. Systemic disorders such as lupus, rheumatoid arthritis, sarcoidosis, histoplasmosis
4. Malignancy (node is often supraclavicular, firm and fixated to skin and underlying tissue; patient often has persistent fever or weight loss)
5. Generalized lymphadenopathy is usually caused by systemic disease (see LYMPHADENOPATHY section)
6. Thyroid nodules occur infrequently in children; if they do occur, there is an 80% chance they are malignant
7. Lipoma is a benign, subcutaneous tumor composed of fat cells that may be located on back of neck or on trunk and extremities; consistency is soft and rubbery

D. Diagnostic Tests
    1. Ultrasound is helpful in establishing whether mass is solid, cystic, or fluctuant
    2. In moderately or severely ill patient, consider CBC, sedimentation rate, throat culture, and blood culture
    3. PPD should be considered if tuberculosis is suspected
    4. Heterophil tests or titers for Epstein-Barr virus, cytomegalovirus, and *Toxoplasma* may be indicated to rule-out specific viral infections
    5. Consider aspiration and culture in patients who have large, fluctuant nodes which do not respond to initial therapy
    6. Biopsy of node is needed when malignancy is suspected

V.   Plan/Management

    A.   For patient who appears well with minimal pain, close observation for 2-3 days and symptomatic treatment may be all that is needed
        1.   Prescribe analgesic such as tylenol or nonsteroidal anti-inflammatory agent
        2.   Warm compresses every 4 hours

    B.   For the patient with moderate to severe adenitis prescribe one of following antibiotics:
        1.   Amoxicillin/clavulanic acid (Augmentin) 500 TID or in children, 40 mg/kg/day in three divided doses. Available 125 mg/5mL or 250mg/5mL suspension for 7-14 days
        2.   Cephalexin (Keflex) 500 mg BID or in children, 75 mg/kg/day in 4 divided doses. Available 250mg/5mL suspension for 7-14 days

    C.   Patient Education
        1.   Emphasize that patient should immediately return if difficulty of swallowing or breathing occurs
        2.   Reinforce that follow-up is important if symptoms persist

    D.   Patients with lymph node enlargement persisting more than 2 weeks without regression with antibiotic therapy need further evaluation and possible referral to a specialist

    E.   Follow Up
        1.   Return to clinic if symptoms do not start to resolve in 2-3 days
        2.   For the patient who appears well and is treated only symptomatically, reevaluate symptoms at 3-5 day intervals; some nodes take many weeks to regress but other nodes regress spontaneously within 2-3 weeks without pharmacological treatment
        3.   Reevaluate patients who are treated with antibiotics after completion of therapy
        4.   Individualize follow-up for of patients who are at risk for systemic or serious disorders

REFERENCES

Alho, O., Laara, E., & Oja, H. (1996). What is the natural history of recurrent acute otitis media in infancy? The Journal of Family Practice, 43, 258-264.

Arjmand, E.M., & Lusk, R.P. (1995). Management of recurrent and chronic sinusitis in children. American Journal of Otolaryngology, 16, 367-382.

American Academy of Pediatrics. (1995). Joint Committee of Infant Hearing 1994 position statement. Pediatrics, 95, 152-155.

American Academy of Pediatrics. (1997). Group A streptococcal infections. In Peter, G. (Ed.) 1997 Red Book: Report of the Committee on Infectious Diseases (24th ed.). Elk Grove Village, IL: American Academy of Pediatrics.

Ash, M.M. (1992). Oral pathology: An introduction to general and oral pathology for hygienists. Philadelphia: Lea & Febiger.

Barnett, E.D. (1997). Comparison of ceftriaxone and trimethoprim-sulfamethoxazole for acute otitis media. Pediatrics, 99, 23-28.

Berman, S., Byrns, P.J., & Bondy, J. (1997). Otitis media-related antibiotic prescribing patterns, outcomes, and expenditures in a pediatric Medicaid population. Pediatrics, 100, 585-592.

Bisno, A.L. (1996). Acute pharyngitis: Etiology and diagnosis. Pediatrics, 97 (Suppl), 949-954.

Bojrab, D.I., Bruderly, T., & Abdulrazzak, Y. (1996). Otitis externa. Otolaryngologic Clinics of North America, 29(5), 761-782.

Brookhouser, P.E. (1996). Sensorineural hearing loss in children. Pediatric Clinics of North America, 43, 1195-1216.

Brunton, S. (1997). Allergic rhinitis: Breaking the cycle of disease and treatment. Family Practice Recertification, 19, 14-32

Burgett, F. (1993). Periodontal disease. In J.A. Regezi & J. Sciubba (Eds.), Oral pathology: Clinical-pathologic correlations. Philadelphia: Saunders.

Clement, P.A.R., Bluestone, C.D., Gordts, F., Lusk, R.P., Otten, F.W.A., Goosens, H., Scadding, G.K., Takahashi, H., van Buchem, F.L., Van Cauwenberge, P. & Wald, E.R. (1998). Management of rhinosinusitis in children: Consensus meeting, Brussels, Belgium, September 13, 1996. Archives of Otolaryngology--Head, Neck, and Surgery, 124, 31-34

Consensus Conference Proceedings. (1995). The chronic airway disease connection: Redefining rhinitis. Los Angeles: UCCLA School of Medicine, Office of Continuing Medical Education.

Connolly, A.A.P., & MacKenzie, K. (1997). Paediatric neck masses--a diagnostic dilemma. Journal of Laryngology and Otology, 111, 541-545.

Culpepper, L., & Froom, J. (1997). Routine antimicrobial treatment of acute otitis media: Is it necessary? JAMA, 278, 1643-1645.

Dowell, S.F., Marcy, S.M., Phillips, W.R., Gerber, M.A., & Schwartz, B. (1998). Otitis media--principles of judicious use of antimicrobial agents. Pediatrics, 101, 171-174.

Eden, A.N., Fineman, P., & Stool, S.E. (1996). Managing acute otitis: A fresh look at a familiar problem. Contemporary Pediatrics, 13,(3), 64-65,70,73-85.

Ferguson, B.J. (1997). Allergic rhinitis: Recognizing signs, symptoms, and triggering allergens. Postgraduate Medicine, 101, 110-131.

Forzley, G.J. (1994). Cerumen impaction removal. In J.L. Pfenninger, & G.C. Fowler (Eds.), Procedures for primary care physicians. St. Louis: Mosby.

Friedman, E.M. (1999). Epistaxis. In R.A. Dershewitz (Ed.), Ambulatory pediatric care. Philadelphia: Lippincott.

Goodheart, H.P. (1998). "Lumps" and "bumps." Cysts and lipoma. Women's Health in Primary Care, 1, 725-726.

Goroll, A.H., May, L.A., & Mulley, A.G., Jr. (1995). Management of aphthous stomatitis. In A.H. Goroll, L.A. May, & A.G. Mulley, Jrs. (Eds.), Primary care medicine. Philadelphia: Lippincott.

Gwaltney, J.M., Jones, J.G., & Kennedy, D.W. (1997). Medical management of sinusitis: Educational goals and management guidelines. Annals of Otology, Rhinology, and Laryngology, Suppl. 167, 22-30.

Gungor, A., & Corey, J.P. (1997). Pediatric sinusitis: A literature review with emphasis on the role of allergy. Otolaryngology, Head, and Neck Surgery, 116, 4-15.

Hathaway, T.J. (1994). Acute otitis media: Who needs posttreatment follow-up? Pediatrics, 94, 143-147.

Haynes, J.H., & Newkirk, G.R. (1994). Removal of foreign bodies from the ear and nose. In J.L. Pfenninger, & G.C. Fowler (Eds.), Procedures for primary care physicians. St. Louis: Mosby.

Hays, G.L. (1997). Diseases of the mouth. In R.E. Rakel (Ed.), 1997 Conn's current therapy. Philadelphia: Saunders.

Heikkinen, T. (1999). Prevalence of various respiratory viruses in the middle ear during acute otitis media. New England Journal of Medicine, 340, 260-264.

Herendeen, N.E., & Szilagyi, P.G. (1997). Cystic and solid masses of the face and neck. In R.A. Hoekelman et al., (Ed.). Primary pediatric care, St. Louis: Mosby.

Herzon, F.S. (1995). Peritonsillar Abscess: Incidence, current management practices, and a proposal for treatment guidelines. Laryngoscope, 105, 1-17.

Isaacson, G. (1996). Sinusitis in childhood. Pediatric Clinics of North America, 43, 1297-1318.

Isaacson, G., & Rosenfel, R.M. (1996). Care of the child with tympanostomy tubes. Pediatric Clinics of North America, 43, 1183-1193.

Kaiser, H.D., Kay, G.G., & Palakanis, K. (1998). Contemporary issues in the management of allergic disorders: A focus on respiratory and dermatologic manifestations. Clinical Courier, 16(46), 1-7.

Kraus, I. (1999). Gingivostomatitis. In R.A. Dershewitz (Ed.), Ambulatory pediatric care (3rd ed.). Philadelphia: Lippincott.

LaRosa, S. (1998). Primary care management of otitis externa. Nurse Practitioner, 23(6), 125-133.

Little, D.R., Mann, B.L., & Sherk, D.W. (1998). Factors influencing the clinical diagnosis of sinusitis. The Journal of Family Practice, 46, 147-153.

Low, D.E., Desrosiers, M., McSherry, J., Garber, G., & other Canadian Sinusitis Symposium Panel. (1997). A practical guide for the diagnosis and treatment of acute sinusitis. Canadian Medical Association Journal, 156 (6 suppl.), S1-S14.

MacLeod, D.K. (1995). Common problems of the teeth and oral cavity. In L.R. Barker, J.R. Burton, & P.D. Zieve (Eds.), Principles of ambulatory medicine. Baltimore: Williams & Wilkins.

Meltzer, E.O. (1998). Treatment options for the child with allergic rhinitis. Clinical Pediatrics, 37, 1-10.

Mirza, N. (1996). Otitis externa: Management in the primary care office. Postgraduate Medicine, 99(5), 153-158.

Noble, S.L., Forbes, R.C., & Woodbridge, H.B. (1995). Allergic rhinitis. American Family Physician, 51,837-846.

Nodar, R.H. (1999). Audiology: Testing hearing function. In R.A. Dershewitz (Ed.), Ambulatory pediatric care (3rd ed..). Philadelphia: Lippincott.

O'Brien, K.L., Dowell, S.F., Schwartz, B., Marcy, S.M., Phillips, W.R., & Gerber, M.A. (1998). Acute sinusitis--principles of judicious use of antimicrobial agents. Pediatrics, 101, 174-177.

O'Connor, J.M. (1999). Dentistry for the pediatrician. In R.A. Dershewitz (Ed.), Ambulatory pediatric care. Philadelphia: Lippincott.

Otitis Media with Effusion in Young Chidren Guideline Panel. (1994). Otitis Media with Effusion in Young Children: Clinical Practice Guideline, No. 12. (ACHPR Publication No. 94-0622) Rockville, MD.

Paradise, J. L., Rockette, H.E., Colborn, D.K., Bernard, B.S., Smith, C.G., Kurs-Lasky, M., & Janosky, J.E. (1997). Otitis media in 2253 Pittsburgh-area infants: prevalence and risk factors during the first two years of life. Pediatrics, 99, 318-331.

Parsons, D.S. (1996). Chronic sinusitis: A medical or surgical disease? Otolaryngologic Clinics of North America, 29, 1-9.

Parsons, D.S., & Van Leeuwen, R.N (1997). Otitis externa. In Rakel, R. E. (Ed.), Conn's current therapy. Philadelphia: W.B. Saunders.

Pellett, F.S., Cox, L.C., & MacDonald, C.B. (1997). Use of acoustic reflectometry in the detection of middle ear effusion. Journal of American Academy of Audiology, 8, 181-187.

Perkins, A. (1997). An approach to diagnosing the acute sore throat. American Family Physician, 55, 131-138.

Peterson, M.J., & Baughman, R.A. (1996). Recurrent aphthous stomatitis: Primary care management. Nurse Practitioner, 21, 36-47.

Roark, R., & Berman. S. (1997). Continuous twice daily or once daily amoxicillin prophylaxis compared with placebo for children with recurrent acute otitis media. Pediatric Infectious Disease Journal, 16, 376-381.

Root, P., & Paul, D. (1996). Hearing loss. In M.B. Mengel and L.P. Schwiebert, (Eds.). Ambulatory medicine: The primary care of families (3rd ed.). Stamford, CT: Appleton & Lange.

Rosenfeld, R.M. (1996). An evidence-based approach to treating otitis media. Pediatric Clinics of North America, 43, 1165-1181.

Ruckenstein, M.J. (1995). Hearing loss: A plan for individualized management. Postgraduate Medicine, 98, 197-214.

Ruppert, S.D. (1996). Differential diagnosis of common causes of pediatric pharyngitis. Nurse Practitioner, 21, 38-48.

Schantz, N.V. (1994). Management of epistaxis. In J.L. Pfenninger, & G.C. Fowler (Eds.), Procedures for primary care physicians. St. Louis: Mosby.

Schwartz, B., Marcy, S.M., Phillips, W.R., Gerber, M.A., & Dowell, S.F., (1998). Pharyngitis--principles of judicious use of antimicrobial agents. Pediatrics, 101, 171-174.

Smith, L.J. (1995). Diagnosis and treatment of allergic rhinitis. Nurse Practitioner, 20, 58-66.

Swanson, J. A., & Hoecker, J. L. (1996). Concise review for primary-care physicians: Otitis media in young children. Mayo Clinical Proceedings, 71, 178-183/

Wald, E.R. (1995). Chronic sinusitis in children. The Journal of Pediatrics, 127, 339-347.

Wald, E.R. (1999). Sinusitis. In R.A. Dershewitz (Ed.), Ambulatory pediatric care (3rd ed.). Philadelphia: Lippincott.

Weiss, J.C., Yates, G.R., & Quinn, L.D. (1996). Acute otitis media: making an accurate diagnosis. American Family Physician, 43, 1200-1206.

Williams, J.W., & Simel, D.L. (1993). Does this patient have sinusitis? Diagnosing acute sinusitis by history and physical examination. JAMA, 270, 1242-1246.

Williams, M.A. (1999). Hearing loss. In R.A. Dershewitz (Ed.), Ambulatory pediatric care (3rd ed.). Philadelphia: Lippincott.

Zitelli, B.J. (1999). Neck masses. In R.A. Dershewitz (Ed.), Ambulatory pediatric care (3rd ed.). Philadelphia: Lippincott.

CHAPTER 10

Problems of the Upper Airways, Lower Respiratory System

ASTHMA

I. Definition: Chronic inflammatory disorder of the airways which causes bronchial hyperresponsiveness to stimuli and recurrent episodes of respiratory symptoms which are usually associated with reversible airflow obstruction

II. Pathogenesis

   A. Inflammation plays a central role
      1. Results from complex interactions among many cells and cellular elements (mast cells, eosinophils, T lymphocytes, macrophages, neutrophils, and epithelial cells)
      2. Inflammation is associated with airway obstruction, airway hyperresponsiveness, respiratory symptoms, and disease chronicity

   B. Airway obstruction leads to airflow limitation and is usually widespread, recurrent, variable and reversible either with treatment or spontaneously; obstruction is due to the following:
      1. Acute bronchoconstriction results from airway hyperresponsiveness after exposure to a variety of stimuli such as allergens, drugs (aspirin, nonsteroidal anti-inflammatory drugs), stimuli (exercise, cold air, irritants) and possibly stress
      2. Airway wall edema and mucosal thickening are caused by increased microvascular permeability and leakage
      3. Chronic mucus plug formation sometimes occurs in severe, intractable cases
      4. Airway wall remodeling may develop in severe cases, causing persistent abnormalities in lung function which are unresponsive to treatment

   C. Factors contributing to asthma severity:
      1. Inhaled allergens such as animal allergens, house-dust mites, outdoor allergens, indoor fungi, and cockroaches
      2. Occupational exposures
      3. Irritants such as tobacco smoke and pollution
      4. Rhinitis/sinusitis
      5. Gastroesophageal reflux
      6. Sensitivity to aspirin, other nonsteroidal anti-inflammatory drugs, and sulfites
      7. Topical and systemic beta-blockers
      8. Viral respiratory infection

   D. In children, there usually is a strong history of atopy; allergy or family history of allergy is the factor most strongly related to continuing asthma throughout childhood

III. Clinical Presentation

   A. Underdiagnosis and inappropriate therapy are major factors in morbidity and mortality

   B. Typically, symptoms begin in childhood or adolescence, but can develop in adulthood; 50-80% of asthmatic children develop symptoms before fifth birthday
      1. Most common, chronic illness of childhood; affects 5-10% of children < 20 years
      2. In children, two general patterns of disease progression exist: remission of symptoms in preschool years or symptoms persist throughout childhood
      3. The prevalence, hospitalization, and death rates for children with asthma have increased dramatically in the last ten years

   C. Exercise-induced bronchospasm occurs with loss of heat and/or water from lung during exercise; cough, shortness of breath, chest pain or tightness, wheezing or endurance problems may develop during exercise

   D. Spectrum ranges from few mild episodes in a lifetime to daily debilitating symptoms; classification of asthma severity is based on symptoms and lung function before treatment (see following table)

CLASSIFICATION OF THE SEVERITY OF ASTHMA*

Step/Category	Symptoms**	Nighttime Symptoms	Lung Functions
STEP 4 Severe Persistent	◆Continual symptoms ◆Limited physical activity ◆Frequent exacerbations	Frequent	◆FEV_1 or PEF ≤60%predicted ◆PEF variability >30%
STEP 3 Moderate Persistent	◆Daily symptoms ◆Daily use of inhaled short-acting beta$_2$-agonist ◆Exacerbations affect activity ◆Exacerbations are ≥2 times a week	>1 time a week	◆FEV_1 or PEF >60%-<80% predicted ◆PEF variability >30%
STEP 2 Mild Persistent	◆Symptoms >2 times a week but <1 time a day ◆Exacerbations may affect activity	>2 times a month	◆FEV_1 or PEF ≥80% predicted ◆PEF variability 20-30%
STEP 1 Mild Intermittent	◆Symptoms ≤2 times/week ◆Asymptomatic & normal PEF between exacerbations ◆Exacerbations brief (from a few hours to few days) intensity may vary	≤2 times a month	◆FEV_1 or PEF ≥80% predicted ◆PEF variability <20%

*The presence of one of the features of severity is sufficient to classify patient in that category. A patient should be assigned to the most severe grade in which any feature occurs.

**Patients at any level of severity can have mild, moderate, or severe exacerbations.

Adapted from National Institutes of Health. National Heart, Lung, and Blood Institute. (1997). The Expert Panel Report 2: Guidelines for the Diagnosis and Management of Asthma. National Asthma Education Program. NIH Publ. #97-4051. Bethesda, MD.

IV. Diagnosis/Evaluation

    A. History
        1. Identify the symptoms likely to be due to asthma (see table on KEY INDICATORS)

KEY INDICATORS OF ASTHMA

✔ Wheezing

✔ History of any of the following:
    ◆ Cough worse at night or in early morning
    ◆ Recurrent difficulty breathing
    ◆ Recurrent tightness in chest

✔ Reversible airflow limitation and diurinal variation as measured by peak flow meter

✔ Symptoms occur or are worsened by any of the following:
    ◆ Exercise, viral infection, animals, house-dust mites, mold, smoke, pollen, changes in weather, laughing, hard crying, airborne chemicals or dusts, menses

✔ Symptoms occur or worsen at night, awakening the patient

Adapted from National Institutes of Health. National Heart, Lung, and Blood Institute. (1997). The Expert Panel Report 2: Guidelines for the Diagnosis and Management of Asthma. National Asthma Education Program. NIH Publ. #97-4051. Bethesda, MD.

        2. Assess onset and duration of symptoms (number of days/nights per week/month)
        3. Determine whether symptoms are seasonal, continuous, episodic, or diurnal
        4. Determine profile of asthma attacks or exacerbations
        5. Assess past and present management strategies and responses
        6. Inquire about factors known to be related to asthma
        7. Determine family history of asthma, allergy, sinusitis, rhinitis, or nasal polyps
        8. Assess impact of disease such as effects on family, finances, school, work, activity, sleep, behavior, and in children, growth and development
        9. Assess patient's and family's perceptions such as knowledge level, understanding of treatments, sociocultural beliefs
      10. For persons with occupational asthma, inquire about number of sick days taken from work per month
      11. At each follow-up visit assess whether the goals of therapy are being met

B. Physical Examination
1. In children it is especially important to determine pulse rate and respiratory rate (>40 respirations per minute is worrisome)
2. Assess for signs of dehydration such as delayed capillary refill, poor skin turgor, and dry mucous membranes
3. Observe for use of accessory respiratory muscles, retractions, nasal flaring, diaphoresis, and cyanosis.
4. Observe for hyperexpansion of thorax (hunched shoulders or chest deformity)
5. Observe for flexural eczema or other manifestations of allergic skin conditions
6. Assess for nasal discharge, mucosal swelling, frontal tenderness, postnasal discharge, nasal polyps, and allergic shiners (dark discoloration beneath both eyes)
7. Auscultate and percuss lungs
   a. Wheezing during forced exhalation is no longer believed to be a reliable indicator
   b. In mild, intermittent asthma, wheezing may be absent between attacks; in severe asthma wheezing may be absent due to diminished breath sounds
8. Perform a complete cardiac examination

C. Differential Diagnosis: underdiagnosis of asthma, especially in children, is common; remember that recurrent episodes of coughing and wheezing are usually due to asthma; the following should be included in the differential diagnosis:
1. Bronchiolitis
2. Cystic fibrosis
3. Bronchopulmonary dysplasia
4. Heart disease
5. Laryngotracheomalacia, tracheal stenosis or bronchostenosis
6. Foreign body
7. Vascular rings or laryngeal webs
8. Aspiration from swallowing dysfunction
9. Vocal cord dysfunction can cause recurrent wheezing
10. Enlarged lymph nodes, tumors
11. Pulmonary infections such as pneumonia, tuberculosis, mycoplasma and respiratory syncytial virus disorder
12. Gastroesophageal reflux

D. Diagnostic Tests; regular monitoring of pulmonary function is essential, particularly for patients who do not perceive their symptoms until airways are severely obstructed
1. Spirometry tests
   a. Recommended at following intervals:
      (1) Time of diagnosis
      (2) After treatment when symptoms and peak flow reading are stabilized to document attainment of normal airway function
      (3) Every 1-2 years to monitor maintenance of airway function
   b. More frequent testing is needed in the following cases: to check accuracy of peak flow, when precision is needed to determine treatment response, and when peak flow readings may be unreliable such as when patients are young or have neuromuscular problems
2. Order an exercise challenge test to confirm exercised-induced bronchospasm
3. Other tests to consider: chest x-ray or CBC if infection is suspected; skin testing or in vitro testing for patients with persistent asthma exposed to perennial indoor allergens
4. Peak expiratory flow (PEF) meters
   a. **Should be used to monitor lung function not to confirm diagnosis**
   b. Daily monitoring is not mandatory for all patients, but is important for patients after an exacerbation and for patients with moderate-to-severe, persistent asthma
   c. Teach patients to determine their best PEF (see table that follows)

PATIENT EDUCATION OF THE PEAK FLOW METER

1. Demonstrate and have return demonstration of use of peak flow meter
   - Stand, do not sit
   - Place indicator at bottom of numbered scale
   - Take deep breath
   - Close lips around mouthpiece
   - Blow out as hard and fast as possible in a single blow

2. Teach patient to repeat #1 two more times and record the best of the three blows

3. Instruct patients how to determine their personal best peak flow number
   - Take readings twice a day for 2-3 weeks: upon awakening or between 12 noon & 2:00 p.m.
   - Take readings before and after inhaling beta$_2$-agonist

4. Explain that personal best peak flow numbers are categorized into zones to help patients self-manage their illness and to assess progression of disease and need for additional therapy
   - Green Zone: 80% of patient's personal best and denotes good control
   - Yellow Zone: 50-<80% of patient's personal best and denotes caution and the need to take a short-acting inhaled beta$_2$-agonist
   - Red Zone: <50% of patient's personal best and denotes severe asthma exacerbation and the need to take short-acting inhaled beta$_2$agonist and call health care provider or emergency room or go directly to hospital

5. Explain to patient that once their personal best peak flow is documented they may decrease peak flow readings to once a day in the morning. If morning reading is <80% of personal best, instruct patient to monitor more frequently

6. Teach parents of children with moderate-to-severe persistent asthma that determination of personal best readings should be done every 6 months due to changes that occur with growth

Adapted from National Institutes of Health. National Heart, Lung, and Blood Institute. (1997). The Expert Panel Report 2: Guidelines for the Diagnosis and Management of Asthma. National Asthma Education Program. NIH Publ. #97-4051. Bethesda, MD.

V.   Plan/Management

    A.   Referral to an asthma specialist is recommended in the following situations:
        1.   Life-threatening or severe, persistent asthma (step 4) is present
        2.   Goals of asthma therapy are not fulfilled after 3 to 6 months of treatment
        3.   Signs and symptoms are atypical or diagnosis is uncertain
        4.   Other illnesses such as sinusitis, gastroesophageal reflux, of chronic obstructive pulmonary disease complicate the airway disease
        5.   Immunotherapy is a treatment consideration
        6.   Continuous oral corticosteroids or high-dose inhaled corticosteroids or two bursts of oral steroids in 1 year are needed
        7.   Patient is <3 years and needs step 3 or step 4 care

    B.   Control of the factors contributing to asthma severity is important
        1.   Instruct patient to avoid the following:
            a.   Allergens (see table: MEASURES OF ENVIRONMENTAL CONTROL in section: ALLERGIC AND NONALLERGIC RHINITIS)
            b.   Environmental tobacco smoke
            c.   Exercise when levels of pollution are high
            d.   Beta-blockers
            e.   Foods containing sulfite and other foods to which they are sensitive
        2.   Caution patients with severe, persistent asthma, nasal polyps, or a history of sensitivity to aspirin or nonsteroidal anti-inflammatory drugs that there is risk of severe and possibly fatal exacerbations when using these drugs
        3.   Treat patients for rhinitis, sinusitis, and gastroesophageal reflux if present
        4.   Recommend annual influenza vaccination

    C.   General pharmacological principles; a stepwise pharmacological approach is recommended (see Table on Stepwise Approach in Individuals >5 years)

STEPWISE APPROACH FOR MANAGING ASTHMA IN INDIVIDUALS OLDER THAN 5 YEARS OF AGE: TREATMENT		
Preferred treatments are in bold print.		
	Long-Term Control	**Quick Relief**
STEP 4 Severe Persistent	Daily medications: ■ **Anti-inflammatory: inhaled corticosteroid (high dose)** **AND** ■ Long-acting bronchodilator: either **long-acting inhaled beta₂-agonist**, sustained-release theophylline, or long-acting beta₂-agonist tablets AND ■ Corticosteroid tablets or syrup long term	■ Short-acting bronchodilator: **inhaled beta₂-agonists** as needed for symptoms.

STEP 3
Moderate
Persistent
	Daily medication: (Initial Plan)
	■ Either
	  Anti-inflammatory: inhaled corticosteroid (medium dose)
	OR
	  Inhaled corticosteroid (low-medium dose) and add a long-acting bronchodilator, especially for nighttime symptoms; either **long-acting inhaled beta₂-agonist**, sustained-release theophylline, or long-acting beta₂-agonist tablets.
	
	(Additional Plan)
	■ If needed
	  Anti-inflammatory: **inhaled corticosteroids (medium-high dose)**
	AND
	  Long-acting inhaled beta₂-agonist, sustained-release theophylline, or long-acting beta₂-agonist tablets.
		■ Short-acting bronchodilator: **inhaled beta₂-agonists** as needed for symptoms.

STEP 2 Mild Persistent	One daily medication: ■ **Anti-inflammatory**: either **inhaled corticosteroid** (low doses) or **cromolyn or nedocromil** (children usually begin with a trial of cromolyn or nedocromil). ■ Sustained-release theophylline to serum concentration as alternative, but not preferred, therapy. Zafirlukast or zileuton may also be considered for patients ≥ 12 years of age.	■ Short-acting bronchodilator: **inhaled beta₂-agonists** as needed for symptoms.
STEP 1 Mild Intermittent	■ No daily medication needed.	■ Short-acting bronchodilator: **inhaled beta₂-agonists** as needed for symptoms.

 Step down
Review treatment every 1 to 6 months; a gradual stepwise reduction in treatment may be possible.

 Step up
If control is not maintained, consider step up. First, review patient medication technique, adherence, and environmental control (avoidance of allergens or other factors that contribute to asthma severity).

1. The dose and dosing interval are dictated by the asthma severity with the goal of suppressing airway inflammation and preventing exacerbations
2. Begin therapy at a high level (short course of systemic corticosteroids plus inhaled corticosteroids or use of medium-to-high dose of inhaled corticosteroids) to promptly control symptoms and then lower level
3. Cautiously and very gradually step down therapy after control is achieved and sustained for several weeks or months
   a. Generally, the last medication added should be the first medication reduced
   b. Inhaled corticosteroids may be reduced 25% every 2-3 months to the lowest dose possible to maintain control
4. Continual monitoring is imperative; control is indicated by the following:
   a. Peak expiratory flow (PEF) less than 10-20% variability
   b. PEF consistently greater than 80% patient's personal best

306

c. Minimal symptoms
d. Minimal need for short-acting inhaled beta$_2$-agonist
e. Absence of nighttime awakenings
f. No activity limitations
5. Other actions needed if control is not achieved and sustained at any step
a. Assess patient adherence and technique in using medication
b. Step up to next higher step of care or temporarily increase anti-inflammatory therapy such as with a burst of prednisone
c. Reassess for factors that diminish control
d. Consult a specialist
6. Long-term control drugs are used daily to maintain control of persistent asthma; quick-relief drugs treat acute symptoms and exacerbations (see following tables)

LONG-TERM CONTROL MEDICATIONS

1. Corticosteroids are the most potent and effective anti-inflammatory agents
   ✓ Oral/systemic form used for prompt control when initiating long-term therapy
   ✓ Inhaled form is preferred for long-term control
   ✓ Benefits outweigh risk of adverse effects; to reduce adverse effects, the following are recommended:
      * Use with spacers/holding chambers
      * Rinse mouth after use
      * Use lowest possible dose to maintain control
      * Consider a long-acting beta$_2$-agonist rather than a higher dose inhaled corticosteroid
      * In children, periodically monitor growth
      * Do not give varicella vaccine to patients receiving ≥2 mg/kg or 20 mg/day of oral prednisone
   ✓ In children with episodic therapy with systemic corticosteroids who have not had clinical chickenpox give varicella vaccine

2. Cromolyn sodium and nedocromil are mild to moderate anti-inflammatory medications
   ✓ May be initial choice for long-term therapy in children
   ✓ Comparison of nedocromil and cromolyn
      * Nedocromil is more potent in inhibiting bronchospasm due to exercise, cold dry air and bradykinin aerosol; more effective in nonallergic patients using inhaled corticosteroids
      * Nedocromil may help reduce dose requirements of corticosteroids

3. Long-acting beta$_2$-agonists are used with anti-inflammatory medications; helpful for nocturnal symptoms
   ✓ Salmetrol **is not used for treatment of acute symptoms or exacerbations** and some experts do not recommend it in children
   ✓ Daily use of these drugs should not exceed 84 mcg (salmeterol: 4 puffs)
   ✓ Even if symptoms improve, patients should **not** stop anti-inflammatory medication

4. Methylxanthines (mainly sustained-release theophylline) are used as adjuvant to inhaled corticosteroids for prevention of nocturnal symptoms
   ✓ Although not preferred, sustained-release theophylline may be alternative for long-term preventive therapy when cost or adherence in using inhaled medications is problematic
   ✓ Essential to monitor serum concentration levels
   ✓ Smoking increases metabolism of theophylline

5. Leukotriene modifiers are alternatives to low doses of inhaled corticosteroids or cromolyn or nedocromil for persons with mild persistent asthma (need more research & experience)
   ✓ Zafirlukast has an interaction effect with warfarin; essential to closely monitor prothrombin times and adjust appropriately (not recommended for children <12 years old)
   ✓ Zileuton (not recommended for children <12 years old)
      * May infrequently cause liver toxicity; essential to monitor liver enzymes
      * May inhibit metabolism of terfenadine, warfarin, and theophylline
   ✓ Montelukast sodium (Singular)
      * Can be used in children ≥6 years old

QUICK-RELIEF MEDICATIONS

1. Therapy of choice is a short-acting beta$_2$-agonist
   ✓ Use of >1 canister in 1 month signifies poor control & need to begin or increase anti-inflammatory drug
   ✓ Regularly scheduled, daily use of these drugs is **not** recommended

2. Anticholinergics (ipratropium bromide) may provide additive benefit to inhaled beta$_2$-agonist or may be alternative quick-relief drug for patients unable to tolerate inhaled beta$_2$-agonist

3. Oral/systemic corticosteroids are used for moderate-to-severe exacerbations and can speed resolution of airflow obstruction and reduce rate of relapse

D. Treatment of **Step 1: Mild intermittent asthma in Individuals >5 years**
   1. Prescribe short-acting inhaled beta$_2$-agonist on an as-needed basis (see table)

DOSAGES FOR INHALED BETA$_2$-AGONISTS

Medication	Dosage Form	Adolescent Dose	Child Dose	Comments
Short-Acting Inhaled Beta$_2$-Agonists				
	Metered-Dose Inhaler			
Albuterol (Ventolin)	90 mcg/puff, 200 puffs	■ 2 puffs TID-QID prn	■ 2 puffs TID-QID prn	■ Increasing or regular use on a daily basis indicates the need for additional long-term-control therapy.
Pirbuterol (Maxair Autohaler)	200 mcg/puff, 400 puffs			
	Dry Powder Inhaler			
Albuterol Rotacaps (Ventolin)	200 mcg/capsule	1-2 capsules Q 4-6 hours prn	1 capsule Q 4-6 hours prn	
	Nebulizer solution			
Albuterol (Ventolin)	5 mg/mL (0.5%)	1.25-5 mg (.25-1 cc) in 2-3 cc of saline Q 4-8 hours	0.05 mg/kg (min 1.25 mg, max 2.5 mg) in 2-3 cc of saline Q 4-6 hours	May mix with cromolyn or ipratropium nebulizer solutions.
Bitolterol (Tornalate)	2 mg/mL (0.2%)	0.5-3.5 mg (.25-1 cc) in 2-3 cc of saline Q 4-8 hours	Not established	May not mix with other nebulizer solutions.

Adapted from National Institutes of Health. National Heart, Lung, and Blood Institute. (1997). The Expert Panel Report 2: Guidelines for the Diagnosis and Management of Asthma. National Asthma Education Program. NIH Publ. #97-4051. Bethesda, MD.

2. Treatment of **exercise-induced bronchospasm**; use one of following:
   a. Short-acting inhaled beta$_2$-agonist 1-2 puffs 5 minutes prior to exercise
   b. Inhaled cromolyn sodium (Intal) or nedocromil (Tilade) 2 puffs 10 minutes prior to exercise
3. Treatment of **mild exacerbations** due to viral respiratory infections: prescribe short-acting beta$_2$-agonist every 4-6 hours for approximately 24 hours
4. **Treatment of moderate-to-severe exacerbations:**
   a. Use both of the following:
      (1) Give short-acting beta$_2$-agonist by nebulizer or MDI (with close supervision can give 3 treatments spaced every 20-30 minutes)
      (2) Also, prescribe systemic corticosteroid; patients with history of severe exacerbations should start corticosteroids at first sign of infection (see Table on SYSTEMIC CORTICOSTEROIDS)
   b. Oxygen is recommended for most patients
   c. Careful, vigilant monitoring of patient's condition is paramount

DOSAGES FOR SYSTEMIC CORTICOSTEROIDS				
Medication	**Dosage Form**	**Adolescent Dose**	**Child Dose**	**Comments**
Methylprednisolone (Medrol) Prednisolone (Pediapred) (Prelone) Prednisone (Deltasone)	2, 4, 8, 16, 24, 32 mg tablets 5 mg tabs, 5mg/5cc, 15 mg/5 cc 1, 2.5, 5, 10, 20, 50 mg tabs	■ Short course "burst": 40-60 mg/day as single or 2 divided doses for 3-10 days	■ Short course "burst": 1-2 mg/kg/day, maximum 60 mg/day for 3-10 days	■ The burst should be continued until patient achieves 80% PEF personal best or symptoms resolve. This usually requires 3-10 days but may require longer. ■ Give first dose in AM and last dose by 6 PM

Adapted from National Institutes of Health. National Heart, Lung, and Blood Institute. (1997). The Expert Panel Report 2: Guidelines for the Diagnosis and Management of Asthma. National Asthma Education Program. NIH Publ. #97-4051. Bethesda, MD.

E. Treatment of **Step 2: Mild Persistent Asthma in Individuals > 5 years**: Use inhaled short-acting beta$_2$-agonist on an as-needed basis as well as one of the following:
1. Inhaled corticosteroids at a low dose (see Table on DOSAGES OF INHALED CORTICOSTEROIDS); when taking several inhaled medications simultaneously, always use beta$_2$-agonist first to open airway and then use steroid inhaler for greater penetration of medication
2. Cromolyn (Intal) or Nedocromil (Tilade): a trial of one of these drugs is recommended in children, because of their good safety profile
   a. Cromolyn
      (1) Metered-Dose Inhaler (MDI) (1 mg/puff): For adolescents, use 2-4 puffs TID or QID; for children use 1-2 puffs TID or QID
      (2) Nebulizer (20mg/ampule); for all ages use 1 ampule TID or QID
   b. Nedocromil (MDI 1.75 mg/puff)
      (1) 2-4 puffs BID-QID; for children use 1-2 puffs BID-QID
      (2) Also available in a 0.5% strength nebulizer solution
3. Sustained-release theophylline is an alternative, but is not preferred because of modest effectiveness and potential for toxicity; prescribe drug to achieve a serum concentration of between 5 and 15 mcg/mL (periodic monitoring is necessary to maintain a therapeutic level)
   a. Adolescents: Begin dose at 10 mg/kg/day up to 300 mg maximum; usual maximum is 800 mg/day
   b. Children: Begin dose at 10 mg/kg/day; usual maximum is following:
      (1) <1 year: 0.2 (age in weeks) + 5 = mg/kg/day
      (2) ≥1 year: 16/mg/kg/day
4. Zafirlukast or zileuton is alternative drug for patient >12 years and motelukast sodium is alternative drug for patient ≥6 years; lack of research and clinical experience makes the role of these drugs in long-term treatment uncertain
   a. Zafirlukast (Accolate): One 20 mg tablet BID (take 1 hour before or 2 hours after meals)
   b. Zileuton (Zyflo): 600 mg QID (Available 300 mg and 600 mg tablets); regularly monitor hepatic enzymes
   c. Montelukast sodium (Singular): 10 mg tab QD in evening for individuals >14 years; one 5 mg chewable tab in evening for children 6-14 years
5. For exacerbations, see V.D.3.4 and V.K.

DAILY DOSAGES OF INHALED CORTICOSTEROIDS

Adolescents

Drug	Low Dose	Medium Dose	High Dose
Beclomethasone dipropionate 42 mcg/puff 84 mcg/puff	168-504 mcg (4-12 puffs--42 mcg) (2-6 puffs--84 mcg)	504-840 mcg (12-20 puffs--42 mcg) (6-10 puffs--84 mcg)	>840 mcg (>20 puffs--42 mcg) (>10 puffs--84 mcg)
Budesonide DPI: 200 mcg/dose	200-400 mcg (1-2 inhalations)	400-600 mcg (2-3 inhalations)	>600 mcg (>3 inhalations)
Flunisolide 250 mcg/puff	500-1,000 mcg (2-4 puffs)	1,000-2,000 mcg (4-8 puffs)	>2,000 mcg (>8 puffs)
Fluticasone MDI: 44, 110, 220 mcg/puff	88-264 mcg (2-6 puffs--44 mcg) OR (2 puffs--110 mcg)	264-660 mcg (2-6 puffs--110 mcg)	>660 mcg (>6 puffs--110 mcg) OR (>3 puffs--220 mcg)
Fluticasone DPI: 50, 100, 250 mcg/dose	(2-6 inhalations--50 mcg)	(3-6 inhallations--100 mcg)	(>6 inhalations--100 mcg) OR (>2 inhalations--250 mcg)
Triamcinolone acetonide 100 mcg/puff	400-1,000 mcg (4-10 puffs)	1,000-2,000 mcg (10-20 puffs)	>2,000 mcg (>20 puffs)

Children

Drug	Low Dose	Medium Dose	High Dose
Beclomethasone dipropionate 42 mcg/puff 84 mcg/puff	84-336 mcg (2-8 puffs--42 mcg) (1-4 puffs--84 mcg)	336-672 mcg (8-16 puffs--42 mcg) (4-8 puffs--84 mcg)	>672 mcg (>16 puffs--42 mcg) (>8 puffs--84 mcg)
Budesonide DPI: 200 mcg/dose	100-200 mcg	200-400 mcg (1-2 inhalations--200 mcg)	>400 mcg (>2 inhalations--200 mcg)
Flunisolide 250 mcg/puff	500-750 mcg (2-3 puffs)	1,000-1,250 mcg (4-5 puffs)	>1,250 mcg (>5 puffs)
Fluticasone MDI: 44, 110, 220 mcg/puff	88-176 mcg (2-4 puffs--44 mcg	176-440 mcg (4-10 puffs--44 mcg) OR (2-4 puffs--110 mcg)	>440 mcg (>4 puffs--110 mcg) OR (>2 puffs--220 mcg)
Fluticasone* DPI: 50, 100, 250 mcg/dose	(2-4 inhalations--50 mcg)	(2-4 inhallations--100 mcg)	(>4 inhalations--100 mcg) OR (>2 inhalations--250 mcg)
Triamcinolone acetonide 100 mcg/puff	400-800 mcg (4-8 puffs)	800-1,200 mcg (8-12 puffs)	>1,250 mcg (>12 puffs)

*First U.S. FDA approved inhaled anti-inflammatory corticosteroid medication approved for children as young as 4 years.

Adapted from National Institutes of Health. National Heart, Lung, and Blood Institute. (1997). The Expert Panel Report 2: Guidelines for the Diagnosis and Management of Asthma. National Asthma Education Program. NIH Publ. #97-4051. Bethesda, MD.

F.   Treatment of **Step 3: Moderate Persistent Asthma in Individuals >5 years:** consultation with an asthma specialist is advised

   1.   Initial plan: Choose one of the following three options for initiating step 3 therapy:

      a.   Option 1: Increase inhaled corticosteroid to medium dose (see table)

      b.   Option 2: Add a long-acting bronchodilator to a low-to-medium dose of inhaled corticosteroid; add one of the following long-acting bronchodilators:

         (1)   Inhaled beta$_2$-agonist, salmeterol (Serevent) MDI 21 mcg/puff: In adolescents use 2 puffs every 12 hours and in children use 1-2 puffs every 12 hours; (sustained-release albuterol tablets may be considered but are not preferred)

         (2)   Alternatively, may add sustained-release theophylline (see V.E.3)

      c.   Option 3 is least preferred: Establish control with medium-dose inhaled corticosteroid, then lower the dose (but still within the medium-dose range) and add inhaled nedocromil (Tilade) (MDI 1.75 mg/puff): 2-4 puff BID-QID; for children use 1-2 puffs BID-QID

2. Additional plan: if symptoms are not optimally controlled with initial plan in step 3, the following two strategies are recommended:
    a. Increase inhaled corticosteroid to a high dose
    b. Add a long-acting bronchodilator (an evening dose may control nocturnal symptoms)
3. For exacerbations, see V.D.3.4 and V.K.

G. Treatment of **Step 4: Severe Persistent Asthma in Individuals >5 years:** Prescribe oral systemic corticosteroids (see preceding table) and consult specialist
    1. Prescribe lowest possible dose (single daily dose on alternate days)
    2. Carefully monitor for adverse side effects such as secondary infections, electrolyte imbalances, hypertension, peptic ulcers, dermal atrophy, carbohydrate intolerance, osteoporosis, cataracts, glaucoma, and psychological effects such as euphoria and depression
    3. Conscientiously try to reduce systemic corticosteroids once symptoms are controlled; high doses of inhaled corticosteroids have less adverse effects and are preferable to systemic corticosteroids
    4. For exacerbations see V.D.3.4 and V.K.

H. Treatment of **Infants and young children ≤5 years** (see following table on Stepwise Approach for Managing Infants and Young Children)
    1. Consultation with a specialist should be considered for infants and young children requiring step 2 care; consultation is recommended for all children requiring step 3 and step 4 care
    2. Infants and young children who consistently require symptomatic treatment >2 times per week should be prescribed daily anti-inflammatory medication
    3. Daily long-term-control therapy should begin with a trial of cromolyn or nedocromil
    4. In children <2 years, nebulizers may be preferred delivery system for cromolyn and for high doses of beta$_2$-agonists during exacerbations; children between 3-5 years may use MDI and spacer/holding chamber alone, but they may require a nebulizer or an MDI plus spacer/holding chamber and face mask (see table on AEROSOL DELIVERY DEVICES)

I. Special considerations in school-age children and adolescents
    1. Involve this age group in establishing goals and plans
    2. Active participation in physical activities should be encouraged
    3. A written asthma management plan should be given to student's school

J. Treatment of exercise-induced bronchospasm (EIB) (see V.D.2)

K. Home management exacerbations
    1. Increase inhaled beta$_2$-agonist (up to three treatments of 2-4 puffs by MDI at 20 minute intervals or a single nebulizer treatment)
        a. If good response: continue beta$_2$-agonist every 3-4 hours for 24-48 hours; patients on inhaled corticosteroids should double dose for 7-10 days; contact clinician for followup instructions
        b. If response is incomplete: Add oral corticosteroid and continue beta$_2$-agonist and contact clinician within the day
        c. If poor response: Add oral corticosteroid, repeat beta$_2$-agonist immediately; if distress is severe go to emergency department or call 911
    2. Continue more intensive treatment for several days as recovery from exacerbations is often slow

STEPWISE APPROACH FOR MANAGING INFANTS AND YOUNG CHILDREN (5 YEARS OF AGE AND YOUNGER) WITH ACUTE OR CHRONIC ASTHMA SYMPTOMS

	Long-Term Control	Quick Relief

STEP 4
Severe
Persistent
	■ Daily anti-inflammatory medicine
	  ■ High-dose inhaled corticosteroid with spacer/holding chamber and face mask
	  ■ If needed, add systemic corticosteroids 2 mg/kg/day and reduce to lowest daily or alternate-day dose that stabilizes symptoms
		■ Bronchodilator as needed for symptoms (see step 1) up to 3 times a day

STEP 3
Moderate
Persistent
	■ Daily anti-inflammatory medication. Either:
	  ■ Medium-dose inhaled corticosteroid with spacer/holding chamber and face mask
	OR, once control is established:
	  ■ Medium-dose inhaled corticosteroid and nedocromil
	OR
	  ■ Medium-dose inhaled corticosteroid and long-acting bronchodilator (theophylline)
		■ Bronchodilator as needed for symptoms (see step 1) up to 3 times a day

STEP 2
Mild
Persistent
	■ Daily anti-inflammatory medication. Either:
	  ■ Cromolyn (nebulizer is preferred; or MDI) or nedocromil (MDI only)
	  ■ Infants and young children usually begin with a trial of cromolyn or nedocromil
	OR
	  ■ Low-dose inhaled corticosteroid with spacer/holding chamber and face mask
		■ Bronchodilator as needed for symptoms (see step 1)

STEP 1
Mild
Intermittent
	■ No daily medication needed.	■ Bronchodilator as needed for symptoms ≤2 times a week. Either:
		  ■ Inhaled short-acting beta$_2$-agonist by nebulizer or face mask and spacer/holding chamber
		OR
		  ■ Oral beta$_2$-agonist for symptoms
		■ With viral respiratory infection
		  ■ Bronchodilator Q 4-6 hours up to 24 hours (repeat no more than once every 6 weeks)
		  ■ Consider systemic corticosteroid if
		    • Current exacerbation is severe
		    OR
		    • Patient has history of previous severe exacerbations

↓ **Step down**
Review treatment every 1 to 6 months. If control is sustained for at least 3 months, a gradual stepwise reduction in treatment may be possible.

↑ **Step up**
If control is not achieved, consider step up. But first: review patient medication technique, adherence, and environmental control (avoidance of allergens or other precipitant factors).

Adapted from National Institutes of Health. National Heart, Lung, and Blood Institute. (1997). The Expert Panel Report 2: Guidelines for the Diagnosis and Management of Asthma. National Asthma Education Program. NIH Publ. #97-4051. Bethesda, MD.

L.   Route of administration: inhaled route more effectively delivers medication to lung, has reduced side effects, and the onset of action is shorter than oral medications (see following tables on descriptions and how to use various delivery devices)

AEROSOL DELIVERY DEVICES

Device/Drugs*	Population	Therapeutic Issues
Metered-dose inhaler (MDI) Beta$_2$-agonists Corticosteroids Cromolyn sodium and nedocromil Anticholinergics	>5 years	Takes coordination to actuate and inhale. Mouth washing is effective in reducing systemic absorption.
Breath-actuated MDI Beta$_2$-agonists	>5 years	Best for patients unable to coordinate inhalation and actuation. Cannot be used with currently available spacer/ holding chamber devices.
Dry powder inhaler (DPI) Beta$_2$-agonists Corticosteroids	May be used in children 4 years old; effects more consistent in children >5 years	Delivery may be ≥MDI depending on device and technique. Mouth washing is effective in reducing systemic absorption.
Space/holding chamber	>4 years ≤4 years with face mask	Easier to use than MDI alone. Decrease oropharyngeal deposition. Reduce potential system absorption of inhaled corticosteroid preparations that have higher oral bioavailability; recommended for all patients on medium-to-high doses of inhaled corticosteroids. May be as effective as nebulizer in delivering high doses of beta$_2$-agonists during severe exacerbations.
Nebulizer Beta$_2$-agonists Cromolyn Anticholinergics Corticosteroids	≤2 years	Method of choice for cromolyn in children and for high-dose beta$_2$-agonists and anticholinergics in moderate-to-severe exacerbations in all patients. Less dependent on patient coordination or cooperation.

*See additional tables for directions on how to use metered-dose inhaler, dry powder capsules, and nebulizers

Adapted from National Institutes of Health. National Heart, Lung, and Blood Institute. (1997). The Expert Panel Report 2: Guidelines for the Diagnosis and Management of Asthma. National Asthma Education Program. NIH Publ. #97-4051. Bethesda, MD.

DIRECTIONS ON HOW TO USE AN INHALER*

▲ Remove the cap, hold the inhaler upright and shake it

▲ Tilt your head back slightly and slowly exhale

▲ Put the inhaler 1-2 inches from your mouth (open mouth technique) -- OR -- Enclose mouthpiece with your lips (closed mouth technique); do **not** use closed mouth technique for corticosteroids — OR — Use spacer/holding chamber** (slowly inhale or tidal breathe immediately after actuation; actuate only once into chamber per inhalation or if face mask is used, allow 3-5 inhalations per actuation)

▲ Press down on the plunger and take a full, deep, slow, even breath (breathe in through mouth, not through nose)

▲ Hold your breath for 10 seconds, then exhale slowly through your nose

▲ Wait one minute before taking next puff

▲ Rinse your mouth afterward to prevent possible fungal infection

▲ Keep mouth piece clean

Counsel regarding danger of overuse of inhaler. Patients should be using no more than 1 canister (200 metered dose inhalations of a β-agonist) in a month
**Spacers/holding chambers are particularly recommended for young children and patients using inhaled corticosteroids

Adapted from National Institutes of Health. National Heart, Lung, and Blood Institute. (1997). The Expert Panel Report 2: Guidelines for the Diagnosis and Management of Asthma. National Asthma Education Program. NIH Publ. #97-4051. Bethesda, MD.

DIRECTIONS ON HOW TO USE DRY POWDER CAPSULES

● Close mouth tightly around mouthpiece
● Inhale deeply and rapidly
● Minimally effective inspiratory flow is device dependent

DIRECTIONS ON HOW TO USE A NEBULIZER

- ✦ Measure correct amount of normal saline solution and place into cup (if medicine is premixed, go to step 3)
- ✦ Measure correct amount of medicine and put into cup with saline solution
- ✦ Fasten mouthpiece to the T-shaped part and then fasten this unit to the cup OR fasten mask to cup (use mouthpiece for persons >2 years)
- ✦ Put mouthpiece in mouth and seal lips tightly around OR place mask on face
- ✦ Turn on the air compressor machine
- ✦ Take slow, deep breaths through mouth
- ✦ Hold breath 1-2 seconds before exhaling
- ✦ Continue until medicine is depleted from cup (approximately 10 minutes)
- ✦ Don't forget to clean nebulizer; cleaning removes germs and prevents infection as well as keeps nebulizer from clogging

Adapted from National Institutes of Health. (1992). Teach Your Patients about Asthma: A Clinician's Guide. National Asthma Education Program, Office of Prevention, Education and Control. Publication #92-2737. Bethesda, MD.

M. Patient Education: establish a partnership with patient and include patient in developing goals and plan; important components of patient education include the following:
   1. Basic facts about asthma
   2. Roles of medications
   3. Discuss asthma triggers and ways to avoid or control them (see V.B.)
   4. Review techniques and ask patient to demonstrate use of inhaler, spacer, or nebulizer (many drug failures are due to improper use of equipment)
   5. Counsel regarding overuse of inhalers which could result in tachyarrhythmias and death
   6. Teach how to recognize symptom patterns that indicate poor asthma control; may need to keep a daily diary of symptoms, peak flow readings, and medications
   7. Develop a written action plan based on peak flow readings (see Expert Panel Report 2, 1997, page 131, 138-143)
   8. Extensive teaching on exacerbation management is needed
      a. Discuss indicators of worsening asthma, specific recommendations for using beta$_2$-agonist rescue therapy, early administration of systemic corticosteroids, and directions on seeking medical care
      b. Patients at high risk of asthma-related death include those using >2 canisters per month of beta$_2$-agonists, difficulty perceiving airflow obstruction, co-morbidity, severe psychiatric or psychosocial problems, low socioeconomic status, illicit drug use, and prior history of severe exacerbations, intubation, hospitalizations, frequent ER visits

N. Follow Up
   1. For acute exacerbations with incomplete or poor responses see patient within 24 hours and then reevaluate in 3-5 days
   2. After exacerbation has resolved completely, schedule follow up visits every 1-3 months
   3. For patients on theophylline, check serum drug levels after 2 weeks from initiation of therapy; then every 4 months; in children, need more frequent monitoring during growth spurts
   4. Follow up for other patients depends on symptom severity, symptom control, knowledge level, social support and other resources; for new asthmatics, frequent visits are important to monitor disease as well as for patient education

BRONCHIOLITIS

I. Definition: Inflammation of the bronchioles resulting in small airway obstruction

II. Pathogenesis

    A. Due to necrotizing desquamation and subsequent deposition of debris along epithelium of bronchioles, lumina becomes partially obstructed resulting in air trapping and hyperinflation of lungs

    B. Usually caused by one of the following viruses: respiratory syncytial virus (RSV) (majority of cases), parainfluenza type III, adenovirus, and enterovirus; *Mycoplasma pneumoniae* is less common pathogen but may occur in older children

    C. RSV is transmitted by direct contact or in aerosolized nasal secretions; eyes and nose are common sites of inoculation; fomite transmission is also possible
        1. Virus may be shed for one to two days before symptoms appear and for 3-4 days or up to four weeks or longer after the symptoms have disappeared; infants shed for longest time period
        2. Incubation period is approximately three to five days

III. Clinical Presentation

    A. Factors contributing to increased risk include male gender, low socioeconomic status, crowded living conditions, passive cigarette smoke exposure, attendance in day care, presence of older siblings in home, and lack of breastfeeding

    B. Yearly epidemics usually occur in late winter and early spring

    C. Criteria which are helpful for diagnosing bronchiolitis include the following:
        1. First episode of wheezing
        2. Infant 24 months of age or younger
        3. Associated physical findings of viral infection such as coryza, cough, and low-grade fever
        4. Elimination of atopy or pneumonia as cause of wheezing

    D. Although wheezing is the prominent sign, child may have diffuse crackles and rhonchi

    E. Child may have respiratory distress with flaring nares, intercostal and subcostal retractions, and may use accessory muscles of respiration; because of hyperinflated lungs, liver and spleen may be pushed down and palpable; dehydration may occur with increased respiratory effort

    F. Most children improve substantially within several days; upper respiratory symptoms gradually improve over 1-2 weeks

    G. Fatality rate is less than 1%:
        1. Emergent cases may have cyanosis, listlessness, apnea or decreased breath sounds
        2. Infants, children with underlying cardiopulmonary disease, those born prematurely, and immunodeficient children are at increased risk for complications

    H. Children with RSV bronchiolitis have increased risk of persistent bronchial reactivity and asthma

IV. Diagnosis/Evaluation

    A. History
        1. Determine activity level and presence of any breathing problems
        2. Explore fluid/food intake
        3. Question about number of wet diapers, or frequency of voiding in older child

4. Question about onset and characteristics of URI symptoms (especially describe cough and wheeze)
5. Inquire about duration of any temperature elevation
6. Ask about any periods of apnea or cyanosis
7. Question about gastroesophageal reflux, choking, and vomiting
8. Explore family history of asthma and allergies
9. Explore past history of previous respiratory distress, cyanosis, weight loss, and fatigue
10. Explore history of other cardiac or pulmonary diseases as these conditions predispose children to dangerous sequelae from bronchiolitis

B. Physical Examination
1. Determine respiratory rate and color (An increasing respiratory rate is the sign best correlated with poor oxygenation)
2. Observe for nasal flaring, accessory muscle use, intercostal or subcostal retractions
3. Observe chest wall and abdominal motion (an ominous sign is failure of abdomen to move outward with inspiration)
4. Assess degree of alertness and fatigue (eye contact with mother, crying, ability to suck or drink)
5. Assess hydration status: capillary refill time, skin turgor, moisture of mucous membranes
6. Auscultate lungs (children with bronchiolitis may have fine crackles, wheezes, and prolonged expiratory phase)
7. Ascertain that breath sounds are equal bilaterally
8. Percuss chest which usually has a hyperresonant ring with bronchiolitis
9. Auscultate heart and determine pulse
10. Palpate for organomegaly

C. Differential Diagnosis
1. Asthma is difficult to differentiate from bronchiolitis; asthma usually has the following:
   a. Strong family history of asthma
   b. Marked positive response to bronchodilators
   c. Symptoms which are episodic and precipitated by exercise, allergens, weather changes, or irritant exposure
   d. Wheezes occurring without predisposing viral respiratory infection
   e. Fine inspiratory crackles are usually NOT present as in bronchiolitis
2. Pneumonia
3. Cystic fibrosis is characterized by the following:
   a. Frequent respiratory infections
   b. Failure to thrive
   c. Chronic cough
   d. Malabsorption; symptoms include diarrhea and foul-smelling bowel movements
4. Anatomic abnormalities such as tracheomalacia
   a. Hypercompliant tracheal cartilage that collapses during expiration and may vibrate during inspiration
   b. Symptoms are continuous and do not go away
5. Gastroesophageal reflux (chronic symptoms)
6. Aspiration of foreign body (unilateral wheezing)
7. Congenital heart disease
8. Alpha, antitrypsin deficiency, immunodeficiency, dysmotile cilia syndrome
9. Croup (prolonged inspiratory stridor, hoarseness, and barky cough)

D. Diagnostic Tests
1. Diagnosis is usually made on characteristic clinical presentation
2. Pulse oximeter may be used to determine degree of hypoxemia
3. Gold standard for detecting RSV infection is cell culture but it is rarely recommended because it is costly, requires technical expertise and facilities, and takes at least 2 -21 days to detect virus

4. Rapid antigen tests using enzyme-linked immunosuppressive assay or rapid fluorescent antibody studies are acceptable alternatives for cell culture
    a. Usually not performed except when confirmation of diagnosis will change clinical management
    b. Nasopharyngeal wash specimens are superior to nasal or pharyngeal swabs
5. Collection of urine for determination of specific gravity may be helpful in determining hydration status
6. Order chest x-ray if diagnosis is unclear; suspect bronchiolitis if x-ray reveals the following:
    a. Hyperinflation
    b. Increased anterior-posterior diameter of chest
    c. Flat or depressed diaphragm
    d. Scattered areas of atelectasis and interstitial infiltrates which may be difficult to differentiate from pneumonia
7. Arterial blood gases may be needed in severe cases

V. Plan/Management

A. Children with respiratory distress need immediate transport to hospital for oxygen and ventilatory support.
    1. Usually hospitalization is not required unless child is a small infant or has underlying cardiac or pulmonary disease
    2. Hospitalized children may be treated with the antiviral drug, ribavirin, delivered by aerosol; in 1996, the Committee on Infectious Disease of the American Academy of Pediatrics revised its previous recommendation and stated that providers should decide whether ribavirin is appropriate based on the particular clinical situation and their preferences

B. Carefully and frequently observe child's respiratory rate and status in outpatient settings

C. If oxygen saturation measures <95% with pulse oximetry, humidified oxygen with nasal prongs, face mask, or via a hood is recommended

D. Treatment for uncomplicated cases is supportive and symptomatic
    1. Encourage parents to frequently offer clear fluids or dilute milk
    2. Vigorous and frequent suctioning of nasal secretions is important, particularly in infants who become easily fatigued when breathing through a mucous obstruction
    3. Mist treatment with vaporizer is no longer recommended
    4. Administer antipyretics if necessary

E. Although the effects of bronchodilators are questionable, consider a trial of one of the following:
    1. Beta$_2$-agonist
        a. For severe bronchiolitis prescribe nebulized albuterol (Ventolin) 5 mg/5 mL solution: 0.1-0.15 mg/kg in 2 cc of saline every 20 minutes for 1 hour and continually assess clinical condition. Consider consultation with a specialist if respiratory rate is still elevated or other signs of respiratory distress are present after treatments
        b. For moderate bronchiolitis, prescribe nebulized albuterol (Ventolin) 5 mg/5 mL solution; 0.1-0.15 mg/kg in 2 cc of saline every 4-6 hours OR oral albuterol 2 mg/5mL solution; 0.1-0.15 mg/kg every 4-6 hours
    2. Nebulized epinephrine in saline (3-5 mL of a standard 1:1000 preparation); three recent clinical trials found epinephrine superior to beta$_2$-agonists

F. Ineffective medications include corticosteroids, decongestants, antihistamines, antibiotics, and nebulized ipratropium

G. Prevention of respiratory syncytial virus infections: Recommendations of the American Academy of Pediatrics (1998)
    1. Palivizumab (Synagis) or respiratory syncytial immune globulin (RSV-IGIV) (RespiGam) prophylaxis should be considered for infants and children <2 years with chronic lung disease (CLD) who have required medical therapy for their CLD within 6 months prior to the anticipated RSV season; prophylaxis should be considered for two RSV seasons in children with more severe CLD

a. Palivizumab is preferred for most high-risk children
   (1) It is easy to administer, safe, and effective and does not interfere with vaccine administration
   (2) Recommended dose is 15 mg/kg IM injection once a month during the RSV season
b. RSV-IGIV
   (1) Disadvantages: Must be given intravenously and must defer administration of measles-mumps-rubella vaccine and varicella vaccine for 9 months after last dose of RSV-IGIV
   (2) The maximum recommended total dosage per infusion is 750 mg/kg; give monthly infusion during RSV season

2. Infants born at 32 weeks gestation or earlier without CLD or who do not meet the criteria in the above recommendation (V.G.1.) may also benefit from RSV prophylaxis; consider major risk factors such as gestational age and chronologic age at the start of RSV season
   a. Infants born at 28 weeks gestation or earlier may benefit from prophylaxis up to 12 months of age
   b. Infants born at 29-32 weeks of gestation may benefit from prophylaxis up to 6 months of age
3. Because of the large number of infants born between 32-35 weeks of age and the cost of the drugs, prophylaxis in this population should be reserved for patients with additional risk factors
4. Palivizumab and RSV-IGIV prophylaxis are not FDA licensed for infants with congestive heart disease; however, patients with CLD and/or who are premature who meet the criteria in above recommendations (V.G.1. and 2.) and who also have asymptomatic acyanotic congestive heart disease (e.g., patent ductus arteriosus or ventricular septal defect) may benefit from prophylaxis
5. Limited data are available on prophylaxis with immunocompromised infants; however, children with severe immunodeficiencies may benefit from prophylaxis
6. Begin RSV prophylaxis at onset of RSV season and terminate it at the end of the season
   a. In most regions of the U.S., the usual RSV season is from October to December and ends in March to May
   b. In the southern states, the RSV season occurs earlier than in the northern states
   c. Contact health department to determine optimal time for RSV prophylactic administration

H. Patient Education
   1. Teach parents to assess child for signs of respiratory distress and changes in level of activity and signs of dehydration
   2. Remind parents about the highly contagious nature of viral infections
      a. Family members need good handwashing techniques
      b. Eliminate exposure of other small children to ill patient
   3. Teach ways to possibly prevent episodes: avoid tobacco smoke and air pollutants such as wood stoves

I. Although trials of an effective vaccine to prevent bronchiolitis are underway, no safe vaccines are currently available

J. Follow Up: Close monitoring of child's condition is needed
   1. Phone call to child's home in 2-8 hours often is warranted
   2. Consider return visit next morning
   3. After this initial follow up, schedule return visit for 10-14 days or sooner if symptoms have not improved

BRONCHITIS, ACUTE

I. Definition: Infection of the tracheobronchial tree that causes reversible bronchial inflammation

II. Pathogenesis

   A. Mucous membrane of tracheobronchial tree becomes hyperemic, edematous, with increased bronchial secretions and destruction of epithelium and impaired mucociliary activity

   B. Pathogens
       1. In approximately 95% of cases, the infection is due to a virus such as common cold virus, influenza, adenovirus
       2. *Bordetella pertussis* is the second leading cause
       3. *Mycoplasma pneumonia, Chlamydia pneumoniae, Moraxella catarrhalis* are other less common pathogens
       4. Secondary bacterial invasion by *Streptococcus pneumoniae* and *Haemophilus influenzae* type b may occur but is uncommon in nonsmokers and patients without chronic obstructive pulmonary disease

III. Clinical Presentation

   A. Cough, particularly at night, is hallmark symptom; sputum may be clear or purulent

   B. Most patients are afebrile with mild symptoms

   C. Severe symptoms such as fever, substernal pain, and possibly mucoid sputum production, dyspnea, or bronchospasm with wheezing occur occasionally

   D. Symptoms typically last 7-14 days but may continue for 3-4 weeks

   E. Smokers have more frequent, longer, and more severe episodes than nonsmokers

   F. Some patients with acute bronchitis have an underlying predisposition to bronchial reactivity which may turn into more chronic bronchial inflammation which characterizes asthma; untreated chlamydial infections may have a role in this transition to asthma

   G. Adults with acute bronchitis due to pertussis typically have a chronic cough which is often paroxysmal ("whooping"); adults with unrecognized pertussis may transmit pathogen to nonimmune children

IV. Diagnosis/Evaluation

   A. History
       1. Determine onset, duration and characteristics of cough, particularly ask about night coughing
       2. Inquire about frequency and pattern of previous episodes of coughing
       3. Ask about associated symptoms such as fever, pharyngitis, dyspnea, chest pain
       4. Questions about the appearance of the sputum are not considered helpful as purulent sputum is most often related to viral infections
       5. Inquire about infectious illnesses of other household members
       6. Always ask if patient or household members smoke
       7. Inquire about past medical history, particularly respiratory diseases
       8. Determine immunization history of patient and household members

B. Physical Examination
1. Assess eyes, ears, nose and throat for signs of inflammation
2. Palpate and transilluminate sinuses
3. Perform a heart examination
4. Perform a complete lung examination; inspect, palpate, percuss, and auscultate
5. Palpate for lymph nodes

C. Differential Diagnosis
1. Pneumonia and acute bronchitis are extremely difficult to differentiate. The following characteristics are more consistent with <u>pneumonia</u> than bronchitis:
   a. High fever
   b. Increased respiratory rate
   c. Rigors and constitutional symptoms
   d. Pleuritic chest pain
   e. Rusty/bloody sputum
   f. Focal crackles on auscultation
   g. X-ray abnormalities
2. Upper respiratory infection and sinusitis
3. Tuberculosis
4. Asthma should be considered in patients who have repetitive episodes of acute bronchitis
5. Allergies
6. Cystic fibrosis
7. Nonpulmonary causes of cough such a congestive heart failure, reflux esophagitis, and bronchogenic tumors

D. Diagnostic Tests: Acute bronchitis is a diagnosis of exclusion
1. Order a chest x-ray if the patient has severe symptoms to confirm or rule out the diagnosis of pneumonia
2. Consider PPD if patient is at risk for tuberculosis
3. Consider diagnostic pulmonary function testing or provocative testing with a methacholine challenge test when asthma is suspected; to diagnose asthma, abnormalities in tests must persist after the acute phase
4. Order culture or antigen detection from nasopharyngeal secretions if diagnosis of pertussis is suspected
5. CBC and sputum cultures are not necessary unless diagnosis is uncertain

V. Plan/Management

A. Antibiotic treatment is recommended in only a few clinical situations because most cases of acute bronchitis are viral; even patients who have a persistent cough (>10days) usually do not need antibiotics
1. Although there is only preliminary evidence, treatment of persistent wheezing with agents effective against Chlamydia species may prevent development of asthmatic symptoms
   a. For children ≥8 years and adolescents, prescribe doxycycline (Vibramycin) 100 mg BID for 2 to 3 weeks
   b. Prescribe macrolide such as clarithromycin (Biaxin) for children <8 years 7.5 mg/kg every 12 hours; available 125 mg/5mL and 250 mg/5 mL liquid
2. For patients with secondary bacterial infections who have a change in color, consistency, and amount of sputum, prescribe 10-day course of erythromycin (E-Mycin) 250-500 QID or in children, erythromycin ethyl succinate (Eryped) 20-40 mg BID-TID. Trimethoprim-sulfamethoxazole 800/160 (Bactrim DS) BID or in children 8 mg/kg/day trimethoprim and 40 mg/kg/day sulfamethoxazole in two divided doses is an alternate medication
3. Children with cystic fibrosis and underlying severe chronic lung disease and a persistent cough (>10 days) may benefit from antibiotic treatment; treatment must be tailored to each child
4. Consider prescribing erythromycin for 14 days for patients in frequent contact with small infants who are nonimmunized due to risk of pertussis infection; careful surveillance of infant is probably more beneficial than treating contagious patient

B. Although controversial, bronchodilators may relieve symptoms. Consider a trial of inhaled albuterol (Ventolin) 2 puffs every 6 hours for 7 days, especially for patients who have wheezes or rhonchi

C. Only symptomatic treatment is needed in most cases

D. Antihistamines should be avoided because they dry out secretions; expectorants have not been found to relieve symptoms

E. Cough suppressants should be avoided except if patient is unable to sleep due to irritating cough

F. Encourage smoking cessation

G. Follow Up
    1. Return to clinic if symptoms persist longer than 7-14 days or if condition worsens; although previously patients with symptoms lasting over one week were treated with antibiotics for a bacterial etiology; today it is recognized that even viral infections may persist for 3 or 4 weeks
    2. Patients who do not improve after 4 to 6 weeks need further evaluation (see section on COUGH)

COMMON COLD

I. Definition: An acute, mild and self-limiting syndrome caused by a viral infection of the upper respiratory tract mucosa

II. Pathogenesis

    A. Inflammation of all or part of the mucosal membranes from the nasal mucosa to the bronchi

    B. Etiology is usually rhinoviruses, coronaviruses, or other viruses; respiratory syncytial virus (RSV) is common pathogen in young children

    C. Incubation period averages 48 hours with a range of 12 hours to 5 days; maximum viral shedding occurs in first 2-4 days

    D. Transmission occurs through direct contact with infectious secretions on skin and environmental surfaces and air-borne droplets

III. Clinical Presentation

    A. Adults average 2-4 colds per year; children average 3-8 colds per year

    B. Characterized by one or more of the following symptoms:
        1. General malaise with low grade or no fever
        2. Nasal discharge, obstruction or congestion
        3. Sneezing/coughing, sore throat and hoarseness
        4. Conjunctivae may be watery and inflamed

    C. Usually self-limited (lasting approximately 5-7 days), but can predispose patient to bacterial infections such as otitis media, sinusitis, pneumonia and exacerbation of chronic conditions such as asthma

IV.   Diagnosis/Evaluation

    A.   History: Question about the following:
       1.   Respiratory distress (wheezing, dyspnea, stridor), inability to swallow, drooling and severe headaches which indicate the need for immediate evaluation
       2.   Fever, chills, anorexia, nausea, vomiting and diarrhea
       3.   Duration, character, and timing (day and/or night) of cough
       4.   Facial, head, ear, throat, or chest pain
       5.   Number and seasonal pattern of previous colds within 1 year
       6.   Exposure to others with similar symptoms
       7.   Medication use
       8.   Past medical and family history; particularly history of allergies, asthma, or other respiratory problems
       9.   History of tobaccos use and passive tobacco exposure

    B.   Physical Examination
       1.   Measure temperature, pulse and blood pressure
       2.   Examine conjunctivae, ears, nose and throat
       3.   Sinus percussion and transillumination
       4.   Palpate cervical lymph nodes for enlargement and tenderness
       5.   Perform a complete lung examination

    C.   Differential Diagnosis
       1.   Allergic rhinitis (nasal mucosa may be pale and boggy rather than erythematous and swollen as in common cold)
       2.   Foreign body (especially if nasal discharge is unilateral, purulent and malodorous)
       3.   Sinusitis
          a.   Thick, opaque, and discolored nasal discharge are typical of the common cold and do not indicate a more severe, sinus infection
          b.   Symptoms persisting or worsening for >10-14 days with facial swelling and tenderness and mucopurulent sputum are suggestive of sinusitis
       4.   Influenza (arthralgias are usually present)
       5.   Streptococcal pharyngitis
       6.   Otitis media
       7.   Pneumonia

    D.   Diagnostic Tests
       1.   Usually none are indicated
       2.   Throat culture or quick strep test if symptomatic or history of streptococcal exposure

V.   Plan/Management

    A.   Decongestants cause vasoconstriction and reduce nasal secretions and congestion; topical decongestants are effective for short-term therapy and provide rapid decrease in airway resistance whereas oral decongestants are best when treatment is needed for more than 3-4 days
       1.   Topical decongestants should be used no longer than 3-4 days because of potential for rebound congestion. Suggest one of the following:
          a.   Individuals over 6 years of age: oxymetazoline hydrochloride 0.05% (Afrin 12-Hour Nasal Spray) 2-3 sprays each nostril BID or phenylephrine hydrochloride 1% (Neo-Synephrine Spray) 1 sprays each nostril every 3-4 hours as needed
          b.   Children 2-6 years: Oxymetazoline hydrochloride (Afrin 12-hour Children's nasal spray), 2-3 drops each nostril every 12 hours
          c.   Children <2 years should not use topical decongestant; instead, use nasal saline drops (see below V.G.1)
       2.   Oral decongestants (not as effective); suggest one of the following:
          a.   In adolescents, prescribe pseudoephedrine hydrochloride (Sudafed) 60 mg, 1 tablet every 4-6 hours or pseudoephedrine sulfate (Afrin 12-Hour Tablets) 120 mg, 1 tablet every 12 hours.

      b.   In children 2-6 years, prescribe pseudoephedrine hydrochloride (Sudafed) 5mL every 4-6 hours (available 15 mg/5 mL liquid); 6-12 years, 30 mg tablets or 10mL liquid every 4-6 hours.

      c.   In infants less than 4 months of age, oral decongestants are not recommended. For older infants, can cautiously prescribe pseudoephedrine hydrochloride 7.5mg/0.8mL dropperful (Triaminic Infants Oral Decongestant): 12-17 lbs, 1 dropper; 18-23 lbs, 1½ droppers; 24-35 lbs, 2 droppers; every 4-6 hours; maximum 4 doses per day

B.   Intranasal ipratropium bromide (Atrovent) 2 puffs per nostril TID or QID reduces nasal discharge, severity of rhinorrhea and sneezing; not recommended as first-line agent for these symptoms but may prove useful in patients with disease-state contraindications to oral decongestants such as severe hypertension or angle-closure glaucoma

C.   Conflicting research is available on the benefits of zinc gluconate lozenges
     1.   Dosage is 1 lozenge (Halls Zinc Defense) every 2 hours for 4 days while awake
     2.   Therapy should be initiated within 24 hours of symptom onset
     3.   Adverse effects of bad taste and nausea limit use of lozenges
     4.   Zinc is not safe in pregnancy

D.   Although controversial, some researchers found a decrease in the duration and severity of cold symptoms with the use of Vitamin C

E.   Cough suppressants such as dextromethorphan or codeine may be beneficial when patient is unable to sleep due to irritating cough; but suppression of cough may lead to complications such as pneumonia because the body is unable to clear lungs and airways of unwanted material; recommend that cough suppressant be given only at bedtime

F.   Acetaminophen or nonsteroidal antiinflammatory agents (NSAIDS) such as ibuprofen and naproxen are effective in reducing cough and relieving fever and headaches

G.   Nonpharmacologic approaches to relieve symptoms
     1.   Saline nose drops or sprays: 2-3 drops in each nostril BID to QID of commercial products (Ocean, SalineX) or homemade solution (1/4 tsp salt in 8 oz boiled water)
     2.   Steamy showers or inhalation of steam
     3.   Fluids or hydration help loosen secretions and prevent upper airway obstruction; warm fluids such as tea and chicken soup can increase the rate of mucous flow
     4.   Salt-water gargle for sore throat
     5.   Hard candy or throat lozenge for sore throat and cough

H.   Treatments that are not recommended
     1.   Antihistamines are ineffective because nasal congestion in colds is not mediated by histamine receptors; antihistamines may increase upper airway obstruction by impairing flow of mucus
     2.   With exception of increased water intake, expectorants such as guaifenesin provide no benefit in cold management

I.   Patient Education
     1.   Review the etiology, course, and proper treatment of the common cold
          a.   Explain that colds are caused by viruses which are not eradicated with antibiotics
          b.   Reinforce that the indiscriminate use of antibiotics can cause adverse effects such as diarrhea, yeast infection, and drug resistance
     2.   Emphasize that cold remedies are to relieve symptoms and prevent complications rather than cure infection
     3.   Demonstrate use of nasal bulb syringe and saline drops to help clear nasal discharge in infants
     4.   Advise rest and increased oral fluid intake.
     5.   Increase humidity of the air at home; place a cool-mist humidifier in the child's room

6. Discuss ways to prevent the spread of colds
   a. All household members should frequently wash hands
   b. Since complications are more common in children during the first year of life, try to avoid undue exposure of infants to other people with colds and limit visits to areas with large crowds such as shopping malls

J. Follow Up: None indicated unless symptoms worsen after 3-5 days, new symptoms develop, or symptoms do not improve or resolve after 10-14 days

COUGH, PERSISTENT

I. Definition: Host defense mechanism to clear airway of secretions and inhaled particles which lasts at least 3 weeks or longer

II. Pathogenesis

A. In infancy, persistent coughs are often abnormal and may be due to any of the following: Congenital malformations (e.g., tracheoesophageal fistula or tracheobronchomalacia), cystic fibrosis, tuberculosis, infections (e.g., bronchiolitis, chlamydial pneumonia or HIV infection), gastroesophageal reflux, or congestive heart failure

B. In toddlers and preschool children, the most common causes are viral bronchitis, hyperactive airway disease such as asthma or foreign body aspiration

C. In school age children, mycoplasma infection may be the etiology

D. In adolescents, the most common causes are postnasal drip from chronic sinusitis or allergic rhinitis, asthma, gastroesophageal reflux, chronic bronchitis due to cigarette smoking or environmental irritants

E. Other causes have no age predilection such as physical irritants, foreign body aspiration, tuberculosis, and psychogenic factors

F. Worrisome causes of coughing include mediastinal or pulmonary masses such as tumors or nodes

G. In 25% of patients, multiple disorders contribute to a persistent cough

III. Clinical presentation of important causes of persistent cough

A. Cystic fibrosis
   1. Genetic disorder usually occurring in Caucasian children
   2. Cough is often productive, purulent, and paroxysmal
   3. Associated symptoms include recurrent respiratory infections, poor weight gain, large and foul-smelling, steatorrheic bowel movements

B. Tuberculosis
   1. Initially cough is minimally productive of yellow or green mucus which is worse upon arising in morning
   2. As disease progresses, cough becomes more productive
   3. Associated symptoms include fatigue, night sweats, dyspnea, and hemoptysis

C. Gastroesophageal reflux
   1. May have history of heartburn, dysphagia, sour or bitter taste in mouth, and frequent use of antacids
   2. Symptoms are often aggravated by meals and relieved by sitting up

D. Asthma
1. Often occurs at night or after exercise, laughing, or exposure to cold air
2. May be seasonal in occurrence and have a strong family history
3. Cough may be nonproductive or productive but not purulent nor yellow or green in color
4. Associated symptoms include wheezing and intercostal retractions

E. Aspirated foreign body
1. Cough may persist for weeks or even months
2. Fixed, localized wheezing audible when chest is auscultated

F. Viral infections infrequently last beyond 2 weeks
1. Often occur during the winter
2. Cough is often nonproductive
3. Usually accompanying symptoms are mild and include rhinitis and nasal congestion

G. Bacterial infections such as pneumonia
1. Cough may be productive and purulent but this is not always the case
2. Associated symptoms may include fever and respiratory distress

H. Postnatal drip from chronic sinusitis or allergic rhinitis
1. Involved in approximately 41% of patients with chronic cough
2. Patient often complains of clear nasal discharge, nasal congestion, tickle in throat, and frequent throat clearing

I. Chronic bronchitis: Patient often has dry, hacking cough which is worse in the morning

J. Carcinoma of the lung
1. Cigarette smoking accounts for the majority of cases
2. Characteristic of the cough depends on location of the primary tumor

K. Cough related to psychogenic factors
1. Disappears during sleep and is worse when attention is drawn to it and during times of emotional stress
2. Lacks other associated physical symptoms

IV. Diagnosis/Evaluation

A. History
1. Determine type of onset and duration of cough
2. Determine characteristics of cough
   a. Productive (white, purulent, bloody) or nonproductive
      (1) Productive cough usually suggests infection
      (2) Thick, tenacious sputum in children may indicate cystic fibrosis
   b. Quality (raspy, barking, harsh, wet)
      (1) Barking cough suggests croup
      (2) Paroxysms of cough occur in pertussis, cystic fibrosis, and foreign body aspiration
   c. Temporal occurrence (night, morning, or seasonal)
      (1) Nighttime cough suggests asthma, sinusitis with postnasal drip
      (2) Cough associated with exercise may indicate asthma, cardiac disease (rare), and bronchiectasis
3. Ask about associated symptoms such as fatigue, rhinitis, epistaxis, tickle in throat, pharyngitis, night sweats, dyspnea, fever, heartburn, hemoptysis, weight loss
   a. Hemoptysis signals concern for tuberculosis, cancer, or foreign body (see section on HEMOPTYSIS)
   b. Weight loss and fever suggest tuberculosis or HIV infection
4. Ask if the cough is preceded by feeding or choking episodes
5. Inquire about precipitating factors such as exercise, cold air, laughing
6. Explore environmental and occupational exposure
7. Inquire about infectious illness of other household members

8. Always ask about smoking or the exposure to passive smoking
9. Ask about medications, particularly angiotensin-converting enzyme (ACE) inhibitors
10. Explore family history of cystic fibrosis, malabsorption, asthma, and allergies
11. Inquire about past medical history such as allergies, frequent infectious diseases, obstructive airway disease, cardiac disease

B. Physical Examination
1. Observe patient for signs of respiratory distress such as cyanosis, shortness of breath on ambulating, intercostal retractions, accessory muscle use
2. Observe general appearance, noting whether patients appear robust or fatigued and wasted
3. In children, always plot height and weight, noting any growth changes
4. Listen for the quality of spontaneous coughing during the interview
5. Assess eyes, ears, nose and throat
   a. Conjunctivitis, rhinitis and pharyngitis suggest infection
   b. Cobblestoning in oropharynx suggests allergies or chronic sinusitis
6. Check for tenderness of sinuses
7. Palpate lymph nodes
8. Observe for tracheal deviation which suggests mediastinal mass or foreign body aspiration
9. Perform a complete lung exam including inspection, palpation, percussion, and auscultation
10. Perform a complete cardiac exam as chronic cardiovascular problems may present with persistent coughs

C. Differential Diagnosis: See pathogenesis section

D. Diagnostic Tests
1. Order tuberculin skin test (PPD) and chest x-ray for unexplained persistent cough
2. If diagnosis is unclear after PPD and chest x-ray, order spirometry to detect airway obstruction as in asthma
3. In young children, consider ordering a sweat chloride test to rule-out cystic fibrosis
4. Consider a CBC with differential if infection, anemia, carcinoma are likely possibilities
5. Cough that is productive should have Wright and gram stains of sputum as well as cultures
6. If asthma is suspected, a methacholine bronchoprovocation challenge should be considered
7. To uncover silent, pathologic gastroesophageal reflux, 24-hour pH probe monitoring may be needed
8. Oximetry may be helpful to quickly evaluate the patient's respiratory status and later may be used to assess response to treatment
9. Other possible tests to order depend on characteristics of patient and include sinus x-rays, immunologic testing, allergy testing, or a barium swallow for detecting structural lesions
10. More invasive tests such as bronchoscopy may be needed

V. Plan/Management

A. Treat all known causes such as antibiotic therapy for bacterial infections, bronchodilators for asthma, and antihistamines for allergies

B. Discuss need to stop cigarette smoking and avoid environmental irritants

C. Air humidification and keeping the throat moist are simple suggestions that may be beneficial

D. Cough suppressants such as dextromethorphan or codeine may be beneficial in improving sleep and rest (use only at bedtime)

E. Expectorants and mucolytic agents are ineffective

F. For parents who hear wheezing in their children at night, encourage a visit to the emergency department for documentation

G. A stepwise approach may be beneficial by progressing from simple to more aggressive diagnostic tests and treatments in patients with persistent mild-to-moderate coughing of unknown etiology
1. Initial screen: eliminate environment irritants (smoking, cough-producing medications, etc.)
2. Step 1: Treat empirically for postnasal drip with first generation antihistamine-decongestant combination; add nasal steroids or order CT of sinuses if symptoms persist
3. Step 2: Evaluate and treat possible asthma with inhaled cromolyn, steroids, and bronchodilators
4. Step 3: Order chest radiographs and CT of sinuses if asthma is not confirmed; treat specific, identified disease
5. Step 4:
   a. Treat for GERD if no abnormalities found in step 3: Antireflux measures and high-dose proton-pump inhibitor
   b. Order endoscopy or 24-hour esophageal pH monitoring
6. Step 5
   a. Perform bronchoscopic examination if no abnormalities are found and previous treatments are unsuccessful
   b. Repeat course of antihistamine-decongestant combination
   c. Consider less common diagnoses such as cancer, tuberculosis, congestive heart failure, sarcoidosis, bronchiectasis, etc.

H. In undiagnosed patients with risk factors for cancer such as smoking or occupational exposure consider referral to specialist

I. Follow Up
1. Frequency of return visits will depend on patient's condition
2. Patients who have a complete work-up with no abnormalities should be seen at least every 1-3 months if their coughing persists

CROUP

I. Definition

A. Clinical syndromes characterized by laryngeal obstruction caused by subglottic edema

B. Two most common croup syndromes are spasmodic croup and laryngotracheobronchitis
1. Differentiation of the two syndromes is difficult and is of questionable value because the management of the syndromes is similar
2. Typically, patients with spasmodic croup improve quickly whereas patients with laryngotracheobronchitis have a longer course; an allergy may be a predisposing factor in spasmodic croup

II. Pathogenesis

A. Pathogens
1. Parainfluenza is most common agent in all age groups
2. Younger children may be infected with *Respiratory syncytial virus*
3. Influenza virus and *Mycoplasma pneumoniae* are present in children >5 years

B. Symptoms are due to inflammation and narrowing of the subglottic region of the larnyx

III. Clinical Presentation

  A. Epidemiology
    1. Most common in children 3 months to 5 years of age with a peak at 2 years
    2. Higher incidence in males than females
    3. Occurs in fall and winter months with peak in November

  B. Symptoms are usually preceded by coryza, cough, and nasal congestion

  C. Characterized by inspiratory stridor, a barking cough, and hoarseness which are usually worse at night; prolonged inspiration and coarse rales are often present

  D. Most children have mild symptoms and look ill but not toxic; a few children require hospitalization and have cyanosis, hypoxemia, rales, and retractions

  E. Symptoms typically resolve within 3-7 days

IV. Diagnosis/Evaluation

  A. History
    1. Determine if child has any change in activity level, alertness, fluid intake, and voiding
    2. Explore whether child has had episodes of apnea or difficulty with breathing
    3. Question about duration and onset of any upper respiratory infection
    4. Ask parents to describe the cough
    5. Determine what helps or worsens the symptoms
    6. Explore family medical history, particularly asking about allergies or asthma
    7. Inquire about *hemophilus influenza* immunization status to eliminate a diagnosis of epiglottitis

  B. Physical Examination
    1. Measure respiratory rate and observe for signs of respiratory distress such as cyanosis, nasal flaring, accessory muscle use, and retractions
    2. Assess for hydration status such as capillary refill time, skin turgor, and moisture of mucous membranes
    3. Assess degree of alertness and fatigue
    4. Observe for signs of drooling or difficulty swallowing
    5. Assess ears, nose, throat, and sinuses (do not examine throat with tongue blade; do not place in supine position until epiglottitis can be ruled out as a diagnosis)
    6. Perform complete lung examination
    7. Auscultate heart

  C. Differential Diagnosis
    1. Epiglottitis, a pediatric emergency, is characterized by inspiratory and expiratory stridor, drooling, and a toxic appearance
    2. Bacterial tracheitis, a pediatric emergency, is characterized by respiratory stridor, high fever, and frequently copious purulent secretions; caused by infection secondary to streptococcus species, staphylococcus species, or *Haemophilus influenzae* type b pathogens
    3. Congenital subglottic stenosis presents as prolonged or recurrent episodes of croup
    4. Aspirated foreign body presents with unequal breath sounds
    5. Laryngeal edema can occur from an allergic reaction
    6. Diphtheria is characterized by gray, exudative, pharyngeal membrane and acute dysphagia
    7. Retropharyngeal or peritonsillar abscess presents with severe sore throat, drooling, and unilateral tonsillar swelling

D. Diagnostic Tests
   1. Usually diagnosis is made on clinical presentation without diagnostic tests
   2. Pulse oximetry is beneficial in determining degree of hypoxemia
   3. In cases where the diagnosis is questionable, consider ordering a lateral inspiratory and expiratory chest x-ray and a posteroanterior x-ray of the neck which will reveal a steeple sign due to subglottic swelling if diagnosis of croup is correct
   4. If brachial tracheitis is suspected, a sputum culture is helpful

V. Plan/Management

A. Consider hospitalization for children with severe symptoms such as dehydration, fatigue, increasing respiratory rate, retractions, nasal flaring, and use of accessory muscles

B. Outpatient management is acceptable for children with moderate symptoms who have reliable families and available transportation to the hospital if needed

C. Drug therapy for outpatients is controversial
   1. No therapy or 1-3 saline aerosol treatments are usually recommended for children with mild symptoms; however, a few experts advise prescribing a corticosteroid (see V.C.2.b. below) to prevent complications
   2. For children with moderate symptoms, epinephrine plus corticosteroids or corticosteroids alone are recommended with close follow up and comprehensive health education (see V.E. that follows)
      a. Nebulized racemic epinephrine is often recommended but recent studies have found nebulized L-epinephrine to be equally effective but less expensive
         (1) Administer nebulized racemic epinephrine (0.5 mL of 2.25% racemic epinephrine hydrochloride in 3-5 mL of normal saline) or nebulized L-epinephrine (5 mL of 1:1000 solution)
         (2) Action of epinephrine lasts approximately 2 hours and children may have rebound mucosal vasodilation and dyspnea; **observe patients in outpatient setting for 3 hours after administration**
         (3) Children requiring two epinephrine treatments need hospitalization
      b. Because of rebound phenomena, corticosteroids which are longer acting are often given alone, concurrently or after epinephrine
         (1) Single dose of dexamethasone (Decadron) either orally (which is more convenient) or in an intramuscular injection (which has been most studied) is recommended
            (a) Oral dexamethasone may be given 0.15, 0.3 or 0.6 mg/kg (0.6 mg/kg dose has been most studied)
            (b) IM dexamethasone is given 0.6 mg/kg; available 4 mg/mL
            (c) Avoid giving if child has been exposed to varicella in the preceding 3 weeks or if child has received varicella virus vaccine in preceding 2 weeks
            (d) Medication may increase child's appetite and aggressiveness
         (2) Nebulized budesonide 2 mg (4 mL) is currently an investigational drug, but was effective in several studies

D. Symptomatic treatment for outpatients
   1. Administer oxygen if oximetry results are less than 88% to 92%
   2. Cool-mist humidifer or breathing of cool, dry, night air
   3. Control of fever with acetaminophen 5-15 mg/kg/dose
   4. Encourage fluids (offer fluids every 5 to 10 minutes)

E. Patient Education
   1. For the child with moderate symptoms, explain to parents that any disturbance may result in hyperventilation and respiratory distress so they should remain calm and hold and comfort their child

2. Teach parents to count respirations, to assess child's levels of alertness and fatigue, monitor fluid intake and output, and degree of respiratory distress such as observing for retractions, use of accessory muscles and nasal flaring; explain that if symptoms intensify, they should go to emergency room or health care provider

F. Follow Up
1. For children with moderate croup who are discharged to home, contact parents by phone in 8-24 hours; frequent monitoring is needed thereafter
2. Return visit is needed if there is no improvement in symptoms within 48 hours

EPIGLOTTITIS (SUPRAGLOTTITIS)

I. Definition: Inflammation of the soft tissues above the glottis

II. Pathogenesis

A. Caused almost exclusively by *Haemophilus influenzae* type b

B. Involves rapid and pronounced inflammation of the epiglottis and surrounding areas which results in edema and subsequent mechanical obstruction to the flow of air

C. The swollen epiglottis may be pulled down into the larynx during inspiration and create complete airway obstruction

D. The inflammation may also result in increased secretions and exudate which can compound the airway obstruction

III. Clinical Presentation

A. HIB vaccine can prevent invasive *H. influenzae* infections such as epiglottitis and meningitis

B. Usually occurs in children age 2-8 years but may occur in adults; increasing in children <24 months of age; most common in males and African Americans

C. Classic symptoms are an abrupt onset of severe sore throat, fever, and toxicity in a previously active child

D. Children do not have hoarseness and brassy cough as with croup; instead their voice sounds muffled

E. Usual appearance is a child in sitting position, leaning forward with head extended, jaw thrust forward, mouth open, tongue protruding, and drooling

F. As the condition progresses may have dysphagia, stridor, respiratory distress, anxiety and later exhaustion and limpness with diminished breath sounds

G. Signs include a "beefy red" pharynx with copious secretions

IV. Diagnosis/Evaluation

A. History: Quickly question parents about onset and characteristics of symptoms and level of alertness

B. Physical Examination
  1. Quickly assess vital signs and respiratory status such as respiratory rate, cyanosis, retractions, use of accessory muscles, nasal flaring
  2. Quickly auscultate lungs
  3. If epiglottitis is suspected, do **NOT** attempt to examine pharynx with a tongue depressor because occlusion of airway may result

C. Differential Diagnosis
  1. Croup
  2. Bacterial tracheitis
  3. Aspiration of foreign body
  4. Diphtheria
  5. Peritonsillar abscess
  6. Angioneurotic edema

D. Diagnostic Tests
  1. Tentative diagnosis must be made quickly on the basis of the history and clinical presentation
  2. After admission to hospital the following are performed:
     a. Lateral x-ray of the neck will confirm diagnosis ("thumb sign" or swelling of epiglottis)
     b. Blood and surface cultures are obtained after intubation to confirm the presence of *H. influenzae*

V. Plan/Management

  A. Immediate transport to the hospital

  B. Have oxygen, emergency airway, and equipment available; empiric treatment for *H. influenzae* infection is recommended for children <13 years who have serious infections

  C. Attempt to keep patient calm

  D. Child's family needs prophylaxis with rifampin (Rifadin) when there is *H. influenzae* type b infection
  1. Infant 0-1 month: 10 mg/kg/day QD for 4 days
  2. Child >1 month to adult: 20 mg/kg/day QD for 4 days (maximum of 600 mg/day QD for 4 days)

  E. Follow up after discharge from the hospital will depend on the child's condition

HEMOPTYSIS

I. Definition: Expectoration of both blood-tinged and grossly bloody sputum

II. Pathogenesis

  A. Infection and inflammation of the tracheobronchial mucosa are the most common causative factors in children
  1. Minor mucosal erosions can occur from upper respiratory infections and bronchitis
  2. Bronchiectasis
  3. Tuberculosis (TB)
  4. Endobronchial inflammation due to sarcoidosis

  B. Foreign body aspiration is the second most common cause in children

331

C. Congenital defects such as heart defects, absent pulmonary artery and arteriovenous malformation are associated with hemoptysis

D. Autoimmune hemosiderosis, Wegener granulomatosis, milk allergy, and collagen-vascular diseases can cause hemophysis

E. Bronchogenic carcinoma may injure the mucosa whereas metastatic lung cancer rarely results in hemoptysis; hemoptysis is an uncommon symptom in children with malignancies

F. Injury to the pulmonary vasculature is an important cause
   1. Cystic fibrosis
   2. Lung abscess
   3. Necrotizing pneumonias such as those caused by *Klebsiella*
   4. Aspergillomas
   5. Pulmonary infarction secondary to embolization

G. Elevations in pulmonary capillary pressure can result in hemoptysis
   1. Pulmonary edema
   2. Mitral stenosis

H. Bleeding disorders and excessive anticoagulant therapy are additional causes

I. Chest trauma is a less common cause

J. Cryptogenic hemoptysis is hemoptysis in which the patient has a normal or nonlocalizing chest radiograph and nondiagnostic fiberoptic bronchoscopy; 90% of patients experience resolution of hemoptysis by 6 months

III. Clinical presentation of important causes of hemoptysis

A. Blood that is coughed is bright red, frothy, has an alkaline pH, and is mixed with sputum rather than hematemesis that is darker brown, has an acid pH, and may be mixed with food particles

B. Blood-streaked sputum is common, usually occurs with nonthreatening conditions, and often arises from the nasal mucosa and oropharynx rather than the lower respiratory tract

C. Foreign body
   1. Most common in children <4 years old
   2. Presents with coughing, localized wheezing and locally diminished or absent breath sounds

D. Bronchitis and bronchiectasis
   1. Occasional, blood-tinged sputum is characteristic
   2. Patient usually has chronic cough and dyspnea which may be worse in the morning

E. Lung tumors account for about 20% of the cases of hemoptysis in adults but are uncommon in children
   1. Occur most frequently in persons over age 40 and in smokers
   2. Patient often has a change in cough pattern
   3. Chest ache may be an accompanying symptom

F. Pneumonia
   1. Sputum appears red-brown or red-green and is mixed with pus
   2. May have fever, pleuritic chest pain, and malaise

G. Pulmonary infarction secondary to pulmonary emboli
   1. Characterized by a sudden onset of pleuritic pain in conjunction with hemoptysis
   2. Diaphoresis and syncope often are present

3. Signs include tachypnea, tachycardia, rales, fever, shock, fourth heart sound, pleural rub, or cyanosis
4. Frequently patient has a history of phlebitis, calf pain, or immobilization of the legs

H. Pulmonary edema
1. Characteristically has pink, frothy sputum
2. Diaphoresis, tachypnea, tachycardia are present
3. Jugular venous distention, hepatomegaly, and ankle edema may be present

IV. Diagnosis/Evaluation

A. History
1. Inquire about onset and whether hemoptysis is a recurrent problem
2. Explicitly determine that the bleeding is originating from the lungs rather than from vomiting blood or expectorating blood from nasopharyngeal bleeding
3. Ask patient to describe the color, consistency, and characteristics of sputum
   a. Pink sputum is suggestive of pulmonary edema fluid
   b. Putrid sputum suggests a lung abscess
   c. Currant-jelly-like sputum may indicate necrotizing pneumonia
   d. Copious amounts of purulent sputum mixed with blood points toward bronchiectasis
4. Ask patient to quantify amount of bleeding or if possible collect the sputum
5. Inquire about associated symptoms such as recent weight loss, fatigue, persistent cough, dyspnea, wheezing, fever, night sweats, excessive bruising, hematuria
6. Determine whether patient has had recent respiratory inflammation or infection
7. Inquire about past medical history, particularly ask about previous lung, cardiac, hematological, and immunological problems
8. Inquire about exposure to tuberculosis
9. Ask about patterns of cigarette smoking
10. Inquire about history of chest trauma
11. Ask about use of anticoagulant drugs
12. Explore environmental exposure to such things as asbestos
13. Ask about family history of hemoptysis, respiratory, cardiac, and hematological problems
14. Inquire about date of last chest x-ray and tuberculin skin test

B. Physical Examination
1. Assess vital signs, particularly noting fever and tachypnea
2. Observe skin for ecchymosis, telangiectasis and nails for clubbing; clubbing is consistent with neoplasm, bronchiectasis, lung abscess and other severe respiratory problems
3. Examine nose, sinuses and pharynx for source of bleeding
4. Inspect neck for jugular venous distention which is suggestive of heart failure
5. Palpate for lymph nodes; lymphadenopathy is associated with TB, sarcoidosis, and malignancy
6. Perform a complete lung and cardiovascular exam
7. Check for ankle edema

C. Differential Diagnosis: Hemoptysis is a symptom. See pathogenesis for possible causes.
1. Most cases of blood-tinged sputum are upper-respiratory in nature and do not need extensive workup
2. Differentiate hemoptysis from epistaxis, hematemesis and bleeding from nasopharyngeal sources

D. Diagnostic Tests
1. Order chest x-ray
   a. Inspiratory and expiratory films may demonstrate local air trapping if foreign body aspiration is suspected
   b. Fluoroscopy of chest can increase rate of detecting foreign body
2. Administer tuberculin skin test (PPD) unless there has been a positive PPD in the past
3. Consider gram stain of sputum for suspected infections, an acid-fast stain for suspected tuberculosis, and cytologic examination of three sputum samples for malignant cells

4. Consider bronchoscopy for patients who smoke, who have normal chest x-rays, and children who have possibly aspirated a foreign body; also consider for patients with persistent, recurrent hemoptysis or massive bleeding
5. Consider ventilation-perfusion scanning or angiography when pulmonary embolization is suspected
6. Computed tomography and magnetic resonance imaging may detect additional abnormalities unrecognized on chest x-ray
7. PT, PTT, platelet count and bleeding time are necessary when more than one site of bleeding is present
8. Consider CBC, erythrocyte sedimentation rate, urinalysis and blood gas measurements
9. Consider sweat electrolyte count (cystic fibrosis) and milk precipitins in serum (milk allergy, hemosideros)
10. If collagen-vascular disease is a possibility, order antinuclear antibody, lupus erythematosus (LE) cell preparation and rheumatoid factor

V. Plan/Management

A. Consider consultation with a specialist for patients who are at increased risk for malignancy and those cases in which bronchoscopy is indicated

B. Patients expectorating more than 25-50 mL of blood in 24 hours require hospitalization

C. Treat any underlying illness or infection

D. Foreign body
1. Life threatening, complete airway obstruction in persons >12 months is to deliver 6-10 abdominal thrusts (Heimlich maneuver) until foreign body is expelled; if unsuccessful, deliver 4 sharp blows to back
2. Infant <12 months: Support in prone position with head lower than trunk and deliver 5 back blows; if unsuccessful, turn to supine position and give 5 chest thrusts
3. After stabilized refer to skilled endoscopy team

E. Because blood is irritating to the tracheobronchial tree and triggers a cough response, consider prescribing a mild cough suppressant. However, instruct patient to continue expectorating as mucus and blood can accumulate and cause additional problems

F. Patient Education
1. Instruct patient to record episodes of hemoptysis and collect all blood that is expectorated
2. Instruct patient to return to clinic or emergency room if bleeding increases, has clots, or if patient has respiratory distress, diaphoresis, chest pain, or tachypnea

G. Follow Up
1. For mild blood-streaking of sputum with respiratory infection, all blood streaking should resolve in 2-3 days. If blood-streaking of sputum persists, patient needs a reevaluation
2. Patients with hemoptysis which involves expectoration of blood, not just minimal amounts of blood-streaked sputum, should have follow up visit within 12-48 hours

PNEUMONIA

I. Definition: Acute respiratory infection of the lung parenchyma including the interstitial tissue and the alveolar spaces

II. Pathogenesis

A. Mainly results from aspiration of pathogens into the lower respiratory tract from oropharyngeal contents

B. Less commonly, pathogens spread to lungs hematogenously from distant foci such as bacterial endocarditis or from aerosolized particles

C. Aspirated pathogens are usually cleared before infection develops unless there are alterations in the normal protective mechanisms such as depressed mucociliary transport by obstruction of bronchus by mucus or tumors, or preexisting clearance abnormalities such as bronchopulmonary dysplasia or cystic fibrosis

D. Bacterial pneumonia is often aided by concurrent viral infection which may suppress the immune system and disrupt the respiratory tract mucosa

E. In infants 3-11 weeks of age suspect infection due to *Chlamydia trachomatis*; in addition, infants less than three months of age may have infection from respiratory syncytial viruses, genital mycoplasmas, although bacterial pneumonia must also be considered

F. In the older infant (3 months) to the young child (4-5 years) viruses are the most common cause with respiratory syncytial being the most common virus peaking at 2-5 months of age; parainfluenza and influenza viruses also play important roles; one third of children in this group have bacterial infection usually due to *Streptococcus pneumoniae* or *Haemophilus influenzae* type b

G. In children older than 5 years and adolescents, *Mycoplasma pneumoniae, Streptococcus pneumoniae, Chlamydia pneumoniae*, and viruses are most common causes

H. Children with congenital or acquired immunodeficiency may have cytomegalovirus infection or *Pneumocystis carinii.*

III. Clinical Presentation

A. Even though pneumonia accounts for only 10-15% of respiratory infections in children, it causes significant morbidity and mortality

B. Chlamydial infection in the infant is characterized by a staccato cough, rales, wheezes, and possibly a history of conjunctivitis in the first 2 weeks of life

C. Viral infections often begin gradually with rhinorrhea, low-grade fever, cough, wheezing, followed by progressive increase in respiratory rate and intercostal retractions

D. Bacterial pneumonia is characterized by acute onset of fever, productive cough, pleural pain, rales or diminished breath sounds, tachypnea and toxic appearance
    1. Infants and young children may not have these classical findings and may present with lethargy, vomiting, diarrhea and poor feeding; often rales are not present when initially examined
    2. Other children may have right-sided abdominal pain due to right lower lobe pneumonia

E. In pneumonia due to *Mycoplasma pneumonia*, cough and fever, but not coryza, are usually the first symptoms followed by malaise, headache, rales, pharyngitis, and wheezing

F. The older child and adolescent with pneumonia due to *Chlamydia pneumoniae* have symptoms and disease courses similar to pneumonia due to *M. pneumoniae*

G. Children with underlying pulmonary obstruction such as cystic fibrosis, cleft palate, and anatomic abnormalities are at increased risk for developing bacterial pneumonia and complications of pneumonia

H. Empyema, lung abscess, and bacteremia are complications of bacterial pneumonia; death occurs almost exclusively in patients with underlying diseases

IV.   Diagnosis/Evaluation

    A.   History
        1.   Determine whether onset was gradual involving mild upper respiratory symptoms or abrupt with rapid onset of fever and cough
        2.   Inquire about attentiveness and consolability
        3.   Question about fluid intake and number of wet diapers or voiding patterns
        4.   Inquire about associated symptoms such as conjunctivitis, rhinorrhea, fever, chills, myalgias, pharyngitis, nausea, and diarrhea
        5.   Ask patient or parents to describe cough and any sputum that is produced
        6.   Inquire about recent infectious illnesses in the patient's household
        7.   Ascertain that child has not missed any immunizations which may indicate susceptibility to measles, pertussis or *Haemophilus influenzae* type b infection
        8.   Question about choking which may indicate foreign body aspiration
        9.   Ask about birth history and whether mother had a history of sexually transmitted diseases during pregnancy if child is an infant
     10.   Inquire about past medical history such as acquired immunodeficiency, asthma, tuberculosis, cystic fibrosis

    B.   Physical Examination
        1.   Observe general appearance as well as attentiveness to the environment, ability to drink, ability to sustain sucking, vocalization, color, and consolability
        2.   Assess vital signs, paying particular attention to respiratory rate and hydration status (see table on normal respiratory rates in section, FEVER WITHOUT LOCALIZING SOURCE)
        3.   Observe for respiratory distress such as cyanosis, tachypnea, intercostal retractions, accessory muscle use, nasal flaring, and grunting
        4.   Auscultate lungs; typical findings are the following:
            a.   Localized diminished breath sounds
            b.   Rales and tubular breath sounds
            c.   Egophony (changes child's "ee" to what sounds like "ay")
            d.   Bronchophony (voice sounds are louder and clearer than usual)
            e.   Whispered pectoriloquy (whispered sounds are louder and clearer than normal)
        5.   Palpate chest for tactile fremitus (palpate for increased areas of vibration as child cries or says "ninety-nine")
        6.   Percuss chest for dullness which is typical over consolidated lung tissue
        7.   Perform a cardiac examination

    C.   Differential Diagnosis: the best individual sign for ruling out pneumonia is absence of tachypnea; chest indrawing and other findings of increased work of breathing increases the likelihood of pneumonia
        1.   Upper respiratory infections (URI); pneumonia can usually be distinguished from URIs by presence of lower respiratory tract signs (tachypnea, cyanosis, rales, hypoxemia) and area of infiltration on chest x-ray
        2.   Differentiating viral and atypical pneumonias from bacterial pneumonia is difficult; typically, patients with viral and atypical pneumonias have fever less than 40°C., gradual onset of symptoms, and nonproductive cough; WBCs are normal or slightly elevated and chest x-ray may reveal an interstitial infiltrate in a diffuse or perihilar distribution
        3.   Bronchiolitis
        4.   Asthma
        5.   Croup
        6.   Bronchitis
        7.   Tuberculosis
        8.   Noninfectious diseases: gastroesophageal reflux, aspiration, tracheoesophageal fistula with aspiration

    D.   Diagnostic Tests
        1.   Order PA and lateral chest x-ray; although not always present, in bacterial pneumonia, x-ray often reveals hyperaeration with alveolar infiltrate in a patchy or consolidated lobar or subsegmental distribution

2. Order CBC; elevated WBCs with left shift in bacterial pneumonia
3. Consider ordering serum cold agglutinins for diagnosing *M. pneumoniae*
4. Gram stain of sputum is helpful but difficult to obtain in young children
5. Enzyme-linked immunosorbent assay (ELISA), latex agglutination, or counterimmunoelectrophoresis are being used more frequently to detect antigens
6. Blood and sputum cultures should be ordered for patients with severe symptoms
7. Urine cultures should be obtained on all seriously ill children with fever
8. Administer purified protein derivative (PPD) if tuberculosis is suspected

V. Plan/Management

A. Consider hospitalization if child appears toxic, has underlying deficiencies in host defenses, has concomitant chronic cardiac or pulmonary disease, is in respiratory distress, or is dehydrated

B. Refer to specialist, patients who fail to recover from first episode of pneumonia or who have recurrent disease; patients should respond to antibiotics within 48-72 hours

C. Treatment for viral pneumonia is usually symptomatic
1. Hospitalized child may be prescribed ribavirin therapy
2. If the likely diagnosis is influenza pneumonia consider prescribing amantadine (Symmetrel) 50mg/5ml syrup: children aged 1-9 years give 4.4-8.8 mg/kg/day in two or three divided doses for maximum of 150 mg/day; children age 9-12 years 100 mg caps BID; continue dose for 24-48 hours after all symptoms have subsided

D. Empiric drug therapy for pneumonia not caused by viruses is based on age of child, clinical presentation, and x-ray findings (modifications in antibiotics should be made when susceptibility profile is known)
1. Neonates are usually treated in a hospital with ampicillin plus an aminoglycoside
2. In the infant with signs and symptoms of chlamydial infection prescribe one of the following for a 10 day course:
   a. Erythromycin ethylsuccinate (EES) available in 200 mg/5 mL, 400 mg/5 mL liquid; 40 mg/kg/day in divided doses every 6 hours
   b. Erythromycin/sulfisoxazole (Pediazole), available in erythromycin 200 mg and sulfisoxazole 600 mg/5 mL liquid; 40 mg/kg/day of erythromycin component in divided doses every 6 hours
3. For children with suspected bacterial infection from *Streptococcus pneumoniae* and *Haemophilus influenzae* type b prescribe one of the following for a 10 day course:
   a. Amoxicillin (Amoxil), available in 125 mg/5 mL and 250 mg/5 mL liquid or 125 mg and 250 mg chewable tablets and regular tablets; 40 mg/kg/day in divided dosages every 8 hours.
   b. If suspect infection due to ß-lactamase producing organism or if child has severe infection, prescribe amoxicillin/clavulanic acid (Augmentin), available in 125 mg/5 mL and 250 mg/5 mL liquids or 125 mg and 250 mg chewable and regular tablets; 40 mg/kg/day in divided dosages every 8 hours. To avoid side effect of diarrhea suggest that child eat cultured yogurt
   c. Alternative ß-lactamase inhibiting drug is trimethoprim/ sulfamethoxazole (Septra), available in sulfamethoxazole 200 mg and trimethoprim 40 mg per 5 mL in liquid; 40 mg/kg/day of sulfamethoxazole component in 2 divided doses every 12 hours
   d. Alternative therapy for severe infections: Administer ceftriaxone (Rocephin) IM (50-100mg/kg) as single dose then give one of following regimens:
      (1) Oral amoxicillin/clavulanic acid or trimethoprim/sulfamethoxazole for 10 days
      (2) If child is severely ill, administer daily IM injections of ceftriaxone until the child has been afebrile for 24 hours and then switch to oral antibiotic
4. For older child and adolescent who has suspected mycoplasma pneumonia or chlamydial pneumonia prescribe one of the following:
   a. Erythromycin ethylsuccinate (EES) available in 200 mg/5 mL, 400 mg/5 mL liquid; 40 mg/kg/day in divided doses every 6 hours for 10 days. Also available as (Eryped) 200 mg chewable tablets for older children
   b. For adolescents, prescribe erythromycin (E-Mycin) 250 mg TID or QID or doxycycline (Vibramycin) 100 mg BID for 10 days

      c.   Erythromycin/sulfisoxazole (Pediazole), available in erythromycin 200 mg and sulfisoxazole 600 mg/5 mL liquid; 40 mg/kg/day of erythromycin component in divided doses every 6 hours for 10 days

      d.   Azithromycin (Zithromax)

          (1)   Adolescent >16 years: 500 mg daily for 1 day, then 250 mg daily for 4 days

          (2)   Children ≤16 years: 10mg/kg once daily for 1 day; then 5 mg/kg once daily for 4 days; Available 100mg/5mL and 200mg/5mL oral suspension; Oral suspension but not tablets must be taken one hour before or two hours after meals

E.   Prevention

    1.   Routine immunizations for pertussis, measles and *H. influenzae* type b have reduced incidence of pediatric pneumonia

    2.   Consider vaccines for influenza and *streptococcus pneumoniae* in children with enhanced susceptibility

    3.   Administer palivizumab or respiratory syncytial immune globulin (RSV-IGIV) in infants with chronic lung disease (see section on BRONCHIOLITIS)

F.   Patient Education

    1.   Teach parents to watch for signs of respiratory distress such as changes in level of activity and signs of dehydration

    2.   Increase child's fluid intake

    3.   Avoid giving child cough medications, particularly cough suppressants

G.   Follow Up

    1.   Evaluate patient within 48-72 hours or sooner if condition is not improving

    2.   Consider hospitalization if child fails to respond to therapy in 48-72 hours

    3.   After initial follow up, schedule return visit for 2 weeks

    4.   Repeat chest-rays are needed for children with recurrent pneumonia, but remember that after acute pneumonia x-rays can remain abnormal for 4-6 weeks

TUBERCULOSIS

I.   Definition: Necrotizing bacterial infection most commonly infecting the lungs; other important definitions include the following:

A.   Exposure: Applies to persons who have recent contact with an individual with suspected or confirmed, contagious pulmonary tuberculosis (TB) and whose tuberculin skin test is nonreactive and who has a normal physical examination and chest x-ray

B.   TB infection: Positive tuberculin skin test in an individual with absent physical findings of disease and has a chest x-ray which is either normal or has only granulomas or calcifications in lung and/or regional lymph nodes

C.   TB disease: Individual with infection who has signs, symptoms, and x-ray manifestations which are apparently caused by *M. tuberculosis*; disease may be pulmonary or extrapulmonary

II.   Pathogenesis

A.   Primary or initial infection occurs by inhalation of the etiologic agent, *Mycobacterium tuberculosis*, which is dispersed as droplet nuclei (small airborne particles) from persons with sputum-smear-positive pulmonary tuberculosis (TB) when they cough or sneeze

B.   Approximately 90% of primary TB infections remain in a latent or dormant infection stage; persons in this stage are not infectious

C. Active TB may develop after periods of stress or at times when the body is undergoing change or fighting an infection

D. The duration of infectivity is variable, but the majority of adult and adolescent patients are noncontagious within a few weeks of starting appropriate therapy; children < 12 years are usually not contagious because their lesions are small and cough is minimal

E. Incubation period from infection to development of a positive reaction to tuberculin skin test is 2-12 weeks

F. Current classification system (see Table that follows) is based on pathogenesis

G. The lungs are the most common sites for clinical TB (85% of cases), but TB is a systemic disease and can result in, disseminated TB (miliary TB), or infections in the bones and joints as well as in the lymphatic, genitourinary, and central nervous systems

	CLASSIFICATION SYSTEM FOR TB	
Class	Type	Description
0	No TB exposure Not infected	No history of exposure Negative reaction to tuberculin skin test
1	TB exposure No evidence of infection	History of exposure Negative reaction to tuberculin skin test
2	TB infection No disease	Positive reaction to tuberculin skin test Negative bacteriologic studies (if done) No clinical or radiographic evidence of TB
3	Current TB Disease	*M. tuberculosis* cultured (if done) or Positive reaction to tuberculin skin test and Clinical or radiographic evidence of current disease
4	Previous TB disease	History of episode(s) of TB or Abnormal but stable radiographic findings Positive reaction to the tuberculin skin test Negative bacteriologic studies (if done) and No clinical or radiologic evidence of current disease
5	TB suspected	Diagnosis pending

Source: US Department of Health and Human Services, Public Health Service, Centers for Disease Control. (1994). Core Curriculum on Tuberculosis.

III. Clinical Presentation

A. From 1985-1993 reported TB cases increased by 14% due to such factors as the HIV epidemic, deterioration in the health-care infrastructure, number of cases among foreign-born individuals, and transmission of TB in congregate shelters

B. Outbreaks of multidrug-resistant TB (MDR-TB) -- resistant to both isoniazid (INH) and rifampin (RIF) -- are a serious concern; these outbreaks have been associated with a high prevalence of HIV infection among the outbreak cases, a high mortality rate, and a high transmission rate of MDR-TB to heath-care and correctional facility workers

C. Presenting symptoms of TB in adolescents are often vague and may include the following:
  1. Productive, prolonged cough over 3 weeks' duration
  2. Chest pain
  3. Hemoptysis
  4. Increased fatigue, malaise, anorexia, weight decrease
  5. Periodic fever, night sweats

D. Children are usually asymptomatic with normal chest x-rays; the infection is usually self-limited, but clinical manifestations can occur 1-6 months after the initial infection and include the following:
   1. Fever, weight loss, cough, night sweats, chills
   2. Lymphadenopathy of hilar, mediastinal, cervical, or other lymph nodes
   3. Atelectasis or pleural effusion
   4. In approximately 25% of children <15 years who are not treated in early stages of disease, extrapulmonary disease occurs
   5. Disseminated TB
   6. TB meningitis

E. Symptoms of extrapulmonary TB depend on the site affected: hematuria may occur in TB of the kidney and back pain may occur in TB of the spine

F. Certain persons are more likely to become infected with *M. tuberculosis* (see table)

INDIVIDUALS AT RISK FOR TB INFECTION

✦ Anyone in close contact with an infectious case

✦ Anyone with associated COPD, diabetes, malignancy, alcoholism, end-stage renal disease, poor nutrition, gastrectomy, stomach bypass surgery for weight loss, chronic malabsorption syndromes, steroid treatment, 10% or more below ideal body weight

✦ Minority groups, homeless, institutionalized groups, persons living in correctional facilities, migrant farm workers, users of intravenous or other street drugs or children who are frequently exposed to adults from the preceding groups

✦ Patients who are HIV positive

Source: U.S. Department of Health & Human Services, Public Health Service, Centers for Disease Control. (1994). Core Curriculum on Tuberculosis.

IV. Diagnosis/Evaluation

A. History
   1. Inquire about onset and duration of weight loss, fatigue, fever, night sweats, anorexia, cough, hemoptysis, chest pain as well as localized symptoms in other body organs such as hematuria, enlarged lymph nodes
   2. Ask about history of exposure to TB at home, work, school, or social events
   3. Determine whether patient has had previous TB or active disease; inquire about previous TB treatments
   4. Ask about risk factors
   5. Ask about results and dates of TB skin tests and chest x-rays
   6. Inquire about travel to developing countries where TB is common

B. Physical Examination
   1. Observe for skin pallor
   2. Palpate for lymphadenopathy
   3. Inspect, palpate, percuss, and auscultate chest (rales in upper posterior chest, bronchovesicular breathing and whispered pectoriloquy are often positive findings in patients with TB)
   4. Complete physical exam is needed if disseminated TB is suspected

C. Differential Diagnosis
   1. Malignancy
   2. Silicosis
   3. Chronic obstructive pulmonary disease
   4. Asthma
   5. Bronchiectasis
   6. Pneumonia

D. Diagnostic Tests
    1. Screening is performed to identify infected individuals at high risk for developing TB and to identify individuals with TB disease who need treatment; regular tuberculin testing of high risk groups is recommended (no need to repeat PPD on person with a known positive tuberculin skin test)
       a. Preferred method of screening is the Mantoux tuberculin skin test 5 TU-PPD
           (1) The skin test is the only way to diagnosis TB infection before the infection has progressed to TB disease; generally, takes 2 to 10 weeks after infection for person to react positively to skin test
           (2) Administer intradermal injection of 0.1 mL of purified protein derivative (PPD) tuberculin containing 5 tuberculin units (TU) into volar or dorsal surface of forearm which should produce a discrete pale wheal 6 mm to 10 mm in diameter
               (a) Monitor for reactions 48 hours after application
               (b) Measure only the area of induration and record in millimeters
           (3) Interpretation of PPD: PPD is considered positive and indicating primary, latent or active TB in the following cases:

POSITIVE PPDs
✦ ≥5 mm if patient is one of the following: Known or suspected HIV+, had close contact with person with infectious TB, has chest x-ray suggestive of previous TB, injects IV drugs (if HIV status is unknown), and is a child with symptoms suggestive of TB or is immunosuppressed from causes other than HIV infection
✦ ≥10 mm if patient is one of the following: foreign born from area where TB is common, lives in medically underserved area, member of low-income population (including high-risk racial and ethnic groups), lives in long-term care residence, is an IV drug user (if HIV status negative), has medical risk factor, is health care worker in facility where TB patients receive care, is from locally identified high-prevalence group (migrant farm worker or homeless person), is a child <4 years of age
✦ ≥15 mm: all persons with no known risk factor for TB

Adapted from U.S. Department of Health & Human Services, Public Health Service, Centers for Disease Control. (1994). Core Curriculum on Tuberculosis.

           (4) Anergy
               (a) Although routine anergy testing is no longer recommended for HIV positive persons, consider anergy on an individual basis in persons with negative skin tests who have the following: HIV infection, severe or febrile illness, overwhelming immunosuppressive therapy, severe or febrile illness or overwhelming TB infection
               (b) Determine anergy by administering two delayed-type hypersensitivity antigens such as mumps, or *Candida* by the Mantoux technique; persons with a reaction ≥3mm are not anergic
               (c) If anergy is present, probability of infection should be evaluated and persons judged at high risk of exposure should be considered for preventive therapy
           (5) Two-step testing is used to differentiate boosted reactions from reactions due to new infection and should be performed in adults who will be retested periodically such as health care workers
               (a) Some individuals with TB infection may have a negative skin test when tested several years after an infection; however, the skin test may stimulate their ability to react to tuberculin and cause positive reactions to subsequent tests (boost) which may be misinterpreted as new infections
               (b) To distinguish a boosted reaction from a new infection when the first test is negative, administer a second skin test 1-3 weeks after first test.
                   i) If second test is negative: person is uninfected and any subsequent positive test should be classified as a new infection
                   ii) If second test is positive: person is infected and should be treated accordingly

b. Chest radiograph or sputum smears may be the recommended first screening test in populations where risk of transmission is high and difficulties in administering and reading tests exist such as jails or homeless shelters

2. Screening in Children; all children need routine health care evaluations and assessments of their risk for TB (see Table REVISED TUBERCULIN SKIN TEST RECOMMENDATIONS FOR CHILDREN)

REVISED TUBERCULIN SKIN TEST RECOMMENDATIONS FOR CHILDREN*

Immediate Skin Testing
- ❖ Contacts of persons with confirmed or suspected infectious tuberculosis in the last 5 years
- ❖ Children with radiographic or clinical findings suggesting tuberculosis
- ❖ Children immigrating from countries where TB is endemic
- ❖ Children with travel histories to endemic countries and significant contact with indigenous persons from such countries

Annual Skin Testing†
- ❖ Children infected with HIV
- ❖ Incarcerated adolescents

Skin Testing Every 2-3 Years†
- ❖ Children exposed to the following individuals: HIV-infected, homeless, residents of nursing homes, institutionalized adolescents or adults, users of illicit drugs, incarcerated adolescents or adults, and migrant farm workers; this would include foster children with exposure to adults in the above high-risk groups

Consider for Tuberculin Skin Testing at Ages 4-6 and 11-16 Years
- ❖ Children whose parents immigrated from endemic areas; continued potential exposure by travel to the endemic areas and household contact with persons from the endemic areas
- ❖ Children without specific risk factors who reside in high-prevalence areas

Risk for Progression to Disease
- ❖ Children with other medical risk factors, including diabetes mellitus, chronic renal failure, malnutrition, and congenital or acquired immunodeficiencies deserve special consideration; initial histories of potential exposure to tuberculosis should be included in all these patients; if these histories or local epidemiologic factors suggest a possibility of exposure, immediate and periodic tuberculin skin testing should be considered in these patients

---

*BCG immunization is not contraindication to tuberculin skin testing.
†Initial tuberculin skin testing initiated at the time of diagnosis or circumstance.

Adapted from American Academy of Pediatrics. (1996). Committee on infectious diseases: Update on tuberculosis skin testimg of children. Pediatrics, 97, 282.

3. Diagnosis of active disease
   a. Order three sputum specimens for **both** smear examination and culture in patients suspected of pulmonary or laryngeal TB
      (1) A presumptive diagnosis of TB can be made with detection of acid-fast bacilli (AFB); results can usually be obtained in 24 hours
      (2) A positive sputum culture for *M. tuberculosis* is essential to confirm diagnosis, but often takes several weeks for results to be obtained
      (3) Drug susceptibility testing should be done on the initial *M. Tuberculosis* isolate; testing should also be performed on additional isolates from patients whose cultures fail to convert to negative within 3 months of beginning therapy, or if there is clinical evidence of failure to respond to therapy
      (4) Aerosol induction to stimulate sputum production, bronchoscopy, or gastric aspiration should be done if the patient cannot produce a sputum specimen and there is suspicion of TB
   b. A tuberculin skin test is helpful in making diagnosis and should be applied, but absence of a reaction to the test does not exclude diagnosis
   c. Order posterior-anterior chest x-ray
      (1) Abnormalities are suggestive, but are not diagnostic of TB; x-rays may rule out possibility of pulmonary TB in an asymptomatic person with a positive skin test
      (2) In pulmonary TB, abnormalities are often present in apical or posterior segments of upper lobes or superior segments of lower lobes; in HIV infected persons, other abnormalities are often present

4. Other tests are ordered after TB is diagnosed. Order baseline measurements of hepatic enzymes, bilirubin, serum creatinine, blood urea nitrogen (BUN), CBC, and platelet count; serum uric acid if pyrazinamide will be prescribed (see V.C. for additional tests needed when drug therapy is used)

V. Plan/Management

A. Preventive therapy reduces the risk that TB infection will progress to actual disease
   1. Preventive therapy is needed for certain groups of people (see following table)

CANDIDATES FOR PREVENTIVE THERAPY
❖ Skin test positive for persons in the following high-risk groups, regardless of age:
✔ Persons with known or suspected HIV infection
✔ Close contacts of infectious TB cases
✔ Recent tuberculin skin-test converters
✔ Previously untreated or inadequately treated persons with abnormal chest radiographs
✔ Intravenous drug users
✔ Persons with medical conditions which increase the risk of TB
❖ Skin test positive persons in the following high-risk groups who are <35 years of age:
✔ Foreign-born persons from high prevalence countries
✔ Medically underserved, low income populations, including high-risk minorities
✔ Residents of long-term care facilities (including prisons)
✔ Locally identified high-prevalence groups (migrant farm workers or homeless persons)
✔ Children younger than 4 years of age
❖ Other candidates:
✔ Infected persons <35 years of age with no additional risk factors should be evaluated for preventive therapy if reaction to tuberculin test ≥15 mm (priority is lower than groups already listed)
✔ Persons who are close contacts with infectious cases should have X-ray regardless of skin test reaction and considered for preventive therapy in following cases: persons in circumstances with high probability of infection, children or adolescents, immunosuppressed persons (close contacts with negative initial reaction should be retested 10 weeks after last exposure to TB)
✔ Infants exposed to person with TB should be given a skin test and chest x-ray and started on preventive therapy even if tests are negative because infants <6 months may be anergic; retest again in 3-4 months and at 6 months if initial tests are negative
❖ Consult specialist for pregnant females

Table adapted from U.S. Department of Health & Human Services. (1994). Core Curriculum on Tuberculosis.

2. Before beginning preventive therapy:
   a. Exclude possibility of current TB which would require multiple drug therapy
   b. Question history of previous preventive therapy
   c. Explore characteristics of person (preventive therapy might **not** be indicated in the following persons: persons at high risk for adverse reactions to isoniazid (INH) such as those with acute or active liver disease, persons who cannot tolerate INH, persons likely to be infected with drug-resistant *M. tuberculosis*, persons who are highly unlikely to complete course of preventive therapy)
3. Drug therapy for prevention of disease is recommended for persons <35 years with positive PPD and no evidence of active disease but is **not** recommended for persons who are ≥35 years unless they are at high risk for developing TB disease because the risk of isoniazid-related hepatitis outweighs the benefits of preventive therapy in this age group (see Table DOSAGES FOR PREVENTIVE THERAPY)
   a. Dispense only a 1-month supply of drug at a time
   b. Monthly question for the following: compliance, symptoms of neurotoxicity (paresthesias of hands and feet), signs of hepatitis

DOSAGES FOR PREVENTIVE DRUG THERAPY

Type of Patient	Dosage[†]
❖ All infants and children	Isoniazid (INH) 10-15 mg/kg (maximum 300 mg) QD for 9 months
❖ Adults	INH 300 mg QD for 6 months
❖ Adults with HIV infection	INH 300 mg QD for 12 months
❖ Adults with positive skin test and either silicosis or chest x-ray demonstrating old fibrotic lesions	INH 300 mg QD for 12 months or 4 months of INH and rifampin 10 mg/kg/day
❖ Adults with close contacts of infectious patients who have INH-resistant TB	Rifampin 10 mg/kg/day QD for 6 months or Rifampin 300 mg tab BID; 1 hour before meals or 2 hours after meals
❖ Children with close contacts of infectious patients who have INH-resistant TB	Rifampin 10mg/kg/day QD for 9 months

[†] INH can also be given 2x weekly in dose of 15 mg/kg when compliance is doubtful and direct observation is needed

      c.   Take special precautions in patients who are at high risk of adverse reactions to INH such as persons ≥35 years, or who have chronic liver disease, peripheral neuropathy (or are predisposed to developing neuropathy such as diabetics), abuse alcohol, are pregnant or inject drugs
          (1)   Frequently monitor liver enzymes; if measurements exceed 3-5 times upper limit of normal, discontinue INH
          (2)   In patients prone to developing neuropathy, prescribe pyridoxine (10-15mg/day)
      d.   New, short-course preventive treatment regimens are currently being investigated

   B.   Treatment of active disease (uncomplicated, intrathoracic TB): The initial treatment should include four drugs: isoniazid (INH), rifampin (RIF), pyrazinamide (PZA), and either ethambutol (EMB) or streptomycin (SM)
      1.   See Tables that follow for regimens and dosages of initial drug therapy in children and adolescents and in patients with special considerations; when drug susceptibility results are available, the regimen should be altered as appropriate

REGIMEN OPTIONS FOR INITIAL TREATMENT OF PULMONARY AND EXTRAPULMONARY TB AMONG CHILDREN AND ADOLESCENTS

TB without HIV Infection

Option 1	Option 2	Option 3
Administer daily INH, RIF, PZA, and EMB or SM for 8 wks, followed by 16 wks* of INH and RIF daily or 2-3 times/ week** In areas where the INH resistance rate is <4%, EMB or SM may not be necessary for patients with no individual risk factors for drug resistance. Consult a TB medical expert if the patient is symptomatic or smear or culture positive after 3 months.	Administer daily INH, RIF, PZA, and SM or EMB for 2 wks followed by 2 times/week** administration of the same drugs for 6 weeks (by DOT[‡]), and subsequently, with 2 times/week** administration of INH and RIF for 16 weeks (by DOT).* Consult a TB medical expert if the patient is symptomatic or smear or culture positive after 3 months.	Treat by DOT, 3 times/week** with INH, RIF, PZA, and EMB or SM for 6 months.[†] Consult a TB medical expert if the patient is symptomatic or smear or culture positive after 3 months.

*For infants and children with miliary TB, bone and joint TB, or TB meningitis, treatment should last 12 months; for older adolescents with these forms of extrapulmonary TB, response to therapy should be closely monitored and treatment should be altered accordingly.
**All regimens administered 2 times/week or 3 times/week should be monitored by DOT for the duration of therapy.
[†]The strongest evidence from clinical trials is the effectiveness of all four drugs administered for the full 6 months. There is weaker evidence that SM can be discontinued after 4 months if the isolate is susceptible to all drugs. The evidence for stopping PZA before the end of 6 months is equivocal for the 3 times/week regimen, and there is no evidence on the effectiveness of this regimen with EMB for less than the full 6 months.
[‡]DOT = Directly observed therapy.

Table adapted from U.S. Department of Health & Human Services. (1994). Core Curriculum on Tuberculosis.

OPTIONS FOR INITIAL TREATMENT OF PULMONARY AND EXTRAPULMONARY TB AMONG CHILDREN AND ADOLESCENTS IN SPECIAL CIRCUMSTANCES

Smear-and culture negative pulmonary TB in adolescents	Pulmonary and extrapulmonary TB in adults and children when PZA is contraindicated
Administer INH, RIF, PZA, and EMB or SM following options 1, 2, or 3 for initial therapy in table above for 8 weeks followed by INH, RIF, PZA, and EMB or SM daily or 2-3 times per week (DOT) for 8 weeks. If drug resistance is unlikely, EMB or SM may be unnecessary and PZA may be discontinued after 2 months	Administer INH, RIF, and EMB or SM daily for 8 weeks followed by INH and RIF daily or 2 times per week (DOT) for 24 weeks. If drug resistance is unlikely, EMB or SM may be unnecessary

DOSAGE RECOMMENDATION FOR FIRST-LINE DRUGS IN INITIAL TREATMENT OF TB AMONG CHILDREN* AND ADOLESCENTS

	Dosage					
	Daily		2 times/week		3 times/week	
Drugs	Children	Adolescents	Children	Adolescents	Children	Adolescents
Isoniazid	10-20 mg/kg Max 300 mg	5 mg/kg Max 300 mg	20-40 mg/kg Max 900 mg	15 mg/kg Max 900 mg	20-40 mg/kg Max 900 mg	15 mg/kg Max 900 mg
Rifampin	10-20 mg/kg Max 600 mg	10 mg/kg Max 600 mg	10-20 mg/kg Max 600 mg	10 mg/kg Max 600 mg	10-20 mg/kg Max 600 mg	10 mg/kg Max 600 mg
Pyrazinamide	15-30 mg/kg Max 2 gm	15-30 mg/kg Max 2 gm	50-70 mg/kg Max 4 gm	50-70 mg/kg Max 4 gm	50-70 mg/kg Max 3 gm	50-70 mg/kg Max 3 gm
Ethambutol[†]	15-25 mg/kg Max 2.5 gm	15-25 mg/kg Max 2.5 gm	50 mg/kg Max 2.5 gm	50 mg/kg Max 2.5 gm	25-30 mg/kg Max 2.5 gm	25-30 mg/kg Max 2.5 gm
Streptomycin	20-40 mg/kg Max 1 gm	15 mg/kg Max 1 gm	25-30 mg/kg Max 1.5 gm	25-30 mg/kg Max 1.5 gm	25-30 mg/kg Max 1.5 gm	25-30 mg/kg Max 1 gm

*Children ≤12 years of age.
[†]Ethambutol is generally not recommended for children whose visual acuity cannot be monitored (<6 years of age). However, ethambutol should be considered for all children with organisms resistant to other drugs, when susceptibility to ethambutol has been demonstrated, or susceptibility is likely.

Source: Initial therapy for tuberculosis in the era of multi resistance: Recommendations of the Advisory Council for the Elimination of Tuberculosis. MMWR 42 (No. RR-7) (1993).

2. Second-line TB drugs may be prescribed after consulting a specialist: capreomycin, kanamycin, ethionamide, para-aminosalicylic acid, cycloserine, ciprofloxacin, ofloxacin, amikacin, clofazimine
3. Treatment of persons with additional medical conditions must be individualized
   a. For patients with impaired renal function avoid streptomycin, kanamycin and capreomycin if possible
   b. In patients with HIV infection duration of treatment is the same as HIV-negative adults; HIV positive adults should be aggressively assessed for response to treatment and treatment should be prolonged if response is slow or suboptimal
4. Treatment of children and infants
   a. Treat with same regimens as adults; avoid EMB in children too young to be monitored for visual acuity
   b. In infants, treat as soon as diagnosis is suspected because disseminated TB is more likely
5. Treatment of drug-resistant TB
   a. In patients with documented INH resistance during initial four-drug therapy, discontinue INH and continue RIF, PZA, and EMB or SM for entire 6 months -or- treat with RIF and EMB for 12 months
   b. Consult specialist for multidrug-resistant TB
6. Directly observed therapy (DOT) is one method to ensure adherence
   a. DOT requires that a health-care provider or other designated person observe patient while ingesting anti-TB medications
   b. All patients with TB caused by organisms resistant to either INH or RIF and all patients receiving intermittent therapy should receive DOT

C. Monitoring of patients on drug therapy includes the following:
1. Patients treated for TB should have baseline measurements of hepatic enzymes, bilirubin, serum creatinine or BUN, CBC and platelet count; measure serum uric acid if pyrazinamide is used; test visual acuity if EMB is used; test hearing function if SM is used
2. At minimum, patients should be seen monthly by provider and assessed for adverse reactions to drugs
3. Drug interactions: Current literature and package inserts should be consulted
   a. INH and phenytoin interact; monitor serum level of phenytoin
   b. Rifampin may increase the clearance of drugs metabolized by the liver: methadone, coumadin derivatives, glucocorticoids, estrogens, oral hypoglycemic agents, digitalis, anticonvulsants, ketoconazole, fluconazole, cyclosporin; females should use birth control method other than oral contraceptives or Norplant while on rifampin
4. Specific guidelines for drug monitoring
   a. INH: baseline hepatic enzymes; then, repeat measurements if abnormal or at risk for adverse reactions
   b. Rifampin: baseline CBC, platelets, hepatic enzymes; repeat as needed
   c. PZA: Baseline uric acid and hepatic enzymes; repeat as needed
   d. Ethambutol: baseline and monthly visual acuity and color vision tests
   e. Streptomycin: Baseline hearing test and kidney function; repeat as needed
5. Monitoring response to therapy includes the following:
   a. Sputum exam at least monthly until conversion to negative; then, at least one sputum at completion of therapy
   b. For patients with multi-drug resistant TB, monthly sputum evaluation should continue for entire course of treatment
   c. Chest radiographs are less important than sputums but chest film at completion of treatment provides a baseline for future comparisons
   d. Patients with sputum that remains culture positive beyond 3 months should be evaluated for disease due to drug-resistant organisms
   e. When waiting for drug susceptibility results, continue the original drug regimen or augment regimen with at least three new drugs; **never** add one drug to a failing regimen

D. BCG vaccination
1. Vaccination is used in many countries, but is not generally recommended in U.S.
2. BCG vaccination should be considered for an infant or child who has a negative tuberculin skin-test result in the following circumstances
   a. Child is exposed continually to an untreated or ineffectively treated patient and cannot be separated from this patient or given long-term preventive therapy
   b. Child is exposed continually to a patient with infectious pulmonary TB caused by strains resistant to INH and rifampin, and child cannot be separated from this patient
3. BCG vaccination should be considered on an individual basis among health care workers (HCW) in high-risk settings; HCWs should be informed of variable data about efficacy of BCG vaccination, the interference of BCG vaccination with diagnosing newly acquired TB infection, and possible serious complications of BCG vaccine in immunocompromised persons
4. BCG vaccination is **not** recommended for HCWs in low-risk settings and is **not** recommended for HIV-infected children or adults
5. In persons vaccinated with BCG, sensitivity to tuberculin is highly variable; there is no reliable method for distinguishing tuberculin reactions caused by BCG from those caused by natural infections; all BCG-vaccinated persons who have positive skin test should be further evaluated to determine need for preventive therapy

E. Patient Education: Teach about possible reactions to medicines
1. INH
   a. Hepatic toxicity is the most common adverse reaction
   b. Peripheral neuropathy may be prevented by taking 25 mg of pyridoxine QD

2. Rifampin
    a. GI upset, hepatitis, bleeding problems, flu-like symptoms, and rash
    b. Warn patient that tears, urine, saliva, etc., may turn orange-red; may permanently stain contact lenses
3. Pyrazinamide: hyperuricemia, gout, hepatitis, joint aches, rash, and GI upset
4. Ethambutol: Optic neuritis
5. Streptomycin: Hearing and balance changes and renal toxicity

F. Patient education also includes discussion of mode of transmission and need to cover nose and mouth when coughing or sneezing; no sharing of eating utensils

G. Follow Up
1. Patient must have sputum examination at least monthly until conversion to negative
2. Patients with multi-drug resistant TB need monthly sputum evaluations for entire course of therapy
3. Monthly monitoring of adverse reactions to drugs and response to treatment while on drug therapy is essential
4. Chest films are helpful at completion of therapy

REFERENCES

Advisory Committee on Immunization Practices. (1997). Prevention of pneumococcal disease: Recommendations of the Advisory Committee on Immunization Practices (ACIP). MMWR, 46(RR-8), 1-21.

Advisory Council for the Elimination of Tuberculosis (1993). The initial therapy for tuberculosis in the era of multidrug resistance: Recommendations of the Advisory Council for the Elimination of Tuberculosis. MMWR, 42(RR-7), 1-7

Advisory Council for the Elimination of Tuberculosis and the Advisory Committee on Immunization Practices. (1996). The role of BCG vaccine in the prevention and control of tuberculosis in the United States. MMWR, 42(RR-4), 1-17

American Academy of Pediatrics, Committee on Infectious Disease. (1996). Reassessment of the indications for ribavirin therapy in respiratory syncytial virus infections. Pediatrics, 97, 137-140.

American Academy of Pediatrics, Committee on Infectious Disease. (1996). Update on tuberculosis skin testing of children. Pediatrics, 97, 282.

American Academy of Pediatrics, Committee on Infectious Disease and Committee on Fetus and Newborn. (1998). Prevention of respiratory syncytial virus infections: Indications for the use of palivizumab and update on the use of RSV-IGIV. Pediatrics, 102, 1211-1216.

American Academy of Pediatrics. 1997. In G. Peter (Ed.). Red Book: Report of the Committee on Infectious Disease. 24th ed. Elk Grove Village, IL: Academy of Pediatrics.

Bar-on, M.E., & Zanga, J.R. (1996). Bronchiolitis. Primary Care, 23, 805-818.

Baum, V.C. (1999). Foreign body aspiration. In R.A. Dershewitz (Ed.), Ambulatory pediatric care (3rd ed.). Philadelphia: Lippincott-Raven.

Bergh, K.D. (1998). The patient's differential diagnosis: Unpredictable concerns in visits for acute cough. The Journal of Family Practice, 46, 153-158.

Campbell, P.W. & Hazinski, T.A. (1997). Acute pneumonia. In R.A. Hoekelman, (Ed.), Primary pediatric care. (3rd edition). St. Louis: Mosby.

Carney, I.K., Gibson, P.G., Murree-Allen, K., Saltos, N., Olson, L.G., & Hensley, M.J. (1997). A systematic evaluation of mechanisms in chronic cough. American Journal of Respiratory Critical Care Medicine, 156, 211-216.

Churgay, C.A. (1996). The diagnosis and management of bacterial pneumonias in infants and children. Primary Care, 23, 821-835.

Cruz, M.N., Steward, G., & Rosenberg, N. (1995). Use of dexamethasone in the outpatient management of acute laryngotracheitis. Pediatrics, 96, 220-223.

DeMuri, G.P. (1996). Afebrile pneumonias in infants. <u>Primary Care, 23,</u>849-860.

Dershewitz, R.A., & Dorkin, H.L. (1999). Persistent cough. In R.A. Dershewitz (Ed.), <u>Ambulatory pediatric care</u> (3rd ed.). Philadelphia: Lippincott-Raven.

Folland, D.S. (1997). Treatment of croup: Sending home an improved child and relieved parents. <u>Postgraduate Medicine, 101,</u> 271-273, 277-278.

Glaser V. (Ed.). (September 30, 1997). Bracing for the cold and flu season. <u>Patient Care,</u> 47-62.

Goodman, M. & Brady, M. (1996). Respiratory disorders. In C.E. Burns, N. Barber, M.A. Brady, & A.M. Dunn. (Eds.), <u>Pediatric primary care: A handbook for nurse practitioners.</u> Saunders: Philadelphia.

Goroll, A.H., May, L.A., & Mulley, A.G., Jr. (1995). Evaluation of hemoptysis. In A.H. Goroll, L.A. May & A.G. Mulley, Jr. (Eds.), <u>Primary care medicine: Office evaluation and management of the adult patient.</u> Philadelphia: J.B. Lippincott.

Hayden, F.G., Diamond, L., Wood, P.B., Korts, D.C., & Wecker, M.T. (1996). Effectiveness and safety of intranasal ipratropium bromide in common colds: A randomized, double-blind, placebo-controlled trial. <u>Annals of Internal Medicine, 125,</u> 89-97.

Hemila, H. , & Herman, Z.S. (1995). Vitamin C and the common cold: A retrospective analysis of Chalmers' Review. <u>Journal of American College of Nutrition, 14,</u> 116-123.

Hueston, W.J., & Mainous, A.G. (1998). Acute bronchitis. <u>American Family Physician, 57,</u> 1270-1276.

Iseman, M.D. (1993). Treatment of multidrug-resistant tuberculosis. <u>New England Journal of Medicine, 329</u>(11), 784-790.

Jaffe, D.M. (1998). The treatment of croup with glucocorticoid. <u>New England Journal of Medicine, 339,</u> 553-554.

Klassen, T.P. (1997). Recent advances in the treatment of bronchiolitis and laryngitis. <u>Pediatric Clinics of North America, 44,</u> 249-261.

Klassen, T.P., Craig, W.R., & Moher, D. (1998). Nebulized budesonide and oral dexamethasone for treatment of croup: A randomized controlled trial. <u>JAMA, 279,</u> 1629-1632.

Ledwith, C.A., Shea, L.M., & Mauro, R.D. (1995). Safety and efficacy of nebulized racemic epinephrine in conjunction with oral dexamethasone and mist in the outpatient treatment of croup. <u>Annals of Emergency Medicine, 25,</u> 331-337.

Levy, B.T., & Graber, M.A. (1997). Respiratory syncytial virus infection in infants and young children. <u>The Journal of Family Practice, 45,</u> 473-480.

Margolis, P. & Gadomski, A. (1998). Does this infant have pneumonia? <u>JAMA, 279,</u> 308-313.

Mello, C.J., Irwin, R.S., & Curley, F.J. (1996). Predictive values of the character, timing, and complications of chronic cough in diagnosing its cause. <u>Archives of Internal Medicine, 156,</u> 997-1003.

Meyer, A.A., & Aitken, P.V. (1996). Evaluation of persistent cough in children. <u>Primary Care, 23,</u> 883-892.

Millan, S.B. & Cumming, W.A. (1996). Supraglottic airway infections. <u>Primary Care, 23,</u> 741-757.

Mossard, S.B., Macknin, M.L., Medendorp, S.V., & Mason, P. (1996). Zinc gluconate lozenges for treating the common cold. <u>Annals of Internal Medicine, 125,</u> 81-88.

National Institutes of Health. (1992). <u>Teach your patients about asthma: A clinician's guide.</u> National Asthma Education Program, Office of Prevention, Education and Control. Publication #92-2737. Bethesda, MD.

National Institutes of Health. National Heart, Lung, and Blood Institute. (1997). <u>The Expert Panel Report 2: Guidelines for the Diagnosis and Management of Asthma.</u> National Asthma Education Program, Office of Prevention, Education and Control. NIH Publication #97-4051. Bethesda, MD.

O'Brien, K.L., Dowell, S.F., Schwartz, B., Marcy, S.M., Phillips, W.R., & Gerber, M.A. (1998). Cough illness/bronchitis--principles of judicious use of antimicrobial agents. <u>Pediatrics, 101,</u> 178-181

Philip, E.B. (1997). Chronic cough. <u>American Family Physician, 56,</u>1395-1402.

Rosenstein, B.J. (1997). Hemoptysis. In R.A. Hoekelman (Ed.)., <u>Primary pediatric care</u> (3rd ed.). St. Louis: Mosby.

Rosenstein, N., Phillips, W.R., Gerber, M.A., Marcy, M., Schwartz, B., & Dowell, S.F. (1998). The common cold--principles of judicious use of antimicrobial agents. <u>Pediatrics, 101,</u> 181-184.

Rowe, P.C., & Klassen, T.P. (1996). Corticosteroids for croup: Reconciling town and gown. <u>Archives of Pediatric and Adolescent Medicine, 150,</u> 344-346.

Schwartz, R. (1995). Respiratory syncytial virus in infants and children. Nurse Practitioner,20, (9), 24-29.

Sitzman, S.J., & Fiechtner, H.B. (1998). Treatment of croup with glucocorticoid. Annals of Pharmacotherapy, 32, 973-974.

Starke, J.R. (1996). Tuberculosis in children. Primary Care, 23, 861-881.

Turner, R.B. (1997). Epidemiology, pathogenesis, and treatment of the common cold. Annals of Allergy, Asthma, & Immunology, 78, 531-537.

Uba, A. (1996). Infraglottic and bronchial infections. Primary Care, 23, 759-791.

U.S. Department of Health & Human Services, Public Health Service, Centers for Disease Control. (1994). Core Curriculum on Tuberculosis: What the Clinician Should Know (3rd ed.). Publication number 00-5763. Atlanta.

U.S. Department of Health & Human Services, Public Health Service, Centers for Disease Control. (1997). Anergy skin testing and preventive therapy for HIV-infected persons: Revised recommendations. MMWR, 46,(RR-15), 1-10.

Cardiovascular Problems

CHEST PAIN

I.   Definition: Unpleasant sensation in the chest associated with actual or potential tissue damage

II.   Pathogenesis

A.   Chest pain may emanate from the chest wall and can be associated with musculoskeletal causes such as muscle strain due to exercise and coughing, muscle spasm, costochondritis, and trauma (i.e., rib fractures)

B.   Pain originating from the chest wall may also be secondary to neurological disorders such as herpes zoster and nerve root compression

C.   Distention of the pleura may produce pain (called pleurisy) and is commonly due to inflammation, infection, and neoplasm

D.   Cardiac causes of pain are least common but most severe; structural heart lesions, infection and arrhythmias are possible causes

E.   Gastrointestinal problems due to structural defects such as gastroesophageal reflux (GERD), esophageal spasm, and hiatal hernia or abdominal organ problems resulting from inflammation and infection such as cholecystitis and pancreatitis may produce chest pain

F.   Psychogenic disorders due to anxiety, depression, or cardiac neurosis are possible causes

G.   Idiopathic causes of chest pain are common, particularly in the pediatric population

III. Clinical Presentation

A.   Chest pain in children and adolescents
      1.   Idiopathic causes of chest pain are common in children and not associated with any abnormal finding in the history or physical examination; symptoms usually are self-limited and resolve within one year
      2.   Musculoskeletal pain often occurs and is related to exercise of infrequently used muscle groups
      3.   Psychogenic causes are also common in this age group

B.   Chest pain due to musculoskeletal factors is variable and may last from a few seconds to several days or even a month or more and may be sharp, dull or aching
      1.   Pain is aggravated by deep inspiration and cough; the chest is tender on palpation
      2.   Costochondritis is characterized by sharp, anterior chest pain at the costochondral junction (junction at the anterior ribs and sternum); may have warmth, erythema, and swelling at junction as well

C.   Nerve irritation or compression has characteristic types of chest pain (see section on HERPES ZOSTER)
      1.   Herpes zoster causes pain along dermatomes and typically precedes a persistent, vesicular rash; commonly affects immunosuppressed patients; patient may have pain along the dermatomes long after the rash has healed
      2.   Nerve root compression results in pain and motor and sensory deficits (numbness or tingling) in the neck, chest and upper arm

D.   Pleural causes of chest pain typically present as pain worsened by deep inspiration and coughing; pleural spasm secondary to cold weather and increased activity may occur
      1.   Bacterial pneumonia is one of the most common causes of pleuritic pain and is characterized by abrupt onset of fever, chills, leukocytosis, and purulent sputum (see section on PNEUMONIA)

352

2. Pulmonary embolus (PE) is another common cause of pleuritic pain; patients present with sudden onset of dyspnea, tachypnea, tachycardia, hypotension, and possibly hemoptysis; remember, however, that many patients with PE may be asymptomatic
   a. Rales and a pleural rub may be present; may exhibit decreased or absent breath sounds distal to PE
   b. May progress to acute right failure, pulmonary hypertension, or respiratory arrest
   c. Typically associated with risk factors such as immobility, surgery, pregnancy, oral contraceptives, pelvis or lower extremity trauma
   d. Patents with history of malignancy, deep venous thrombosis, previous pulmonary embolus, congestive heart failure, chronic obstructive pulmonary disease, obesity, and hypercoagulability conditions are more prone to developing a PE
3. Spontaneous pneumothorax or hemothorax secondary to trauma can cause acute, unilateral, stabbing pain with dyspnea
   a. Typically, there is decreased breath and voice sounds over the involved lung or lobe
   b. Be on the alert for mediastinal shift and cardiopulmonary compromise in these patients

E. Chest pain due to cardiac diseases may be mild to severe, transient and exertional related or constant
   1. Pericarditis may present with pleuritic pain or with steady retrosternal or left precordial pain that resembles angina
      a. Typically, the pain decreases upon sitting and leaning forward
      b. Characterized by a two- or three-component friction rub
      c. Associated signs are fever, tachycardia, pulsus paradoxus, tamponade, elevated sedimentation rate, and leukocytosis
      d. Risk factors include infection, autoimmune disease, recent myocardial infarction, cardiac surgery, malignancy, uremia, drugs such as procainamide, hydralazine, isoniazid
   2. Left ventricular outflow tract obstructive lesions (valvular aortic stenosis and pulmonic stenosis), cardiomyopathies (idiopathic hypertrophic subaortic stenosis), and coronary arterial anomalies have varying degrees of chest pain; signs of myocardial infarction and congestive heart failure may occur
      a. Patients with myocardial infarction (MI) typically complain of sudden onset of substernal pain which may radiate and is associated with dyspnea, diaphoresis, nausea, vomiting, and anxiety; pain is unrelieved by nitroglycerin and usually lasts 30 minutes or longer
      b. Patients with congestive heart failure have dyspnea, edema, and electrocardiogram changes
   3. Patients with mitral valve prolapse (MVP) are often asymptomatic, but chest pain, fatigue, palpitations (especially when lying supine on left side), lightheadedness, shortness of breath, headaches, and mood swings may be present; only 15% of patients experience moderate to severe symptoms
      a. Pain is usually fleeting and sharp and localized over the central or left chest wall; rarely radiates
      b. Pain is not relieved by nitroglycerin; usually pain is unrelated to exertion
      c. Pain may be brief or last for several days
      d. In rare cases, MVP can progress to mitral insufficiency with enlargement of left atrium and left ventricle, and congestive heart failure
      e. Hallmark diagnostic sign is a mid- to late-systolic click and late systolic murmur
      f. Echocardiogram will reveal extent of regurgitation and may reveal an abnormally thickened, redundant mitral valve
   4. Supraventricular tachycardia may cause chest pain and hypotension
   5. Cocaine-induced chest pain may present with severe, sharp, pressure-like or squeezing substernal pain
      a. Associated symptoms include euphoria, mydriasis, hyperstimulation, paranoia, delusions, followed by depression, nausea, vomiting, and muscle twitching
      b. Complications include myocardial ischemia and infarction, arrhythmias, respiratory failure, and circulatory collapse

F. Pain from disorders of the gastrointestinal system can mimic cardiovascular symptomatology
   1. Gastroesophageal reflux (uncommon in children) presents with burning, substernal pain which is related to consuming a large meal, lying down or bending over; pain is usually relieved by ingestion of antacid or food (see section on GASTROESOPHAGEAL REFLUX DISEASE)
   2. Esophageal spasm often is substernal, radiating to neck, shoulder, arm and relieved by nitroglycerin

G. Although infrequent in childhood, other gastrointestinal problems such as cholecystitis, peptic ulcer disease, and pancreatitis sometimes resemble cardiac pain, but often they can be distinguished by their association with eating and their relief from antacids

H. Chest pain may be due to psychiatric or mental health disorders
   1. Patients with psychogenic problems often describe pain as generalized, constantly present and aggravated by any effort
      a. Associated symptoms include dyspnea, fatigue, and other somatic symptoms
      b. Common in childhood and may be similar to pain described by an adult in the child's family
   2. Patients with panic disorders often have chest pain which is accompanied by intense fear, tachypnea, palpitations, diaphoresis, trembling, nausea, dizziness, and chills or hot flashes

IV. Diagnosis/Evaluation

A. History (length of history will depend on patient's clinical presentation; perform a rapid history for any patient with a suspected emergent condition)
   1. Determine whether onset was sudden, gradual, recurrent, or new
   2. Ask patient to describe the pain's location, regions of radiation, quality, intensity, and duration
   3. Determine the quantity of pain, possibly on a scale from 0 to 10 with 10 being the worst pain ever experienced and 0 indicating no pain which is the ultimate goal
   4. Inquire about aggravating factors such as exercise, stress, food intake, movement, coughing
   5. Inquire about relieving factors such as rest, use of nitroglycerin, antacids, intake of food
   6. Ask about associated symptoms such as dyspnea, hemoptysis, fever, chills, sputum production, exanthem, diaphoresis, dizziness, syncope, nausea, diarrhea
   7. Determine whether patient has a coexistent viral illness or if other members of the household have a viral disease
   8. Explore stress-related factors in the patient's school, work or home environments
   9. Ask about risk factors for ischemic heart disease
   10. Explore past medical history
   11. Inquire about family history of chest pain and cardiovascular disease

B. Physical Examination
   1. Observe general appearance of patient, assessing for level of distress and anxiety
   2. Measure vital signs. Take blood pressure in both arms; if unable to detect, use Doppler and/or take thigh pressure to assess presence and compare with arm pressures
   3. Measure height and weight (growth delays suggest a serious organic problem)
   4. Inspect skin for pallor, cyanosis, jaundice, or herpetic rash
   5. Examine eyes, including funduscopy
   6. Auscultate carotid pulse for bruits
   7. Assess neck for lymphadenopathy, thyromegaly, midline trachea, jugular venous distention, bruits
   8. Perform a complete examination of the heart, noting extra heart sounds, murmurs, clicks, rubs, or irregular irregularities
   9. Examine chest wall for herpes lesions and signs of trauma
   10. Palpate chest wall noting tenderness and swelling
   11. Auscultate lungs for equal breath sounds, a pleural rub, and crackles and wheezes
   12. Auscultate abdomen for bowel sounds and bruits

13. Palpate abdomen for tenderness and masses (particularly in the right upper quadrant and epigastrium), organomegaly, bounding pulses, and ascites
14. Palpate for femoral pulses (with absent pulses suspect dissecting abdominal aortic aneurysm)
15. Assess lower extremities for cyanosis, diminished pulses, unilateral swelling, and other signs of phlebitis
16. Patients who present with pain that changes with movement should have a musculoskeletal and neurological exam performed, focusing on focal tenderness, muscular weakness, and motor and sensory deficits

C. Differential Diagnosis: All conditions listed under pathogenesis should be included in the differential diagnosis; generally, pain should be considered cardiovascular and life threatening until proven otherwise
1. The type of pain pattern is helpful at arriving at a diagnosis
   a. Pain brought on by exertion and relieved with rest suggests cardiac or psychogenic pain (psychogenic pain, however, usually is accompanied by a myriad of noncardiac symptoms such as headache, hyperventilation)
   b. Pain which worsens upon deep inspiration or cough suggests a pleural, pericardial or chest wall source; focal tenderness along with pain on inspiration suggests costochondritis
   c. Pain relieved by leaning forward and aggravated by lying supine suggests pericarditis
   d. Pain with a sudden onset and dyspnea suggests pneumothorax or pulmonary edema (PE); lean towards diagnosis of PE if patient has a risk for thrombophlebitis or has had a recent fracture
   e. Pain occurring with eating suggests esophageal, biliary, pancreatic, and peptic disease
   f. Risk factors provide important information to arrive at a diagnosis
   g. Quality, location, radiation, and intensity of pain are nonspecific symptoms and are usually not helpful in arriving at a diagnosis

D. Diagnostic tests are based on the information collected in the history and physical examination; not every patient needs a routine chest x-ray and electrocardiogram (ECG)
1. Consider pulse oximetry to assess for either oxygen desaturation or oxygen saturation in patients with suspected cardiac and pulmonary problems
2. Order an ECG in patients with suspected cardiac disease
3. Echocardiography is helpful in diagnosing mitral valve prolapse, pericarditis, and to assess for wall motion and ejection fraction
4. Consider ordering a chest x-ray in the following cases:
   a. Suspected chest trauma such as rib fractures
   b. Suspected pulmonary diseases such as pneumonia or tuberculosis
   c. Suspected pneumothorax or pulmonary embolus
5. Consider a lung scan or ventilation scan for a patient with suspected PE
6. Consider gram stain of sputum for suspected pulmonary infections and acid-fasts stains for suspected tuberculosis

V. Plan/Management

A. Relief of pain is based on the etiology

B. Treatment of musculoskeletal problems such as costochondritis is usually symptomatic (see sections within MUSCULOSKELETAL topic)
1. Apply local heat
2. For adolescents, prescribe nonsteroidal anti-inflammatory drugs such as ibuprofen (Motrin) 400-800 mg every 4-8 hours. Prescribe acetaminophen 10 mg/kg/dose for children

C. Treatment of pulmonary problems
1. Pneumonia (see section on PNEUMONIA)
2. Pulmonary embolus requires hospitalization and intravenous anticoagulation; typically patient is then placed on long-term anticoagulation

3. Carefully assess vital signs and watch for mediastinal shift in patients with a pneumothorax
   a. A small, stable pneumothorax without evidence of respiratory compromise requires only observation for several days until stabilization and resolution
   b. Hospitalization and insertion of chest tubes is needed for a large, expanding tension pneumothorax

D. Treatment of cardiac pain
   1. Referral to cardiologist is recommended for structural heart problems, myopathies, infections, and arrhythmias
   2. Mitral valve prolapse
      a. No specific treatment is indicated for most patients, except for reassurance about a good prognosis
      b. The major therapeutic dilemma is whether to recommend antibiotic prophylaxis for infective endocarditis when certain invasive procedures are performed
         (1) Patients with MVP who have mitral regurgitation and/or thickened leaflets should have prophylaxis (see procedure for prophylaxis of bacterial endocarditis in section on RHEUMATIC HEART DISEASE)
         (2) Prophylaxis is also recommended for patients with MVP who have a murmur of mitral regurgitation, but not in those who have only a click
         (3) If there is uncertainty about the diagnosis of mitral regurgitation refer to cardiologist
      c. Patients with severe mitral regurgitation may require valve surgery
      d. Patients with annoying arrhythmias may benefit from a beta-blocker such as atenolol (Tenormin)

E. Treatment of abdominal problems (see section on GASTROINTESTINAL PROBLEMS)

F. Patient Education
   1. To avoid cardiac neurosis carefully explain to the patient or parents that a thorough history and physical exam revealed no abnormality
   2. Allow time for the patient to express concerns and questions
   3. Teach risk factors for cardiac and ulcer disease and strategies to reduce risks

G. Follow up is variable depending on diagnosis and patient's condition

HYPERTENSION IN CHILDREN

I. Definitions:

   A. Normal blood pressure (BP): systolic and diastolic BP less than the 90th percentile for age and sex

   B. High-normal BP: average systolic or diastolic BP greater than or equal to the 90th percentile but less than 95th percentile

   C. Hypertension: average systolic or diastolic BP greater than or equal to the 95th percentile for age and sex measured on at least three separate times

II. Pathogenesis

   A. Primary or essential hypertension has no identifiable cause
      1. A familial influence on BP occurs early in life
      2. Mild to moderate hypertension in children older than 10 years is usually essential hypertension

356

B. Secondary hypertension is the usual cause of high blood pressure in children younger than 10 years
    1. Approximately 80% of cases of secondary hypertension are related to renal disorders
    2. Hyperthyroidism, sleeping apnea, or hypercalcemia are less common causes

C. Transient hypertension or an acute, short-lived elevation of blood pressure is often related to acute illness or ingestion of oral contraceptives or anabolic steroids

D. Labile hypertension occurs predominantly in adolescents and is due to stressful events

E. Severe, abrupt onset of elevated blood pressure is usually a result of poor control of the chronically hypertensive patient but can be due to head trauma, drug reactions, acute glomerulonephritis, pregnancy, and pheochromocytoma

III. Clinical Presentation

A. Hypertension in childhood is a risk factor for the development of true hypertension in adulthood

B. A direct relationship between weight and BP has been documented as early as 5 years of age; most children and adolescents with hypertension are overweight and have family histories of hypertension

C. Height is independently related to BP at all ages

D. African-American and Asian-American children have higher BPs than Caucasian children

E. Primary hypertension is often asymptomatic and detected by routine screening

F. Secondary hypertension occurs most frequently during infancy and late childhood; symptoms include dizziness, headaches and changes in vision

G. Severe, abrupt onset of elevated blood pressure can lead to encephalopathy, cardiac failure, acute renal failure, and loss of vision if not corrected immediately

IV. Diagnosis/Evaluation

A. History
    1. Inquire about associated symptoms such as headaches, dizziness, visual changes and other neurological problems
    2. Explore risk factors for developing cardiovascular disease such as family history, obesity, diet, smoking and physical inactivity
    3. In adolescents, explore use of oral contraceptive, anabolic steroids, alcohol, cocaine or other addictive substances
    4. Obtain a complete medical history, focusing on cardiac, renal and genetic disorders
    5. Obtain a complete family history of both first- and second-degree relatives
    6. Explore psychosocial and environmental factors that might affect BP control

B. Physical Examination
    1. Measure blood pressure in all extremities; measure blood pressure lying, sitting, and standing (in infants and very young children use automated devices for measurement)
        a. For consistency and comparison use the right arm for measurement
        b. Use the appropriate cuff size: choose a cuff with a bladder width that is approximately 40% of arm circumference midway between the olecranon and the acromion
        c. Measure BP in controlled environment, after 3-5 minutes of rest, in seated position with cubital fossa supported at heart level
        d. Record at least twice on each occasion and arrive at an average of each of the systolic and diastolic BP measurements
        e. The fifth Korotkoff sound (K5), or the disappearance of Korotkoff sounds is used as the definition of diastolic pressure

2.   Measure height and weight and plot on growth charts
3.   Do a complete eye exam, including funduscopy
4.   Assess the neck for thyromegaly, bruits, and distended veins
5.   Palpate, percuss, and auscultate the heart
6.   Auscultate the lungs
7.   Assess for abdominal bruits
8.   Palpate abdomen for hepatomegaly, splenomegaly and enlarged kidneys or masses
9.   Inspect and palpate extremities, noting edema, decreased femoral and pedal pulses, and temperature and color changes
10. Perform a complete neurological exam
11. For infants and neonates determine BP level percentiles (see table that follows)

NEONATES AND CHILDREN <1 YEAR: BLOOD PRESSURE CLASSIFICATION		
Age Group	Significant Hypertension mm Hg	Severe Hypertension mm Hg
Newborn - 7 days	Systolic BP ≥96	Systolic BP ≥106
Neonate - 8 days -30 days	Systolic BP ≥104	Systolic BP ≥110
Infant (<1 year)	Systolic BP ≥112 Diastolic BP ≥74	Systolic BP ≥118 Diastolic BP ≥82

Adapted from National, Heart, Lung, and Blood Institute. (1987). Report of the second task force on blood pressure control in children--1987. Pediatrics, 79, 1-19.

12. For children >1 year old determine BP level percentiles: after documenting height percentile from standard growth charts, child's measured systolic and diastolic BP is compared with numbers in the following tables (boys or girls) for age and height percentiles (see following tables)

C.   Differential Diagnosis
1.   Goal is to differentiate essential or primary hypertension from elevated blood pressure due to secondary causes
2.   The younger the child and the higher the blood pressure, the greater the possibility of secondary hypertension

D.   Diagnostic Tests
1.   Order complete blood count, serum creatinine, electrolytes, blood urea nitrogen, serum uric acid, urinalysis, urine culture, and plasma renin activity
2.   Optional, baseline tests are echocardiogram, chest x-ray, and cholesterol level
3.   Less frequently ordered are renal imaging tests, 24-hour urine collection for creatinine clearance and protein, computerized tomography and hormone studies
4.   Genetic types of hypertension such as glucocorticoid-remediable aldosteronism can be detected from blood sent to centers which perform genetic testing

V.   Plan/Management

A.   Treat all causes of secondary hypertension

B.   Life style modifications should be introduced and used as initial therapy in children with essential hypertension
1.   Dietary recommendations
     a.   Weight reduction in obese children
     b.   Increase fresh fruits and vegetables in diet; eliminate added salt to home-cooked meals, and reduce foods with high sodium content
     c.   Decrease fat in diet; decrease access to "fast food" restaurants
2.   Regular exercise is recommended. Uncomplicated, primary hypertension should not prevent asymptomatic children from participating in physical activity
3.   Identification and reduction of stressors are important
4.   Counsel about other risk factors for cardiovascular disease such as smoking

BOYS AGED 1-17 YEARS: BLOOD PRESSURE LEVELS FOR THE 90TH AND 95TH PERCENTILES OF BLOOD PRESSURE BY PERCENTILES OF HEIGHT

Age, y	Blood Pressure Percentile	Systolic Blood Pressure by Percentile of Height, mm Hg							Diastolic Blood Pressure by Percentile of Height, mm Hg						
		5%	10%	25%	50%	75%	90%	95%	5%	10%	25%	50%	75%	90%	95%
1	90th	94	95	97	98	100	102	102	50	51	52	53	54	54	55
	95th	98	99	101	102	104	106	106	55	55	56	57	58	59	59
2	90th	98	99	100	102	104	105	106	55	55	56	57	58	59	59
	95th	101	102	104	106	108	109	110	59	59	60	61	62	63	63
3	90th	100	101	103	105	107	108	109	59	59	60	61	62	63	63
	95th	104	105	107	109	111	112	113	63	63	64	65	66	67	67
4	90th	102	103	105	107	109	110	111	62	62	63	64	65	66	66
	95th	106	107	109	111	113	114	115	66	67	67	68	69	70	71
5	90th	104	105	106	108	110	112	112	65	65	66	67	68	69	69
	95th	108	109	110	112	114	115	116	69	70	70	71	72	73	74
6	90th	105	106	108	110	111	113	114	67	68	69	70	70	71	72
	95th	109	110	112	114	115	117	117	72	72	73	74	75	76	76
7	90th	106	107	109	111	113	114	115	69	70	71	72	72	73	74
	95th	110	111	113	115	116	118	119	74	74	75	76	77	78	78
8	90th	107	108	110	112	114	115	116	71	71	72	73	74	75	75
	95th	111	112	114	116	118	119	120	75	76	76	77	78	79	80
9	90th	109	110	112	113	115	117	117	72	73	73	74	75	76	77
	95th	113	114	116	117	119	121	121	76	77	78	79	80	80	81
10	90th	110	112	113	115	117	118	119	73	74	74	75	76	77	78
	95th	114	115	117	119	121	122	123	77	78	79	80	80	81	82
11	90th	112	113	115	117	119	120	121	74	74	75	76	77	78	78
	95th	116	117	119	121	123	124	125	78	79	79	80	81	82	83
12	90th	115	116	117	119	121	123	123	75	75	76	77	78	78	79
	95th	119	120	121	123	125	126	127	79	79	80	81	82	83	83
13	90th	117	118	120	122	124	125	126	75	76	76	77	78	79	80
	95th	121	122	124	126	128	129	130	79	80	81	82	83	83	84
14	90th	120	121	123	125	126	128	128	76	76	77	78	79	80	80
	95th	124	125	127	128	130	132	132	80	81	81	82	83	84	85
15	90th	123	124	125	127	129	131	131	77	77	78	79	80	81	81
	95th	127	128	129	131	133	134	135	81	82	83	83	84	85	86
16	90th	125	126	128	130	132	133	134	79	79	80	81	82	82	83
	95th	129	130	132	134	136	137	138	83	83	84	85	86	87	87
17	90th	128	129	131	133	134	136	136	81	81	82	83	84	85	85
	95th	132	133	135	136	138	140	140	85	85	86	87	88	89	89

Source: National High Blood Pressure Education Program Working Group on Hypertension Control in Children and Adolescents. (1996). Pediatrics, 98, 649-658.

GIRLS AGED 1-17 YEARS: BLOOD PRESSURE LEVELS FOR THE 90TH AND 95TH PERCENTILES OF BLOOD PRESSURE BY PERCENTILES OF HEIGHT

Age, y	Blood Pressure Percentile	Systolic Blood Pressure by Percentile of Height, mm Hg							Diastolic Blood Pressure by Percentile of Height, mm Hg						
		5%	10%	25%	50%	75%	90%	95%	5%	10%	25%	50%	75%	90%	95%
1	90th	97	98	99	100	102	103	104	53	53	53	54	55	56	56
	95th	101	102	103	104	105	107	107	57	57	57	58	59	60	60
2	90th	99	99	100	102	103	104	105	57	57	58	58	59	60	61
	95th	102	103	104	105	107	108	109	61	61	62	62	63	64	65
3	90th	100	100	102	103	104	105	106	61	61	61	62	63	63	64
	95th	104	104	105	107	108	109	110	65	65	65	66	67	67	68
4	90th	101	102	103	104	106	107	108	63	63	64	65	65	66	67
	95th	105	106	107	108	109	111	111	67	67	68	69	69	70	71
5	90th	103	103	104	106	107	108	109	65	66	66	67	68	68	69
	95th	107	107	108	110	111	112	113	69	70	70	71	72	72	73
6	90th	104	105	106	107	109	110	111	67	67	68	69	69	70	71
	95th	108	109	110	111	112	114	114	71	71	72	73	73	74	75
7	90th	106	107	108	109	110	112	112	69	69	69	70	71	72	72
	95th	110	110	112	113	114	115	116	73	73	73	74	75	76	76
8	90th	108	109	110	111	112	113	114	70	70	71	71	72	73	74
	95th	112	112	113	115	116	117	118	74	74	75	75	76	77	78
9	90th	110	110	112	113	114	115	116	71	72	72	73	74	74	75
	95th	114	114	115	117	118	119	120	75	76	76	77	78	78	79
10	90th	112	112	114	115	116	117	118	73	73	73	74	75	76	76
	95th	116	116	117	119	120	121	122	77	77	77	78	79	80	80
11	90th	114	114	116	117	118	119	120	74	74	75	75	76	77	77
	95th	118	118	119	121	122	123	124	78	78	79	79	80	81	81
12	90th	116	116	118	119	120	121	122	75	75	76	76	77	78	78
	95th	120	120	121	123	124	125	126	79	79	80	80	81	82	82
13	90th	118	118	119	121	122	123	124	76	76	77	78	78	79	80
	95th	121	122	123	125	126	127	128	80	80	81	82	82	83	84
14	90th	119	120	121	122	124	125	126	77	77	78	79	79	80	81
	95th	123	124	125	126	128	129	130	81	81	82	83	83	84	85
15	90th	121	121	122	124	125	126	127	78	78	79	79	80	81	82
	95th	124	125	126	128	129	130	131	82	82	83	83	84	85	86
16	90th	122	122	123	125	126	127	128	79	79	79	80	81	82	82
	95th	125	126	127	128	130	131	132	83	83	83	84	85	86	86
17	90th	122	123	124	125	126	128	128	79	79	79	80	81	82	82
	95th	126	126	127	129	130	131	132	83	83	83	84	85	86	86

Source: National High Blood Pressure Education Program Working Group on Hypertension Control in Children and Adolescents. (1996). Pediatrics, 98, 649-658.

C. Pharmacologic therapy (consultation with a specialist is recommended)
    1. Goal is to reduce BP to below the 95th percentile
    2. Diuretics and beta-blockers were recommended almost exclusively in the first task force report and these drugs are helpful; other classes of drugs are considered beneficial in the 2nd task force report
        a. ACE inhibitors
            (1) Do not prescribe in patients with bilateral renal artery stenosis or renal artery stenosis in a solitary or transplanted kidney
            (2) ACE inhibitors (and angiotensin II receptor blockers) have teratogenic risks with fetal exposure; use these drugs with extreme caution in adolescent girls who may be sexually active
        b. Calcium channel blockers: Use cautiously because of possible adverse cardiac effects that have occurred in adults
    3. Individualize therapy based on level of BP, degree of response, occurrence of adverse effects, and child's medical history (see following table)

ANTIHYPERTENSIVE MEDICATIONS IN CHILDREN

Medication	Dose mg/kg/day Initial-Maximum	Dosing Interval	Route
Diuretics			
Hydrochlorothiazide	1-3	q 12 hours	oral
Furosemide	1-12	q 4-12 hours	oral
Metolazone	0.1-3	q 12-24 hours	oral
Triamterene	2-3	q 6-12 hours	oral
Spironolactone	1-3	q 6-12 hours	oral, intravenous
Adrenergic Blocking			
β Adrenergic blockers			
Metoprolol	1-4	q 12 hours	oral
Propranolol	1-8	q 6-12 hours	oral
Atenolol	1-8	q 12-24 hours	oral
α blocker, Prazosin	0.05-0.5	q 6-8 hours	oral
α/β blocker, labetalol	1-3	q 6-12 hours	oral, intravenous
α-Agonist, Clonidine	0.05*-0.5**	q 6 hours	oral
Angiotensin-converting enzyme inhibitor			
Captopril			
Neonates	0.03-2	q 8-24 hours	oral
Children	1.5-6	q 8 hours	oral
Enalapril	0.15-not established	q 12-24 hours	oral
Calcium antagonists			
Nifedipine	0.25-3	q 4-6 hours	oral
Nifedipine XL	0.25-3	q 12-24 hours	oral
Vasodilators			
Hydralazine	0.75-7.5	q 6 hours	oral, intravenous
Minoxidil	0.1-1	q 12 hours	oral

*Total initial dose in milligrams
**Total daily dose in milligrams

Adapted from National High Blood Pressure Education Program Working Group on Hypertension Control in Children and Adolescents. (1996). Update on the 1987 task force report on high blood pressure in children and adolescents. Pediatrics, 98, 649-658.

D. Children with associated diabetes mellitus may benefit from antihypertensive drug therapy to maintain BP below the 90th percentile

E. Acute hypertensive therapy consists of one of the following medications: oral nifedipine, IV sodium nitroprusside, IV labetalol, IV esmolol, IV diazoxide, IV hydralazine, oral minoxidil; consult specialist in pediatric hypertension for dosage

F.   Follow Up
1.   Children with elevated blood pressure detected on screening, should have blood pressure measured 2 more times before the diagnosis of hypertension is made; time intervals between measurements are dependent on degree of elevation
2.   Frequency of follow up is variable depending on patient characteristics and physiological status

INNOCENT HEART MURMURS

I.   Definition: Vibrations of normal structures within the heart which occur in the absence of structural or physiologic cardiac disease; other synonymous terms are normal, functional, benign, innocuous, or physiological murmur

II.   Pathogenesis: Caused by turbulent blood flow in the normal heart

III. Clinical Presentation

A.   Innocent heart murmur occurs in almost 50% of all school-aged children

B.   Approximately 80% of all children with murmurs have one of the following innocent murmurs:
1.   Classic vibratory murmur (Still's)
a.   Most common functional murmur
b.   Characteristic feature is the vibratory, buzzing quality
c.   Nonradiating, midsystolic, short, low-pitched murmur
d.   Heard best with the bell of the stethoscope and along the lower, left sternal edge, at the third to fourth left interspace
e.   Heard best when child is supine, diminishes in upright position
f.   When child holds breath or performs a Valsalva maneuver the murmur usually disappears
g.   Accompanied with normal first and second heart sounds and no extra sounds or other cardiac abnormalities
h.   Most typically heard in children 2-6 years old; uncommon before age 2 years, but heard in 50% of healthy children by age 3 or 4
2.   Venous hum
a.   Continuous humming murmur heard above and sometimes below the clavicle on one or both sides; louder in diastole
b.   Normal second heart sound
c.   Best heard in sitting or standing position
d.   Can be obliterated by having child turn head to side, compressing external jugular vein, or assumption of supine position
e.   Commonly occurs between 3 and 6 years of age
3.   Pulmonic flow murmur
a.   Heard best at upper left sternal border
b.   Short, midsystolic murmur with 3/6 or less intensity and rough sound
c.   Normal second heart sound
4.   Pulmonary flow murmur of newborn or peripheral pulmonary murmur
a.   Vibratory
b.   Heard best in pulmonic area and radiates to both axilla and possibly, back
c.   Frequently heard in infants and small children; usually disappears by 4-6 months of age
5.   Carotid bruit
a.   Grade 3/6 or less intensity
b.   Systolic murmur with normal second heart sound
c.   Heard over carotid artery

6. Pulmonary souffle or mammary arterial souffle
   a. Soft, blowing, early to midsystolic murmur heard best in the pulmonic area
   b. Occurs in adolescence and in young adult females who are pregnant or lactating
   c. Heard in high cardiac output states such as fever, anemia, or hyperthyroidism

IV. Diagnosis/Evaluation

A. History
   1. Ask about symptoms related to cardiovascular dysfunction such as failure to thrive, syncope, chest pain, palpitation, and shortness of breath
   2. Question regarding child's activity level and endurance; in an infant, question about ability to vigorously suck when feeding
   3. Carefully take comprehensive prenatal and perinatal histories
   4. Obtain a complete medical history including past hospitalizations, frequency of infections, and previous illnesses
   5. Inquire about family history, particularly explore history of hypertrophic cardiomyopathy, congenital cardiac disease, and unexplained death at any age

B. Physical Examination
   1. Observe for general body habitus and nutritional status; chromosomal disorders are associated with structural cardiac disease
   2. Inspect skin for color; differentiate central from peripheral cyanosis
      a. Central cyanosis denotes an elevated percentage of reduced hemoglobin in arterial blood and usually requires referral to cardiologist: observe for cyanosis in inner portion of lips, tongue and nail beds
      b. Peripheral cyanosis or acrocyanosis is related to a normal level of reduced hemoglobin and normal oximetry readings; cyanosis may be present in healthy children around mouth and on hands and feet
   3. Assess temperature and moisture of skin
   4. Measure temperature, pulse rate, and respiratory rate
   5. Measure blood pressure in both arms and leg
   6. Examine neck for thyromegaly, distended veins
   7. Auscultate neck for bruits; palpate the cardiac apex while simultaneously listening to bruit to differentiate a bruit from a murmur; a radiating murmur will be synchronous with apical impulse whereas a bruit will occur later
   8. Inspect chest for precordial bulge and observe for asymmetry of chest which reflects long-standing enlargement of the heart
   9. Palpate chest for thrill, heave and locate point of maximal impulse (PMI)
   10. Auscultate heart
   11. Perform techniques to elicit murmurs
      a. Compare murmur when patient is standing versus sitting (standing reduces systemic venous return to the heart and lowers both right and left ventricular diastolic filling volume and may reduce intensity of murmur)
      b. Listen to murmur when child squats for 30 seconds and then when child quickly rises to a standing position
      c. Place patient on left, lateral side which brings the heart closer to the lateral wall which may increase murmurs
      d. Ask child to perform Valsalva maneuver by exhaling and holding breath midway through cycle
      e. In young children, passive raising of the legs to about 45° is helpful

12.   Assess the murmur for following characteristics (see table below)

CHARACTERISTICS OF CARDIAC MURMURS	
Characteristic	**Examples**
Timing	Relative position within cardiac cycle; relationship to S1 and S2 (systolic, diastolic, continuous)
Quality	Presence of harmonics and overtones (harsh, soft, vibratory, musical)
Intensity	Loudness (see table below on grades of murmurs): Systolic graded on scale of I to VI Diastolic graded on scale of I to IV
Duration	Length (midsystolic, holosystolic)
Location	Area where murmur is loudest (point of maximal impulse)
Radiation of sound	Direction of murmur
Configuration	Dynamic shape
Pitch	Frequency range (low, medium, high)

13.   Grade the murmur based on degree of loudness and presence of a thrill (palpable sensation)

GRADES OF HEART MURMURS	
Grade I	Very faint; may not be heard in all positions
Grade II	Quiet, but heard immediately upon placing stethoscope on chest
Grade III	Moderately loud but not associated with a thrill
Grade IV	Loud and may be associated with a thrill
Grade V	Very loud and associated with a thrill
Grade VI	Heard with stethoscope off the chest; accompanied with thrill

14.   Perform a complete lung exam
15.   Palpate abdomen for organomegaly
16.   Examine extremities for pulses, edema, color, and clubbing of nails

C.   Differential Diagnosis:
1.   Crucial to distinguish a pathological murmur from an innocent murmur; quality and characteristics of murmur do not always provide reliable criteria for diagnosis (atrial septal defects, hypertrophic cardiomyopathy, and coarctation of aorta produce relatively unimpressive murmurs); however, innocent murmurs are more likely to have the following characteristics
    a.   Systolic in timing (except venous hum)
    b.   Quality is often vibratory or blowing and low pitched
    c.   Intensity is often grade II or less
    d.   Localized without radiation
    e.   Short in duration
    f.   Heard most commonly either at the second left interspace or halfway between the lower left sternal border and apex
    g.   Presence and intensity vary or disappear with change in positions
    h.   Accompanied with no extra heart sounds
2.   Patient's age at onset of mumur and physical findings help to differentiate pathological murmurs from innocent murmurs
    a.   Consider all murmurs in infants less than one year as pathological until proven otherwise
    b.   In first year of life, poor feeding, excessive irritability, tachypnea, and central cyanosis are signs suggestive of cardiovascular instability

3. The following table illustrates the differential diagnosis of abnormal murmurs

DIFFERENTIAL DIAGNOSIS OF ABNORMAL MURMURS*		
Timing of Murmur	Pathology	Characteristics
Midsystolic	Pulmonic stenosis	Variable click, left sternal border
	Aortic stenosis	Loud, harsh, constant click, apex
	Atrial septal defect	Diastolic rumble, wide fixed S2, left lower sternal border
	Ventricular septal defect (small)	Blowing, left lower sternal border
	Coarctation	Weak femoral pulses
Late systolic	Mitral valve prolapse	Murmur may or may not be present, variable apical click
	Hypertrophic cardiomyopathy	Biphasic carotid pulse
Holosystolic	Ventricular septal defect	Apical diastolic rumble, loud S2
	Mitral regurgitation	Blowing murmur, radiates to left axilla, heard best in apex
Diastolic	Aortic regurgitation	High pitch, left third ICS, radiates down
	Atrial septal defect or ventricular septal defect	Diastolic rumble due to high flow across AV valve
Continuous	Patent ductus arteriosus	Systolic-diastolic murmur

* Patients with abnormal murmurs are usually referred to a cardiologist;
See section on RHEUMATIC HEART DISEASE for prevention or prophylaxis recommendations for bacterial endocarditis

D. Diagnostic Tests: Innocent heart murmurs often do not need diagnostic tests. If there is any question about the type of murmur consider the following:
   1. Echocardiogram is ordered if child is thought to have cardiac disease or if diagnosis is uncertain (American Academy of Pediatrics recommends that all echocardiograms be evaluated by a pediatric cardiologist)
   2. Consider ordering electrocardiogram and chest x-ray [whereas previous studies found these tests unreliable in determining murmur type, a recent study (Swenson, et al., 1997) found them to be valuable in the initial assessment of children with murmurs and/or chest pain]
   3. In some cases, consider hemoglobin level to determine anemia or polycythemia which is a sensitive indicator for chronic hypoxemia
   4. Once diagnosis of innocent murmur is made, no further diagnostic tests are needed

V. Plan/Management

   A. If it is uncertain whether the murmur is innocent, studies have found that the most cost-effective approach is referral to a pediatric cardiologist

   B. Emphasize to the parents that the child does not have heart disease and that nearly half of all children have an innocent murmur during childhood; inform parents that the murmur may become louder when the child has a fever or strenuously exercises; stress that the child does not need antibiotic prophylaxis against infective endocarditis when visiting the dentist nor should child limit activities due to risk of sudden death

   C. Follow Up: Assess child, at each health maintenance visit, carefully documenting the characteristics of the murmur

PRESYNCOPE/SYNCOPE

I.   Definitions:

    A.   Presyncope: Sensation of dizziness, lightheadedness and an impending loss of consciousness

    B.   Syncope: Sudden transient loss of consciousness with concurrent loss of postural tone with spontaneous recovery

II.   Pathogenesis

    A.   Usually due to any mechanism that decreases cerebral blood flow; results in decreased delivery of oxygen and nutrients to brain

    B.   Pathophysiologic abnormalities underlying syncope
        1.   Reflex-mediated vasomotor instability associated with a decrease in vascular resistance and/or venous return
            a.   Conditions are usually benign and include vasovagal episodes, situational syncope, orthostatic hypotension, drugs, carotid sinus disorder, and psychiatric illnesses
            b.   Vasovagal episodes are most common cause of presyncope/syncope; simple faint accounts for majority of syncopal episodes in children
        2.   Cardiac causes associated with decreased cardiac output or obstruction of blood flow within heart or pulmonary circulation
            a.   Electrical etiology such as arrhythmias and heart block
            b.   Mechanical etiology such as idiopathic hypertrophic subaortic stenosis, valvular diseases, myxoma, myocardial infarction, and aortic dissection
        3.   Neurologic causes such as cerebrovascular diseases, subclavian steal syndrome, seizures, and migraines
        4.   Metabolic causes such as hypoglycemia, hypoxia, and hyperventilation; these disorders usually lead to somnolence and coma rather than syncope

    C.   Most common causes are vasovagal episodes, heart disease and arrhythmias, orthostatic hypotension and seizures

    D.   Approximately 48% of all patients who have syncope have an unexplained cause

III. Clinical Presentation of Important Causes of Presyncope/Syncope; in children most syncopal episodes are vasovagal in origin but other causes must be ruled out

    A.   Vasovagal syncope or the common faint (psychological activation of the autonomic system which causes an intense vagal drive)
        1.   Results in transient decrease in cardiac output
        2.   Often precipitated by fear, anxiety, alcohol, a large meal, or prolonged standing
        3.   Symptoms occur in the standing or seated position
        4.   Typically patient has prodromal symptoms such as nausea, warmth, lightheadedness, weakness, diaphoresis, constriction of visual fields, epigastric discomfort and a sensation of impending faint
        5.   At first, patient has increased heart rate, but then becomes bradycardic
        6.   In recovery stage the patient may have weakness, lightheadedness, fatigue but no confusion or signs of injury; usually after the episode, the patient remembers the event and does not have loss or bowel and bladder
        7.   Occasionally, hypotension and hypoperfusion are so profound that cerebral hypoxia and seizure activity occur, but there is no loss of consciousness

B. Orthostatic hypotension
1. Reflex vasoconstriction and increase in heart rate fail to occur when the patient stands, leading to inadequate cerebral perfusion
2. Defined as systolic blood pressure fall of 20 mm Hg or more on standing
3. Possible etiologic factors
   a. Condition may be idiopathic; often this type occurs after patient has been exposed to a warm environment
   b. Medications such as diuretics and autonomic blocking agents
   c. Blood loss often due to a gastrointestinal bleed
   d. Dehydration

C. Drug-induced syncope is most likely when patients are taking nitrates, vasodilators, β-blockers, antidepressants, analgesics, and central nervous system antidepressants

D. Psychological distress often involves circumoral numbness and digital paresthesia
1. Patients often have a history of generalized anxiety disorder, panic disorder, somatization, or depression
2. Estimated that up to 20% of patients presenting with syncope have psychiatric illness

E. Typical presentation of syncope due to cardiac disease
1. Symptoms often worsen on standing and improve with lying down; although patients with arrhythmias may have symptoms when supine
2. May have generalized weakness, fatigue, and pallor; some patients are asymptomatic

F. Arrhythmia often present with brief loss of consciousness, lack of prodrome, and palpitations

G. Seizures may have signs and symptoms of blue face, frothing at mouth, and disorientation after the event which are not common with other types of syncope

IV. Diagnosis/Evaluation (see also section on VERTIGO)

A. History; it is important to determine whether patient has a cardiac disease with a possible poor prognosis or a more benign condition
1. Ask patient to briefly describe in own words the sensation he/she experiences.
2. If possible obtain a description of the episode and events preceding the episode from a witness
3. Differentiate feelings of fainting from vertigo, imbalance, fatigue, weakness, or anxiety; specifically ask the following types of questions:
   a. Is there a sensation of movement or rotation? (vertigo)
   b. Is the sensation similar to when you get out of bed too quickly? (orthostatic hypotension)
   c. Does it feel like you can't keep your balance? (disequilibrium)
4. Ascertain that patient did not actually lose consciousness which may indicate an emergent problem
5. Ask about frequency of syncopal or near syncopal episodes, even though frequency does not correlate well with specific causes
6. Ask about duration of episode; brief duration is more common with vestibular disorders
7. Inquire about associated symptoms such as hearing loss, heart palpitations, neurological problems
8. Determine if sensation occurs after exertion and when one arises to sitting or standing position, which suggests cardiac disease
   a. Disequilibrium occurs primarily when one is standing or walking
   b. Benign positional vertigo often occurs with a change of position or when lying down
9. Determine precipitants such as cough with loss of consciousness (post-tussive syncope), emptying of distended bladder (postmicturition syncope), warm, crowded environment (simple faint), or shaving or tight collar (carotid sinus hypersensitivity)

10. Ask about symptoms occurring after episode; disorientation after an event is most common in patients who have seizures
11. Inquire about past medical history including history of cardiac disease or risk factors, trauma, infection, seizures, thyroid disease, metabolic problems, anxiety and medication/drug use

B. Physical Examination
1. Vital signs should include check for orthostatic hypotension (see following table)

DETERMINING ORTHOSTATIC HYPOTENSION
• Measure in lying position first.
• After patients stands for 2-5 minutes, measure again.
• Normally, systolic pressure falls no more than 10 mm, diastolic pressures rises 2-5 mm, and heart rate increases 5-20 beats (if there is no increase in heart rate, consider a cardiac problem).

2. Measure blood pressure in both arms; differences in pulse intensity and blood pressure (more than 20 mm Hg) in two arms suggests aortic dissection
3. Perform careful cardiac examination noting forceful left ventricular impulse, murmurs, or arrhythmias
4. Auscultate neck for carotid bruits
5. Perform thorough neurological examination.
6. Dizziness simulation tests such as following:
   a. Valsalva maneuvers
   b. Carotid sinus massages help to determine autonomic impairment; tests should be done cautiously in facilities where cardiac monitoring and emergency equipment are available; if patient has bruits or history of cardiac or cardiovascular disease, massage should be performed by a specialist
7. Determine if hyperventilation evokes symptomatology by asking patient to breathe rapidly for 1-3 minutes
8. Complete psychiatric examination is often needed

C. Differential Diagnosis: One way to sort out the many causes of dizziness is to differentiate the sensations the patient experiences into 3 categories:
1. Presyncope/syncope: feeling of lightheadedness or feeling that one is about to faint
2. Vertigo: Sensation of abnormal movements of the body or surroundings (see section on VERTIGO)
3. Disequilibrium or imbalance due to multiple sensory deficits: Sensation of feeling drunk, seasick, or unsteady on one's feet; subtle, enduring symptom that one cannot quite keep balance and might fall

D. Diagnostic Tests; routine laboratory testing is not recommended; instead, laboratory testing should be done based on results of history and physical examination
1. Electrocardiogram (ECG) should be core of the workup for patients with suspected cardiac problems
2. Consider pregnancy testing in female adolescents, especially those for whom tilt table or electrophysiologic testing is being considered
3. Tilt-testing may be frightening to the patient and some patients may not be able to tolerate
   a. Upright tilt testing at 60 degrees for 45 minutes is ordered in patients in whom cardiac causes of syncope have been excluded who have infrequent syncopal episodes
   b. Tilt-table testing with isoproterenol is recommended for patients with negative results on passive tilt-table test who have a high pretest probability of neurally mediated syncope
4. Order 24-hour Holter monitor or prolonged ambulatory continuous-loop ECG recordings (patient activates a system when a syncopal episode occurs) in following cases
   a. Patients with normal heart who have frequent episodes of syncope
   b. Patients who have heart disease or an abnormal ECG or symptoms suggestive of arrhythmias

5. Echocardiogram is useful for detecting suspected heart disease such as valve dysfunction
6. Exercise stress testing is important in patients experiencing exertional syncope
7. Intracardiac electrophysiologic studies are needed when symptoms are suggestive of cardiac syncope, but no abnormality is uncovered with noninvasive tests
8. Computerized tomography (CT) scan or magnetic resonance imaging (MRI) is warranted if intracranial abnormalities (patient has focal neurologic signs) are suspected
9. Electroencephalogram (EEG) may be indicated to detect seizure disorder
10. Order carotid and transcranial Doppler ultrasonography for patients with bruits and who experience drop attacks (sudden loss of postural tone without a clear-cut loss of consciousness)
11. Lung ventilation-perfusion is reserved for patients with suspected pulmonary embolism
12. Consider other tests such as fasting blood glucose, hematocrit/hemoglobin, electrolytes, toxicology screens, thyroid function tests, and stool for occult blood based on patient symptomatology

V. Plan/Management

A. Admit to hospital the patients with known serious cardiovascular disease or new findings of cardiovascular disease, significant ECG changes, and patients who have chest pain; consider hospitalization for patients with disabling episodes of syncope, patients who have symptoms suggestive of coronary disease or pulmonary embolus, patients who have sudden loss of consciousness with injury, rapid pulses, or exertional syncope

B. Depending on etiological factors, consultation with a specialist is often needed; surgical procedures are considered for some conditions such as valvular and cerebrovascular diseases

C. Simple faint may resolve rapidly by elevating patient's feet and legs.

D. Adolescents with recurrent, disabling episodes of vasovagal syncope may benefit from the following:
   1. Medications such as β-blockers [Atenolol (Tenormin) 25-50 mg/day] or anticholinergic agents (Transdermal scopolamine, one patch every 2-3 days)
   2. If symptoms are not relieved by first-line drugs, consider the following:
      a. Fludrocortisone acetate (Florinef) 0.1 to maximum of 0.3 mg/day; contraindicated in patients with congestive heart failure
      b. Fluoxetine (Prozac) 10 mg/day
   3. Measures to expand volume such as increased salt intake, custom-fitted counter pressure support garments from ankle to waist
   4. Atrioventricular pacing can be considered in patients with clinically important bradycardia in response to upright tilt testing

E. Orthostatic hypotension prevention
   1. Wear elastic stocking
   2. Change positions slowly
   3. Sleep with head of bed elevated
   4. Exercise legs before standing
   5. Eat multiple small meals
   6. Avoid alcohol
   7. Avoid hot environments and hot showers or baths

F. Follow up is variable depending on diagnosis

REFERENCES

Allen, H.D., Golinko, R.J., & Williams, R.G. (1994). Heart murmurs in children: When is a workup needed? Contemporary Pediatrics, 11(11), 29-52.

American Academy of Pediatrics. (1997). Echocardiography in infants and children. Pediatrics, 99, 921.

Benditt, D.G., et al., (1996). Tilt table testing for assessing syncope. Journal of American College of Cardiology, 28, 263-275.

Bowen, J. (January, 1998). Dizziness: A diagnostic puzzle. Hospital Medicine, 39-44.

Cohn, H.E. (1999). Chest pain. In R.A. Dershewitz (Ed.), Ambulatory pediatric care (3rd ed.). Philadelphia: Lippincott-Raven.

Driscoll, D., Allen, H.D., Atkins, D.L., Brenner, J., Dunnigan, A., Franklin, W., Gutgesell, P., et al. (1994). Guidelines for evaluation and management of common congenital cardiac problems in infants, children, and adolescents: A statement for healthcare professionals from the Committee on Congenital Cardiac Defects of the Council on Cardiovascular Disease in the Young, American Heart Association. Circulation, 90, 2180-2188.

Epperly, T.D., & Fogarty, J.P. (1996). Syncope. In M.B. Mengel & L.P. Schwiebert (Eds.). Ambulatory medicine: The primary care of families (2nd ed.). Stamford, CT: Appleton & Lange.

Feit, L.R. (1997). The heart of the matter: Evaluating murmurs in children. Contemporary Pediatrics, 14(10), 97-122.

Fleet, R.P., & Beitman, B.D. (1997). Unexplained chest pain: When is it panic disorder? Clinical Cardiology, 20, 187-194.

Freed, L.A., Eagle, K.A., Mahjoub, ZA., et al. (1997). Gender differences in presentation, management, and cardiac event-free survival in patients with syncope. American Journal of Cardiology, 80, 1183-1187.

Goroll, A.H., May, L.A., & Mulley, A.G. (1995). Evaluation of chest pain. In A.H. Goroll, L.A. May, & A.G. Mulley (Eds.), Primary Care Medicine (3rd ed.), Philadelphia: Lippincott.

Gutgesell, H.P., Barst, R.J., Humes, R.A., Franklin, W.H., & Shaddy, R.E. (1997). Common cardiovascular problems in the young: Part I. Murmurs, chest pain, syncope, and irregular ryhthms. American Family Physician, 56, 1825-1830.

Heydemann, P.T. (1999). Pediatric nonepileptiform disorders. In R.A. Dershewitz (Ed.), Ambulatory pediatric care (3rd ed.). Philadelphia: Lippincott-Raven.

Hill, B., & Geraci, S.A. (1998). A diagnostic approach to chest pain based on history and ancillary evaluation. Nurse Practitioner, 23(4), 20-37.

Hobbs, J. (1996). Chest pain. In M.B. Mengel & L. P. Schwiebert (Eds.), Ambulatory medicine: The primary care of families (2nd ed.), Stamford, Connecticut: Appleton & Lange.

Hoefnagels, W.A.J., Padberg, G.W., Overweg, J., van der Velde, E.A., & Roos, R.A.C. (1997). Transient loss of consciousness: The value of the history for distinguishing seizure from syncope. Journal of Neurology, 238, 39-43.

Hupert, N., & Kapoor W. N. (March 15, 1997). Syncope: A systematic search for the cause. Patient Care, 136-152.

Kapoor, W.N. (1997). Syncope. In L. Dornbrand, A.J. Hoole, & R.H. Fletcher (Eds.), Manual of clinical problems in adult ambulatory care (3rd ed.). Philadelphia: Lippincott-Raven.

Katz, J.R., Krafft, P., & Fox, K. (1996). Assessing a murmur, saving a life: Current trends in the management of hypertrophic cardiomyopathy. Nurse Practitioner, 21(11), 62-75.

Kroenke, D. (August, 1996). Dizziness: A focused 5-minute workup. Consultant, 1715-1721.

Linzer, M., Yang, E.H., Estes III, N.A.M., Wang, P., Vorperian, V.R., & Kapoor, W.N. (1997). Diagnosing syncope: Part 1: Value of history, physical examination, and electrocardiography. Annals of Internal Medicine, 126, 989-996.

Linzer, M., Yang, E.H., Estes III, N.A.M., Wang, P., Vorperian, V.R., & Kapoor, W.N. (1997). Diagnosing syncope: Part 2: Unexplained syncope. Annals of Internal Medicine, 127, 76-86.

McCrindle, B.W., Shaffer, K.M., Kan, J.S., Zahka, K.G., Rowe, S.A., & Kidd, L. (1996). Cardinal clinical signs in the differentiation of heart murmurs in children. Archives of Pediatric and Adolescent Medicine, 150, 169-174.

Moller, J.H., Taubert, K.A., Allen, H.D., Clark, E.B., & Lauer, R.M. (1994). Cardiovascular health and disease in children: Current status. Circulation, 89(2), 923-930.

National Heart, Lung, and Blood Institute. (1987). Report of the second task force on blood pressure control in children--1987. <u>Pediatrics, 79,</u> 1-19.

National High Blood Pressure Education Program, National Institutes of Health, National Heart, Lung, and Blood Institute. (1997). <u>The Sixth Report of the Joint National Committee on Detection, Evaluation, and Treatment of High Blood Pressure</u> (NIH Publication no. 98-4080). Bethesda, MD: US Government Printing Office.

National High Blood Pressure Education Program Working Group on Hypertension Control in Children and Adolescents. (1996). Update on the 1987 task force report on high blood pressure in children and adolescents: A working group report from the National High Blood Pressure Education Program. <u>Pediatrics, 98,</u> 649-658.

Pelech, A.N. (1998). The cardiac murmur: When to refer? <u>Pediatric Clinics of North America, 45,</u> 107-122.

Sinaiko, A.R. (1996). Hypertension in children. <u>New England Journal of Medicine, 335,</u> 1968-1973.

Swenson, JM., Fischer, DR., Miller, SA., et al. (1997). Are chest radiographs and electrocardiograms still valuable in evaluating new pediatric patients with heart murmurs or chest pain? <u>Pediatrics, 99,</u> 1-3.

Zalenski, R.J., McCarren, M., Roberts, R., Rydman, R.J., Jovanovic, B., Das, K., Mendez, J., El-Khadra, M., Fraker, L., & McDermott, M. (1997). An evaluation of a chest pain diagnostic protocol to exclude acute cardiac ischemia in the emergency department. <u>Archives of Internal Medicine, 157,</u> 1085-1091.

CHAPTER 12

Gastrointestinal Problems

ACUTE AND RECURRENT ABDOMINAL PAIN IN CHILDREN

I. Definition: Acute pain is defined as recent onset of severe abdominal pain; recurrent pain is three or more discrete episodes of debilitating abdominal pain over at least a three-month period

II. Pathogenesis

    A. Common causes of acute pain for different age groups
        1. Gastroenteritis is the most common cause in all age groups with viral agents predominating
        2. Children <2 years of age: trauma, intussusception, incarcerated hernia, urinary tract infection, and intestinal malrotation
        3. Children 2-5 years of age: sickle cell anemia, right lower lobe pneumonia, and urinary tract infections
        4. Children >5 years: appendicitis (peak incidence is between 10-15 years)
        5. Adolescents: mittelschmerz (ovulatory pain), ectopic pregnancy, tubo-ovarian pathologic conditions
        6. Less common occurrences in all age groups: pancreatitis, cholecystitis, renal stones, peptic ulcer disease

    B. Common causes of recurrent pain
        1. Chronic constipation is the most common cause
        2. Lactose intolerance
        3. Musculoskeletal pain
        4. Parasitic infection
        5. Peptic ulcer disease
        6. Dysmenorrhea
        7. Dysfunctional abdominal pain
        8. Psychogenic pain

    C. In over 90% of cases of recurrent abdominal pain in children, no organic basis for the symptoms can be found

III. Clinical Presentation

    A. Approximately 15% of school-age children present to a primary care setting each year because of abdominal pain

    B. Gastroenteritis is characterized by crampy pain with associated symptoms of diarrhea, vomiting, malaise, and sometimes fever (see section on DIARRHEA)

    C. Intussusception presents as paroxysmal, colicky pain and the infant often has currant jelly stools, a palpable right upper quadrant abdominal mass, and ultimately distention

    D. Incarcerated hernias do not have to be strangulated to cause discomfort; a tender abdominal mass at any of the hernia orifices may be present

    E. Urinary tract infections (UTI) can cause abdominal pain and often the child with a UTI does not complain of dysuria and frequency as adults typically do (see section on URINARY TRACT INFECTION)

    F. Intestinal malrotation must be considered when a healthy infant suddenly refuses to eat, vomits, becomes inconsolable, and develops abdominal distention

G. Appendicitis
1. Often begins with symptoms of dull, steady periumbilical pain and anorexia
2. After approximately 4-6 hours, the pain localizes in the right lower quadrant
3. Patient often complains of associated constipation but can also have diarrhea
4. Vomiting and diarrhea present after the pain whereas with gastroenteritis the vomiting and diarrhea occur before the pain
5. May cause urinary frequency, urgency, and pyuria, making appendicitis difficult to distinguish from a UTI
6. In one study, 50% of the children with diagnosed appendicitis did not appear sick or in severe pain

H. Mittelschmerz is characterized by sudden onset of localized right or left lower quadrant pain which persists for less than 14-36 hours

I. Girls with ruptured ectopic pregnancies have acute onset of unilateral lower quadrant pain which usually is continuous and crampy with some degree of vaginal bleeding and a low-grade fever

J. Chronic stool retention
1. Child may have history of ineffective toilet training
2. Often a family history of constipation
3. Child may have encopresis (see section on ENCOPRESIS)

K. Lactose intolerance
1. If child is genetically programmed to become lactase deficient, the symptoms usually begin around 4-6 years of age; prevalence is highest in African blacks, Indians, and Asians
2. Symptoms include intestinal dilatation, bloating, increased flatulence, pain, and eventually diarrhea
3. Symptoms often do not appear until 2 hours after ingestion of milk or milk products; sometimes symptoms do not occur until as long as 12 hours after ingestion of lactose
4. Lactose intolerance is often confused with cow's milk intolerance which occurs in infancy and has symptoms of blood in the stools and often manifestations of allergies such as eczema, hives or asthma

L. Musculoskeletal pain is usually sharp and triggered by various activities or body movements

M. Parasitic infection
1. Symptoms vary depending of type of infection
2. Most common symptom is diarrhea which is often accompanied with nausea, vomiting, and abdominal pain

N. Peptic ulcer disease
1. Less typical symptoms in children than in adults
2. May have pain 1-3 hours after meals, nocturnal pain, recurrent vomiting, and relief of pain with food or antacids; may have a positive family history

O. Nonspecific dysfunctional abdominal pain
1. Occurs more commonly in children 5-10 years of age
2. Involves periumbilical pain which is often severe enough to modify the child's activity
3. Pain is often irregular in timing, duration, and intensity
4. Child may have pallor, nausea, vomiting, headache, and perspiration
5. On examination, the child may complain of tenderness, but there should be no muscle guarding or rebound tenderness
6. Child should be growing and developing normally and the abdominal pain should not be explainable by any structural or biochemical abnormalities

IV. Diagnosis/Evaluation

    A. History
        1. Determine onset and course of pain
        2. Question about timing, location, character, radiation, and severity of pain
        3. Determine whether pain disrupts normal activities and awakens child from sleep
        4. Ascertain whether pain is related to food or milk ingestion
        5. Ask about other aggravating or relieving factors such as pain with micturition which suggests a urogenital cause
        6. Inquire about associated symptoms such as fever, jaundice, change in stools, vomiting, anorexia, weight loss
        7. Inquire about history of abdominal trauma, abdominal surgery, or recent excessive exercise
        8. Explore history of predisposing disease such as diabetes, sickle cell disease, hemophilia, inflammatory bowel disease, recurrent pneumonia, or urinary tract infections
        9. In adolescent females, always ask dates of last two normal menstrual periods, whether sexually active, condom use, and type of contraceptive use
        10. Obtain past medical history, family history, and medication history

    B. Physical Examination
        1. Observe general appearance: Resisting movement or lying still on one side with legs flexed suggests acute, emergent abdominal pain
        2. Assess vital signs to determine if child is febrile and to assess for volume depletion/impending shock; measure height and weight and compare with previous measurements
        3. Complete abdominal exam is essential (Position child with hips flexed)
            a. Inspect for scars and shape of abdomen
            b. Inspect the inguinal and femoral areas for evidence of hernia or (in males) testicular torsion
            c. Auscultate for decreased bowel sounds which suggest intestinal obstruction or possibly appendicitis
            d. Percuss abdomen, beginning in nonpainful region, and note gastric distention with intestinal obstruction; tympany with fluid accumulation or a solid mass
            e. Palpate abdomen, evaluating for organomegaly, masses (including retained stool), tenderness, rebound tenderness, and guarding
        4. Check for peritonitis which is marked by a tense, hard abdomen
            a. Evaluate for rebound tenderness

ASSESSING FOR REBOUND TENDERNESS

After thorough exam of the abdomen, evaluate for peritoneal irritation as follows

✦ Using the flat of your hand, press on the area identified by the patient as most painful

✦ Press sufficiently to depress the peritoneum. The patient will experience pain with this maneuver

✦ Keep pressing with a constant pressure and, as the patient adjusts to the constant pressure over a 30 to 60 second period, the pain lessens in intensity and may even subside

✦ Then, without warning, remove your hand suddenly to just above skin level

✦ Observation of the patient's face may be the best index of a complaint of pain and peritoneal irritation

---

b. May additionally check for obturator and psoas signs

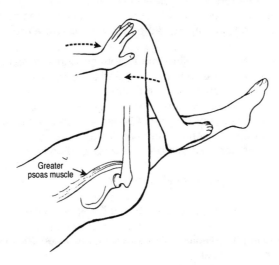

Figure 12.1. Psoas Sign.

With the patient in the supine position, instruct him/her to lift the right thigh against the resistance of the examiner's hand which is placed just above the patient's knee. Increased pain with the maneuver is a positive test, indicating irritation of the psoas by an inflamed appendix

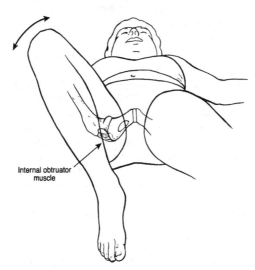

Figure 12.2. Obturator Sign.

Passively flex the right hip and knee and internally rotate the leg at the hip, stretching the obturator muscle. Right-sided abdominal pain is a positive sign, indicating irritation of the obturator muscle by an inflamed appendix

    5. Check back for costovertebral angle (CVA) tenderness
    6. In the older girl, may need to do a pelvic exam
    7. Rectal exam with guaiac testing is recommended
    8. Because abdominal pain is often referred pain, examination of the heart, lungs and other body systems may be needed

C. Differential Diagnosis
    1. Rule out all emergent conditions such as appendicitis, volvulus, bowel obstruction, ruptured ectopic pregnancy, trauma, ovarian hernia and torsion which require surgical intervention
    2. Pain which is progressive, localized, steady for >6 hours with rebound tenderness and guarding suggests an emergent condition
    3. Nonspecific dysfunctional abdominal pain and psychogenic abdominal pain are diagnoses of exclusion

D.	Diagnostic Tests
1.	Order CBC, differential, and platelet count
2.	Order urinalysis to rule out genitourinary conditions and diabetes
(Note: Children with appendicitis may have some red and white blood cells in their urine)
3.	Order urine pregnancy test (human chorionic gonadotropin or HCG)
4.	Order abdominal ultrasound or computed tomography
a.	If conditions such as ovarian torsion, ectopic pregnancy, or pelvic abscess are suspected, transvaginal ultrasonography is more sensitive than transabdominal
b.	CT scan is the procedure of choice for diagnosing such conditions as appendicitis, abscess formation and diverticular disease
5.	Other laboratory tests should be ordered based on H&P

V.	Plan/Management for common causes of abdominal pain

A.	Consultation with a specialist is recommended if diagnosis is unclear and the patient is unstable

B.	Emergency transport and hospitalization are required when child has acute abdominal pain related to an emergent condition

C.	Chronic stool retention problems or if child has overflow of liquid stool: See sections on CONSTIPATION or ENCOPRESIS

D.	Lactose Intolerance
1.	Teach parents to give child a lactose-free diet for 2 weeks (if pain disappears suspect lactose intolerance); gradually introduce regular diet noting emergence of symptoms (instruct parents to go through 2 cycles)
2.	Remind parents that cake mixes, milk chocolate, salad dressings, canned meats, pancakes, breads, and cereals often contain lactose
3.	If child is intolerant to lactose, teach parents and child which food are high in lactose such as soft cheeses with exception of cream cheese; hard cheeses such as cheddar and Swiss are low in lactose and may be tolerated
4.	Lactose intolerance is a dose-related phenomenon so children may be able to tolerate gradual introduction of lactose-containing foods after several weeks of a lactose-free diet
5.	Advise child to drink milk with meals to minimize the occurrence of symptoms
6.	Tablets and capsules containing lactose-digesting enzyme (Dairy Ease, Lactaid) can be taken 30 minutes before ingestion of a milk product to reduce symptoms
7.	If child is unable to tolerate most lactose-containing foods, give calcium supplements; yogurt with live and active cultures can provide an excellent substitute for milk

E.	Nonspecific dysfunctional abdominal pain
1.	Consider asking parents to keep a diary or calendar of the child's pain to help uncover possible triggers (this strategy may have negative consequences because it focuses the family's attention on the pain which is not recommended)
2.	Provide support to parents, explaining that child's pain is real and that child is not fabricating pain
3.	Explain that a thorough exam was done and no serious organic disease exists; emphasize that the child is in no physical danger
4.	Explain that recurrent abdominal pain is common in children and that many different causes exist
5.	Explain that child may have many reoccurrences of pain and will need to learn ways to cope with symptoms just as adults with recurrent headaches must learn to function at work and perform activities of daily living
6.	Encourage normalization of the family's life-style with immediate return to school and try to minimize the importance of the pain episodes
7.	During severely painful episodes, teach parents to allow child to rest; medications are usually not indicated
8.	Teach parents to assess child for signs of emergent abdominal problems such as fever, pallor, sweating, vomiting, diarrhea, rigid and tender abdomen

9. Reevaluate child periodically to provide support and assess for other problems
10. Consider referral to mental health specialist if underlying stress or family difficulties are suspected

F. Management and follow up of other causes of abdominal pain is variable depending on diagnosis

COLIC

I. Definition: Episodes of intense fussing and crying in an otherwise healthy infant lasting for several hours a day, most often in the early evening

II. Pathogenesis: Possible etiologies include normal variant, discomfort between parent and infant, family tensions, immaturity of the gastrointestinal tract, stimulus sensitivity (infant easily startled and awakened), temperamental disposition in the infant, food allergy or intolerance

III. Clinical Presentation

A. Affects 10-30% of infants worldwide

B. Occurs equally in breast fed and formula fed infants, males and females

C. Onset is usually at 3 weeks of age and condition resolves by about 3 months of age

D. Virtually all 4 month old infants are free of symptoms

E. During the attack, infant appears hypertonic with entire body stiffened, hands clenched, and legs flexed rigidly over abdomen

IV. Diagnosis/Evaluation

A. History
1. Determine age at onset and pattern of crying (time of day, duration, and so on); type, quantity, and frequency of feeding, satisfaction with feeding, and elimination patterns
2. Inquire about interventions tried and their effectiveness
3. Ask how the infant is doing otherwise in terms of behavior and activity

B. Physical Examination
1. Take vital signs; measure and plot length, weight, and head circumference to determine growth patterns
2. Assess for developmental milestones
3. Look for conditions that would increase irritability
4. Use exam to reassure parents

C. Differential Diagnosis
1. Colic is a diagnosis of exclusion used to explain recurrent, prolonged crying episodes in healthy appearing infants
2. Must exclude acute causes of infant crying such as infection, obstruction/gastrointestinal dysfunction, and injury

D. Diagnostic Tests: None indicated if child is gaining weight, achieving developmental milestones, has a normal physical exam, and nothing in the history indicates a need for further evaluation

V.   Plan/Management

   A.   Intervention should focus on four general areas:

FOUR AREAS OF INTERVENTION FOR COLIC	
Educate parents	Regarding infant colic and the self-limited nature of the condition
Provide support	To the family through empathic listening and assurance to the family that there will be follow up (allows parents to know that they are not alone in dealing with this)
Emphasize normality	Baby is growing and developing as expected (based on history and physical exam)
Suggest home remedies	That parents may try with recognition that such treatments are of questionable value and may fail

   B.   Home remedies that <u>may</u> work with some babies are summarized in the table below:

ADVICE TO PARENTS ON HOW TO SOOTHE A CRYING BABY
✿ Use rhythmic rocking motions, such as infant swing, car ride, carrying baby in body carrier
✿ Try continuous monotonous noise such as a fan, vaporizer, or clothes dryer
✿ Encourage sucking using pacifier
✿ Try slow feedings with infant held in vertical position during feeding
✿ Burp infant in upright position after every 1-2 ounces of formula/5-10 minutes of breast feeding
✿ Place infant face down across knees with tummy on warm hot water bottle (wrapped in towel) and rub gently on back; pressure on abdomen may relieve discomfort
✿ Use swaddling, cuddling, and soothing methods to create restful environment
✿ Advise parent to have someone else look after baby every few days for a few hours if parent is feeling very tense and anxious
✿ Caution parent to never shake the baby!
✿ Finally, parents should understand that none of these strategies may work, and that putting a crying infant in his/her crib is permissible for short periods of time

   C.   Watchful waiting may be the best approach
      1.   No pharmacologic interventions are recommended
      2.   Formula changes have not been shown to be an effective remedy for colic and may suggest to the parents that the infant has a medical problem when none exists
         a.   Allergy to cow's milk protein during infancy is very uncommon
         b.   Infants who have cow's milk allergy present with persistent diarrhea and /or blood in stool
         c.   Change to soy formulas are usually not helpful and about 25% of infants with a true allergy to cow's milk protein are also allergic to soy formula
      3.   If mother is breast feeding, she should continue

   D.   Follow up by telephone in a few days and again in a week or two to determine progress

CONSTIPATION

I. Definition: Diminished frequency of defecation, incomplete evacuation, or stools that are too hard or too small

II. Pathogenesis

  A. Fecal continence is defined as the ability to control defecation voluntarily and requires normal contractions of the anal sphincters, normal sensory receptors in the rectum and anus to identify the rectal contents as liquid, solid, or gaseous, and a normal rectal reservoir

  B. Movement of a fecal bolus into the rectum stimulates several automatic, coordinated reflexes
    1. The lower colon, including the rectum, contracts and the internal sphincter relaxes
    2. The external sphincter initially contracts, but the initial contraction is followed by a total inhibition of both the external and internal sphincters
    3. Intraabdominal pressure is voluntarily increased (Valsalva maneuver), the pelvic floor descends and stool is expelled

  C. Defecation can be delayed until it is convenient
    1. Retention of stool over prolonged periods of time can result in a stretching of the rectal wall and the subsequent development of megarectum
    2. When the whole colon is dilated and full of stool, the condition is referred to as megacolon

  D. Common causes of constipation in children and adolescents are the following
    1. Ignoring urge to defecate
    2. Inadequate ingestion of fluids and fiber in diet
    3. Sedentary lifestyle
    4. Medications

  E. Constipation is **most commonly functional** with no underlying pathology

III. Clinical Presentation

  A. Constipation accounts for 2.5 million health care visits per year

  B. About 4% of all pediatric office visits are for constipation

  C. In children, constipation represents a complex interaction between parental expectations, and the child's gastrointestinal physiology, development, and nutritional and fluid intake

  D. Despite the high incidence of constipation, only a small minority of children with constipation have a significant abnormality

  E. Vomiting, excessive urination, blood on stool, soiling of underclothes (encopresis), and behavioral problems may occur with constipation

IV. Diagnosis/Evaluation

  A. History
    1. Determine what the patient/parent means by constipation (Is it small stools, infrequent stools, a feeling of fullness, or difficulty/pain with passing stools?) [see PATTERN OF STOOLING IN INFANTS AND YOUNG CHILDREN table]
    2. Assess stooling pattern, dietary intake, and activity level
    3. Determine if any recent changes in pattern (acute or chronic process)
    4. Inquire about current medications and laxative use

❖ Pattern of stooling in most infants is a bowel movement after each feeding for the first weeks of life

❖ By 3-4 months of age, most infants have 1-2 stools per day

❖ By 4 years of age, an adult pattern of stooling is achieved

❖ Note that the infrequent passage of stool in contented breast-fed babies in the first few weeks and months is normal so long as the stools are soft

❖ Parents should keep in mind that stooling patterns vary in children just as they do in adults

❖ Parents should be aware of their child's normal bowel pattern and typical size/consistency of stools

---

B. Physical Examination
1. Determine if there is a weight loss
2. Assess abdomen for tenderness, masses
3. Rectal exam for anal fissures, hemorrhoids, or irritation; obtain stool for guaiac
4. Check for fecal impaction, especially in children in whom encopresis is suspected

C. Differential Diagnosis
1. Partial bowel obstruction (tumor)
2. Irritable bowel syndrome
3. Rectal fissures

D. Diagnostic Tests: None indicated in an otherwise healthy child

V. Plan/Management

A. Infants between 6-12 months of age
1. Continue on present formula/breast milk. **Do not place infant on low iron formula!**
2. Advise parent
   a. To increase daily consumption of water by offering water frequently (**Note:** Infants ≤6 months of age who are being exclusively fed formula or breast milk (and no solid foods) do not require additional water as they receive adequate water from formula or breast milk; children >6 months may be offered water as they are usually receiving solid food beginning at 6 months)
   b. To add high fiber food to diet in the form of prunes, apricots, plums, peas, and beans (pureed at 6 months and progressing to chopped by 12 months of age)

B. Toddlers and preschoolers
1. Offer child whole fruits instead of juice
2. Offer child water frequently
3. Provide dietary fiber in both soluble (dried beans/peas, oats, barley, fruits) and insoluble forms (whole wheat products, wheat bran, skins of fruits and root vegetables) [see HOW MUCH FIBER DO CHILDREN AND ADOLESCENTS NEED and FIBER CONTENT OF SELECTED FOODS tables]
4. Choose cereals with 5 or more grams of fiber per serving

C. Children over 5 and adolescents
1. Retrain in proper bowel habits
   a. Never ignore urge to defecate, even though it may not be convenient
   b. Allow adequate time for bowel movements; learn to sit on toilet and relax
   c. Capitalize on the gastrocolic reflex by establishing a routine for bowel movements that coincides with after having eaten a meal such as breakfast
2. Increase daily fluid intake (1.5-2.0 liters per day in adolescents)
3. Increase dietary fiber with bran cereal, raw fruits and vegetables, whole wheat breads, oats, barley (see HOW MUCH FIBER DO CHILDREN AND ADOLESCENTS NEED and FIBER CONTENT OF SELECTED FOODS tables)
4. Skip orange juice in the morning and eat a whole orange instead
5. Choose cereals with 5 or more grams of fiber per serving

6. Increase activity level using easy, no-cost approaches such as spending more time in outdoor play and walking to do errands that are just a few blocks away

7. Continue these measures for at least one month before effects on bowel function are determined

HOW MUCH FIBER DO CHILDREN AND ADOLESCENTS NEED?

Children ages 3 to 15	**Just Add 5!** Add 5 to the child's age (Child's age + 5 = number of grams of fiber needed/day) **Example:** A six year old child needs 6 + 5 = 11 grams of fiber each day
Children >15	Need about 20-35 grams of fiber in their diet each day **Increase fiber intake gradually over a 2 week period to reduce abdominal discomfort sometimes associated with high fiber intake!**

Note: There is no Recommended Dietary Allowance (RDA) for daily intake of fiber, but most experts agree that the above intakes of fiber for children are appropriate

FIBER CONTENT OF SELECTED FOODS

Fruits

Food	Amount	Fiber (grams)	Food	Amount	Fiber (grams)
apple (with skin)	1 medium	3	orange	1 medium	3
banana	1 medium	2	orange juice	3/4 cup	<1
blueberries	1/2 cup	2	pear (with skin)	1 medium	4
grapes	1/2 cup	1	strawberries	1 cup	4

Vegetables, raw

Food	Amount	Fiber (grams)	Food	Amount	Fiber (grams)
carrots	1 medium	2	lettuce, romaine	1 cup	1
celery	1 stalk	<1	tomato	1 medium	2

Vegetables, cooked

Food	Amount	Fiber (grams)	Food	Amount	Fiber (grams)
broccoli	1/2 cup	2	spinach	1/2 cup	2
potato, baked (with skin)	1 medium	4	zucchini	1/2 cup	1

Legumes, cooked

Food	Amount	Fiber (grams)	Food	Amount	Fiber (grams)
baked beans	1/2 cup	3	kidney beans	1/2 cup	3

Breads, grains, and pasta

Food	Amount	Fiber (grams)	Food	Amount	Fiber (grams)
bagel	1 medium	1	white bread	1 slice	<1
brown rice (cooked)	1/2 c	2	whole wheat bread	1 slice	2
wheat germ	1 tablespoon	1			

Breakfast Cereals

Food	Amount	Fiber (grams)	Food	Amount	Fiber (grams)
bran flakes	3/4 cup	5	oatmeal, cooked	3/4 cup	3
cornflakes	3/4 cup	1	raisin bran	3/4 cup	5

Snack Foods

Food	Amount	Fiber (grams)	Food	Amount	Fiber (grams)
peanuts, dry roasted	1/4 cup	3	popcorn, air popped	1 cup	1

D. If general measures fail, may try the following alternatives:

1. Bulk-forming agents (adolescents) : psyllium (Effersyllium), methylcellulose (Citrucel), and polycarbophil (Fibercon)

        a.   Start with 1 tbsp daily and increase to 3 tbsp

        b.   Must drink plenty of fluids for product to work (**Note:** 16 oz water with each dose)

        c.   Must be used on regular basis

2.   Stool softeners (children and adolescents): docusate sodium (Colace) and docusate calcium (Doxidan)

        a.   Can be used for short-term constipation only (few days to 2 weeks)

        b.   Do not use in chronic constipation

3.   Osmotic agents (infants >6 months): Corn syrup (Karo syrup)

        a.   Breast-fed: 5-10 mL in 2 to 4 oz of water or fruit juice BID

        b.   Bottle-fed: 5-10 mL in every second feeding

4.   Osmotic agents (infants): Malt soup extract (Maltsupex); use same dosage as that of corn syrup

5.   Agents such as milk of magnesia can be used occasionally (every 2-3 weeks) to treat constipation in otherwise healthy adolescents

E.   For children with chronic constipation (see section on ENCOPRESIS)

F.   Advise parents/patients to avoid chronic laxative use

G.   Follow Up: Unnecessary unless there is failure to improve which may indicate serious underlying cause and need for referral

DIARRHEA

I.   Definition: A change in bowel habits characterized by increased stool volume, looseness, and frequency

II.   Pathogenesis

A.   Pathophysiology of diarrhea involves one or a combination of three basic mechanisms

1.   Increased fluid secretion

2.   Decreased water absorption

3.   Abnormal intestinal motility

B.   Diarrhea that is produced via increased fluid secretion can be caused by inflammation (such as occurs with viral and bacterial infections) and enterotoxins (such as are produced with *Staphylococcus aureus* infection)

C.   Damage to the bowel mucosa (such as occurs with some infectious agents or inflammatory conditions such as inflammatory bowel disease and sprue [sprue is a malabsorption syndrome that causes inflammation of the bowel mucosa]) or the presence of poorly absorbable, osmotically active substances in the lumen (such as lactose in a lactase deficient patient) cause diarrhea via the mechanism of decreased reabsorption of fluid

D.   Abnormal intestinal motility (such as occurs in irritable bowel syndrome and with the ingestion of such medications as erythromycin) can decrease contact time with the bowel mucosa, limiting reabsorption of fluids, and producing diarrhea

III.   Clinical Presentation

A.   Most diarrheal illness is acute, lasts only a day or two and resolves spontaneously

B.   By far the most common cause of **acute diarrhea** in both children and adults is infection of the gastrointestinal tract by a variety of pathogens with viral etiologies being most common

C.   Distinguishing features of commonly occurring infectious causes of acute diarrhea are summarized in the table that follows

COMMONLY OCCURRING INFECTIOUS CAUSES OF ACUTE DIARRHEA: DISTINGUISHING FEATURES

Infectious Agent	Mode of Transmission	Incubation Period	Associated Signs and Symptoms	Characteristics of Stool	Laboratory Examination of Stool	Important to Remember
Viral Rotaviruses and Norwalk virus	Fecal-oral; fomites may have a role	24-72 hours	Nausea, vomiting, abdominal cramps Fever	Watery No occult or gross blood	No WBCs in stool	By far the most common cause of acute diarrhea in both children and adults In children, rotavirus infection is more common; in adults Norwalk virus is more common Vomiting most prominent symptom in children; diarrhea most prominent in adults
Bacterial *Staphylococcus aureus*	Ingestion of food containing a preformed toxin produced by enterotoxicogenic staphylococci Food products most commonly involved are ham, poultry, filled pastries, egg/potato salads Contamination is via food handlers Not transmissible from person-to-person	Very short--30 minutes to 6 hours	Nausea, vomiting, abdominal cramps Fever is uncommon	Soft, but not watery No occult or gross blood	No WBCs in stool	Onset is abrupt Look for a common source pattern
Clostridium perfringens	Ingestion of food contaminated by the organism Once ingested, an enterotoxin is produced in the lower intestine of the host, producing symptoms Beef, poultry, Mexican-style foods are common sources Not transmissable from person-to-person	8-12 hours	Nausea, vomiting, moderate-to-severe mid-epigastric pain Fever is uncommon	Watery No occult or gross blood	No WBCs in stool	Onset is not as abrupt as in staphylococcal food poisoning because enterotoxin is not preformed, but is produced in host's intestine Look for a common source pattern Look for recent ingestion of foods served from steam tables
Campylobacter jejuni	Ingestion of contaminated food, including unpasteurized milk and untreated water OR by direct contact with fecal material from infected persons/animals Main vehicles of transmission: Improperly cooked poultry, untreated water, unpasteurized milk Person-to-person spread is not common	1-7 days	Nausea, vomiting, abdominal pain, malaise Fever	Watery Occult and gross blood	WBCs in stool Positive culture	Abdominal pain can mimic that produced by appendicitis Mild infection lasts 1-2 days with most patients recovering in <7 days Outbreaks in child care centers are uncommon

(continued)

COMMONLY OCCURRING INFECTIOUS CAUSES OF ACUTE DIARRHEA: DISTINGUISHING FEATURES--CONTINUED

Infectious Agent	Mode of Transmission	Incubation Period	Associated Signs and Symptoms	Characteristics of Stool	Laboratory Examination of Stool	Important to Remember
Salmonella	Major modes: Ingestion of food of animal origin, including poultry, red meat, eggs, and unpasteurized milk Other modes: Ingestion of contaminated water, contact with infected animals such as pet turtles/reptiles Direct person-to-person transmission (fecal-oral) are less common than other modes	6-72 hours; usually <24 hours	Nausea, vomiting, abdominal cramping Fever	Watery Occult and gross blood	WBCs in stool Positive culture	Most likely to occur in children <5 (peaks in first year of life) and adults >70 Outbreaks of this infection are rare in day care centers Report all confirmed cases to local public health department
Shigella	Ingestion of contaminated food or water and homosexual transmission most common routes in adults Fecal-oral transmission is most common route in children Feces of infected humans are source of infection No animal reservoir known	1-7 days; usually 2-4 days	Abdominal pain Fever	Watery Occult blood No gross blood	WBCs in stool Positive culture	Most common in children 1-4 years of age Important problem in child care centers in US Report all confirmed cases to the local health department
Escherichia coli (ETEC)	One of at least 5 different groups of diarrhea-producing strains of *E. coli* Most commonly from food or water contaminated with human or animal feces Most common cause of "travelers' diarrhea," acquired by travelers to developing countries	10 hours to 6 days	Abdominal cramps Usually no fever	Watery No occult or gross blood	No WBCs (usually); can be present Positive culture	The enterotoxin that is produced by the organism promotes fluid secretion in the small bowel which results in a watery diarrhea History of recent travel to a developing country is important epidemiologic information
Protozoal *Giardia*	Main route of spread is fecal-oral transfer of cysts from feces of an infected person Many common source outbreaks are traced to contaminated drinking water Humans are principle reservoir but organism can infect animals such as dogs, cats, beavers	1-4 weeks	Abdominal pain associated with flatulence, distention, and anorexia Passage of foul-smelling stools No fever	Soft, watery No occult or gross blood	Positive stool for O & P (see IV.D.3 DIAGNOSTIC TESTS)	Most often represents an acute presentation of chronic or recurrent diarrhea

D.   Drugs such as laxatives, antibiotics, caffeine, magnesium containing antacids and alcohol also cause diarrhea

E.   Chronic diarrhea (lasting at least 2 weeks or frequent recurrences after initial attack) also often presents in primary care settings

F.   Some of the more common causes of chronic diarrhea along with their associated signs and symptoms are listed here:
1.   Irritable bowel syndrome: recurrent abdominal pain, diarrhea alternates with constipation; the most common of the motility disorders causing chronic diarrhea (see IRRITABLE BOWEL SYNDROME section for a discussion of this condition)
2.   Inflammatory bowel diseases: destruction of the bowel wall compromises absorption of electrolytes; characterized by bloody stools, abdominal pain, fever, and extraintestinal manifestations involving skin, joints, liver, and heart
3.   Malabsorption of fat or carbohydrate
a.   With fat malabsorption, there are foul, bulky, greasy stools and the signs and symptoms are those associated with the resultant caloric and vitamin deficiencies (weight loss, ecchymosis, glossitis, peripheral neuropathy)
b.   With carbohydrate malabsorption, patients report bloating, abdominal cramps and diarrhea after intake of dairy produces
4.   Chronic laxative abuse can also cause diarrhea; occurs often in patients with bulimia; substances appear in the stool and the stool can be tested if laxative abuse is suspected

IV.   Diagnosis/Evaluation

A.   History
1.   Determine if acute or chronic process; recent relatively sudden onset of non-bloody diarrhea in otherwise healthy persons is usually due to infectious causes and likely to be self-limited
2.   Question regarding stool volume, frequency, and consistency; ask if stool contains blood, mucus
3.   Ask about the presence of associated signs and symptoms including abdominal pain, vomiting, fever, malaise
4.   Ask about intake of fluids and urine output
5.   In infants, ask about feeding, irritability, activity level, number of wet diapers, and if general behavior is significantly changed since onset of diarrhea
6.   Obtain past medical history and medication history
7.   Question regarding similar illness in others. Viral etiology likely when secondary cases develop in household suggesting person-to-person spread rather than one-time exposure to a common food or drink
8.   Ask appropriate questions to identify if patient is at risk of being HIV positive

B.   Physical Examination
1.   Determine if patient is febrile and assess cardiovascular status (pulse, blood pressure; check for postural changes, a reflection of significant volume depletion)
2.   Weigh patient and determine if there has been a weight loss (more of an issue in infants and in chronic diarrhea)
3.   In infants and young children, assess hydration status based on criteria in ASSESSMENT OF DEHYDRATION IN INFANTS AND CHILDREN in the following table
4.   Examine abdomen for tenderness, rigidity, abnormal tympany, bowel sounds, liver/spleen enlargement
5.   Perform rectal exam for tenderness, masses; obtain stool for occult blood
6.   Look for extraabdominal causes of diarrhea such as otitis media and urinary tract infection which often are associated with diarrhea in children through an unknown mechanism

ASSESSMENT OF DEHYDRATION IN INFANTS AND CHILDREN			
Indicator	Mild, 3-5%	Moderate, 6-9%	Severe, ≥10%
Blood pressure	Normal	Normal	Normal to reduced
Quality of pulses	Normal	Normal or slightly decreased	Moderately decreased
Heart rate	Normal	Increased	Increased (Brachycardia may occur also)
Skin turgor	Normal	Decreased skin elasticity	Decreased with tenting
Fontanelle	Normal	Somewhat depressed	Depressed
Mucous membranes	Sl dry lips, Thick saliva	Dry lips, buccal mucosa	Very dry lips, buccal mucosa
Eyes	Normal	Sunken orbits	Deeply sunken orbits
Capillary refill time (In seconds)	Normal (<1.5)	Delayed (1.5-3.0)	Delayed (>3.0)
Mental status	Normal	Normal to listless	Normal to lethargic or comatose
Urine output	Slightly Decreased	<1 mL/kg/h	<<1 mL/kg/hr
Thirst	Slightly Increased	Moderately increased	Very thirsty or too lethargic to indicate

Adapted from Duggan, C., Santosham, M., & Glass, R.I. (1992). The management of acute diarrhea in children: Oral rehydration, maintenance, and nutritional therapy. MMWR, 41(RR-16), 1-20.

    C.   Differential Diagnosis: Diarrhea is a symptom. Refer to common causes of acute and chronic diarrhea under section III. above

    D.   Diagnostic Tests
        1.   If no systemic signs and symptoms and duration 24-48 hours, no lab studies indicated
        2.   Obtain stool culture if any of the following are present:
             a.   Fever over 24 hours
             b.   Diarrhea persistent over several days with no improvement
             c.   Family or close population outbreak
             d.   Stool positive for blood (either occult or gross)
             e.   Gram's stain of stool positive for WBCs
        3.   If *Giardia* is suspected
             a.   Obtain stool specimens on 3 separate days for O&P (excretion of organism is intermittent)
             b.   Identification of either trophozoite or cysts on direct smear examination is diagnostic
             c.   Detection of *G. lamblia* antigens in stool specimen by enzyme immunoassay (EIA) is also diagnostic; enzyme immunoassay techniques for antigen detection in stool specimens are available commercially and have greater sensitivity than microscope detection
             d.   Examination of duodenal contents for trophozoites via commercially available string test (Entero-test) is also diagnostic

V.   Plan/Management

    A.   Management of acute diarrhea in all age groups involves identification of causes that need specific treatment and restoring and/or maintaining hydration status while waiting for the resolution of the symptoms
        1.   See TREATMENT OF ACUTE DIARRHEA CAUSED BY COMMONLY OCCURING INFECTIOUS AGENTS in the table that follows
        2.   Whether or not the cause of the diarrhea is determined, supportive therapy should be instituted immediately to rehydrate (if necessary) and maintain hydration status in the patient (see ASSESSMENT OF DEHYDRATION IN INFANTS AND CHILDREN table above)

TREATMENT OF ACUTE DIARRHEA CAUSED BY COMMONLY OCCURRING INFECTIOUS AGENTS

Infectious Agent	Pharmacologic Management	Counseling and Control Measures
Viral Rotavirus Norwalk virus	✓ No specific antiviral therapy is available	✓ Emphasize importance of good hand washing ✓ Advise to clean all surfaces where diapering is done with chlorine-based disinfectants ✓ Infected children should be excluded from child-care centers until diarrhea resolves
Bacterial *Staphylococcus aureus*	✓ Antibiotics are not recommended	✓ Proper cooking and refrigeration of food helps prevent the disease ✓ Persons with staphylococcal infections should be excluded from handling food
Clostridium perfringens	✓ Antibiotics are not recommended	✓ *C. perfringens* should not be allowed to proliferate in food (beef, poultry, gravies, and Mexican-style foods are common sources) ✓ Foods should never be held at room temperature to cool, but should be refrigerated promptly, and reheated thoroughly before serving ✓ Foods should not be kept in warming devices or serving tables for long periods of time
Campylobacter infections	✓ Erythromycin, given early in the course of infection, shortens duration of illness and prevents relapse * Adolescents: 250 mg PO QID x 5-7 days * Children: 20-50 mg/kg/day divided into 4 doses for 5-7 days	✓ Persons who prepare food should practice frequent handwashing, wash surfaces that have been exposed to raw poultry, and thoroughly cook poultry ✓ Pasteurization of milk and chlorination of water supplies are essential ✓ Infected food handlers who are asymptomatic need not be excluded from work if proper personal hygiene measures are maintained ✓ Outbreaks are uncommon in child care centers
Salmonella infections (nontyphoidal)	✓ Antimicrobial therapy is not indicated for uncomplicated gastroenteritis caused by nontyphoidal *Salmonella* species because it can prolong excretion of the organism ✓ Treatment of patients at an increased risk of invasive disease such as persons with HIV infection and patients with severe colitis is recommended. Consult specialists for treatment recommendations	✓ Emphasis should be on good hand-washing and personal hygiene ✓ There must be proper sanitation in food processing and preparation; **infected persons should be excluded from handling food** ✓ Eggs and other foods of animal origin should be cooked thoroughly before ingestion ✓ Raw eggs as well as food containing raw eggs should not be eaten ✓ Handwashing when handling pet turtles and other reptiles is important ✓ Outbreaks of *Salmonella* infection are rare in child care centers ✓ Vaccination for typhoid is recommended only for international travelers ✓ Report all cases of *Salmonella* infection to local public health department so that proper investigation of outbreak can be conducted
Shigella	✓ To shorten course and prevent further spread, may treat with trimethoprim-sulfamethoxazole * Adolescents: 1 DS tab BID x 5 days * Children: 1 mL/kg/day in two divided doses (Q 12 hours) x 5 days (Available as Bactrim suspension 200 mg sulfamethoxazole and 40 mg trimethoprim per 5mL) ✓ Intestinal motility patterns are considered important in recovery from infection, therefore anti-diarrhea drugs should not be given	✓ Emphasis should be on good hand-washing and personal hygiene, particularly among workers in group care settings such as child care and group living facilities ✓ There must be proper sanitation in food processing and preparation; **infected persons should be excluded from handling food** ✓ Prevention of contamination of food by flies during preparation and serving ✓ Insuring that water supply is not contaminated is important ✓ Outbreak of Shigella infection must be reported to the local health department for investigation
Escherichia coli infection (entero-toxigenic) [ETEC], major cause of Travelers' Diarrhea	✓ May treat with trimethoprim-sulfamethoxazole * Adolescents: 1 DS tab, BID x 3 days * Children: 1 mL/kg/day in two divided doses (Q 12 hours) x 3 days (Available as Bactrim suspension 200 mg sulfamethoxazole and 40 mg trimethoprim per 5 mL)	✓ When traveling in developing countries or in any area where water supply is questionable, drink only bottled water ✓ Avoid all raw fruits and vegetables that may not have been properly washed (unless can peel and eat)

(continued)

Infectious Agent	Pharmacologic Management	Counseling and Control Measures

Protozoal
Giardia
	✓ Drug of choice is metronidazole
	  * Adolescents: 250 mg TID x 5 days
	  * Children: Not recommended
	✓ Alternative drug is furazolidone
	  * Adolescents: 100 mg QID x 7-10 days
	  * Children: 6 mg/kg/day in 4 divided doses x 7-10 days
	✓ In pregnant females, panomycin is recommended for treatment of symptomatic infections. Consult PDR for dosing recommendations
		✓ Emphasize sanitation and personal hygiene, especially in group care settings
		✓ Hand washing after diaper changes and after personal toilet use by workers cannot be overemphasized; persons with diarrhea (both workers and children) should be excluded from day care until problem resolves
		✓ Adequate filtration of municipal water supply prevents water-borne outbreaks in metropolitan areas
		✓ Boiling of water by campers, backpackers will eliminate cysts; drinking from streams is risky
		✓ Treatment of asymptomatic carriers is not recommended except for prevention of household transmission by toddlers to pregnant females
		✓ Outbreaks in day care centers require reporting to local public health department for epidemiological investigation

B. Because infants are at higher risk for development of **dehydration and malnutrition, the two major consequences of diarrhea**, management must be very aggressive in this age group (see TREATMENT OF DIARRHEA IN INFANTS > ONE MONTH AND CHILDREN ≤5 YEARS table)

C. Neonates (infants ≤ one month of age) who present with diarrhea should be referred to a specialist for management because of the greater likelihood of severe infection in this age group

D. Treatment of infants >one month of age and children ≤ 5 years of age with acute diarrhea is determined by the degree of dehydration that is present

TREATMENT OF INFANTS >ONE MONTH OF AGE AND CHILDREN ≤ 5 YEARS OF AGE

Degree of Dehydration	Management
Infants and children who have mild diarrhea and who are not dehydrated	✧ Continue to feed age appropriate diet ✧ Children in this category do not require glucose-electrolyte solutions but they should be given more fluids than usual during episode of diarrhea

Children who are mildly dehydrated (3-5%)	✧ Give 50 mL/kg of ORT plus replacement of continuing losses during a 4-hour period
	  ✦ Replacement of continuing losses from stool is achieved by providing 10mL/kg for each stool
	  ✦ Emesis volume should also be estimated and replaced each time the child vomits
	  ✦ At least every 2 hours, the hydration status of the child should be reevaluated and replacement of losses should occur
	  ✦ Children who require rehydration should be fed age-appropriate diet as soon as they have been rehydrated
	  ✦ Special diets such as the **BRAT are no longer recommended** as such diets are not calorie dense enough and lack adequate amounts of protein and fat

Children who are mildly dehydrated and who have vomiting	✧ Can be successfully treated with ORT with the administration of small volumes of the solution on a frequent basis
	  ✦ Administer 5 mL every 2-3 minutes
	  ✦ Using this technique, 150/300 mL/h can be given
	  ✦ Once dehydration and electrolyte imbalance are corrected, vomiting often decreases and ends
	  ✦ When rehydration is achieved, age appropriate diet should be reinstated

(continued)

TREATMENT OF INFANTS >ONE MONTH OF AGE AND CHILDREN ≤ 5 YEARS OF AGE (CONTINUED)	
Degree of Dehydration	**Management**
Infants and children who are moderately dehydrated (6-9%)	✧ Give 100 mL/kg of ORT plus replacement of continuing losses during a 4-hour period ✦ Every hour during the period of rehydration, hydration status should be assessed; continuing stool and emesis losses should be calculated with the total added to the amount remaining to be given over the 4-hour period ✦ These children are best managed in an emergency department or urgent care facility ✦ Children who require rehydration should be fed age-appropriate diet as soon as they have been rehydrated
Infants and children who are severely dehydrated (≥10%)	✧ **Require immediate emergency management**
Solutions Appropriate for Oral Rehydration Therapy (ORT) for Infants and Children ≤5 Years	
♦ Pedialyte ♦ Infalyte (formerly Ricelyte) ♦ Rehydralyte ♦ Naturalyte ♦ Pediatric electrolyte	

Adapted from American Academy of Pediatrics, Provisional Committee on Quality Improvement, Subcommittee on Acute Gastroenteritis. (1996). Practice parameter: The management of acute gastroenteritis in young children. Pediatrics, 97, 424-433.

E. Supportive therapy for older children and adolescents should focus on attaining and maintaining adequate hydration status through appropriate fluid intake
   1. Water or sports drinks may be used for hydration as well as the commercial rehydration products such as those listed above
   2. Children may also like products such as Pedialyte Freezer Pops
   3. Normal diet should be resumed as soon as the patient can tolerate it; special diets such as the BRAT are no longer recommended as they are not calorie dense enough, and lack adequate amounts of protein and fat

F. As a general rule, pharmacologic agents should not be used to treat diarrhea in children ≤5 years of age

G. The following anti-diarrheal agents are available and may be used in selected cases where there are no contraindications

ANTI-DIARRHEAL AGENTS FOR ACUTE DIARRHEA			
Agents	**Medication**		**Dosage**
Antimotility agents	Loperamide (Immodium), available as 2 mg caps	Adolescents: Children:	4 mg initially, then 2 mg after each unformed stool. Maximum 16 mg/day; use for 2 days Not recommended
	Immodium A-D (OTC), available as I mg/5mL syrup and 2 mg caplets	Adolescents: Children:	4 mg initially, then 2 mg after each unformed stool. Maximum 8 mg/day; use for 2 days 6-8 years (48-59 lbs), 2 mg initially, then 1 mg after each loose stool Maximum 4 mg/day for 2 days 9-11 years (60-95 lbs) Same as for younger child EXCEPT maximum of 6 mg/day for 2 days
	Lomotil, available as 2.5 mg tabs and liquid, 2.5 mg/5 mL	Adolescents: Children:	2 tabs QID (maximum 20 mg/day) for 2-3 days ≥6 years of age, 0.3 -0.4 mg/kg/day in 4 divided doses for 2 days
Adsorbents	Kaolin-pectin mixture (Kaopectate) liquid	Adolescents: Children:	30-120 mL after each loose stool ≥6 years of age, see label for dosing
Antisecretory agents	Bismuth subsalycilate, available as 262 mg chewable tabs and 262 mg/15 mL liquid	Adolescents: Children:	2 tabs or 30 mL Q 30-60 minutes (Maximum 8 doses/day) 6-9 years of age, 2/3 tab or 10 mL Q 30-60 minutes (Maximum 8 doses/day) 9-12 years of age, 1 tab or 15 mL Q 30-60 minutes (Maximum 8 doses/day)

H. Patients with chronic diarrhea require treatment of the underlying cause
   1. Refer to sections on HIV/AIDS and IRRITABLE BOWEL SYNDROME for management of patients with these conditions
   2. If Giardia is suspected, obtain appropriate diagnostic tests

3. If a medication that the patient is taking is producing the diarrhea, change medication if possible
4. If inflammatory bowel disease or a malabsorption syndrome such as sprue or lactase deficiency is suspected, refer to a specialist for management

I. Follow Up
1. Infants and small children: In 24 hours
2. Older children and adults: In 48 hours if diarrhea has not resolved

GASTROESOPHAGEAL REFLUX IN INFANTS

I. Definition: Effortless regurgitation of a portion of the feeding

II. Pathogenesis

A. There are three main physiological barriers for preventing reflux of gastric contents into the esophagus:
1. Functional esophageal sphincter
2. Normal distal esophageal motility
3. Efficient gastric emptying

B. Reflux in infants appears to be caused by a delay in maturation of one or more of the three barriers and is considered a multifactorial disorder

III. Clinical Presentation

A. Reflux is a common condition, occurring to a significant degree in about 18% of all infants

B. More common in premature babies

C. Most often occurs during or soon after feeding

D. Self-limited; resolves rapidly with time. Many affected infants have normal function by 6 weeks; by 6 months almost all have improved or resolved; 90% have complete resolution by 18 months

E. Infants with physiologic reflux are otherwise healthy with appropriate growth and development

F. Choking during feedings (except on a very occasional basis) should not be attributed to reflux

G. Infants with significant regurgitation or vomiting might be responding to disease process outside the gastrointestinal tract

IV. Diagnosis/Evaluation

A. History
1. Question regarding type, amount, and frequency of feeding; timing, frequency, and amount of reflux
2. Ask if coughing or frequent choking during feedings occurs
3. Question regarding bloody or bilious vomiting, regurgitation of entire feedings
4. Question about signs or symptoms such as fever, irritability, poor feeding, or diarrhea that might be associated with an infectious, metabolic, or neurologic cause for the reflux
5. Question regarding attainment of developmental milestones
6. Ask about any illnesses or hospitalizations since birth
7. Ask about family history of dietary protein intolerance

B. Physical Examination
1. Height, weight, and head circumference to document normal growth
2. Perform a complete head-to-toe exam, making sure to check gag and sucking reflexes
3. Observe child being fed
4. Determine if developmental milestones are present

C. Differential Diagnosis
1. Partial upper-intestinal obstruction
2. Infections such as otitis media, pneumonia, urinary tract infections

D. Diagnostic Tests: None indicated if history and physical exam are normal and infant is growing and developing normally

V. Plan/Management

A. Uncomplicated GER in infants is usually self-limiting and resolves spontaneously by 12-18 months of age

B. Rationale for the indiscriminate treatment of reflux with pharmacologic therapy in infants under 2 years of age has received little justification in the medical literature and is therefore discouraged

C. Management should be aimed at reassuring the parents and counseling them about postural placement and feeding techniques

D. Recommended postural placement: Instruct parents to hold infant upright after feeding for 15-30 minutes
1. Because the prone position is associated with SIDS, placing infant prone, flat, with the entire body tilted 30° (reverse Trendelenburg) is no longer recommended
2. Furthermore, once the infant reaches 3-4 months of age and can turn over, it is almost impossible to maintain infant in any specific position when placed in a crib

E. Dietary measures: Instruct parent in these feeding techniques
1. Avoid overfeeding and provide smaller, more frequent feedings to decrease stomach distention and reduce the volume available for reflux
2. Use of thickening agents such as rice cereal is not recommended because this is believed to delay gastric emptying, thereby increasing the time period when food is in stomach and available to be refluxed

F. With postprandial regurgitation of a small amount of feeding, no specific treatment other than reassurance to parent is indicated

G. Refer the patient to a specialist if abnormalities of the upper-gastrointestinal tract are suspected, if there is failure to gain weight at an appropriate rate, or if developmental delays are noted

H. Follow Up: In 4 weeks to evaluate if reflux is resolving

VIRAL HEPATITIS

I. Definition: An inflammatory process of the liver caused by infection by one of the five distinct viruses (A, B, C, D, and E); other causes of hepatitis are not considered here

II. Pathogenesis

   A. Hepatitis A (HAV): RNA virus which is classified as a member of the picornavirus group; replication appears to be limited to the liver; only one serotype of HAV has been recognized in humans

   B. Hepatitis B (HBV): DNA-containing hepadenavirus; important components include HbsAg, hepatitis B core antigen, and hepatitis B e antigen

   C. Hepatitis C (HCV): Small, single-stranded RNA virus of the Flavivirus family; multiple HCV genotypes exist

   D. Hepatitis D (HDV): Small particle consisting of an RNA genome and a delta protein antigen, both of which are coated with hepatitis B surface antigen; requires HBV as a helper virus; cannot produce infection in absence of HBV

   E. Hepatitis E (HEV): Single-stranded RNA virus that is structurally similar to a calicivirus

III. Clinical Presentation

   A. Hepatitis A
       1. In US, HAV infection is endemic with periodic outbreaks occurring in certain groups such as Native Americans, Alaskan natives, Hispanic communities
       2. **Mode of transmission** is primarily through fecal-oral route; spreads readily in households and child care centers, with risk of spread in such centers increasing with the number of children who wear diapers
       3. Common source **outbreaks** from food and water contaminated with human sewage also occur
       4. Unlike other infectious diseases that spread in child care centers, children who are infected are either asymptomatic or have very mild, nonspecific symptoms; adult contacts of infected children who themselves become infected, on the other hand, usually are symptomatic
       5. Illness is self-limited and includes jaundice, anorexia, nausea, vomiting, malaise, and fever
       6. When acquired during infancy and early childhood, infections are likely to be mild without jaundice; adult infections are likely to be quite severe
       7. Viral shedding and the contagious period last 1-3 weeks, with the infected person being most contagious 1-2 weeks before the onset of illness; risk of transmission diminishes and is minimal in the week after onset of jaundice (if present)
       8. **Incubation period** is 15-50 days, with an average of 25-30 days
       9. **Chronic infection does not occur**
       10. **Diagnosis**: Anti-HAV IgM appears early in the disease, diminishes after several weeks; Anti-HAV IgG develops and usually persists for life. (Thus, Anti-HAV IgM is a marker of acute infection, while anti-HAV IgG persists throughout life and is a reliable marker of past infection)
       11. Presence of serum anti-HAV IgG in unvaccinated persons indicates lifelong immunity to HAV
       12. Children vaccinated with HAV only rarely have detectable anti-HAV IgM titers

B. Hepatitis B
1. Approximately 300,000 persons are infected with HBV each year with most infected persons acquiring the disease as adolescents or adults
2. **Transmission** occurs via contact with infected blood or body fluids such as semen, cervical secretions, wound exudates, and saliva
3. **Modes of transmission** include
    a. Transfusion of blood or blood products (rare in US today)
    b. Needle-sharing
    c. Percutaneous or mucous membrane exposures to blood or body fluids
    d. Heterosexual and homosexual activity
    e. Vertical transmission (during perinatal period)
    f. More than 30% of infected persons do not have a readily identifiable risk factor
    g. Not transmitted via fecal-oral route
4. The primary reservoir for infection is the HBV chronic carrier (defined as person with serum HBsAg-positive for 6 months or more)
5. Hepatitis B causes a spectrum of illness ranging from an asymptomatic seroconversion, to acute illness with anorexia, nausea, malaise, and jaundice, to fatal hepatitis
6. Arthralgias, arthritis, and a macular skin eruption can also occur as part of the illness
7. Asymptomatic infection is most common in young children
8. Age of the person at initial HBV infection is the major determinant of chronicity; chronic HBV infection is much more likely to develop after prenatal or perinatal exposure than after exposure later in life
9. To illustrate the effect of age on chronic disease, chronic HBV infection develops in
    a. Up to 90% of infants infected by perinatal transmission
    b. Thirty percent of children 1-5 years of age
    c. Five to ten percent of older children, adolescents, and adults
10. **Incubation period** is 45-160 days, with an average of 120 days
11. **Diagnosis**: During acute illness, two detectable factors in serum are hepatitis B surface antigen (HBsAg) and antibody to the viral core proteins (Anti-HBc); when the patient recovers, HBsAg usually disappears and evidence of surface antibody (anti-HBs) can be found; the finding of coexistent anti-HBs and anti-HBc indicates a state of recovery; the e antigen (HBeAg) can also be detected during the acute phase; the presence of HBeAg in conjunction with HBsAg in the serum indicates a more serious prognosis than the presence of HBsAg alone (see INTERPRETATION OF THE HEPATITIS B PANEL table)

INTERPRETATION OF THE HEPATITIS B PANEL

Tests	Results	Interpretation
HBsAg anti-HBc anti-HBs	negative negative negative	susceptible
HBsAg anti-HBc anti-HBs	negative negative or positive positive	immune
HBsAg anti-HBc IgM anti-HBc anti-HBs	positive positive positive negative	acutely infected
HBsAg anti-HBc IgM anti-HBc anti-HBs	positive positive negative negative	chronically infected
HBsAg anti-HBc anti-HBs	negative positive negative	four interpretations possible*

* 1. May be recovering from acute HBV infection
2. May be distantly immune and test not sensitive enough to detect very low level of anti-HBs in serum
3. May be susceptible with a false positive anti-HBc
4. May be undetectable level of HBsAg present in the serum and the person is actually a carrier

Laboratory Diagnosis of Chronic Hepatitis B and C

Hepatitis B	HBsAg. If positive, obtain IgM anti-HBc to differentiate acute hepatitis B (IgM anti-HBc is positive) from chronic hepatitis B (IgM anti-HBc is negative). Chronic hepatitis B is also defined by 2 HBsAg-positive tests separated by at least 6 months
Hepatitis C	Anti-HCV. Verify a positive test with a supplemental assay such as RIBA or nucleic acid detection of HCV RNA, depending on the clinical situation

For More Information about Hepatitis B including guidelines for the management of the hepatitis B carrier, contact the Hepatitis B Coalition, 1573 Selby Avenue, St. Paul, MN 55104,

Source: Immunization Action Coalition. (1997.) Basic facts about adult hepatitis B. St. Paul, MN: Author

C. Hepatitis C
1. Prevalence of HCV infection among all age groups is estimated at 1.8%; accounts for 21% of cases of acute viral hepatitis and 60% of cases of chronic viral hepatitis in US each year
2. **Mode of transmission** is primarily through parenteral exposure to blood and blood products
3. Highest seroprevalence rates of infection (60-90%) occur in those with repeated exposure to blood or blood products such as IV drug users or patients with hemophilia (**Note**: Current risk of HCV infection following blood transfusion is about 0.1%)
4. Much lower rates (1-10%) are found among persons with inapparent parenteral exposures such as persons with high-risk sexual behaviors and sexual/household contacts of infected person
5. Other body fluids contaminated with infected blood can be source of infection with intranasal cocaine users having high rates of infection believed to be related to epistaxis and shared equipment
6. For most infected children and adolescents, no specific source can be identified
7. Signs and symptoms are often indistinguishable from those of hepatitis A or B infection
8. Acute disease is most often mild in adults and asymptomatic in children with jaundice occurring in only about 25% of those infected
9. Approximately 65-70% of patients develop chronic hepatitis with 20% developing cirrhosis
10. All persons with HCV antibody and/or HCV-RNA in their blood are considered to be contagious
11. **Incubation period** ranges from 2 weeks to 6 months with an average of 6-7 weeks
12. **Diagnosis**: Two types of tests are available for diagnosis of HCV (see following table)

DIAGNOSTIC TESTS FOR HCV

Antibody-based tests
- ➡ Include an enzyme-linked immunosorbent assay (ELISAII) and Recombinant immunoblot assay (RIBA)
- ➡ Diagnosis using antibody assays involves an initial screening enzyme immunoassay (EIA)
  - ✦ Positive results are confirmed by a recombinant immunoblot assay (RIBA)
  - ✦ Both assays detect IgG antibody; no IgM assays are currently available
  - ✦ Within 5-6 weeks after onset of illness, 80% of patients will be positive for serum anti-HCV antibody

PCR and branched chain DNA (bDNA) assays for HCV
- ➡ Are able to identify HCV sooner after infection than the antibody based tests
- ➡ Compared with antibody-based tests, HCV RNA testing
  - ✦ Is more sensitive
  - ✦ Provides a better marker for effectiveness of treatment
  - ✦ Is much more expensive
  - ✦ Is best used for follow-up to help distinguish active from past infection in patients who are anti-HCV positive

Note: Tests for detecting HCV antigen have not yet been developed

D. Hepatitis D
1. Prevalence of HDV in the US is highest among parenteral drug users, hemophiliacs, and immigrants from endemic areas of the world
2. Occurs as either a **coinfection** with HBV (e.g., following inoculation with blood or secretions that contain both agents) or as a **superinfection** in established chronic HBV infection
3. **Mode of transmission** is via blood or blood products, injection drugs, or sexual contact providing HBV also is present
4. Transmission from mother to newborn is uncommon
5. Hepatitis D resembles hepatitis B in terms of when symptoms appear and period of infectivity
6. Hepatitis D can cause hepatitis only in persons with acute or chronic HBV infection
7. **Incubation period** for HDV superinfection is approximately 2-8 weeks; when both viruses (B and D) infect simultaneously, incubation period averages 120 days and ranges from 45-160 days
8. **Diagnosis**: Diagnosis of hepatitis D is made by detecting anti-HDV antibody in the serum

E. Hepatitis E
1. Occurs predominantly in India, South Central Asia, and the Middle East, but also occurs in the Western Hemisphere, including the US (rare)
2. **Mode of transmission** is the fecal-oral route
3. Causes an acute illness with jaundice, malaise, anorexia, abdominal pain, arthralgias, and fever
4. Occurs more commonly in adults than children and is most serious when it occurs in pregnant females
5. **Period of communicability** is unknown, but probably continues for at least 2 weeks after the acute phase
6. **Chronic infection does not occur**
7. **Incubation period** ranges from 15-60 days, with an average of 40 days
8. **Diagnosis**: Serologic testing for hepatitis E is not available; diagnosis rests on excluding other causes of viral hepatitis

F. The following table contains a comparison of the 5 forms of viral hepatitis

COMPARISON OF FIVE FORMS OF VIRAL HEPATITIS			
Form	Primary Route of Transmission	Incubation Period	Chronicity
Hepatitis A	Fecal-oral, contaminated food/water	15-50 days	None
Hepatitis B	Blood/body fluids	45-160 days	Yes
Hepatitis C	Blood/blood products	14-180 days	Yes
Hepatitis D	Blood/body fluids	45-160 days	Yes
Hepatitis E	Fecal-oral	15-60 days	None

G. All five types of viral hepatitis are similar in their clinical expression and therefore cannot be readily distinguished by clinical features

H. Clinical features include the following:
1. Fatigue, lassitude, anorexia, nausea, dark urine, low grade fever, right upper abdominal discomfort, myalgia, and arthralgias
2. Only a minority of persons who are infected develop jaundice
3. Many infected persons are asymptomatic

I. The characteristic laboratory abnormalities are elevated aminotransferase levels that are high early in the prodromal period, peak before jaundice is maximal, and fall slowly during the convalescent period
1. Aspartate aminotransferase (AST) and alanine aminotransferase (ALT) levels are typically 500-2000 IU/L
2. ALT is usually higher than AST (in alcoholic hepatitis, the reverse is usual)
3. Alkaline phosphatase is only modestly elevated
4. Degree of hyperbilirubinemia is variable
5. Urinary bile usually precedes jaundice
6. Increase in prothrombin time is uncommon; if present suggests severe illness
7. WBC count is usually low-normal, and blood smear may show a few atypical lymphocytes

J. Serologic testing determines the specific etiologic diagnosis

IV. Diagnosis/Evaluation

A. History
1. Question about onset and duration of symptoms (usual symptoms are general fatigue, malaise, joint and muscle pain, loss of appetite, nausea, vomiting, diarrhea, and low-grade fever; tenderness of right upper quadrant and jaundice may also occur)
2. Ask about darkened urine, light-colored stools
3. Inquire about similar illness in household contacts
4. Ask about sexual behaviors and similar illness in sexual partners
5. Ask about history of blood transfusions, IV drug use, alcohol abuse
6. Inquire about occupation
7. Obtain travel history, especially travel to Asia or Africa where hepatitis B is especially common
8. Obtain past medical history and medication history

B. Physical Examination
1. Examine skin, mucous membranes, and sclera for jaundice
2. Perform abdominal exam to determine size, surface characteristics, and tenderness of liver; determine if spleen is enlarged

C. Differential Diagnosis: Noninfectious causes of hepatitis including medications, acute alcohol induced injury

D. Diagnostic Tests
1. If acute hepatitis is suspected, order appropriate diagnostic tests recommended above based on type of hepatitis that is suspected (many insurance carriers will not pay for "hepatitis panels")

2. Serologic features of viral hepatitis are summarized in the following table:

SEROLOGIC FEATURES OF VIRAL HEPATITIS		
Form of Infection	**Serologic Markers**	**Interpretation**
Hepatitis A	IgM anti-HAV	Acute disease
	IgG anti-HAV	Remote infection and immunity
Hepatitis B	HBsAg	Acute or chronic disease
	HBeAg	Active replication (If persists beyond first 3 months, likelihood of chronic infection increases; thus more important to test for in chronic disease)
	IgM anti-HBc	Positive in acute infection; negative in chronic infection
	Anti-HBs	Remote infection and immunity
Hepatitis C	Anti-HCV	Acute, chronic, or resolved disease
Hepatitis D	HBsAg and anti-HDV	Acute disease
	● IgM anti-HBc positive	Co-infection
	● IgG anti-HBc positive	Superinfection
Hepatitis E	None commercially available	

Anti-HAV, antibody to hepatitis A virus; anti-HCV, antibody to hepatitis C virus; anti-HDV, antibody to hepatitis D virus; HBeAg, hepatitis B e antigen; HBsAg, hepatitis B surface antigen; anti-HBc, antibody to hepatitis B core antigen; anti-HBs, antibody to HBsAg

3. If HBsAg is present, testing for HBeAg is needed to determine whether active viral replication is present
4. Testing for anti-HDV should be done in all persons with chronic hepatitis B to rule out coexisting hepatitis D
5. If all test results are negative, follow up testing for anti-HCV is appropriate because of delay in appearance of antibody
6. CBC, total and direct bilirubin, prothrombin time, liver function tests, urinalysis should be obtained also
7. All persons with chronic hepatitis should have liver biopsy to determine extent of disease

V. Plan/Management

A. Hepatitis usually resolves spontaneously over 4-8 weeks

B. For acute infections for all types of viral hepatitis (A, B, C, D, E), provide symptomatic treatment for symptoms such as myalgia, nausea, vomiting, and pruritus

C. Bed rest, special diets, vitamin supplements are not required

D. If patient on hepatotoxic drugs, those should be discontinued until recovery has occurred

E. Interferon alpha is the only treatment that has been shown to be effective in treatment of chronic hepatitis infection in adults

VI. Control measures: Hepatitis A

A. Improved sanitation and personal hygiene (especially good hand washing) are the keys to controlling spread of the virus

B. Postexposure prophylaxis for household and sexual contacts: Give 0.02 mL/kg of immune globulin (IG) as soon as possible after exposure (use of IG more than 2 weeks after last exposure in not indicated) **and** give HAV vaccine in dosage and schedule under VI.E. below

C. Newborn infants of infected mothers: If mother's symptoms began 2 weeks before or 1 week after delivery, give IG (0.02 mL/kg) to newborn (**Note:** Perinatal transmission is rare)

D. When there is an index case in a child care center:
1. Report all child care associated hepatitis A cases to local health department
2. Stress importance of good hygiene to prevent fecal-oral spread
3. Children and adults with acute hepatitis should be excluded from child care until one week after onset of illness
4. For use of immune globulin (IG) in child care facilities, consult Red Book (1997) for details of management

E. Hepatitis A vaccine: Havrix and Vaqta, both with pediatric and adult formulations are now available in the US
1. Havrix for children 2-18 years of age has two formulations, one for a 2 dose and the second for a 3 dose schedule
2. Vaqta for children 2-18 years of age is given in a 2 dose schedule only
3. Children ≥19 and adults receive a 2 dose schedule of either Havrix or Vaqta

F. Hepatitis A vaccine should be given to the following groups:
1. International travelers
2. Children ≥2 years living in communities with high endemic rates/periodic outbreaks
3. Patients with chronic liver disease
4. Homosexual and bisexual males
5. Users of injection/illicit drugs
6. Persons with occupational risk of exposure
7. Any healthy person at least 2 years of age at discretion of health care provider (examples, child care center staff/attendees, custodial care workers, hospital workers, food handlers)

VII. Control measures: Hepatitis B

A. **All infants** should receive hepatitis B vaccine as part of their routine immunizations in childhood (series of 3 doses is required for optimal antibody response); all children who have not received the vaccine previously should be immunized by or before 11 or 12 years of age [see IMMUNIZATIONS section]
1. Susceptibility testing before vaccination is not recommended in children and adolescents
2. Testing for previous infection should be considered in adults in high-risk groups

B. Prenatal screening for HBsAg can prevent perinatal transmission (for care of infant whose mother is HBsAg-Positive, consult Red Book (1997), pp. 256-257, as these children do need special care including HBIG within 12 hours after birth)

C. Prevention of HBV transmission to medical personnel is possible through use of universal precautions for blood and body fluids; nonetheless, all health care workers and others with occupational exposure to blood are at high risk and should be immunized

D. Consult Red Book (1997) for complete listing of other high-risk groups who should receive pre-exposure hepatitis B immunization

E. Recommendations for Hepatitis B prophylaxis after percutaneous or permucosal exposure are contained in the following table

RECOMMENDED POSTEXPOSURE PROPHYLAXIS FOR PERCUTANEOUS OR PERMUCOSAL EXPOSURE TO HEPATITIS B VIRUS, UNITED STATES

Vaccination and Antibody Response Status of Exposed Person	Treatment When Source Is		
	HBsAg[1] Positive	HBsAg Negative	Source Not Tested or Status Unknown
Unvaccinated	HBIG[2] x 1; initiate HB vaccine series[3]	Initiate HB vaccine series	Initiate HB vaccine series
Previously vaccinated: Known responder[4]	No treatment	No treatment	No treatment
Known non-responder	HBIG x 2 or HBIG x 1 and initiate revaccination	No treatment	If known high-risk source, treat as if source were HBsAg positive
Antibody response unknown	Test exposed person for anti-HBs[5] 1. If adequate,[4] no treatment 2. If inadequate,[4] HBIG x 1 and vaccine booster	No treatment	Test exposed person for anti-HBs 1. If adequate,[4] no treatment 2. In inadequate,[4] initiate revaccination

[1]Hepatitis B surface antigen [2]Hepatitis B immune globulin; dose 0.06 mL/kg intramuscularly [3]Hepatitis B vaccine [4]Responder is defined as a person with adequate levels of serum antibody to hepatitis B surface antigen (i.e., anti-HBs ≥10 mIU/mL); inadequate response to vaccination defined as serum anti-HBs <10 mIU/mL [5]Antibody to hepatitis B surface antigen
Source: Centers for Disease Control. (1997). Immunization of health care workers. MMWR, 46, No. RR-18.

VIII. Control measures: Hepatitis C

   A.   Should be managed with the universal precautions for blood and body fluids as in Hepatitis B

   B.   Because a high percentage of persons with Hepatitis C develop chronic liver disease, referral to specialist for management is indicated

IX.   Control measures: Hepatitis D

   A.   Transmission is similar to that of HBV, so universal precautions for blood and body fluids should be observed

   B.   Cannot be transmitted in the absence of HBV, so prevention of HBV is key to prevention

   C.   Immunoprophylaxis not available

X.   Control measures: Hepatitis E

   A.   Immunoprophylaxis not available

   B.   Prevention through good sanitation and hygiene

XI.   Follow Up

   A.   Variable depending on type of hepatitis

   B.   Hepatitis A and E do not have a chronic stage, so generally resolve without any long-term effects (Hepatitis E only found in developing countries and rarely in the US at this time)
       1.   Make sure IG prophylaxis is given as described above
       2.   Emphasize control measures to prevent spread
       3.   Recheck patient after 2 weeks to evaluate condition

   C.   Hepatitis B, C, D should be referred for management because of development of high rate of chronic hepatitis

ABNORMAL LIVER FUNCTION TESTS

I. Definition: Elevations in serum values of liver chemistries in asymptomatic patients

II. Pathogenesis:

A. Although these tests are referred to as "liver function tests," they are not a true assessment of liver function but rather markers of hepatic injury

B. Liver function tests provide information on three liver functions: cellular integrity, protein synthesis, and excretory function
    1. Alanine aminotransferase (ALT) and aspartate aminotransferase (AST) are measures of cellular integrity
    2. Prothrombin time (PT) and albumin level reflect the liver's synthetic capacity
    3. Bilirubin, gamma-glutamyl-transpeptidase (GTT) and alkaline phosphatase (ALP) measure hepatic excretory function

C. **Evaluation of cellular integrity**: ALT and AST are enzymes found in many tissues and cellular injury causes these enzymes to leak into the interstitial space and plasma
    1. Serum levels are elevated not only with hepatocellular injury, but also with such conditions as myocardial infarction and musculoskeletal injury
    2. Highest elevations are seen in toxin or drug induced, viral or ischemic hepatitis
    3. Acetaminophen overdose can produce transaminase elevations higher than 10,000 IU
    4. Alanine Aminotransferase (ALT)
        a. High concentrations are located in liver, especially the periportal area; found in muscle to a lesser extent
        b. A more specific marker of hepatocellular damage than AST as elevated ALT level is more likely to reflect damage to liver than to other organ systems
        c. (**Note**: Determination of creatine phosphokinase [CPK] levels can exclude brain and muscle injury as the source of abnormal levels)
        d. Isolated measures not as useful as serial measures because levels change rapidly
    5. Aspartate Aminotransferase (AST)
        a. Predominantly found in liver, cardiac and skeletal muscle, and the kidney
        b. Levels become elevated when injury to hepatocyte occurs, particularly to mitochondria
    6. An AST:ALT ratio >2 is highly correlated with damage from alcohol ingestion

D. **Evaluation of protein synthesis**: Measurement of the hepatic synthetic function is done through measurement of serum albumin level and prothrombin time (Protime) [a reflection of hepatic synthesis of Factors I, II, V, VII, and X]
    1. Albumin is the most abundant serum protein with about 12 g synthesized by the liver each day
    2. Albumin synthesis can be affected by such factors as decreased dietary protein intake, increased alcohol consumption, trauma, and conticosteroids
    3. Elevated Protime can be due to deficiency of one of the Factors, but can also be due to vitamin K deficiency
        a. To differentiate between hypovitamin K and liver disease, administer vitamin K, 10 mg IM and recheck Protime in 24 hours
        b. If the Protime improves by at least 30%, hepatic synthetic function is intact

E. **Evaluation of excretory function**: Alkaline Phosphatase (ALP), bilirubin, and gamma-glutamyl-transpeptidase (GGT) are markers of cholestatic injury/hepatic excretory function
    1. Alkaline Phosphatase has origin in multiple tissues including bone, liver, placenta, intestine, and leukocytes, with more than 80% derived from liver and bone
        a. In late pregnancy, level can double and still be considered normal
        b. Can be normally elevated in childhood/adolescence as it is a measure of osteoblastic activity in bone

    c. Elevations of this enzyme to a degree greater than transaminase elevation is consistent with cholestatic injury (intra- or extrahepatic biliary obstruction)

    d. If the Alkaline Phosphatase is the only abnormality on the LFT screen, consider a GGT (described below) to help differentiate liver versus bone as the source

  2. Bilirubin is elevated in patients with cholestasis and liver damage

    a. Humans produce about 4 mg/kg/day of bilirubin with the majority attributable to red blood cell breakdown

    b. Small contribution comes from degradation of heme containing proteins in the liver and destruction of erythroid cells when erythropoiesis is ineffective

    c. Total bilirubin levels reflect both direct and indirect bilirubin

    d. Pathway of bilirubin metabolism

     (1) About 80% of bilirubin is derived from breakdown of RBCs in the reticuloendothelial system

     (2) Bilirubin is then transported to liver for further metabolism bound to albumin

    e. After arriving in liver, three phases of metabolism occur

     (1) First, uptake-dissociation from albumin takes place

     (2) Second, there is conjugation-addition of one or two molecules of glucuronic acid

     (3) Third, excretion-via bile occurs (the rate limiting step)

    f. Indirect bilirubin is insoluble in water, but is lipid soluble allowing for diffusion across membranes

    g. Direct bilirubin is bilirubin conjugated to glucuronic acid, which is water soluble and allows for intestinal excretion in bile

    h. An excess of unconjugated bilirubin implies a problem in bilirubin metabolism at level of conjugation or any of the other steps

    i. Specifically, this means overproduction of bilirubin

  3. Gamma-glutamyl-transpeptidase (GGT) is found in liver, kidney, pancreas, heart, and brain

    a. Function of enzyme remains unclear but serves as tool in correlation of hepatobiliary disease with abnormal serum alkaline phosphatase (ALP); parallels the activity of ALP, except in the presence of bone disease

    b. A sensitive indicator of hepatic disease (elevated in >95% of all diseases involving liver)

    c. Particularly sensitive to damage caused by drugs and chemicals

    d. Isolated elevation of GGT is a sensitive screening test for excess alcohol use

III. Clinical Presentation

  A. Patient may be asymptomatic and abnormal laboratory findings were unanticipated

  B. Variable presentation depending on the underlying cause

IV. Diagnosis/Evaluation

  A. History

    1. Inquire about any symptoms such as anorexia, weight loss, malaise

    2. Ask about alcohol and drug use

    3. Obtain detailed medication history (always ask about use of vitamins, dietary supplements, herbs)

    4. Ask about previous medical history including any previous acute illnesses that could have been hepatitis, surgical history for any gastrointestinal problems, history of blood transfusions

    5. Obtain detailed sexual history

    6. Question patient about household/work exposures to chemicals such as carbon tetrachloride, vinyl chloride

B. Physical Examination: Focus should be on searching for evidence of liver disease
1. Skin exam for spider angioma, palmar erythema, jaundice
2. Sclera for icterus
3. Abdominal exam, checking for ascites, right upper quadrant tenderness, hepatomegaly, splenomegaly
4. Complete other parts of the exam as necessary

C. Diagnostic Testing
1. If history and physical examination are normal, and patient is completely asymptomatic, repeat testing is the first step with the addition of ancillary tests to confirm liver damage; as part of the repeat blood draw, consider testing for hepatitis B and C
   a. Consultation with a specialist at this point may be helpful in order to determine if imaging studies are indicated
   b. Note: Serum ALP and GGT levels are often abnormal if tumors, granulomas, or cholestasis are present, which would indicate need for imaging studies
2. If history and physical examination are abnormal, refer patient to a specialist for imaging studies, with ultrasound usually being the first choice

D. Differential Diagnosis: Many conditions/diseases affect cellular integrity, protein synthesis, and excretory function

V. Plan/Management

A. Diagnostic testing as outlined above is the first step in management

B. If no underlying cause is found, and the patient remains completely asymptomatic, observation for 3 to 6 months for progressive symptoms and liver dysfunction may be appropriate
1. Further laboratory testing should be done at the end of this period of observation
2. If abnormalities in liver function tests persist, referral to a specialist is indicated

C. Follow up: Should be done by specialist to whom patient was referred

HYPERBILIRUBINEMIA IN THE HEALTHY TERM INFANT

I. Definition: Elevations in bilirubin in the circulating blood, resulting in clinically apparent icterus or jaundice that occurs in infants ≥ 37 weeks of gestation who are otherwise healthy

II. Pathogenesis

A. Jaundice in the newborn period results from an imbalance between the production and excretion of bilirubin and is generally clinically apparent at levels greater than 2.0 to 2.5 mg/dL

B. Nonpathologic causes of hyperbilirubinemia in the neonate are physiologic jaundice and jaundice associated with breast-feeding
1. Physiologic jaundice results from the interaction of a number of complex factors that results in an overproduction of bilirubin as well as delayed conjugation of bilirubin
   a. RBC survival is shortened and catabolism of fetal hemoglobin is increased
   b. There is delayed conjugation of bilirubin that occurs secondary to immaturity of the glucuronyl transferase enzyme
   c. A decrease in cytoplasmic transport proteins delays hepatocellular transport of bilirubin
   d. Increased intestinal reabsorption of unconjugated bilirubin further delays conjugation of bilirubin

2. Jaundice associated with breast-feeding results from causes that have not been clearly established, but the proposed etiologies includes the following
   a. There is competitive inhibition of glucuronyl transferase by long-chain fatty acids within the breast milk leading to impaired conjugation of bilirubin
   b. There is increased absorption from the gastrointestinal tract, and altered bile acid metabolism

C. There are numerous pathologic causes of neonatal jaundice including hemolysis from Rh/ABO incompatibility, hemoglobinopathies, erythrocyte membrane defects, sepsis, hypoxia, and Gilbert syndrome

III. Clinical Presentation

A. Approximately 60% of the 4 million newborns in the US become clinically jaundiced with unconjugated bilirubin levels that peak on average between 5-6 mg/dL

B. Physiologic jaundice is a self-limited clinical state that usually appears on the second or third day of life and resolves in 7-10 days in the full-term infant (pattern in preterm infant is different)
   1. Peak rise in bilirubin occurs at 3 days of age and rarely exceeds 10 mg/dL
   2. Presently, it remains unclear as to what level of bilirubin concentration or under what circumstances significant risk of brain damage occurs or when the risk of damage exceeds the risk of treatment

C. Jaundice associated with breast-feeding occurs in about 1% of breast-fed infants, usually appearing between the 6th and 8th days of life in otherwise healthy infants
   1. Frequently recurs in siblings
   2. The serum concentrations of unconjugated bilirubin is usually ≤15 mg/dL
   3. Approximately 30% of healthy breast-fed infants have persistent jaundice
   4. Breast milk jaundice has never been known to cause kernicterus

D. A mild, gradual caudal progression of yellow skin discoloration is the usual presentation in a neonate with physiologic jaundice or jaundice associated with breast-feeding
   1. Dermal icterus is apparent first in the face and progresses caudally to the trunk and extremities
   2. As the total serum bilirubin (TSB) rises, the extent of cephalocaudal progression may be helpful in quantifying the degree of jaundice; the use of an icterometer or transcutaneous jaundice meter may be helpful
   3. Skin color of the infant may alter the clinical presentation of jaundice but the sclera, mucous membranes, and palmar aspects of the hands and feet are good indicators of the degree of jaundice

IV. Diagnosis/Evaluation

A. History
   1. Question parent about onset of jaundice; ask when was jaundice first noticed and what part of the body was involved initially
   2. Obtain complete feeding history including whether bottle or breast fed, type of formula (if bottle-fed), number and amount of feedings and how infant tolerates feedings
   3. In addition to jaundice, question parent if other signs and symptoms are present such as poor feeding, vomiting, lethargy, irritability, abnormal stooling, decrease in number of wet diapers
   4. Inquire about the course of pregnancy, including history of maternal illnesses, exposure to infection, drug use during pregnancy, and any medications taken during the pregnancy; obtain complete birth history including any maternal complications, weight and Apgar scores of infant at birth
   5. Obtain detailed family history including presence of familial forms of jaundice, whether jaundice was present in sibling (of patient), and whether there have been infant deaths of patient's siblings

B. Physical Examination
    1.   Determine if fever is present, and weigh infant to assess weight gain (or loss) since birth
    2.   A well-lighted room is essential for a proper clinical assessment of jaundice
    3.   Observe overall appearance looking for congenital malformations and dysmorphism
    4.   Observe skin color which may be yellowish; observe conjunctiva for icterus
    5.   Blanch the skin using digital pressure, to reveal the underlying color of the skin and the subcutaneous tissue (experts in the diagnosis and management of neonatal jaundice may use noninvasive measurement instruments such as an icterometer or transcutaneous jaundice meter to help quantify the degree of jaundice)
    6.   Perform complete physical exam, focusing on the abdominal exam; determine size, firmness and texture of the liver

C. Differential Diagnosis: Pathologic versus physiologic/breast-milk jaundice
    1.   Factors that suggest the possibility of hemolytic disease are listed in the following table

FACTORS SUGGESTING HEMOLYTIC DISEASE IN THE NEWBORN
Family history of significant hemolytic disease
Onset of jaundice prior to age 24 hours
A rise in serum bilirubin levels of more than 0.5 mg/dL/hour
Pallor, hepatosplenomegaly
Rapid increase in the TSB level after 24-48 hours
Ethnicity suggestive of inherited disease
Failure of phototherapy to lower the TSB level

    2.   Factors that suggest the possibility of other disease such as sepsis or galactosemia are listed in the following table

FACTORS SUGGESTING OTHER DISEASES
Vomiting, poor feeding, lethargy
Apnea, tachypnea
Hepatosplenomegaly
Weight loss, temperature instability

D. Diagnostic Tests
    1.   A direct Coombs' test, a blood type, and an Rh(D) type on the infant's cord (preferably) or venous blood are recommended when the mother has not had prenatal blood grouping or is Rh-negative
    2.   Measure infant's total serum bilirubin (TSB) with follow up measurements as indicated
    3.   If pathologic jaundice is suspected based on history and physical examination, additional testing will be done by the specialist to whom the infant is referred

V. Plan/Management

A. All infants suspected of having pathologic jaundice, or who have feeding difficulty, behavior changes, apnea, fever, or temperature instability must immediately be referred to an expert for management

B. Management of hyperbilirubinemia in the healthy term newborn has been outlined in a practice parameter issued by the American Academy of Pediatrics (AAP) and provides the basis for the recommendations contained here

C. The practice parameter is based on the underlying belief that therapeutic interventions for hyperbilirubinemia in the healthy term infant may carry significant risk relative to the uncertain risk of hyperbilirubinemia in this population and that there are no simple solutions to management of neonates who are jaundiced

D. Management decisions are based on age of the infant in hours and the total serum bilirubin levels (**Note**: Keep in mind that this discussion involves management of the healthy term infant with physiologic or breast-feeding jaundice only!)
   1. Four options are recommended and are detailed in the four tables that follow: Consider phototherapy, order phototherapy, order exchange transfusion, and order both exchange transfusion and phototherapy
   2. Recommendations are for infants initially seen with elevated TSB levels as well as infants who are being followed up for clinical jaundice
   3. The TSB level is relied on as the relevant criterion; because direct bilirubin measurements vary substantially among various laboratories, it is recommended that the direct bilirubin measurement NOT be subtracted from the TSB level
   4. There is continuing uncertainty regarding what specific TSB levels warrant exchange transfusion

E. Infants ≤24 hours old are excluded from the practice parameter because jaundice occurring before the age of 24 hours is considered pathologic and always requires further evaluation

F. Treatment of jaundice associated with breast-feeding should follow the same guidelines as those outlined in the tables below with the following special considerations
   1. Breast-feeding in healthy term newborns should not be interrupted; continued and frequent breast-feeding (8-10 times every 24 hours) is recommended
   2. Supplementing breast feeding with water or dextrose water does not lower the bilirubin level in jaundiced, healthy, breast-feeding infants and is therefore unnecessary
   3. However, depending upon the mother's preference and the health care provider's judgment, several options are available; breast-feeding can be continued or interrupted and phototherapy administered if indicated based on age of infant in hours and TSB level

INFANTS IN THE FOLLOWING CATEGORY SHOULD BE CONSIDERED* FOR PHOTOTHERAPY	
Age in Hours	**TSB Level, mg/dL (pmol/L)**
25-48	>12 (170)
49-72	>15 (260)
>72	>17 (290)

*This means that treatment with phototherapy is a clinical option that is available and should be used according to the judgment of the clinician in consultation with experts and with the parents

Source: American Academy of Pediatrics, Provisional Committee for Quality Improvement and Subcommittee on Hyperbilirubinemia. (1994). Management of hyperbilirubinemia in the healthy term newborn. Pediatrics, 94, 558-562.

INFANTS IN THE FOLLOWING CATEGORY SHOULD RECEIVE PHOTOTHERAPY	
Age in Hours	**TSB Level, mg/dL (pmol/L)**
25-48	>15 (260)
49-72	>18 (310)
>72	>20 (340)

Source: American Academy of Pediatrics, Provisional Committee for Quality Improvement and Subcommittee on Hyperbilirubinemia. (1994). Management of hyperbilirubinemia in the healthy term newborn. Pediatrics, 94, 558-562.

Age in Hours	TSB Level, mg/dL (pmol/L)
INFANTS IN THE FOLLOWING CATEGORY SHOULD RECEIVE EXCHANGE TRANSFUSION IF INTENSIVE PHOTOTHERAPY FAILS*	
25-48	>20 (340)
49-72	>25 (430)
>72	>25 (430)

* Intensive phototherapy should produce a decline of TSB of 1-2 mg/dL within 4-6 hours and the TSB level should continue to fall and remain below the threshold level for exchange transfusion--if this does not occur, phototherapy is considered a failure

Source: American Academy of Pediatrics, Provisional Committee for Quality Improvement and Subcommittee on Hyperbilirubinemia. (1994). Management of hyperbilirubinemia in the healthy term newborn. Pediatrics, 94, 558-562.

Age in Hours	TSB Level, mg/dL (pmol/L)
INFANTS IN THE FOLLOWING CATEGORY SHOULD RECEIVE EXCHANGE TRANSFUSION AND INTENSIVE PHOTOTHERAPY	
25-48	>25 (430)
49-72	>30 (510)
>72	>30 (510)

Source: American Academy of Pediatrics, Provisional Committee for Quality Improvement and Subcommittee on Hyperbilirubinemia. (1994). Management of hyperbilirubinemia in the healthy term newborn. Pediatrics, 94, 558-562.

G.   Follow Up
    1.   Infants requiring phototherapy and exchange transfusion are best managed by experts
    2.   Many issues must be managed such as selection of method for delivery of phototherapy, intermittent versus continuous phototherapy, role of intensive phototherapy, requirements for hydration and fluid supplementation, and criteria for discontinuation of phototherapy
    3.   Follow up should be with the specialist to whom the infant was referred

ABDOMINAL HERNIAS

I.   Definition: Protrusion of an abdominal viscus or part of a viscus through the abdominal wall

    A.   Incarcerated hernias are hernias that cannot be reduced and the contents of the hernial sac cannot be returned to the peritoneal cavity

    B.   Strangulated hernias are hernias which occur when the blood supply to the viscera lying within the hernial sac is obliterated or cut off

II.   Pathogenesis

    A.   A hernia is a defect in the normal musculofascial continuity of the abdominal wall and is either congenital or acquired

    B.   Acquired hernias may occur from any condition that increases intraabdominal pressure such as obesity, chronic cough, ascites, chronic constipation with straining, and lifting heavy objects

    C.   Distinction between congenital and acquired hernias is often unclear as hernias can be acquired because of a congenital predisposition
        1.   Distinction has little implication for management
        2.   Distinction may be very important when work-related injury is claimed

III.   Clinical Presentation

    A.   The symptoms of reducible hernias are related to the degree of pressure of contents rather than to size

    B.   Most patients with reducible hernias are asymptomatic or complain of only mild pain, whereas patients with strangulated hernias have colicky abdominal pain, nausea, vomiting, abdominal distention, and hyperperistalsis

    C.   Inguinal hernias are classified as direct (portions of the bowel and/or omentum protrude directly through the floor of the inguinal canal and emerge at the external inguinal ring) or indirect (pass through the internal abdominal ring, traverse the spermatic cord through the inguinal canal and emerge at the external inguinal ring) [see Figure 12.3]
        1.   Approximately 75% of abdominal hernias are inguinal; most common type of hernia in both genders but occurs more frequently in males
        2.   Indirect hernias are more common in younger persons since they are due to a congenital defect in which the processus vaginalis remains patent
            a.   However, the incidence of inguinal hernias increases with advancing age and are approximately four times more common after age 50 years than before
            b.   Indirect hernias often enter the scrotum
        3.   Direct hernias occur mainly in the middle and later years of life and are due to a weakness in the abdominal structures. Direct hernias usually reduce and rarely enter the scrotum
        4.   Symptoms of both direct and indirect hernias include a dull ache in the groin and a bulge localized in the groin or extended into the scrotum (referred to as a complete hernia); in females a complete hernia may enter the labia major as a labial hernia

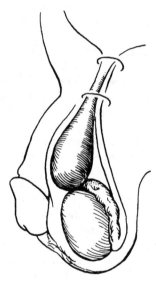

Figure 12.3. Hernia.
Source: Judge, R.D., Zuidma, G.D., &   Fitzgerald, F.T. (Eds.). (1989). <u>Clinical diagnosis</u>. Boston: Little, Brown, & Company, p. 381. Reprinted by permission.

    D.   Femoral hernias: Protrusion of omentum through the femoral canal
        1.   Second most common abdominal hernia in both females and males; rare in children
        2.   Occurs 3-5 times more commonly in females than males
        3.   Incidence increases with age and with increased pressure produced by pregnancy and straining
        4.   Risk of strangulation is high
        5.   In females, may have signs of intestinal obstruction

    E.   Incisional hernias: Protrusion of bowel and/or omentum through a surgical incision
        1.   Risk factors are post-operative wound infection, dehiscence, malnutrition, obesity, and smoking
        2.   Bulge can usually be seen through incision
        3.   If not repaired immediately, an intestinal obstruction can develop

F. Umbilical hernias: Protrusion of bowel and/or omentum through the umbilical ring
    1. So common in infants and young children that it can be considered a normal variation
        a. Incidence varies widely with race, affecting African American children much more often
        b. Low birth weight infants are more often affected; males and females are affected equally
    2. Also occurs in middle-aged multiparous females, patients with cirrhosis and ascites, chronically ill patients and elderly patients
    3. Infrequently, patient may have vague, intermittent pain and tenderness
    4. Most umbilical hernias in infants close spontaneously (many close within the first year of life and the majority are closed by the fifth year); infrequently, these hernias may become incarcerated and/or strangulated

G. Epigastric hernias: Protrusion of fat or omentum through the linea alba between the umbilicus and the xiphoid
    1. Most common in males between the ages of 20-50
    2. Presents as small, painless subcutaneous mass

IV. Diagnosis/Evaluation

A. History
    1. Inquire about circumstances and time of onset of hernia
    2. Ask about presence of **alarm markers**: acute onset of colicky abdominal pain, nausea, vomiting (suggests entrapment/strangulation in person with known hernia)
    3. Inquire about groin pain and swelling
    4. Determine whether patient can reduce hernia
    5. Ask about aggravating and alleviating factors (worse with standing, straining, coughing?)

B. Physical examination is directed at determining type of hernia, distinguishing hernias from other causes of inguinal swelling/pain, and identification of hernias that require no therapy, those that should be referred for elective surgery, and those for which emergency surgery is indicated
    1. Patients with reducible hernias should be examined in both standing and supine positions
    2. Carefully inspect abdomen and groin, with and without patients performing Valsalva maneuver
    3. With hernias that are not reducible, assess for discoloration, edema, elevated temperature, tenderness, and signs of bowel obstruction
    4. Do not try to reduce strangulated hernias, because reduction can cause gangrenous bowel to enter the peritoneal cavity
    5. Examination for inguinal hernias involves the following:
        a. In males, if a suspected hernia is not visible the examiner's finger should gently invaginate the scrotum and advance toward the head and laterally into the inguinal canal to the external inguinal ring; then the patient should cough or strain and the examiner should feel for a bulge at the examining finger (see Figure 12.4)
        b. With a direct hernia, when the finger is inserted through the external canal a bulge will be felt striking the side of the finger
        c. With an indirect hernia, when the finger is inserted through the external canal, the bulge will be felt at the finger tip when the patient coughs
        d. In females, it is more difficult to establish the diagnosis of inguinal hernia; locate the external inguinal ring by identifying the inguinal ligament and os pubic; place hand over inguinal ring and palpate for bulge when patient coughs
    6. Femoral hernias are more difficult to diagnose
        a. The external opening of the femoral canal can be located just medial to the femoral artery and deep to the inguinal ligament
        b. Ask patient to cough and palpate for swelling and impulse within the femoral canal
    7. To detect umbilical and incisional hernias, inspect abdomen while patient lifts head from a supine position while bearing down to tense abdominal wall
    8. Check the groin area for lymphadenopathy and other masses that are unchanged with position or Valsalva; groin pain but no mass suggests a musculoskeletal etiology

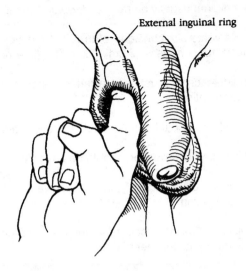

External inguinal ring

Figure 12.4. Technique of Examination for Inguinal Hernia.
Source: Judge, R.D., Zuidma, G.D., & Fitzgerald, F.T. (Eds.). (1989). <u>Clinical diagnosis</u>. Boston: Little, Brown, & Company, p. 383. Reprinted by permission.

    C.   Differential Diagnosis
        1.   Inguinal hernias (see sections on HYDROCELE and VARICOCELE)
            a.   Hydrocele
            b.   Varicocele
            c.   Spermatocele
            d.   Epididymal cysts
            e.   Epididymitis
            f.   Testicular tumor
            g.   In children, undescended testes
        2.   Femoral hernias
            a.   Enlarged lymph node
            b.   Lipoma
            c.   Direct inguinal hernia
            d.   Saphenous varix
            e.   Psoas abscess
        3.   Other causes of groin pain/swelling include muscle strain, inguinal adenopathy, and hip arthritis
        4.   Incisional, umbilical, and to a lesser extent, epigastric hernias are usually not confused with other conditions

    D.   Diagnostic Tests: Often none needed, may order ultrasound if uncertain about abdominal mass

V.   Plan/Management

    A.   Patients with asymptomatic, easily reducible inguinal hernia can be managed with watchful waiting
        1.   Elective surgery should be considered in younger patients
        2.   Obviously, should signs of incarceration develop, the patient should be referred for surgery

    B.   Patients with symptomatic, reducible inguinal hernia should be referred for elective repair

    C.   Patients with nontender incarcerated inguinal hernia of recent onset, with no signs of inflammation/obstruction, can be referred to a specialist for an attempt at reduction before referral to surgeon

    D.   Patients with reducible femoral hernias should be referred for immediate elective repair because of high rate of strangulation

E.   Umbilical hernias in children usually do not need repair; tend to close spontaneously at school age
   1.   For children < 4 years old, consider referral for hernias >4 cm in diameter (internal ring)
   2.   Consider referral for hernias >1.5 cm in diameter (internal ring) in children ≥4 years old

F.   Umbilical hernias in adolescents must be referred for repair because there is a high risk of incarceration and strangulation

G.   Patients with small neck incisional hernias should undergo immediate repair

H.   Factors associated with hernia formation should be corrected, if possible

I.   Patients who are managed conservatively should receive detailed instruction about symptoms of incarceration and strangulation

J.   Follow Up: Return visits will usually occur after surgery; for patients who do not undergo immediate surgery follow up is only needed for problems

ASCARIASIS (ROUNDWORM)

I.   Definition: An intestinal parasitic infection caused by *Ascaris lumbricoides*, a large roundworm of humans

II.   Pathogenesis

A.   Adult worms live in small intestine of humans; ova are excreted in the stool and incubate in soil for 2-3 weeks in order for embryo to form and become infectious

B.   Ingestion of infective eggs from soil that is contaminated leads to infection

C.   Ingestion occurs from eating food that is unwashed or drinking water contaminated by human feces

D.   Interval from ingestion of eggs and development of egg-laying adult worms is about 8 weeks

III.   Clinical Presentation

A.   Most commonly occurs in the tropics, in areas of poor sanitation, and in areas where human waste is used for fertilizer

B.   Worldwide, most common nematode parasite of humans; in US, second only to pinworms in prevalence

C.   Most infections are either asymptomatic infections or so mild that the infected person does not present for treatment

D.   May cause nausea, vomiting, anorexia, weight loss, fever, irritability, diarrhea, and abdominal cramping

E.   Larvae in the lungs may cause cough and wheezing

F.   Adult worms may be vomited or passed in the stool

G.   Eosinophilia is common

IV. Diagnosis/Evaluation

  A. History
     1. Question about anorexia, nausea, vomiting, weight loss, fever, irritability
     2. Ask about pica
     3. Inquire if cough, fever (lung migration) present
     4. Ask if adult worm found in stool

  B. Physical Examination
     1. Measure weight
     2. Perform abdominal exam for tenderness, masses
     3. Obtain stool for occult blood

  C. Differential Diagnosis
     1. Asthma, pneumonia
     2. Poor nutrition
     3. *Giardiasis*

  D. Diagnostic Tests
     1. If worm is visualized, none needed
     2. Three stool specimens for O&P

V. Plan/Treatment

  A. Consult the following table for treatment recommendations

DRUGS FOR TREATMENT OF ASCARIASIS (ROUNDWORM)	
Drug of Choice	**Pediatric Dosage**
Mebendazole OR	100 mg BID x 3 days
Pyrantel pamoate OR	11 mg/kg x 1 dose (Maximum 1 g)
Albendazole	400 mg x 1 dose
In pregnant females, benefits and risks should be considered	

  B. In cases of partial or complete intestinal obstructions by worms, piperazine citrate solution (75 mg/kg/day, not to exceed 3.5 g) may be given through a gastrointestinal tube

  C. Importance of maintaining a clean play area for children and sanitary disposal of feces should be emphasized

  D. Follow Up
     1. Not essential
     2. Re-examination of stools 3 weeks after therapy to determine treatment efficacy may be helpful

PINWORM INFESTATION
(ENTEROBIASIS VERMICULARIS)

I.   Definition: An intestinal parasitic infection caused by *Enterobius vermicularis*, a white, threadlike worm for whom humans are the only hosts

II.   Pathogenesis

    A.   Worms live primarily in the cecum and adjacent bowel

    B.   Adult gravid females, which are about 1 cm in length, migrate to perianal area to deposit eggs on perianal skin and then die

    C.   Infection would be self-limited at that point were it not for re-infestation

    D.   Transmission occurs via various routes, but primarily through fecal-oral route with worm eggs transmitted by fingers and via fomites such as toys, bedding, and toilet seats

    E.   Infection must be acquired from others by ingesting the ova

    F.   Incubation period from ingestion of egg until an adult worm migrates to perianal area is about 1-2 months

    G.   Eggs are fairly hardy and can remain infective in an indoor environment for 2-3 weeks; however, most eggs die within a day

III.   Clinical Presentation

    A.   Occurs worldwide and commonly in family clusters; incidence appears to have declined over past few decades

    B.   Prevalence rates are highest in preschoolers, in school-aged children, in mothers of infected children, and in the institutionalized

    C.   Perianal pruritus with secondary excoriation and dermatitis is common; rarely, pruritus vulvae occurs

    D.   Restlessness, insomnia, and loss of weight and appetite may occur

    E.   Bruxism or teeth grinding is not due to pinworms, contrary to popular opinion

    F.   In general, pinworms cause no serious problems

IV.   Diagnosis/Evaluation

    A.   History
        1.   Inquire about time of and circumstances surrounding onset of symptoms
        2.   Ask if anal pruritus is present
        3.   In females, question about genital irritation
        4.   Ask if others in household have similar symptoms

    B.   Physical Examination
        1.   Focus on exam of anus; may be excoriated from scratching
        2.   In females, also examine for genital irritation

C. Differential Diagnosis
1. Poor hygiene
2. Chemical irritants, such as bubble bath

D. Diagnostic Tests: Technique for detection follows

USING CELLOPHANE TAPE TO DETECT PINWORM EGGS

✔ Instruct parents in the following technique
  ✗ First thing in the morning, either immediately before or immediately after arising, is the best time to obtain specimen
  ✗ Using cellophane tape that is transparent, apply the tape to the perianal skin
  ✗ Cover tape with specimen with a second piece of tape and place in plastic bag for transport to office/lab
✔ Technician affixes specimen to slide (using more tape if necessary)
  ✗ Slide is then scanned under low power for eggs (eggs are 50 x 30 μg, oval, flat on one side, and thin-shelled)
    ✦ A single specimen usually detects 50% of infestations
    ✦ Three tests will detect 90%
    ✦ Five tests will detect almost 100%

V. Plan/Treatment

A. Consult the following table for treatment recommendations

B. No unusual cleaning or hygienic measures are required, but the following common sense recommendations should be followed
1. Keep nails trimmed short as eggs may lodge under nails with scratching
2. Wash hands frequently, and always on arising, before eating, and after toileting
3. Morning showers will wash away any eggs deposited during the night
4. Application of bland ointment such as petroleum jelly to the perianal area may help with dispersion of eggs

C. There is a high incidence of reinfections particularly in child care centers and schools; repeated infections should be treated the same as initial one

DRUGS FOR TREATMENT OF PINWORMS

Drug of Choice		Pediatric Dosage
Pyrantel pamoate		11 mg/kg x 1 dose (Maximum 1 g)
	OR	Repeat in 2 weeks
Mebendazole		100 mg x 1 dose
	OR	Repeat in 2 weeks
Albendazole		400 mg x 1 dose Repeat in 2 weeks
In pregnant females, benefits and risks should be considered		

D. Families may need to be treated as a group

E. Follow Up: None indicated

VISCERAL LARVA MIGRANS (HOOKWORM)

I. Definition: An intestinal parasitic infection caused by *Ancylostoma duodenale* and *Necator americanus*, two worms with similar life cycles

II. Pathogenesis

    A. Larval penetration into skin, usually soles of feet, palms of hands, occurs via contact with contaminated soil

    B. Eggs pass out with the stools of infected persons and hatch into larvae that become infective for humans; contact with contaminated soil for 5-10 minutes results in skin penetration

    C. Larvae are carried by the circulation to the lungs and eventually arrive in their final habitat, the small intestine

    D. Incubation period is about 4-6 weeks

III. Clinical Presentation

    A. Humans are the major reservoir and the disease is prevalent in rural, tropical and subtropical areas where soil is contaminated with human waste

    B. Intense pruritus can occur at the site of larvae penetration into skin; a papulovesicular eruption lasting for 1-2 weeks also commonly occurs

    C. Abdominal pain with diarrhea and eosinophilia may occur about 1 month after onset of infection

    D. Chronic infection can result in anemia secondary to blood loss

    E. Pulmonary infiltration with cough and wheezing can occur in heavily infected individuals

    F. Many infected persons who are otherwise healthy are often asymptomatic

IV. Diagnosis/Evaluation

    A. History
        1. Inquire about episodes of intense pruritus of feet, palms of hands, and buttocks in recent past
        2. Inquire about presence of papulovesicular rash on area of skin where initial penetration was likely
        3. Inquire about transitory chest symptoms (cough, wheezing)
        4. Inquire about abdominal pain, diarrhea, and weight loss

    B. Physical Examination
        1. Examine skin for erythematous papular vesicular lesions that may be excoriated from scratching. Usually located on feet, hands, or upper thighs (from sitting in sand, dirt)
        2. Abdominal exam for masses, tenderness
        3. Chest exam for wheezing

    C. Differential Diagnosis
        1. Asthma, pneumonia
        2. Poor nutrition
        3. *Giardia*

D. Diagnostic Tests:
   1. Stool for O & P x 3
   2. Microscopic examination of stools that reveal hookworm eggs in feces is diagnostic
   3. Potassium iodide saturated with iodine can be used to better visualize the eggs in the fecal smear

V. Plan/Management

   A. Consult the following table for treatment recommendations

DRUGS FOR TREATMENT OF HOOKWORM INFECTION	
Drug of Choice	**Pediatric Dosage**
Mebendazole OR	100 mg BID x 3 days
Pyrantel pamoate OR	11 mg/kg (Maximum 1 g) x 3 days
Albendazole	400 mg x 1 dose
In pregnant females, benefits and risks should be considered	

   B. Sanitary disposal of human waste to prevent contamination of the soil is of paramount importance, particularly in endemic areas; wearing shoes is also helpful

   C. Follow Up
   1. A repeat stool exam should be performed 2 weeks posttreatment
   2. If positive, re-treatment is indicated

IRRITABLE BOWEL SYNDROME

I. Definition: Chronic, benign gastrointestinal disorder characterized by altered bowel habits and abdominal pain in the absence of structural or biochemical abnormalities with no inflammatory component and no underlying identifiable organic cause

II. Pathogenesis:

   A. Considered a functional disorder which by definition is a disorder in which symptoms are not explained by structural or biochemical abnormalities

   B. Abdominal pain that is characteristic of irritable bowel syndrome (IBS) is probably the result of altered sensory perception due to either visceral hypersensitivity or decreased pain threshold

   C. Central nervous system modulation may also be a factor in IBS in view of the effect of stressful stimuli on gastrointestinal motility in some people

III. Clinical Presentation

   A. Irritable Bowel Syndrome (IBS) is a common malady occurring in about 15% of the population, with symptoms most often appearing during late teens, early adulthood

   B. Females are affected more often than males (2:1); IBS accounts for 50% of all referrals to gastroenterologists

C. Most common presentation is that of abdominal pain and altered bowel habits with either diarrhea or constipation predominating

D. Pattern of symptoms varies from person to person but symptoms are generally mild to moderate with little disability

E. Symptoms are most often intermittent, though some patients have daily problems and a small percentage of patients are refractory to treatment, with pain that is disabling

F. The symptom-based diagnostic classification system below can be helpful in evaluating patients

---

SYMPTOMS OF IRRITABLE BOWEL SYNDROME USED AS DIAGNOSTIC CRITERIA

Continuous or recurrent abdominal pain or discomfort for at least a 3 month period that is
- ✦ Relieved with defecation and/or
- ✦ Associated with a change in frequency of stooling and/or
- ✦ Associated with a change in consistency of stool

PLUS

Two or more of the following that occur at least a quarter of the time
- ✦ Altered stool frequency (more than 3 bowel movements/day or fewer than 3 bowel movements/week)
- ✦ Altered stool passage (straining, urgency, feeling of incomplete evacuation)
- ✦ Passage of mucus
- ✦ Feeling of abdominal distension

Adapted from Drossman, D.A. (1995). Diagnosing and treating patients with refractory functional gastrointestinal disorders. Annals of Internal Medicine, 123, 688-697.

IV. Diagnosis/Evaluation

    A. History
1. Ask about onset, duration, location, and severity of abdominal pain and changes over time

2. Ask questions relating to diagnostic criteria outlined above
    a. Has the abdominal pain/discomfort been present for at least 3 months on a continuous or recurrent basis?
      (1) Is pain relieved with defecation?
      (2) Is pain associated with a change in frequency of stool?
      (3) Is pain associated with change in consistency of stool?
    b. Regarding stooling quality and pattern, ask the patient if two or more of the following are present at least 25% of time
      (1) Is there altered stool frequency?
      (2) Is there altered stool form, that is lumpy and hard or loose and watery?
      (3) Is there altered stool passage?
      (4) Is there passage of mucus?
      (5) Is there a feeling of bloating or distension?
3. If diarrhea is present, question about blood in diarrhea, awakening in night because of diarrhea (if positive response to either question, points to inflammatory bowel disease rather than IBS)
4. Question about weight loss (significant weight loss should not occur with IBS)
5. Inquire if any stresses occurred at time the disorder appeared or intensified
6. Obtain diet history to determine usual diet and eating patterns
7. Ask about drug/alcohol use/present medications used
8. Inquire about treatments tried and results
9. In females, take menstrual history

    B. Physical Examination
1. Determine if weight loss has occurred
2. Perform abdominal exam for tenderness (usually present in left lower quadrant), guarding, rigidity, abnormal bowel sounds, masses, liver or spleen enlargement
3. Perform rectal exam for tenderness, masses; stool for occult blood

C. Differential Diagnosis
1. Ulcerative colitis
2. Crohn's disease
3. Lactose intolerance
4. Diverticulitis
5. Gastroenteritis

D. Diagnostic Tests
1. CBC and sedimentation rate
2. Fecal occult blood x 6
3. Stool for O&P x 3
4. Stool for culture leukocytes and fecal fat
5. If symptoms are severe, or diagnosis is uncertain, sigmoidoscopy and barium enema are necessary

V. Plan/Management

A. For patients with typical presentation (no significant weight loss, no occult blood in stool, no abnormal physical findings) symptomatic treatment should be offered with the plan being to evaluate the patient's response in 2 to 3 weeks

B. Approach to management should be based on individual patient characteristics that can be determined by evaluating the patient response to several key questions

---

KEY QUESTIONS TO ASK IN THE EVALUATION OF PATIENTS WITH IBS

Is there a pain history?
Does the patient have a long-standing pattern of pain behaviors, such as frequent headaches, back pain, dysmenorrhea that treatment has been sought for?
✔ If yes, the patient's prognosis is poorer than if response is "no"

What is the patient's understanding of the condition?
Ask "What do you think is causing your symptoms?" and "What do you hope I can do for you?"
✔ Patient's who are not satisfied by negative findings
✔ who are convinced there must be an organic basis for symptoms
✔ who are unrealistic in their expectations for treatment
✔ will continue to seek new diagnostic tests and treatments

Does the patient understand and accept the fact that stress may play a contributing role?
✔ Persons who have a tendency to deny or minimize the psychological effect of stressful life events more often seek care than do those who have insight into the role that mood disturbances have on symptoms such as gastrointestinal pain
✔ Those with insight are often able to manage the condition on their own

Does that patient have abnormal illness behavior?
✔ Patients who are eager to adopt the "sick role," who relentlessly search to validate the existence of disease, and who place responsibility for "cure" on the health care provider have abnormal illness behavior which interferes with optimal management

Is the family's involvement associated with emotional support and oriented toward recovery and health?
✔ Families who pay undue attention to the condition as a mechanism for avoiding family problems that arise need counseling

What is the reason for this visit or referral?
Ask "What led you to come into see me at this time?"
✔ Clarify the reason that patient is seeking help at this time as he/she has had the symptoms for a while (in most cases)

What are the patient's coping mechanisms?
✔ Factors that promote health and buffer the effects of stress need to be identified as these are associated with improved outcomes

Adapted from Drossman, D.A. (1995). Diagnosing and treating patients with refractory functional gastrointestinal disorders. Annals of Internal Medicine, 123, 688-697.

C. Establishment of an effective patient-provider relationship based on patient education and reassurance is important

D. Set realistic treatment goals in which the patient takes responsibility for own care
   1. One approach is to use of a symptom diary for several weeks in which patient records symptom, date/time of occurrence, description of severity (scale of 1-10), factors associated with symptom (diet, activity, menses, stressful event, etc.); emotional responses (what person feels); thoughts and cognition (what person thinks)
   2. Review diary with patient on each return visit as a way of evaluating his/her progress in "gaining control" of the condition

E. Severity of symptoms and degree of disability dictate treatment plan
   1. For patients with predominant diarrhea,
      a. Increasing soluble fiber intake helps to bulk up the stool and improve quality of bowel movements
      b. Use of antidiarrheal agents such as loperamide, 2-4 mg QID can be helpful
   2. For patients with predominant constipation,
      a. Increase dietary fiber to 20-30 grams/day
      b. Laxative use should be strongly discouraged, but if laxatives must be used on an occasional basis, osmotic laxatives such as lactulose are preferred (see section on CONSTIPATION for dosing)
   3. For patients with predominant pain or gas syndromes
      a. Elimination of gas-forming foods may be helpful (lactose, legumes, broccoli, cauliflower, brussel sprouts, onions, cucumbers); if symptoms improve, these foods can be gradually reintroduced
      b. Dicyclomine (Bentyl), 10-20 mg TID or QID acts mainly on smooth muscle and may have fewer side effects than nonselective anticholinergic agents

F. Discuss with all patients modifications in lifestyle that can improve symptoms
   1. Stress reduction is important, and can be accomplished via the use of relaxation tapes, books, or meditation taught by behavioral therapists
   2. Biofeedback can sometimes help decrease stress and reduce gut hypersensitivity
   3. Regular exercise can also reduce stress and increase feelings of well-being; can also improve bowel transit

G. Follow Up: Every 2 weeks until patient's condition is improved, then every month, then every 6 months

NAUSEA AND VOMITING

I. Definition

   A. Nausea: An unpleasant feeling in the throat or epigastric region alerting one that vomiting is imminent

   B. Vomiting: The forceful expulsion of gastric contents through the mouth

II. Pathogenesis

   A. Three consecutive phases of emesis include nausea, retching, and vomiting

   B. Vomiting is triggered by afferent impulses received in the vomiting center (VC) believed to be located in the medulla

C. Sensory centers such as the cerebral cortex, visceral afferents from the pharynx and gastrointestinal tract, and the chemoreceptor trigger zone (CTZ) are responsible for sending the impulses to the vomiting center

D. Once the VC is stimulated, efferent pathways to the salivation center, respiratory center, and the pharyngeal, GI, and abdominal musculature work in concert to produce vomiting

III. Clinical Presentation

A. Nausea and vomiting are among the most common symptoms that children and adults experience and may be associated with a variety of clinical presentations

B. May be evoked by disorders of the gastrointestinal tract and may also be caused by neurologic, endocrine, metabolic, psychogenic, iatrogenic, and toxic conditions

C. Common causes
1. Gastrointestinal mechanisms (examples of common causes only)
   a. Acute gastroenteritis, both viral and bacterial
   b. Peptic ulcer disease/gastritis
   c. Motility disorders such as gastroparesis, drug-induced gastric stasis, irritable bowel syndrome
   d. Intraabdominal emergencies such as appendicitis, obstruction, pancreatitis, cholecystitis
2. Central nervous system causes (examples of common causes only)
   a. Motion sickness
   b. Migraine headache
3. Systemic causes (examples of common causes only)
   a. Pregnancy
   b. Infections/food poisoning
   c. Drug overdose
4. Iatrogenic causes: (examples)
   a. Medications such as antibiotics, theophylline, digitalis, and antineoplastic agents
   b. Bulimia

D. Associated symptoms and signs of some common causes
1. Gastroenteritis: fever, diarrhea, lethargy
2. Nongastrointestinal tract infections such as otitis media and UTIs: lethargy, fever, decreased appetite

E. Associated symptoms and signs of some uncommon causes
1. High bowel obstruction: persistent vomiting and weight loss, green bile in vomitus
2. Lower bowel obstruction: absent bowel sounds, constipation

F. Vomiting rapidly produces dehydration in infants and young children

IV. Diagnosis/Evaluation

A. History
1. Question about onset, duration, quantity and quality of vomitus (undigested food, blood)
2. Ask about timing of vomiting with respect to meals and presence of associated symptoms such as abdominal pain, diarrhea, dizziness, headache
3. Ask if systemic symptoms of fever and malaise are present
4. Ask about past medical history and medication history
5. In infants, ask about feedings, activity level, irritability, lethargy, number of wet diaper
6. Ask if others in household are ill to identify a common source cause

B. Physical Examination
1. Determine if febrile
2. Assess hydration status: Check for dry mucous membranes, decreased skin turgor, tachycardia, and oliguria

3. Assess cardiovascular status (pulse, blood pressure; check for postural hypotension)
4. Examine abdomen for tenderness, rigidity, abnormal tympany, bowel sounds, liver and spleen size
5. Perform rectal exam for tenderness, masses; stool for occult blood

C. Differential Diagnosis: Vomiting is a symptom.; see Pathogenesis for possible causes

D. Laboratory Tests
1. If no systemic signs and symptoms, and duration <24 hours, no lab studies indicated
2. If vomiting persists longer than 24 hours, consider following laboratory tests
   a. Serum chemistries to document acid-base, electrolyte status
   b. Glucose
   c. HCG
   d. Amylase
   e. Drug levels, if indicated

V. Plan/Management

A. Identification of most likely cause dictates therapy

B. Most episodes of nausea and vomiting are self-limiting and supportive therapy is all that is indicated

C. Nonpharmacologic interventions:

NONPHARMACOLOGIC INTERVENTIONS	
Infants >1 month and children ≤5 years of age	✓ Almost all children with vomiting and mild dehydration can be treated with oral rehydration therapy (see section on DIARRHEA which contains very specific and detailed guidelines for managing rehydration in infants and small children as well as guidelines for refeeding)
Children >5, adolescent, and adults	✓ Discontinue solid foods ✓ Encourage clear liquids only (not milk) until at least 4 hours have passed without vomiting ✓ Start with 1 tbsp (15 cc) every 10 minutes ✓ If vomiting does not occur, double the amount each hour ✓ If vomiting does occur, allow stomach to rest briefly and then start again ✓ Key is to gradually increase amount of fluid until taking 8 oz every hour ✓ May use glucose-electrolyte solutions developed for infants/small children such as Pedialyte or Rehydralyte (May combine with flavored gelatin to make more palatable) or sports drinks such as Gatorade ✓ Resume age appropriate diet as soon as tolerated (usually, 4 hours after vomiting stops)

D. Pharmacologic therapy is usually not indicated; however, for selected patients (for example, those with electrolyte disturbances, severe anorexia/weight loss, motion sickness, pregnancy, or with chemotherapy-induced nausea and vomiting) antiemetic therapy may be indicated
1. Emetrol (OTC): Do not dilute or take fluids 15 minutes before or after. Can be used in pregnancy
   a. Adolescents: 15-30 mL at 15 minute intervals as needed
   b. Children: 5-10 mL, same time interval as adults
2. Promethazine (Phenergan) is the agent of choice for n/v from gastroenteritis: Available as 12.5, 25, 50 mg tabs and rectal supp; also available as syrup (6.25 mg/5 mL and 25 mg/5 mL)
   a. Children >2: 12.5-25 mg Q 12 hrs
   b. Children <2: Not recommended
3. Prochlorperazine (Compazine): Available 5, 10 mg tabs; 10, 15, 30 mg spanules; 5 mg/5 mL syrup; 2.5, 5, 25 mg rectal supp
   a. Adolescents who weight >85 lbs: Tabs/5-10 mg 3-4 times day; Spanules/10mg Q 12 hrs; rectal supp/25 mg BID

Children: >2: Tabs or rectal supp, dose by weight: 20-29 lbs/2.5 mg 1-2 x d (max. 7.5 mg/day); 20-39 lbs/2.5 mg 2-3 x d (max. 10 mg/day); 40-85 lbs/5mg 2 x d (max. 15 mg/day)
    c.   Children <2: Not recommended
   4.   Trimethobenzamide (Tigan) works well for gastroenteritis and motion sickness: Available as 100, 250 mg caps and rectal supp--adult/100, 200 mg; pediatric/100 mg
    a.   Adolescents who weigh >90 lbs: 250 mg caps OR 200 mg rectal supp 3-4 x day
    b.   Children: 30-90 lb: Use 100-200 mg caps OR 100 mg rectal supp 3-4 x day
    c.   Children <30 lb: Use 100 mg rectal supp 3-4 x day
    d.   Prematures or Neonates: Not recommended

E.   Follow Up: None needed unless failure to respond to nonpharmacologic or pharmacologic therapy

REFERENCES

American Academy of Pediatrics. (1996). Practice parameter. The management of acute gastroenteritis in young children. Pediatrics, 97(3), 424-633.

American Academy of Pediatrics. (1997). Red book: Report of the committee on infectious diseases (24th ed.). Elk Grove Village, IL: Author.

American Academy of Pediatrics, Provisional committee for Quality Improvement and Subcommittee on Hyperbilirubinemia. (1994). Practice parameter: Management of hyperbilirubinemia in the healthy term newborn. Pediatrics, 94(4), 558-562.

Balon, A.J. (1997). Management of infantile colic. American Family Physician, 55, 235-241.

Berkowitz, C. (1997). Management of the colicky infant. Comprehensive Therapy, 23, 277-280.

Bloom, M.D. (1997). Jaundice. In J. C. Gartner, Jr., & B.J. Zitelli (Eds.), Common and chronic symptoms in pediatrics. St. Louis: Mosby.

Bonis, P.A., & Norton, R.A. (1996). The challenge of irritable bowel syndrome. American Family Physician, 53, 1229-1236.

Brady, W.M. (1997). Controversies in diagnosis and treatment of hepatitis C. Postgraduate Medicine, 102 (5), 201-206.

Centers for Disease Control. (1997). Immunization of health care workers. MMWR, 46, RR-18.

DiPiro, J.T. (1998). Gastrointestinal disorders. In B.G. Wells, J.T. Dipiro, T.L. Schwinghammer, & C.W. Hamilton (Eds.), Pharmacotherapy handbook. Stamford, CT:Appleton & Lange.

Drossman, D.A. (1995). Diagnosing and treating patients with refractory functional gastrointestinal disorders. Annals of Internal Medicine, 123, 688-697.

Duggan, C., Santosham, M., & Glass, R.I. (1992). The management of acute diarrhea in children: Oral rehydration, maintenence, and nutritonal theray. Morbidity and Mortality Weekly Report, (RR-16), 1-20.

Faubion, W.A., & Zein, N.N. (1998). Gastroesophageal reflux in infants and children. Mayo Clinical Proceedings, 73, 166-173.

Graber, M.A. (1998). Dealing with acute abdominal pain: Part 1: Clues to the diagnosis. Emergency Medicine, 30(2), 74-100.

Greenberger, N.J. (1997). Update in gastroenterology. Annals of Internal Medicine, 127, 827-834.

Hart, J.J. (1996). Pediatric gastroesophageal reflux. American Family Physician, 54, 2463-2471.

Hillemeier, A.C. (1996). Gastroesophageal reflux: Diagnostic and therapeutic approaches. Pediatric Clinics of North America, 43(1), 197-210.

Hoofnagle, J.H., & Bisceglie, A.M. (1997). The treatment of chronic viral hepatitis. New England Journal of Medicine, 336, 347-355.

Keith, M.L. (1997). Pediatric diarrhea. <u>Journal of the American Academy of Nurse Practitioners, 9</u> (12), 577-579.

Margolies, M.N. (1995). Approach to the patient with an external hernia. In A.H. Goroll, L.A. May, & A.G. Mulley, Jr. (Eds.), <u>Primary care medicine</u>. Philadelphia: Lippincott.

Marion, R.W. (1997). Umbilical anomalies. In R.A. Hoekelman (Ed.), <u>Primary pediatric care</u>. St. Louis: Mosby.

McColl, I. (1998). More precision in diagnosing appendicitis. <u>New England Journal of Medicine, 338</u>, 190-191.

Meyers, A. (1995). Modern management of acute diarrhea and dehydration in children. <u>American Family Physician, 51</u>, 1103-1115.

Mittal, R.K., & Balaban, D.H. (1997). The esophagogastric junction. <u>New England Journal of Medicine, 336</u>, 924-932.

Moir, C.R. (1996). Abdominal pain in infants and children. <u>Mayo Clinical Proceedings, 71</u>, 984-989.

Perez, E.A., & Hallstone, H.A. (1998). Nausea and vomiting. In R.E. Rakel (Ed.), <u>Conn's Current Therapy</u>. Philadelphia: Saunders.

Stone, R. (1996). Primary care diagnosis of acute abdominal pain. <u>Nurse Practitioner, 21</u>(12), 19-27.

Theal, R.M., & Scott, K. (1996). Evaluating asymptomatic patients with abnormal liver function test results. <u>American Family Physicain, 53</u>, 2111-2119.

Tolia, V. (1997). Evaluaton and management of pediatric gastroesophageal reflux. <u>Family Practice Recertification, 19</u> (6), 35-57.

Verne, G.N., & Cerda, J.J. (1997). Irritable bowel syndrome: Streamlining the diagnosis. <u>Postgraduate Medicine, 102</u>, 197-208.

Wagner, J.M., McKinney, W.P, & Carpenter, J.L. (1996). Does this patient have appendicitis? <u>JAMA, 276</u>, 1589-1594.

Wald, A. (1998). Constipation. In R.E. Rakel (Ed.), <u>Conn's Current Therapy</u>, Philadelphia: Saunders.

Genitourinary Problems

HEMATURIA

I.   Definition: Presence of red blood cells (RBCs) in urine; typically, more than 3 RBCs per high-power field on microscopic examination of a centrifuged specimen is the criteria used to make the diagnosis of hematuria

II. Pathogenesis: RBCs can enter the genitourinary tract at any site from the glomerulus to the urethral meatus and the causes can be categorized as prerenal, renal, postrenal, or false

   A. Prerenal
       1. Coagulopathy such as hemophilia or thrombocytopenic purpura
       2. Drugs such as warfarin sodium, heparin sodium or aspirin
       3. Sickle cell disease or trait
       4. Collagen vascular disease such as systemic lupus erythematosus
       5. Wilm's tumor

   B. Renal
       1. Nonglomerular
           a. Pyelonephritis
           b. Polycystic kidney disease
           c. Granulomatous disease such as tuberculosis
           d. Malignant neoplasm
           e. Congenital and vascular anomalies
       2. Glomerular
           a. Glomerulonephritis
           b. Berger's disease
           c. Lupus nephritis
           d. Benign familial hematuria
           e. Vascular abnormalities such as vasculitis
           f. Alport's syndrome (familial nephritis)

   C. Postrenal
       1. Renal calculi
       2. Ureteritis
       3. Cystitis
       4. Epididymitis
       5. Urethritis
       6. Malignant neoplasm

   D. False
       1. Vaginal bleeding
       2. Recent circumcision
       3. Hemoglobinuria
       4. Intake of certain foods such as beets, rhubarb, blackberries, fava beans
       5. Intake of certain medications such as quinine sulfate, phenazopyridine, phenytoin, phenindione, phenothiazine, rifampin, sulfasalazine
       6. Excretion of porphyries
       7. Newborn urine often has a pinkish color due to presence of urate crystals

   E. Miscellaneous causes
       1. Strenuous exercise
       2. Fever
       3. Trauma
       4. Viral infections

   F. Essential hematuria is present when no definable cause can be found

G.   Hematuria may be a complaint in patients with factitious hematuria such as narcotic seekers complaining of kidney stones or individuals in families with Munchausen's disease

H.   Idiopathic hypercalciuria is the most common cause of isolated hematuria in children of all ages
1.   It is an inherited tubulointerstitial disease with increased urinary calcium excretion
2.   May be accompanied by renal stones or calcification

I.   Most common causes of gross hematuria in pediatric population include urinary tract infection, irritation or ulceration of perineum or urethral meatus, or trauma

J.   Common causes in children by age include the following:
1.   In newborn and infant <1 year: trauma, primarily due to catheterization, ischemic renal injury, coagulopathy, renal malformation, infection
2.   Preschool children (1-5 years): infection, renal malformation, glomerulonephritis, trauma, hypercalciuria
3.   School age children and adolescents: infection, menstruation, trauma, glomerulonephritis, hypercalciuria
4.   Irritation or ulceration of perineum or urethral meatus is common in preschool and older children
5.   Wilm's tumor is the most common malignancy; usually occurs in children <6 years old
6.   In about 10-20% of the cases, no definable cause can be found

III.   Clinical Presentation

A.   Hematuria may be gross (visible to naked eye) or microscopic (detected on dipstick or microscopic exam)

B.   Glomerular disease is often associated with edema, hypertension, proteinuria, and oliguria/anuria

C.   Lower tract infections typically have symptoms of dysuria, frequency, urgency and flank pain

D.   Abdominal or flank mass may be found with obstructive processes such as Wilm's tumor, cystic disease or posterior valves

IV.   Diagnosis/Evaluation

A.   History
1.   Question about timing and appearance of hematuria
a.   Hematuria seen at onset of urination often indicates bleeding in the urethra
b.   Terminal hematuria seen in the last few drops of urine often indicates the bladder neck or prostate as the source
c.   Hematuria seen throughout urination suggests that a lesion could be located anywhere from the upper urinary tract to the bladder
2.   Ask about associated symptoms:
a.   Colicky flank pain radiating to groin suggests a kidney stone
b.   Dysuria and frequency suggest cystitis, especially in females
c.   Hesitancy and dribbling suggest benign prostatic hypertrophy
d.   Hemoptysis, hematuria, and acute renal failure in an anemic patient suggests Goodpasture's syndrome
e.   Loin-pain and hematuria in a young females taking oral contraceptives may indicate small-vessel occlusive vascular disease
f.   In a systemic disease, fever, joint pains, and rash are typical manifestations
3.   Ask patient to describe any blood clots that have occurred
a.   Large, thick clots suggest the bladder as the bleeding source
b.   Specks or thin, stringy clots suggest the upper urinary tract as the source
4.   Determine whether hematuria is transient or persistent; in persons <40 years, transient hematuria is common and seldom secondary to significant disease
5.   Ask whether the patient bruises easily or has extended bleeding after a minor cut or dental work (coagulopathy or bleeding dyscrasia may be present)

6.　In females, inquire about the last menstrual period
7.　Obtain a complete medication history
8.　Inquire about a history of pharyngitis with an impetiginous skin rash followed by hematuria, edema and hypertension (presentation of glomerulonephritis)
9.　Ask about recent trauma and strenuous exercise
10.　Explore previous medical history, making certain to inquire about sickle cell disease and trait, previous urinary tract infections, metabolic and endocrine diseases, and surgeries
11.　Inquire about exposure to tuberculosis
12.　Explore patient's family history; kidney stone disease, Alport's syndrome and familial nephritis are common across generations of families

B.　Physical Examination
1.　Measure vital signs; elevated temperature suggests infection, neoplasm, or systemic disease; elevated blood pressure suggest glomerulonephritis
2.　Observe skin for signs of exanthems, pallor, ecchymosis, or purpura
3.　Examine for systemic infection such as tonsillar enlargement, lymphadenopathy, and exanthems
4.　If Alport's syndrome is suspected, perform a hearing test as this syndrome is associated with hearing defects
5.　Auscultate heart
6.　Perform complete abdominal exam, noting tenderness, organomegaly, bladder distention, masses, or bruits
7.　Assess for costovertebral angle tenderness which suggests pyelonephritis or urinary tract obstruction
8.　Examine extremities for edema which may be associated with glomerulonephritis
9.　In males, examine testes, spermatic cord, and vas deferens for tenderness and masses
10.　In males, examine penis for condyloma acuminatum, meatal stenosis, foreign body
11.　In females inspect vulva and urethral meatus, noting signs of urethral caruncle or urethral irritation; bimanual exam may uncover a uterine or ovarian mass which may secondarily involve the genitourinary tract

C.　Differential Diagnosis
1.　Essential hematuria is a diagnosis of exclusion
2.　The majority of cases of hematuria will present with symptoms, signs, or laboratory test results that pinpoint a specific diagnosis
3.　For those patients with asymptomatic, isolated hematuria for whom a cause cannot be identified consider neoplasm

D.　Diagnostic Tests
1.　Always obtain urinalysis (UA) and a subsequent culture to confirm findings on the UA (best to obtain a freshly voided, morning specimen and examine it within 30 minutes); **dipstick can give false-positive results and should always be used in conjunction with a microscopic examination**
　　a.　Alkaline pH and positive nitrite and leukocyte esterase reactions suggest urinary tract infections
　　b.　Hematuria with pyuria but no bacteria suggest a sexually transmitted disease (chlamydia, gonorrhea), viral infection, or less commonly, tuberculosis
　　c.　Protein suggests glomerulonephritis
　　d.　If the dipstick test is negative for RBCs but the urine appears red, pigmenturia caused by endogenous substances that change color of urine is the likely cause
　　e.　Microscopic examination of urinary sediment can help determine the site of bleeding
　　　　(1)　RBC casts suggest glomerulonephritis
　　　　(2)　Crystals suggest renal calculi
　　f.　If exercise hematuria is suspected, patient should refrain from active participation in sports for at least 48 hours prior to urinalysis
2.　Phase contrast microscopy is being used more frequently to determine the site of bleeding; this test is promising and is recommended early in the evaluation of hematuria after an infection has been excluded

3. A single positive urinalysis in an asymptomatic child should be repeated 2-3 more times in 7-14 days
    a. If follow-up urinalyses are negative, recheck urine in one month; if still negative recheck in 6 months before assuming child has benign process
    b. If follow-up urinalyses are positive, proceed with further evaluation
4. If patient has **macroscopic** hematuria, evaluate for sickle cell trait or disease
    a. If positive, advise bedrest or order intravenous pyelogram if clots are present
    b. If sickle cell test is negative and hematuria is **NOT** accompanied with pain, evaluate for proteinuria:
        (1) If positive for proteinuria, evaluate for nephritis
        (2) If negative, order a CT scan or MRI, serum creatinine, and urine calcium/creatinine ratio; refer if tests are abnormal
    c. If sickle cell test is negative and patient has **painful** hematuria, order abdominal flat plate or renal ultrasound to evaluate for kidney stones; refer to specialist for hospitalization and observation if stones are absent or treatment for presence of stones
5. If patient has **microscopic** hematuria:
    a. In patients with microscopic hematuria and proteinuria
        (1) Evaluate further for benign proteinuria (orthostatic, exercise-induced, or fever-induced) or parenchyma renal disease
        (2) Patients with suspected renal disease should be evaluated for systemic disease and have formal quantitation of urine protein excretion and serum creatinine, BUN, albumin, and imaging of kidneys with an ultrasound or a radionuclide scan; refer if abnormalities found
    b. In patients with **isolated hematuria** and a negative urine culture evaluate for hypercalciuria (calcium/creatinine ratio)
        (1) If hypercalciuria is present, order a renal ultrasound, voiding cystogram, and serum creatinine
        (2) If normal calcium/creatinine ratio, order a renal ultrasound, voiding cystogram, and serum creatinine
            (a) If any of these tests are abnormal, refer to specialist
            (b) If normal, reassure and provide frequent follow-up evaluations
6. Order additional tests depending on the patient's presentation
    a. Order clotting studies (i.e., prothrombin time, partial thromboplastin time, platelet count, bleeding time) if a coagulopathy or a bleeding disorder is suspected
    b. Administer a purified protein derivative (PPD) and order urine culture for acid-fast bacillus when tuberculosis is a possibility
    c. Order erythrocyte sedimentation rate (ESR) for patients with suspected secondary glomerular disease such as endocarditis and systemic lupus erythematosus
    d. An immunologic survey consisting of titers of IgG, IgA, IgM, and IgE are helpful if Schönlein-Henoch purpura or glomerular disease is suspected
7. Consider additional testing
    a. Voiding cystourethrography can reveal congenital anomalies, stone formation or foreign bodies
    b. Computed tomography (CT) can delineate a small mass, but it is not cost-effective in most cases
    c. Magnetic resonance imaging is less sensitive than the CT scan for detecting complicated masses but is helpful in imaging other masses such as renal cysts
    d. Angiography is not usually performed, but is the only test to detect arteriovenous malformations and may be considered in patients with gross, painless hematuria after other studies have excluded carcinoma and other renal disease
    e. A biopsy is performed when no cause is apparent

V. Plan/Management

A. Treat infections with appropriate antibiotics (see sections on URINARY TRACT INFECTIONS)

B. Exercise-induced hematuria requires no treatment as it is self-limited

C.   Children diagnosed with essential hematuria should be periodically evaluated with follow-up diagnostic tests

D.   Other children with hematuria should be referred to a specialist, especially those patients with the following:
1.   Gross hematuria
2.   Risk factors for malignancy
3.   Unexplained hematuria without characteristics of glomerular hematuria such as RBC casts, proteinuria, and with a nondiagnostic IVP
4.   Urologic trauma

E.   Follow Up
1.   Because patients who are treated for uncomplicated infections may also have underlying, noninfectious disorders close follow up is needed; repeat urinalysis 2-3 times in a 4-6 week period to determine that hematuria and all other signs and symptoms have abated
2.   Patients with a negative initial workup will need close monitoring
3.   Patients who may have glomerulonephritis should have blood pressure measurements, serum creatinine concentrations and urinalyses annually

CYSTITIS AND PYELONEPHRITIS IN ADOLESCENTS

I.   Definition: Bacteria in urine which have the potential to injure tissues of the urinary tract and adjacent structures. Urinary tract infections (UTIs) are often classified as upper and lower tract infections

A.   Cystitis, infection of the bladder, is an example of a common lower tract infection

B.   Pyelonephritis is the main upper tract infection and involves infection of the renal parenchyma

II.   Pathogenesis of cystitis and pyelonephritis

A.   In females, the major cause is invasion of the urinary tract by bacteria that have ascended the urethra from the introitus. Females have a short urethra which is in close proximity to the perirectal area making colonization possible

B.   Currently, researchers are exploring whether there is a genetic link for females who are prone to frequent UTIs; studies are underway to develop a blood test to identify high-risk females

C.   In males, cystitis and pyelonephritis are uncommon
1.   In the past, these problems were always considered the result of an underlying urologic abnormality
2.   Currently in young, healthy males with isolated cystitis, the literature suggests that infection may be due to endogenous bacteria without an underlying abnormality or related to a subclinical case of prostatitis

D.   Pathogens: Bacteria adhere to uroepithelial cells
1.   Gram negative bacilli are most common; 80-90% of community-acquired infections are due to *Escherichia coli*
a.   Other gram negative bacilli organisms include *Klebsiella pneumoniae* or *Proteus mirabilis*
b.   A wide range of gram-negative bacilli and other microorganisms may be causative agents in males

2. Gram-positive cocci account for 10-15% of community acquired infections; *Staphylococcus saprophyticus* is the second most common pathogen and often occurs in young, sexually active females

3. In hospital settings, *E. coli* is less prevalent with Proteus, Klebsiella, Enterobacter, Pseudomonas, Staphylococci, and Enterococci species being more common

E. Risk factors in both genders
1. Diabetes mellitus; not necessarily an increased risk for developing infection but often there is a disorder of bladder emptying which makes UTI more difficult to eradicate
2. Urinary instrumentation and catheterization
3. Obstruction of normal flow of urine resulting from calculi, tumors, urethral strictures
4. Neurogenic bladder disease from strokes, multiple sclerosis, spinal cord injuries
5. Vesicoureteral reflux as a result of a congenital abnormality or more often from bladder overdistention from obstruction

F. Risk factors in females
1. Females with increased sexual activity, diaphragm and spermicide use, and failure to void after intercourse
2. Pregnancy
3. History of recent urinary infection
4. Tampons and wiping from back to front after a bowel movement are **not** risk factors
5. Postponing urination or incomplete voiding in females

G. Risk factors in males
1. Homosexuality
2. Lack of circumcision
3. Having a sexual partner with vaginal colonization by uropathogens
4. HIV infection with CD4+ T- lymphocyte counts of less than 200 per cubic millimeter
5. Obstruction of normal flow such as occurs with urethral strictures

III. Clinical Presentation

A. After puberty, the prevalence of UTIs increases significantly in females, but remains low in adolescent and young adult males

B. Cystitis
1. Onset is usually abrupt
2. Adolescents may be asymptomatic
3. Typical symptoms include dysuria, urgency, frequency, nocturia, suprapubic heaviness or discomfort; fever is uncommon
4. Bacturia: 10^2 to >10^5 colony-forming units per milliliter of urine (cfu per ml.)

C. Pyelonephritis
1. Acute onset of chills, fever, flank pain, headache, malaise, costovertebral angle tenderness, and possibly hematuria
2. Often occurs concurrently or after a lower urinary tract infection
3. May be associated with renal calculi, ureteral obstruction, or neurogenic bladder.
4. Urine almost always has white blood cells; urine cultures >10^5 cfu per mL, usually have bacterial casts

IV. Diagnosis/Evaluation

A. History
1. Determine onset and duration of urinary symptoms
2. Ask about strength and character of urine stream when voiding
3. Determine whether dysuria occurs during urination or after urine begins to pass over inflamed labia as with herpes simplex infections
4. Inquire about associated symptoms such as fever, chills, nausea, vomiting, diarrhea, constipation, abdominal and back pain, hematuria
5. Ask about onset, duration, and characteristics of vaginal or urethral discharge

6. Always query females about method of birth control and date of last menstrual period
7. Past medical history should include drug allergies, chronic diseases such as diabetes mellitus or multiple sclerosis, previous genitourinary problems
8. Ask patient to count number of previous UTIs and discuss successes and failures of previous treatments

B. Physical Examination
   1. Assess vital signs, particularly noting elevated temperature and signs of orthostatic hypotension
   2. Perform a complete abdominal exam to detect tenderness, a distended bladder, or a mass
   3. Palpate back for costovertebral tenderness
   4. In females may need to inspect perineum and do complete pelvic, speculum, and rectal exams
   5. In males may need to inspect and palpate external genitalia and scrotum
   6. Consider performing a neurologic examination to detect neurogenic diseases such as multiple sclerosis

C. Differential Diagnosis
   1. Males
      a. Gonococcal and nongonococcal urethritis in males (often asymptomatic, but may have mucoid or purulent urethral discharge)
      b. Prostatitis (a tender prostate on rectal exam is usually present)
      c. Epididymitis (testicular tenderness and erythema are present)
      d. Prostatodynia (presents with perineal or back pain accompanied by unilateral testicular pain or dysuria; urinalysis and urine culture are negative)
   2. Females
      a. Interstitial cystitis
         (1) Painful bladder condition which is most common between 20-60 years of age
         (2) Characterized by suprapubic pain which is relieved by bladder emptying
         (3) Involves inflammation of the bladder which may progress to ulcerations, fibrosis, and decreased bladder capacity
         (4) Diagnosed with cystoscopy, urodynamic studies, and bladder biopsy
         (5) There is no cure; the following treatments may be beneficial:
             (a) Oral medications such as pentosan polysulfate (Elmiron) 100 mg cap one hour before or 2 hours after meals with water, amitriptyline (Elavil), hydroxyzine (Atarax), nifedipine (Adalat), or cimetidine (Tagamet)
             (b) Intravesical therapies such as hydrodistention of the bladder
             (c) Intravesical instillation of dimethyl sulfoxide (DMSO)
         (6) Surgery is the last option
      b. Urethral syndrome
         (1) Patient has irritative voiding symptoms with an absence of objective findings
         (2) There is no cure, treatment is symptomatic
      c. Vulvovaginitis (external dysuria, vulvar erythema, and vulvar lesions are often present)
      d. Vaginitis
         (1) Patients deny urinary urgency and frequency
         (2) Usually there are no WBCs or bacteria in the urine
         (3) Vaginal discharge, odor, and pruritis may be present
      e. Cervicitis (cervix will be abnormal on pelvic exam)
   3. Both genders
      a. Urinary calculi (usually patient has severe pain and hematuria)
      b. Bladder outlet obstruction (changes in urinary stream occur)
      c. Renal tuberculosis (hematuria is common)
      d. Tumors and carcinoma (hematuria is common)

D.   Diagnostic Tests
1.   Urine collection
    a.   Clean catch voided specimens are usually acceptable for adolescents
        (1)   First morning specimen is the best voided specimen
        (2)   If urine specimen is obtained later in the day, bladder should not be emptied for at least 2 hours and patients should avoid high fluid intake which would dilute sample
    b.   Single in-and-out catheterization of the bladder should be done on patients who are unable to give a clean midstream urine specimen
2.   Urinalysis
    a.   Dipstick urinalysis: Findings of UTIs are the following:
        (1)   Leukocyte esterase test is positive and denotes pyuria or WBCs in the urine; false positive esterase tests occur with kidney stones, tumors, urethritis, and poor collection techniques
        (2)   Nitrites are positive with gram negative infections; false negatives occur with use of diuretics, inadequate levels of dietary nitrate or presence of bacteria that do not produce nitrate reductase (*Staphylococcus saprophyticus, Enterococcus, Pseudomonas*)
    b.   Microscopic analysis: Examine urine sediment under high power (40X), to count WBCs and perform gram stain to identify type of bacteria
        (1)   Significant pyuria is >2-5 leukocytes per high power field or if using a counting hemocytometer, 10 or more white blood cell/mm^3 is used as the criterion
        (2)   Gram stain is done to identify whether bacteria are gram negative or positive and the shape and pattern of bacteria; it is not helpful to count bacteria on a gram stain
3.   Urine culture and sensitivity (Urine C&S)
    a.   The traditional standard for significant bacteriuria was 10^5 colony-forming units (cfu) of a uropathogen per mL of urine; today the criterion that is used is 10^2 in symptomatic females or 10^3 in symptomatic males
    b.   Bacterial identification and determination of antibiotic susceptibilities or urine C&S is not necessary in most uncomplicated UTIs
    c.   Bacterial identification or urine C&S is important in infections in males, females who have complicated UTIs, and females who are symptomatic but pyuria is absent
4.   With systemic symptoms order CBC with differential and in severely ill patients order blood cultures; consider ordering erythrocyte sedimentation rate
5.   In females with symptoms associated with sexually transmitted disease (STD), perform wet mount of vaginal secretions and order *N. gonorrhoea* (GC) cultures and chlamydia test; also can gram stain cervical secretions
6.   In a male with a possible STD, gram stain urethral secretion and order GC culture and chlamydia tests
7.   Other studies are usually not needed; consider additional tests such as renal ultrasound, voiding cystourethrogram, intravenous pyelogram (IVP), renal scan, renal biopsy, or cystoscopy in patients with repeat infections, slow resolution of symptoms, and atypical features such as persistent hematuria

V.   Plan/Management (the treatment for females and males differ; treatment of isolated and recurrent infections in females will be discussed first)

A.   Bacterial cystitis:
1.   In females with uncomplicated UTIs (young, nonpregnant, non-diabetic females without structural problems or previous UTIs), urine cultures are generally not indicated before treatment
2.   Choose either the 3-day or 7-day regimen or fosfomycin tromethamine (Monurol) in a single dose if patient has uncomplicated UTI (see following table for ANTIBIOTICS)
3.   The 3-day antibiotic therapy is currently gaining favor as the most cost-effective regimen because it is less expensive and has less side effects than the traditional 7-10 day regimen; females at risk for recurrent or relapsing infections should be treated for 7-10 days

4. Order follow up urinalysis for any patient who is at risk for recurrent or relapsing infections (if urinalysis is abnormal order urine culture)

ANTIBIOTICS FOR TREATING CYSTITIS (3-10 DAYS)			
Trimethoprim/sulfamethoxazole (Bactrim)	160 mg/800 mg	1 DS tab	BID
Trimethoprim (Trimpex)	100 mg	1 tab	BID
Nitrofurantoin (Macrodantin)[†]	100 mg	1 tab	QID
Amoxicillin (Amoxil)*	500 mg	1 tab	TID
Lomefloxacin (Maxaquin)**[§]	400 mg	1 tab	QD
Norfloxacin (Noroxin)**[§]	400 mg	1 tab	BID
Fosfomycin tromethamine (Monurol)	3 g	1 sachet with 3-4 oz. of H_2O	Single dose

*Amoxicillin cure rates are lower because of increasing resistance of *E. coli*
**Avoid if possible, because the fluoroquinolones are expensive and have potential teratogenic effects
[†]Take with food
[§]Take with full glass of water

5. Phenazopyridine HCl (Pyridium) may be prescribed 100 mg TID for three days if the patient is experiencing bladder spasms; warn patient that urine will turn orange

B. Recurrent infections in females (Must repeat urine culture and sensitivity each time patient has symptoms)
1. Relapse (uncommon and caused by original infecting pathogen)
   a. Occurs within two weeks of completion of therapy
   b. Treat for 2-6 weeks longer
   c. Seek occult source of infection or urologic abnormality; consider ordering tests of renal function (BUN & creatinine), an intravenous pyelogram (IVP) and referring to a specialist
2. Reinfection (cystitis): Most recurrent UTIs are due to reinfection with a new organism rather than a relapse of the same initial infection
   a. If patient has 2 or fewer UTIs in one year:
      (1) Recommend patient-initiated therapy for symptomatic episodes (give patient a written prescription which she may fill when symptoms occur)
      (2) Prescribe 3-day regimen (see preceding table on ANTIBIOTICS) based on patient's past culture results and clinical success
   b. If patient has greater than or equal to 3 UTIs in one year:
      (1) If UTIs occur only after intercourse recommend a single-dose antiobiotic after coitus such as trimethoprim/sulfamethoxazole 160 mg/800 mg (2 double strength tablets) or nitrofurantoin (Macrodantin) 200 mg
      (2) If UTIs are not related to intercourse, prophylactic antimicrobials should be used for 6 months after the infection has been eradicated
         (a) Urine cultures should be done every 1-2 months.
         (b) Extend prophylactic therapy to 1-2 years if reinfection occurs at end of 6-month period.
         (c) One of the following prophylactic antimicrobials should be prescribed for 6 months (may take daily or thrice weekly): Nitrofurantoin (Furadantin) 50 mg tablet HS; Trimethoprim/sulfamethoxazole (Bactrim) 40/200 mg tablets, half tablet of regular strength at HS; Cephalexin (Keflex) 250 mg tablet at HS
   c. Explore whether patient is using diaphragms, spermicides, and not voiding after intercourse which may be causing reinfections
3. Vaccines to protect against recurrent *E. coli* infections are being studied

C. Pyelonephritis in females (consider consultation with a specialist)
1. Urine cultures are always indicated to definitively identify the invading organism and its antimicrobial sensitivity before treatment
2. Therapy and hospitalization are needed in all cases suggestive of bacteremia

3. Consider hospitalization for females with pyelonephritis, particularly those who are pregnant, have a chronic disease, are vomiting, and who have a history of nonadherence to therapies

4. Close monitoring of female patients is needed if treated on an outpatient basis

5. Outpatient treatment is one of the following (modifications in the antibiotic should be made once the susceptibility profile is known)
   a. Trimethoprim-sulfamethoxazole (Septra) DS tablet BID for 14 days
   b. Ciprofloxacin (Cipro) 250-500 mg BID for 14 days
   c. Ceftriaxone (Rocephin) IM can be used on an outpatient basis in some patients

6. If the 2-week regimen fails, a longer course of 4-6 weeks should be considered because renal parenchymal disease is more difficult to eradicate than bladder mucosal infections

7. Patient's symptoms should improve within 12-48 hours; if not, consider consultation with a specialist and look for deeper infections (imaging studies are often done to exclude obstruction, calculi, and formation of intrarenal abscesses)

8. Schedule return visits or contact patient by phone in 12-24 hours

9. Follow up cultures should be ordered at 2 weeks and 3 months post-treatment

10. Consult specialist for patients who present with a recurrence of pyelonephritis (recommended that these patients need further urologic investigation such as an excretory urography)

D. Treatment of uncomplicated bacterial cystitis in healthy males
   1. In the past all cases of bacterial cystitis in males were believed to be due to underlying structural problems; today, some, but not all experts, recommend that the first UTI can be treated with 7-10 day regimen of trimethoprim-sulfamethoxazole, trimethoprim or a fluoroquinolone (see preceding table on ANTIBIOTICS for dosages)
   2. Shorter treatments are not recommended
   3. Pretreatment and posttreatment urine cultures are recommended
   4. Some authorities recommend reculturing urine at 4-6 weeks as prostatitis may be a related cause

E. Persistent or recurrent bladder infections in males: Consult urologist

F. Pyelonephritis in males (consultation with a specialist is recommended)
   1. In males, pyelonephritis usually suggests a structural problem and is an indication for hospitalization, parenteral antibiotic therapy, and an IVP
   2. Close follow up is essential

G. Patient education may help prevent future recurrent infections
   1. Avoid a full bladder
   2. Do not postpone urinating or rush during urination
   3. High fluid intake at first signs of infection
   4. For females, void after intercourse
   5. For females, consider other types of birth control if using a diaphragm or spermicides

H. Asymptomatic bacteriuria
   1. Defined as reproducible growth of at least 10^5 cfu of the same species of bacteria per milliliter of urine in a patient who has no signs or symptoms of UTI (need 2 positive urine specimens collected over a period of time)
   2. Treatment is controversial: In pregnant females, patients with diabetes, and patients who are to have urologic surgery prescribe antimicrobial therapy in a similar fashion as other UTIs; a repeat culture should be done at 2 weeks posttreatment and if positive, the treatment regimen for relapse should be followed
   3. A more conservative approach is to rule out any underlying or predisposing pathology and then treat the first episode with antibiotics (based on the urine culture and sensitivity); do not treat subsequent episodes if the patent remains asymptomatic

I. Referral
   1. In females consider referral for upper tract illness, recurrent multiple infections, and infections with unusual organisms
   2. Consider referring all males with UTIs with exception of young, healthy males who do not have recurrent infections

J. Follow up is variable depending on age, gender, and condition of patient
   1. For uncomplicated cystitis in females treated with 3-10 day regimen, no follow up or urine testing is needed
   2. For cystitis in males, follow up urine culture is needed after treatment; some recommend following these patients with repeat urine testing in 4-6 weeks
   3. Reinfections need close follow up with urine cultures every 1-2 months
   4. Patients with pyelonephritis should be contacted within 12-24 hours after treatment is begun; then, reschedule visits 2 weeks and 3 months post-treatment for urine cultures

CYSTITIS AND PYELONEPHRITIS IN CHILDREN

I. Definition: Bacteria in urine which have the potential to injure tissues of the urinary tract and adjacent structures. Urinary tract infections (UTIs) are often classified as upper and lower tract infections

   A. Cystitis or bladder infection is an example of a lower tract infection

   B. Pyelonephritis is the main upper tract infection and involves infection of the renal parenchyma

II. Pathogenesis of cystitis and pyelonephritis

   A. In neonates, hematogenous spread of infection to the kidney is the most common mode of infection

   B. The ascending route of infection is most common in older children.
      1. In females, bacteria can ascend the urethra from the introitus. Females have a short urethra which is in close proximity to the perirectal area making colonization possible
      2. In males, the prepuce may be the main source of the bacteria in ascending infections

   C. Bacterial virulence factors such as bacterial adherence are related to the development of UTIs; some bacteria have p-fimbriae which are hair-like structures that have the ability to adhere to uroepithelial cells and produce an inflammatory response; these p-fimbriae are more common on *E. coli* strains and have a major role in the pathogenesis of pyelonephritis

   D. Pathogens
      1. Gram negative bacilli are most common; 80-90% of community-acquired infections are due to *Escherichia coli*. Other gram negative bacilli include *Klebsiella pneumoniae* or *Proteus mirabilis*
      2. Gram-positive cocci account for 10-15% of community acquired infections; *Staphylococcus saprophyticus* is the second most common pathogen and often occurs in young, sexually active females

   E. The prevalence and etiology of urinary tract infections (UTIs) varies with age and gender
      1. In infants <3 months of age, infections are often associated with bacteremia; infections are more common in males and in premature or low-birth weight infants
      2. By age 3-8 months, male infants only account for 11% of total cases with approximately 95% of the male infants being uncircumcised
      3. Prevalence increases in the preschool years, with infections predominant in females
         a. Infections in males are usually due to congenital abnormalities
         b. Vesicoureteral reflux is a common structural abnormality leading to infections in this age group

4. During the school years and before puberty, prevalence is about 1-5% of females; UTIs are rare in males
5. After puberty, the prevalence of UTIs increases significantly in females, but remains low in males

F. Factors which predispose children to developing UTIs include the following:
1. Vesicoureteral reflux (VUR), a structural abnormality, can result in renal damage
   a. Occurs from an incompetent functional sphincter at the vesicoureteral junction or a defect in the valve-like mechanism at the junction of the ureter and bladder which enables organisms in bladder urine to be directly transmitted to the kidney
   b. VUR is the single most important risk factor in the development of pyelonephritis
   c. Approximately 50% of children <5 years of age who have UTIs and fevers also have VUR; more common in Caucasian children than African American children; common in young girls with dysfunctional voiding
   d. When VUR and infected urine are present, progressive loss of renal function often occurs; however, in the absence of infection, VUR does not result in renal scarring which highlights the importance of preventing infection in children with VUR
2. Urinary tract obstruction such as urinary lithiasis, urethral strictures, retroperitoneal fibrosis and neurogenic bladder
3. Nonobstructive renal malformations such as renal hypoplasia, dysplasia, and polycystic kidney disease
4. Behavioral factors such as voluntary deferral of micturition, chronic constipation, and poor hygiene
5. Noncircumcision in male infants
6. Pinworms
7. Conditions such as hypokalemia, vitamin A deficiency, diabetes mellitus, and uremia
8. Foreign body in introitus
9. Urinary instrumentation and catheterization
10. Neurogenic bladder disease from strokes, multiple sclerosis, spinal cord injuries, myelomeningocele (spina bifida) or other spinal anomalies

III. Clinical Presentation

A. UTIs in children can result in renal scarring and permanent renal damage and thus warrant greater attention and more aggressive management than UTIs in adults

B. Cystitis
1. In infants, signs and symptoms may be fever, irritability, decreased appetite, vomiting, diarrhea, constipation, dehydration, jaundice
2. Toddler and preschool children often present with nonspecific complaints such as anorexia and abdominal discomfort; may also have fever, changes in voiding pattern, and enuresis if they are toilet trained
3. School-aged children and adolescents have signs and symptoms typical of adults which are dysuria, frequency, urgency, and suprapubic pain.

C. Pyelonephritis is important to rapidly diagnose and treat as a delay in treatment increases the risk of renal damage
1. Accurate diagnosis of pyelonephritis based on clinical symptoms is difficult as children may not have typical findings of fever and flank pain as seen in adults
2. In infancy, sepsis is a greater possibility and there is increased likelihood of bladder obstruction marked by abdominal distention, weak urinary stream, infrequent voiding and discolored and malodorous urine
3. Older children sometimes have an acute onset of chills, fever, flank pain, costovertebral angle tenderness, and possibly hematuria
4. Often occurs concurrently or after a lower urinary tract infection

D. Recurrent infections are common and are often associated with severe vesicoureteral reflux and concomitant progressive renal scarring
1. Many children, typically girls, with recurrent lower UTIs have a voiding dysfunction whereby residual volumes of urine are left in the bladder after voiding which provide an environment that facilities growth of bacteria and UTIs; the following are three classification groups of voiding dysfunction
    a. Some children have bladder instability characterized by severe frequency, urgency, urge incontinence, and may have a typical squatting or posturing in response to unstable bladder contractions
    b. Other children have large bladders and emptying is often incomplete; voiding is often only once or twice a day
    c. Other children have dyssynergic voiding due to lack of coordination between the bladder and urethral sphincter which results in a large volume of residual urine, increased pressure in the bladder, and uninhibited bladder contractions
2. Chronic constipation and poor bowel habits are also correlated with recurrent UTIs

E. Asymptomatic bacteriuria:
1. Children with culture-proven bacteriuria who do not have symptoms
2. Children with this condition often have a spontaneous remission within a few months

IV. Diagnosis/Evaluation

A. History
1. Question parents of infants about duration and onset of fever, irritability, decreased appetite, etc.
2. Determine onset and duration of urinary symptoms; ask about strength and character of urine stream when voiding
3. Determine whether dysuria occurs during urination or after urination begins to pass over inflamed labia as with herpes simplex infections
4. Inquire about associated symptoms such as fever, chills, nausea, vomiting, diarrhea, abdominal, back pain, hematuria, and perianal itching
5. Explore normal voiding patterns and frequency of voids
6. Ask about history of constipation and encopresis
7. In older children ask about onset, duration, and characteristics of vaginal or urethral discharge
8. Past medical history should include drug allergies, chronic diseases such as diabetes mellitus or multiple sclerosis, previous genitourinary problems (by history or chart)
9. Count number of previous UTIs and discuss success and failures of previous treatments
10. Family history of VUR and recurrent UTIs is important

B. Physical Examination
1. Observe general appearance noting pallor, diaphoresis and listlessness
2. Assess vital signs, particularly noting elevated temperature and signs of orthostatic hypotension or hypertension
3. Assess for signs of sepsis and dehydration
4. Perform an abdominal exam, assessing for distention, tenderness, and masses
5. Palpate back for costovertebral angle tenderness
6. Inspect genitalia for anomalies, irritation, trauma, and in females, vaginitis and labial adhesions; in males, document circumcision status
7. Perform rectal examination for fecal impaction if there is a history of bowel problems
8. In children with history of voiding dysfunction or associated constipation or encopresis, a neurologic examination should be performed; assess perineal sensation, peripheral reflexes of lower extremities, and examine lower back for sacral dimpling or cutaneous abnormalities suggestive of underlying spinal abnormalities
9. May want to observe urinary stream when voiding

C. Differential Diagnosis
1. Gonococcal and nongonococcal urethritis in older male children
2. Urethral syndrome or dysuria-pyuria syndrome in older female children
3. Urinary calculi

4. Epididymitis
5. Bladder outlet obstruction
6. Previously undiagnosed posterior urethral valves in males
7. Renal tuberculosis
8. Tumors and carcinoma
9. Sexual abuse
10. Encopresis
11. Pinworm infestation
12. Foreign body in urethra and vagina
13. Irritant diaper dermatitis
14. Urethritis due to bubble baths or soap
15. Vaginitis

D. Diagnostic Tests: Because children present with vague symptoms, any child with a fever without a focus or recurrent abdominal pain should be evaluated for UTI
   1. Urine collection
      a. Clean catch urine specimens are usually acceptable for older children (first morning specimen is the best); may be helpful for girls to sit in reverse position on the toilet seat before voiding to spread labia away from urethral meatus
      b. Urine collected from a bag applied to perineum (bagged urine) may be obtained in younger children and infants, but because of high level of contamination only negative results are significant; all positive bagged specimens should be confirmed with a catheterized or aspirated specimen; bag should be removed and replaced if on for more than 30 minutes
      c. May perform single in-and-out catheterization of the bladder with children who are unable to give a clean midstream urine specimen; use a 5-French feeding tube in neonates, infants and toddlers or an 8-French in older children (a Coudé tip or curved tip catheter may be helpful in males who have tight sphincters)
      d. Suprapubic aspiration of the bladder may be necessary for preterm infants, girls who cannot be catheterized because of labial adhesions, and uncircumcised boys with tight foreskins; may not obtain specimen if bladder is empty (see following table for performing a suprapubic aspiration)

STEPS IN PERFORMING A SUPRAPUBIC ASPIRATION

❖ Ascertain that child has not voided within one hour of procedure; do not perform on a child with an empty bladder
❖ Restrain child in a supine, frog-legged position
❖ Cleanse suprapubic region with alcohol and providone-iodine
❖ Find puncture site which is 1-2 cm above the symphysis pubis in the midline
❖ With a 22-gauge, 1 ½-inch needle attached to a 3-mL syringe, make a puncture at a 10°-20° angle of the true vertical, aiming toward the head
❖ Exert gentle suction while advancing needle until urine enters the syringe. Continue to aspirate urine with gentle suction. If no urine is obtained, attempt procedure again, but this time aim needle in a caudal direction. If both attempts fail, further attempts are unlikely to be successful.

---

   2. Urinalysis:
      a. Dipstick has limited value in diagnosing UTI as it can be negative even with a positive culture; nonetheless dipstick helps to raise or lower suspicion of UTI if the following are present:
         (1) A positive leukocyte esterase test denotes white blood cells or pyuria
         (2) A positive nitrite test, denotes bacteria
      b. Microscopic analysis: Examine urine sediment under high power (40X), to count WBCs and gram stain to identify bacteria

3. Urine culture and sensitivity (Urine C&S); this test is mandatory for diagnosis of UTI in children
   a. Criteria for the diagnosis of UTI (see following table)

CRITERIA FOR DIAGNOSIS OF URINARY TRACT INFECTIONS BY URINE CULTURE			
Method of Collection	Suprapubic Aspiration	Catheterization	Clean-Catch Void
Colony Count	Any gram-negative bacilli > few thousand gram-positive cocci	$>10^2$ suspicious $>10^3$ likely	$>10^3$ suspicious $>10^5$ likely

   b. Bacterial identification and determination of antibiotic susceptibilities or a urine C&S are important in infections in children
4. Voiding cystourethrogram (VCUG) is recommended in all children less than 16 years with a documented UTI, particularly the following children:
   a. All children <5 years of age
   b. Boys of any age
   c. Girls >5 years of age who have pyelonephritis
   d. Children with recurrent UTIs
   e. Children who have an infection which is not responsive to antibiotics
5. When the voiding cystogram is abnormal, order a renal ultrasound (see management of reflux, section V.D.)
6. Order dimercaptosuccinic acid (DMSA) renal scan in the following cases: if the diagnosis of pyelonephritis is uncertain, for UTIs with high fevers, if this is the first episode of pyelonephritis, and after some infections to determine degree of renal scarring and damage
7. Urodynamic testing should be considered in patients with suspected neurogenic disorders or in children suspected of dysfunctional voiding who fail behavioral therapy and treatment with medications
8. With systemic symptoms or children with suspected pyelonephritis and infants order CBC and blood cultures; consider ordering erythrocyte sedimentation rate
9. With symptoms associated with sexually transmitted disease, perform wet mount of vaginal secretions and order gonococcal (GC) cultures and chlamydial test; also, can gram stain urethral and cervical secretions

V. Plan/Management

   A. Consider hospitalization for children with complicated UTIs (high fever, toxic appearance, persistent vomiting, dehydration, poor compliance with medications), small infants, and children with moderate-to-severe symptoms of pyelonephritis

   B. Uncomplicated bacterial cystitis in children
      1. Always order a urine culture and sensitivity on children suspected of UTI. However, begin treatment prior to obtaining the results if they are symptomatic and have a positive urinalysis (may need to change treatment later based on results of urine C & S)
      2. First drug of choice is trimethoprim/sulfamethoxazole (Septra) in children >2 months of age; prescribe 40 mg/kg/day of sulfamethoxazole component in 2 divided doses for 10-14 days. Available 40 mg trimethoprim, 200 mg sulfamethoxazole per 5 mL. First-tme, uncomplicated infections can be treated with 3-5 day course of antibiotics
      3. Alternative drugs include nitrofurantoin (Macrodantin) 5-7 mg/kg/day in 4 divided doses with food for 10-14 days (not recommended in infants <1 month old and not available in liquid form) or amoxicillin (Amoxil) 40 mg/kg/day in 3 divided doses for 10-14 days. Available in 125 mg/5 mL and 250 mg/5 mL liquids (associated with increasing development of resistant enteric organisms which may lead to reinfection)
      4. Avoid quinolones in children because of potential arthropathy
      5. Urine should be recultured 2-3 days after starting on therapy and after completion of therapy if a 7-10 day regimen is used; followed by a reculture in 1 month, then every 3 months for a year; and then annually for 2-3 years to screen for recurrent infection (some authorities recommend monthly recultures in the first year after an infection)

6.   A voiding cystourethrogram (VCUG) should be ordered after the first documented UTI in children <5 years of age, boys at any age, girls >5 years of age with pyelonephritis, recurrent UTIs, infections unresponsive to antibiotics (make sure patient is asymptomatic and urine is sterile before tests)
   a.   Inform parents/patients that VCUG is invasive
   b.   Best time to obtain VCUG is 4-6 weeks after completion of treatment (low-dose prophylactic antibiotics should be used until imaging test is completed. See section V.E.)
   c.   Early detection of an anatomical abnormality may prevent recurrent infections and subsequent renal damage
   d.   VCUG detects VUR, ureteroceles, bladder wall thickening, and in boys, posterior urethral valves
7.   Order a renal ultrasound to exclude hydronephrosis or other upper tract malformations
8.   If no abnormality is found on VCUG and ultrasound, no further tests are needed
9.   If reflux is found on VCUG or ultrasound, order a dimercaptosuccinic acid (DMSA) renal scan to detect postinflammatory renal cortical scars (see treatment of reflux in sections V.D. and E.)
10.   If possible urinary obstruction is noted on ultrasound, order an excretory renal scan such as MAG-3 or ^{99m}Tc diethylenetriaminepentaacetic acid (DTPA)

C.   Pyelonephritis (consider consultation with a specialist)
1.   IV therapy and hospitalization are often needed in cases suggestive of bacteremia, in children with complicated UTIs, in children less than 1- 2 years old, and in young children who have parenchymal damage as documented by imaging studies
2.   Close monitoring of patients is needed if treated on an outpatient basis
3.   Outpatient treatment should extend for 14 days and include one of the following:
   a.   Cefixime (Suprax) 4 mg/kg/day every 12 hours, Available 100mg/ mL liquid
   b.   Alternatively, may first administer ceftriaxone intramuscularly followed by 10-14 day treatment of oral antibiotics (see appropriate antibiotics in V.B.2-3)
   c.   Do **not** prescribe Nitrofurantoin because tissue bacteriostatic levels are suboptimal
4.   Therapy should stabilize patient within 12-24 hours; if not, look for deeper infections. Schedule return visits or contact patient by phone in 12-24 hours
5.   Urine should be recultured 2-3 days after start of therapy; followed by a reculture after completion of therapy. Also, continue to monitor the urine, with urine culture and sensitivities in 1 month, then every 3 months for a year; and then annually for 2-3 years to screen for recurrent infection (some authorities recommend monthly cultures in first year)
6.   All children with pyelonephritis should have a VCUG, a renal ultrasound, and a DMSA renal scan [maintain child on prophylactic antibiotics (see V.E.) until these diagnostic tests are completed]

D.   Treatment of vesicoureteral reflux (VUR) (consult specialist)
1.   Mild to moderate reflux (grades I, II, and III) can be medically managed with prophylactic antibiotics (see V.E.) and yearly evaluation of VUR with VCUG, renal ultrasound, and/or DMSA renal scan to monitor renal growth and/or damage as long as VUR persists
2.   Referral to pediatric urologist is needed for children with high grade VUR (usually surgery is recommended)
3.   Siblings <5 years of age of children with VUR should have diagnostic tests because of the high familial incidence

E.   Recurrent infections in children are usually relapses of the same initial infection, rather than reinfection with a new pathogen as is usually the case in adults.
1.   Prophylactic antibiotic therapy is needed for children with recurrent infections (defined as 3 in 6 months or 4 in 1 year) as well as those with VUR, those waiting for further diagnostic tests, and in young children with non-reflux pyelonephritis with acute or chronic renal damage

    a. Duration of treatment depends on condition
     (1) Children with VUR need treatment until reflux spontaneously resolves
     (2) Children with recurrent infections and young children with pyelonephritis should remain on prophylaxis a minimum of 6-12 months with periodic urine specimens for cultures at 3-6 months; medications should be restarted for additional 12 months if infection recurs within 3 months of discontinuation of above therapy
    b. Prescribe one of the following:
     (1) Nitrofurantoin 1-2 mg/kg BID in children >2 months
     (2) Trimethoprim/sulfamethoxazole: 1 mg/kg trimethoprim (T) & 10 mg/kg sulfamethoxazole(S) QD or 1 mg/kgT and 5 mg/kgS BID in children > 2 months
   2. Teach patient to double void (void, wait 3 minutes, void again) if post voiding residual (PVR) is present
   3. Children with recurrent infections who have dysfunctional voiding require antimicrobial prophylaxis, timed voiding, and possibly anticholinergic medications
   4. Children with chronic constipation related to recurrent infections need help in improving their bowel habits (see section on ENCOPRESIS)

  F. Asymptomatic bacteriuria: Although controversial, most authorities recommend no treatment unless the child has urinary tract abnormalities

  G. Follow Up
   1. In children with cystitis and pyelonephritis a reculture of urine should be obtained 2-3 days after treatment is initiated, possibly after treatment is completed, and then in 1 month, followed by every 3 months for a year; and then annually for 2-3 years to screen for recurrent infection (some authorities recommend monthly recultures in first year); VCUG and/or renal ultrasound and possibly DMSA renal scan are usually scheduled 4-6 weeks after infection has cleared
   2. Children with recurrent infections should have cultures every 3-6 months

EPIDIDYMITIS

I. Definition: Inflammation of the epididymis

II. Pathogenesis: Pathogens apparently reach the epididymis through the lumen of the vas deferens from infected urine, the posterior urethra, or seminal vesicles

  A. In infants and children, an underlying genitourinary tract abnormality is often present

  B. In adolescents, infection is often sexually transmitted and 75% of cases are caused by *Neisseria gonorrhoea* or *Chlamydia trachomatis* (most common); underlying structural disorders are rare; in homosexual males *Escherichia coli* may be a pathogen

  C. Epididymitis may be nonsexually transmitted
   1. Typically caused by coliform or *Pseudomonas* species; in most cases of bacterial epididymitis, gram-negative rods are found but gram-positive cocci are also important pathogens
   2. Usually associated with urinary tract infections in males >35 years with urinary tract instrumentation, surgery, or anatomical abnormalities

  D. Uncommon causes are due to trauma or tuberculous epididymitis

III.   Clinical Presentation

   A.   Usually patients have a history of sexual activity and associated urethritis

   B.   Commonly, there is a gradual onset of unilateral testicular pain and tenderness, dysuria, and urethral discharge

   C.   Fever occurs in approximately 50% of patients; nausea and vomiting is unusual

   D.   Scrotum is tender on palpation and usually accompanied with a hydrocele and palpable swelling of the epididymis

   E.   Uncommon complications include testicular necrosis, testicular atrophy, and infertility

IV.   Diagnosis/Evaluation

   A.   History
         1.   Determine onset, duration, and course of symptoms
         2.   Ask about scrotal pain, dysuria, urinary frequency and urgency, and color, amount and consistency of urethral discharge
         3.   Inquire about possible associated symptoms such as fever, nausea, and vomiting
         4.   Explore sexual history; ask about new sexual partners and if sexual partners have complained of dysuria or urinary frequency
         5.   Question about previous urinary tract infections and treatments
         6.   Inquire about previous genitourinary surgery, urinary tract instrumentation and anatomic abnormalities
         7.   Inquire about recent trauma to testes

   B.   Physical Examination
         1.   Inspect scrotum, noting edema and erythema which are typical
         2.   Palpate scrotum
               a.   In epididymitis, testes are tender but the position, size, and consistency of testes is entirely normal
               b.   Palpable swelling of epididymis is usually present
         3.   Passive elevation of testis may relieve pain in epididymitis (Prehn's sign)
         4.   Perform rectal exam (this exam may elicit prostatic tenderness and result in expression of urethral discharge)

   C.   Differential Diagnosis
         1.   Must differentiate testicular torsion which is an emergent condition from epididymitis (see following table)

DIFFERENTIATION OF EPIDIDYMITIS AND TESTICULAR TORSION		
	Epididymitis	**Testicular Torsion**
History		
Onset of pain	Gradual	Acute
Nausea and vomiting	Rare	50%
Voiding symptoms	50%	No
Urethral discharge	50%	No
Physical Examination		
Epididymal swelling only	Early	10%
Scrotal edema	Most	Most
Scrotal erythema	Most	Most
Fever	50%	Rare

443

2. Orchitis (patient usually has recently had parotitis)
3. Testicular tumor (usually not tender)
4. Trauma
5. Skin pathology such as insect bites or folliculitis

D. Diagnostic Tests
1. Obtain urinalysis (in about 20-95% of epididymitis cases there is pyuria compared to 0-30% in cases with testicular torsion)
2. Collect urine culture and sensitivity and gram-stained smear of uncentrifuged urine for gram-negative bacteria
3. In adolescents who may have a sexually transmitted disease obtain the following:
   a. Gram-stained smear of urethral exudate or intraurethral swab specimen to detect urethritis (≥5 polymorphonuclear leukocytes per oil immersion field) and for presumptive diagnosis of gonococcal infection
   b. Culture of urethral exudate or intraurethral swab specimen or nucleic acid amplification test (either by first-void urine or intraurethral swab) for *N. gonorrhoeae* and *C. trachomatis*
   c. Collect first-void urine and examine for leukocytes if the urethral Gram stain is negative; culture and gram-stained smear of uncentrifuged urine should be collected
   d. Syphilis serology and HIV counseling and testing
4. Emergency testing for testicular torsion may be necessary when the onset of pain is sudden and severe or if there is uncertainty about the diagnosis; consult a specialist and consider ordering one of the following: Doppler ultrasound, scrotal ultrasound, or radionuclide scrotal imaging

V. Plan/Management

A. In prepubertal boys, treatment is based on urine culture but typically a broad-spectrum agent can be prescribed. Children >2 months prescribe trimethoprim/sulfamethoxazole (Bactrim) 40 mg/kg/day PO BID for 10-14 days. Available trimethoprim 40 mg/sulfamethoxazole 200 mg per 5 mL

B. For active heterosexual adolescents, most likely cause is a sexually transmitted disease
1. For epididymitis most likely due to gonococcal of chlamydial infection, treat empirically based on clinical diagnosis before culture results are available with the following: doxycycline (Vibramycin) 100 mg PO BID for 10 days and ceftriaxone (Rocephin) 250 mg IM in a single dose
2. For epididymitis most likely caused by enteric organisms or in patients allergic to tetracyclines and/or cephalosporins, treat empirically with ofloxacin (Floxin) 300 mg PO BID for 10 days
3. Treat sexual partners if their contact with the index patient was within 60 days preceding onset of symptoms in the patient
4. Instruct patients to avoid sexual intercourse until they and their sex partners are cured or until treatment is completed and patients and partners are asymptomatic

C. Symptomatic treatment of bed rest, scrotal support, scrotal elevation, sitz baths, pain medication, and ice packs may be beneficial

D. Follow Up
1. For patients whose symptoms fail to improve within 3 days, reevaluate both the diagnosis and treatment
   a. Swelling and tenderness that persist after antimicrobial therapy require comprehensive evaluation
   b. Differential diagnosis includes tumor, abscess, infarction, testicular cancer, and tuberculosis or fungal epididymitis
2. In prepubertal boys repeat urine cultures are needed after completion of the therapy and further diagnostic tests can also be scheduled at this time
3. For postpubertal males, no follow up or test of cure is needed if symptoms resolve

TESTICULAR TORSION

I. Definition: Twisting of spermatic cord which results in compromised testicular blood flow

II. Pathogenesis

   A. Occurs when the free-floating testis rotates on the spermatic cord and occludes its blood supply

   B. May occur spontaneously after activity or trauma

III. Clinical Presentation

   A. Commonly occurs during the newborn period and at puberty, but a significant number of patients with torsion are over the age of 21 years

   B. Torsion during perinatal period usually occurs shortly after birth
   1. Scrotum appears swollen and erythematous or bluish
   2. Typically, a nontender mass is palpable in the affected hemiscrotum

   C. Torsion in older children and adolescents
   1. Many patients have an anatomic defect known as "bell-clapper" deformity
   2. Typical history is sudden onset of testicular pain which radiates to groin; but in some cases there is minimal swelling and little or no pain
   3. May also have lower abdominal pain which leads to erroneous diagnosis of appendicitis or gastroenteritis
   4. Nausea and vomiting occur in about half of the patients; usually there is no fever, urethral discharge or dysuria
   5. If not surgically treated, there will be ischemic injury and necrosis of the testis
   6. Degree of injury is determined by the severity of the arterial compression and the interval between the onset and surgical intervention (for severe torsion, must intervene within 4-8 hours to salvage the testis)

IV. Diagnosis/Evaluation

   A. History: Testicular torsion is an urological emergency so rapidly gather a focused history
   1. Ask about onset and circumstances surrounding onset
   2. Ask about accompanying symptoms such as nausea, vomiting, fever, dysuria, urethral discharge
   3. Determine any occurrence of trauma or unusual physical activity
   4. In older males, to rule out epididymitis, question about recent change in sexual partners and symptoms of dysuria and urethral discharge

   B. Physical Examination: Perform a rapid but systematic exam
   1. Observe general appearance (patients with testicular torsion are in acute distress, have pain on ambulation, and prefer to lie quietly on the examination table)
   2. Inspect scrotal skin (often skin is erythematous, taut, and without normal rugations with torsion)
   3. Palpate testes (testis may be located high in the scrotum as a result of shortening of the cord by twisting)
   4. Palpate the epididymis which normally is located on the posterolateral surface of the testis and is smooth, discrete, and nontender (with testicular torsion the epididymis will not be in this typical position as a result of cord twisting and will be extremely tender)
   5. Palpate vas deferens from the testicle to the inguinal ring (normally vas deferens is smooth, discrete and nontender)
   6. Try to elicit the cremasteric reflex; positive reflex is testicular retraction when the upper, medial thigh is stroked (usually absent in torsion, but present in epididymitis)
   7. Perform a complete abdominal exam

C. Differential Diagnosis
1. Epididymitis is the most difficult condition to differentiate (see table in section on EPIDIDYMITIS, differentiating epididymitis from torsion)
2. Torsion of the testicular appendage
   a. More common in pre-pubertal males
   b. Pain is usually less severe than with torsion of the entire testis; pain and swelling develop gradually
   c. "Blue dot" sign at superior aspect of testis is diagnostic of this problem
   d. Management is bedrest and scrotal elevation
   e. With appropriate management, symptoms resolve within a week
3. Orchitis
4. Incarcerated inguinal hernia
5. Vasculitis
6. Tumor
7. Trauma
8. Henoch-Schölein purpura is a systemic vasculitic syndrome characterized by nonthrombocytopenic purpura, arthralgia, renal disease, gastrointestinal pain and bleeding
9. Idiopathic scrotal edema

D. Diagnostic Tests: When clinical presentation is typical, surgical exploration is usually carried out without further testing. If uncertain, consider consulting a specialist and ordering the following:
1. Urinalysis (will be normal in 90% of patients with testicular torsion, but will often be abnormal in epididymitis)
2. Doppler ultrasound (absent testicular artery pulsations with torsion); the development of color Doppler imaging with pulsed Doppler has improved accuracy of this test
3. Nuclear testicular scanning allows evaluation of blood flow to the scrotal contents (decreased perfusion with torsion)
4. Scrotal ultrasonography can be ordered; does not distinguish torsion from epididymitis but is helpful in evaluating scrotal masses and trauma

V. Plan/Management:

A. Immediate consultation and surgical intervention; this is an urological emergency (torsion in perinatal period is sometimes treated nonsurgically)

B. Follow Up: Surgeon should arrange follow up to determine response to operation

HYDROCELE

I. Definition: Collection of peritoneal fluid trapped in a patent processus vaginalis which is beginning to undergo obliteration

II. Pathogenesis

A. Basic facts of the anatomy and embryology of the inguinal region are helpful in understanding the pathogenesis of a hydrocele
1. During the last months of gestation the testes migrate down from the internal inguinal region to the base of the scrotum
2. During this descent, the lining of the abdominal cavity (processus vaginalis) also descends with the testes
3. Normally, after the testicular descent, the processus vaginalis begins to close which leaves only the most distal portion of the processus, the tunica vaginalis, that surrounds the testis

B. Noncommunicating hydroceles are most common and result when residual peritoneal fluid remains after closure of the processus vaginalis

C. In communicating hydroceles there still is a connection between the peritoneal cavity and the tunica vaginalis and peritoneal fluid can shift through the patent processus vaginalis; abdominal contents (hernia) can also descend

D. Hydroceles may form secondary to testicular pathology such as testicular tumors

III. Clinical Presentation

A. Noncommunicating and communicating hydroceles with and without hernias usually occur at birth or in the neonatal period; they infrequently occur later in life and are then usually associated with underlying pathology such as a testicular neoplasm, torsion, injury or infection

B. Noncommunicating hydroceles
1. Scrotal sac appears full, fluctuant, tense and clear if transilluminated
2. Fluid gradually absorbs during the first year of life
3. Since the processus vaginalis is closed off, there is no danger of a hernia developing

C. Communicating hydroceles
1. History reveals a flat scrotum in the morning with a gradual increase in fluid during the day
2. Rarely resolve and have the potential for herniation of the intestine

D. Trauma to the scrotum may cause hemorrhage into the hydrocele sac

IV. Diagnosis/Evaluation

A. History
1. Determine onset and course of the hydrocele
2. Ask patient/parents if the size of the scrotum remains the same or if enlarges from the morning to evening
3. Ask patient/parents about intermittent bulges in scrotum or abdomen which increase when child cries
4. Ask about scrotal pain, heaviness, and symptoms of intestinal obstruction such as colicky abdominal pain and hyperperistalsis

B. Physical Examination
1. Inspect scrotum for size, shape, symmetry, swelling, lesions and color
2. Any swelling should be assessed further with transillumination
   a. In a darkened room a beam of light is directed from behind the scrotum
   b. The light will appear as a red glow with serous fluid but not with blood or tissue
3. Palpate inguinal area and scrotum, checking for an inguinal hernia or other lesions such as varicocele or spermatocele
4. Palpate testes with thumb and first 2 fingers
   a. Normally testes are sensitive to compression but not tender and feel smooth, rubbery, and free of nodules; size in infant is 1 cm.
   b. If mass is felt, carefully palpate to determine whether the mass is separate from the testis as occurs with a hernia or whether it cannot be delineated from testis as occurs with a tumor
5. Palpate epididymis on posterolateral surface of testis which should feel smooth, discrete, and nontender
6. Palpate vas deferens from testicle to inguinal ring (normally, feels smooth and discrete)
7. Perform a complete abdominal exam

C. Differential Diagnosis (see Figure 13.1): Normal scrotum and hydrocele (see Figure 13.1A and 13.1B).
1. Spermatocele is a cyst containing sperm that presents as circumscribed mass that does not transilluminate and persists when patient is supine (see Figure 13.1C)
2. Testicular tumor is the most important disorder to rule out (see Figure 13.1D)
   a. Most common tumor in males between the ages of 15-30
   b. Commonly occurs after age 15, but there is a small peak in incidence at 2 years of age
   c. Tumor is firm, painless mass that gives a sensation of heaviness in the testis
   d. Mass cannot be delineated from substance of testis; does not transilluminate

3. Epididymitis (see Figure 13.1E) (see section of EPIDIDYMITIS)
4. Orchitis (see Figure 13.1F) is associated with viral parotitis (mumps)
   a. Difficult to distinguish from testicular torsion
   b. Presents with sudden onset of pain, and red, warm, and tender testis or testes
5. Hernia (see section on HERNIAS, ABDOMINAL)
6. Varicocele (see section on VARICOCELE)
7. Undescended testes (see section on (UNDESCENDED TESTES)

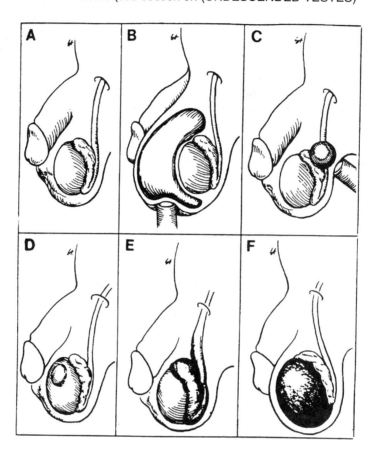

Figure 13.1. Scrotal Lesions.
A. Normal. B. Hydrocele. C. Spermatocele. D. Testicular Tumor. E. Epididymitis. F. Orchitis.

Source: Judge, R.D., Zuidema, G.D., & Fitzgerald, F.T. (Eds.) (1989), <u>Clinical Diagnosis</u> (p. 381). Boston: Little, Brown and Company. Copyright 1989 by A.C. Judge, P.C. Judge, S.M. Judge, N.C. Judge. Reprinted by permission.

D. Diagnostic Tests
   1. Diagnostic tests are often not ordered if the health provider is confident that a hydrocele exists without pathological lesions
   2. Occasionally an abdominal roentogram is helpful because presence of air below the inguinal ligament indicates a hernia
   3. Ultrasound of the inguinal region and scrotum can differentiate a true hernia or another mass (tumor) from a hydrocele with peritoneal fluid

V. Plan/Management

   A. Noncommunicating hydrocele in children
      1. Assure the parents that the scrotum is just enlarged with fluid which will absorb over the next year
      2. No surgical or medical treatment is necessary

448

B. Communicating hydrocele in children
   1. Usually refer to urologist/surgeon
   2. Because of the potential for herniation of the intestine, these hydroceles often are repaired
   3. Boys under 2 years of age should have bilateral exploration because of high incidence of contralateral patent processus vaginalis

C. Hydrocele with inguinal hernia in children
   1. Refer to urologist/surgeon
   2. If the hernia cannot be reduced of if vomiting or signs of intestinal obstruction occur, emergency surgery is indicated

D. Referral to specialist is needed for adolescents with new hydroceles; usually adolescents do not require therapy unless complications exist or there is discomfort from the bulky mass or a tense hydrocele is present that may reduce the circulation and lead to atrophy

E. Follow Up
   1. For patients with noncommunicating hydroceles, closely monitor size of scrotum at each health maintenance visit or at least every 6 months
   2. Confer with urologist/surgeon about follow up for patients with communicating hydroceles and hernias

VARICOCELE

I. Definition: Dilated plexus of scrotal veins situated above the testis in the scrotum

II. Pathogenesis: Due to valvular incompetence of the spermatic vein

A. Varicoceles on left side in adolescents are usually of unknown etiology; new left-sided varicocele in older males may be a renal tumor

B. Varicoceles on the right side may represent acute venous obstruction from a tumor or intra-abdominal pathology

III. Clinical Presentation

A. Usually found in older adolescents but can occur at a any age (onset in prepubertal males and in adult males is often associated with pathology)

B. Approximately, 15% of all adult males have a varicocele

C. Almost always varicoceles occur on left side; a unilateral right varicocele is rare; bilateral varicoceles are more common than previously thought

D. Testis resembles a bag of worms with a bluish discoloration which is visible through the scrotum (see Figure 13.2)

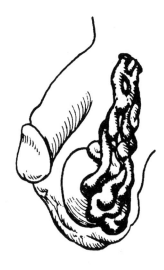

Figure 13.2. Varicocele.
Source: Judge, R.D., Zuidema, G.D., & Fitzgerald, F.T. (Eds.) (1989), <u>Clinical Diagnosis</u> (p. 381). Boston: Little, Brown and Company. Copyright 1989 by A.C. Judge, P.C. Judge, S.M. Judge, N.C. Judge. Reprinted by permission.

E.   Varicocele is most prominent when the patient is standing; tends to collapse when the patient is sitting or supine

F.   Patient is usually asymptomatic and testis is nontender, but may have mild pain or a feeling of heaviness in the scrotum

G.   Varicoceles are associated with a time-dependent decline in testicular function; decreased sperm counts, infertility and testicular atrophy are associated in about 65%-75% of patients with varicoceles

H.   Today, emphasis has shifted to early diagnosis, education and intervention in adolescence to prevent infertility in adulthood

IV.   Diagnosis/Evaluation

A.   History
  1.   Ask when patient first noticed varicocele
  2.   Determine the rate the scrotum is enlarging
  3.   Ask if the varicocele collapses upon sitting or standing
  4.   Inquire about testicular pain or discomfort
  5.   In older males, question about problems with infertility

B.   Physical Examination
  1.   Assess Tanner stage in children and adolescents to determine normal growth and development of testes
  2.   If varicocele is not visible, ask patient to stand and perform a Valsalva maneuver
  3.   Palpate testes, epididymis, and vas deferens in first standing then supine positions
  4.   Perform a rectal examination to assess prostate size since the prostate may shrink with testosterone deficiency that may occur with varicoceles

C.   Differential Diagnosis (see illustration in section on HYDROCELE)
  1.   Hydrocele
  2.   Spermatocele
  3.   Testicular tumor
  4.   Epididymal cyst

D. Diagnostic Tests
1. In adolescents, order testicular ultrasound to assess testicular volume and significant testicular size variations between testes with and without varicocele
2. For right-sided varicoceles and suddenly appearing left-sided varicoceles consider ordering the following:
    a. Venography is the gold standard for diagnosing varicoceles in adults; also used to detect venous obstruction or renal carcinoma associated with varicoceles
    b. Doppler ultrasound, thermography, and scrotal scintigraphy are nonspecific for diagnosing varicoceles, but may be beneficial in some cases
3. Consult specialist about assessing reproductive function in older males with semen analysis, testis biopsy, and fine needle aspiration with flow cytometry

V. Plan/Management

A. Refer the following patients to a surgeon:
1. All prepubertal males
2. All patients with right-sided varicoceles
3. The following adolescent males:
    a. When varicocele is voluminous, rapidly increasing in size, or does not disappear in sitting and supine positions
    b. When pain is present
    c. When there is evidence of testicular atrophy defined as a two standard deviation in testicular size when compared with normal testicular growth curves
    d. When there is greater than a 2 mL difference in testicular volume as noted on serial ultrasonography examination

B. If surgery is not recommended, explain that patient needs to monitor the growth and symptoms related to the varicocele

C. Follow Up: If surgery is not performed, explain to patient the need to return to clinic if he experiences increasing discomfort or if scrotum changes in size and shape

UNDESCENDED TESTES (CRYPTORCHIDISM)

I. Definition: Failure of the testes to descend into the scrotum

II. Pathogenesis:

A. Most undescended testes are a result of a mechanical factor, a hernia sac, or a shortened spermatic artery which impedes the testis descent into the scrotum

B. Failure of testes to descend may be partially due to a lack of gonadotropic and androgenic hormones during fetal development or an inability of the testes to respond to these hormones

III. Clinical Presentation

A. Because the testes descend into the scrotum during approximately the 36th week of fetal life, the incidence of cryptorchidism is much higher in the premature infant than in the full-term infant; about 3% of male term newborns and 20% of premature male infants have undescended testes at birth

B. Testes which are undescended may stop their descent within the canal, in the abdomen (more likely to be abnormal), or descend through the inguinal canal, pass through the inguinal canal and end in a position in the superficial inguinal space, thigh or perineum

C. Approximately 14% of boys with undescended testes have family members who had this condition

D. About 75% of boys with cryptorchidism have a hernia sac associated with the testis and cord structures

E. If testes are undescended by 6 months of age, they are unlikely to spontaneously descend

F. Occasionally, descended testes can ascend spontaneously and occupy a permanent extrascrotal position; thus, it is important to examine the testes on all health maintenance visits, even in those boys who were previously found to have descended testes

G. Deterioration of the undescended testes begins around 1 year of age and may ultimately correlate with poor semen quality and subsequent infertility

H. The risk of developing a testicular malignancy is 40 times higher in an undescended testis than a normal testis

I. Other complications include testicular torsion, emotional stress, hernia, and greater vulnerability to stress

IV. Diagnosis/Evaluation

A. History
1. Determine whether the child was born prematurely
2. Ask about family history of cryptorchidism
3. Ask parents if they have noticed whether the child's testes are in the scrotum during baths or when he is relaxed

B. Physical examination
1. Inspect scrotum; with cryptorchidism the scrotum is not fully developed on the affected side
2. Gently palpate and ascertain that the testis is truly undescended (warm hands before examination); an overactive cremasteric reflex makes palpation difficult
   a. Place child in supine position; sweep hand from the anterior-superior iliac spine over the inguinal canal and toward the pubis, attempting to palpate a testis. Try milking the testis into the scrotum; the older child can help by coughing or straining
   b. If unable to locate testis in a supine position, ask the child to assume a tailor position (sitting cross-legged), kneeling position, or standing position
   c. If unable to locate testis with above methods, search beyond the scrotum and the inguinal canal, palpating as far distant as the inner thigh
   d. Note position, consistency, and size of testis in comparison to the contralateral testis as well as to boys of similar age
   e. Check for inguinal hernias and hydroceles as they are often associated with cryptorchidism; if a hernia is present, the impalpable hernia usually lies just inside the internal inguinal ring
3. Even if there are documented descended testes on previously visits, continue to regularly examine testes because re-ascent is possible

C. Differential Diagnosis
1. Anorchia or the complete absence of a testis which commonly occurs on the right side with the left side of the scrotum being underdeveloped
2. Retractile testis which is a physiologic variation of normal (see physical examination IV.B.2. for how to examine a patient with a retractile testis)
   a. Due to an overactive cremasteric muscular reflex and the incomplete attachment of the testis to the scrotum by the gubernaculum
   b. Usually bilateral
   c. Less of a problem as the child gets older and the cremasteric reflex is less active and the testes become large

D. Diagnostic Tests are ordered when the testes are impalpable
1. Sonography is only helpful with inguinal undescended testes
2. Computed tomography has many false positives, exposes the child to radiation, and requires sedation but is sometimes recommended in older boys
3. Magnetic resonance imaging is sometimes recommended, particularly in adolescents and adult males
4. Laparoscopy is recommended as the initial diagnostic test by some experts
5. A therapeutic trial of human chorionic gonadotropin (HCG) may also be helpful (see V.B.)

V. Plan/Management

A. Refer all children with cryptorchidism to a pediatric urologist; surgical repair, orchidopexy, should be done at 1 year or shortly thereafter to prevent infertility, diminish the possibility of testicular torsion, provide accessible examination (particularly in the event of malignant change), and prevent emotional trauma that often accompanies the disorder

B. If the location of the testis is uncertain, the potential for natural descent can be explored with a therapeutic trial of human chorionic gonadotropin (HCG), 1500 IU/m^2 body surface area intramuscularly twice a week for 4 weeks; surgery is the recommended option if the testis does not descend or re-ascends after the HCG trial

C. Parents are usually anxious; tell parents that after orchidopexy the rate of fertility in these children is about 80% to 90%

D. Follow Up: The optimal timing of follow-up visits after birth is at 3 and 6 months, at which time most testicles descend in response to the postnatal testosterone surge

REFERENCES

Ahmed, Z., & Lee, J. (1997). Asymptomatic urinary abnormalities: Hematuria and proteinuria. Medical Clinics of North America, 81, 641-651.

American Academy of Pediatrics. (1996). Timing of elective surgery on the genitalia of male children with particular reference to the risks, benefits, and psychological effects of surgery and anesthesia. Pediatrics, 97, 590-594.

Anderson, J.E. (1997). Hematuria. In L. Dornbrand, A.J. Hoole, & R.H. Fletcher (Eds.). Manual of clinical problems in adult ambulatory care (3rd ed.). Philadelphia: Lippincott-Raven.

Bacheller, C.D., & Bernstein, J.M. (1997). Urinary tract infections. Medical Clinics of North America, 81, 719-729.

Barber, N. (1996). Genitourinary disorders. In C.E. Burns, N. Barber, M.A. Brady, & A.M. Dunn (Eds.). Pediatric primary care: A handbook for nurse practitioners. Philadelphia: Saunders.

Belman, A.B. (1997). Vesicoureteral reflux. Pediatric Clinics of North America, 44, 1171-1189.

Bock, G.H. (1997). Urinary tract infections. In R.A. Hoekelman (Ed.). Primary pediatric care. St. Louis: Mosby.

Feld, L.G., Wza, W.R., Perez, L.M., & Joseph, D.B. (1997). Hematuria: An integrated medical and surgical approach. Pediatric Clinics of North America, 44, 1191-1211.

Fihn, S.D., et al. (1998). Use of spermicide-coated condoms and other risk factors for urinary tract infection caused by Staphylococcus saprophyticus. Archives of Internal Medicine, 158, 281-287.

Foglia, R.P. (1999). Groin hernias and hydroceles. In R.A. Dershewitz (Ed.). Ambulatory pediatric care (3rd ed.). Philadelphia: Lippincott.

Foglia, R.P. (1999). Undescended testes. In R.A. Dershewitz (Ed.). Ambulatory pediatric care (3rd ed.). Philadelphia: Lippincott.

Gill, B., & Kogan, S. (1997). Crytorchidism: Current concepts. Pediatric clinics of North America, 44, 1211-1227.

Hoberman, A., & Wald, E.R. (1997). UTI in young children: New light on old questions. Contemporary Pediatrics, 14 (11), 140-156.

Junnila, J., & Lassen, P. (1998). Testicular masses. <u>American Family Physician, 57,</u> 685-692.

Kass, E.J., & Lundak, B. (1997). The acute scrotum. <u>Pediatric Clinics of North America, 44,</u> 1251-1266.

Krieger, J.N. (1998). Epididymitis. In R.E. Rakel (Ed.), <u>1998 Conn's current therapy</u>. Philadelphia: Saunders.

Kurgan, A., Nunnelee, J.d., & Ailberman, M. (1994). The importance of the early detection of varicocele in adolescent males. <u>Nurse Practitioner, 19</u> (10), 36-37.

Kurowski, K. (1998). The woman with dysuria. <u>American Family Physician, 57,</u> 2155-2164.

Langman, C.B. (1999). Hematuria. In R.A. Dershewitz (Ed.). <u>Ambulatory pediatric care</u> (3rd ed.). Philadelphia: Lippincott.

Langman, C.B. (1999). Proteinuria. In R.A. Dershewitz (Ed.). <u>Ambulatory pediatric care</u> (3rd ed.). Philadelphia: Lippincott.

Langermann, S., et al. (1997). Prevention of mucosal *Excherichia coli* infection by FimH-adhesion-based systemic vaccination. <u>Science, 276,</u> 607-614.

McCarthy, J.J. (1997). Outpatient evaluation of hematuria: Locating the source of bleeding. <u>Postgraduate Medicine, 101,</u> 125-131.

Neiberger, R.E. (1994). The ABC's of evaluating children with hematuria. <u>American Family Physician, 49</u>(3), 623-628.

Roberts, B.J., & Gibbons, M.D. (May, 1997). Urinary tract infections in children: Causes, effects, and recommendations for management. <u>Advance for Physician Assistants.</u> 26-31.

Ruley, E.J. (1997). Hematuria. In R.A. Hoekelman (Ed.). <u>Primary pediatric care</u>. St. Louis: Mosby.

Rushton, H.G. (1997). Urinary tract infections in children. <u>Pediatric Clinics of North America, 44,</u> 1133-1169.

Seidel, H.M., & Gearhart, J.P. (1997). Hypospadias, epispadias, and cryptorchis. In R.A. Hoekelman (Ed.). <u>Primary pediatric care</u>. St. Louis: Mosby.

Skoog, S.J. (1997). Benign and malignant pediatric scrotal masses. <u>Pediatric Clinics of North America, 44,</u> 12291250.

Skoog, S.J., Roberts, K.P., Goldstein, M. & Pryor, J.L. (1997). The adolescent varicocele: What's new with an old problem in young patients? <u>Pediatrics, 100,</u> 112-121.

Stamm, W.E. & Hooton (1993). Management of urinary tract infections in adults. <u>The New England Journal of Medicine, 329</u>(18), 1328-1334.

US Department of Health and Human Services, Centers for Disease Control. (1998). 1998 guidelines for treatment of sexually transmitted diseases treatment guidelines. <u>Morbidity and Mortality Weekly Report, 47</u>(RR-1).

Wisinger, D.B. (1996). Urinary tract infection: Current management strategies. <u>Postgraduate Medicine, 100,</u> 229-239.

Gynecology

I.   Definition: All classifications of cervicovaginal cytology other than "within normal limits" using the revised Bethesda system

II.   Pathogenesis: An atypical Papanicolaou smear may be due to the following causes

   A.   Infection (fungal, bacterial, protozoal, or viral)

   B.   Reactive and reparative changes (inflammation and miscellaneous factors related to patient history, such as chemotherapy, radiation, use of IUD, and DES exposure)

   C.   Neoplastic (lower genital tract, upper genital tract, extragenital)

III. Clinical Presentation

   A.   Although all sexually active females are at risk for cervical cancer, the disease is more common among females of low socioeconomic status, those with a history of multiple sex partners or early age at first intercourse, and smokers

   B.   Authorities agree that the cause of cervical dysplasia is a DNA mutation in an immature metaplastic cell
      1.   Dysplasia is caused by human papilloma virus (HPV) infection together with other carcinogenic cofactors
      2.   HPV types 16, 18, 31, 33, and 35 have a strong epidemiologic association with cervical dysplasia
      3.   HPV is found in 95% of cervical cancers

   C.   May be asymptomatic, or may have symptoms of fungal, bacterial, protozoan, or viral infection, if the atypia is due to an infectious cause

IV.   Diagnosis/Evaluation

   A.   The cytopathology report is considered a medical consultation

   B.   Every cytopathology report based on Bethesda system has statement on specimen adequacy in the first section of the report. The possible specimen categories are the following
      1.   <u>Satisfactory for evaluation</u>: Provides assurance that sample and preparation were adequate in that the smear had both endocervical and metaplastic ectocervical cells easily visible with ≤ 50% of cells obscured by inflammation, blood or debris (**Note**: The smear can be satisfactory but deficient in other ways, i.e, abnormal cells are present)
      2.   <u>Satisfactory for evaluation but limited by (reason)</u>: Smear may be limited by one or more of four factors which are listed here
         a.   **Lack of metaplastic or endocervical cells**--occurs when transformation zone is not sampled (most common reasons are excessive mucus, a nulliparous, pregnant, or atrophic cervix, or a cervix after an ablative/excisional procedure)
         b.   **Inflammation, blood, or debris** partially obscure >50% but less than 75% of cells on smear (inflammation can be caused by use of douching, tampons, cervical caps, or having sexual intercourse within 48 hours of exam; can also be caused by infection or cellular changes of the cervix that occur with cancer)
         c.   **Air drying** which causes an increased nuclear-cytoplasmic ratio mimicking cell dysplasia
         d.   **Lack of patient information** (name, LMP, history of ablative or excisional therapy)

3. <u>Unsatisfactory for evaluation:</u> Usually means the smear was improperly prepared or that inflammation was so extensive the examination was meaningless (≥75% of cells obscured)
4. **Note**: Two new Pap smear techniques--ThinPrep and MonoLayer--have been shown to increase the detection of abnormal cells by 65%
   a. A cervical broom or brush is used to obtain a cervical specimen that is placed in preservative-filled vial
   b. Specimen is filtered in lab to remove mucus, blood, and inflammatory cells making slides easier to read
   c. Techniques have a lower false negative rate but are more expensive than conventional Pap testing

C. The second section of the Bethesda system report contains three possible categories
   1. Within normal limits
   2. Benign cellular changes; see descriptive diagnoses
   3. Epithelial cell abnormalities; see descriptive diagnoses

D. The descriptive diagnoses section makes up the third part of the report
   1. Benign cellular changes reflect either reactive, reparative changes, or an underlying infection
      a. Reactive changes refer to reparative alterations from inflammation due to such conditions as atrophic vaginitis, mechanical or chemical irritation, or use of an IUD
      b. Infectious causes include common genital infections with pathogens such as *Trichomonas vaginalis*, herpes simplex, *Chlamydia trachomatis, Neisseria gonorrhoeae,* and *Candida* species, among others
   2. Epithelial cell abnormalities are either of squamous or glandular origin
      a. Squamous cell abnormalities are addressed first and these are classified into four categories from the **least to the most serious**

SQUAMOUS CELL ABNORMALITIES

Atypical squamous cells of undetermined significance (ASCUS)
- ❖ A description of cells that have nuclear atypia that are not normal yet are not consistent with low grade squamous intraepithelial lesion (LSIL)
- ❖ Diagnosis of ASCUS should be qualified by indicating whether it favors a reactive or neoplastic process

Low-grade squamous intraepithelial lesion (LSIL)
- ❖ Cellular changes of HPV previously termed koilocytosis, koilocytotic atypia, or condylomatous atypia are included in this category

High-grade squamous intraepithelial lesion (HSIL)
- ❖ Encompasses moderate and severe dysplasia as well as carcinoma in situ

Squamous cell carcinoma

---

b. Glandular cell abnormalities are considered in the next category and are classified from the **least to the most serious**

GLANDULAR CELL ABNORMALITIES

Benign endometrial cells
- ❖ An abnormal finding in post-menopausal females, but insignificant in premenopausal females with normal ovulatory cycling

Atypical glandular cells of undetermined significance (AGUS)
- ❖ Includes a spectrum of findings ranging from minimally abnormal cells to adenocarcinoma in situ
- ❖ The diagnosis should include the origin of the atypical glandular cells, whether endometrial or endocervical

Adenocarcinoma in situ (AIS) and Adenocarcinoma

---

c. Other, less common malignant neoplasms of the genital tract are then considered
3. Finally, a hormonal evaluation (applies to vaginal smears only) is provided in the last part of the descriptive diagnoses section
   a. Hormonal pattern compatible with age and history
   b. Hormonal pattern incompatible with age and history (specify)
   c. Hormonal evaluation not possible due to (specify)

V.   Plan/Management

    A.   Pap smear report of "Satisfactory for evaluation" and "Within normal limits": Counsel female regarding findings and repeat the Pap smear in 1-3 years, depending on patient risk factors and history

    B.   Pap smear report of "Specimen unsatisfactory for evaluation." Obtain a second specimen in 6-8 weeks, preferably when female is at midcycle and has not had intercourse or used vaginal products for at least 24 hours; if poor specimen quality is due to atrophy in postmenopausal female, consider prescribing a topical estrogen cream for 4-6 weeks, then repeat the test no earlier than one week after completing the medication

    C.   Pap smear report of "Satisfactory but no endocervical cells." Repeat the test if the female has any risk factors, if she has had no prior screening, or has a history of abnormal test in past

    D.   Pap smear report of benign cellular changes: Consult descriptive diagnoses section to determine possible cause
        1.   If report of *Trichomonas vaginalis* or other specific infection
            a.   Review chart to determine if patient was treated at time Pap smear was obtained
            b.   If no treatment at that time, contact patient to return for evaluation by pelvic exam and appropriate diagnostic tests before treatment
        2.   If report of reactive changes with inflammation
            a.   Evaluate the patient for possible infection including gonorrhea and chlamydia
            b.   Repeat the Pap test in 3-6 months
            c.   Colposcopy is indicated if the inflammation persists and remains unexplained
        3.   If report of reactive changes associated with atrophy--prescribe a topical estrogen cream if the female has symptomatic atrophic vaginitis (not necessary for the asymptomatic female)
        4.   If report of reactive changes associated with an intrauterine device or radiation therapy-- continue with the routine screening schedule

    E.   Pap smear report of atypical squamous cells of undetermined significance (ASCUS) should be managed as follows

---

INTERPRETATION OF ASCUS

If ASCUS is not qualified or if a reactive process is favored
- A repeat Pap test should be conducted every 4-6 months for 2 years; the pattern should be continued until 3 consecutive smears are negative
- A routine testing schedule should be returned to at that point
- If ASCUS is reported a second time, the patient should be referred for colposcopy

When ASCUS is associated with severe inflammation
- Infection must be ruled out, but treatment is not indicated without a specific diagnosis
- Pap testing should be repeated in 2-3 months
- Colposcopy is indicated if the repeat test is abnormal

When ASCUS is associated with vaginal atrophy (postmenopausal females not using HRT)
- Consider prescribing a topical estrogen cream, unless contraindicated
- Repeat the Pap smear in 2-3 months
- Some experts recommend that patients use the topical estrogen cream even if they are taking the hormone orally
- A colposcopy is indicated if the diagnosis remains equivocal

When ASCUS is qualified as favoring a neoplastic process
- For low-risk compliant patient, repeat Pap smears every 4-6 months for 2 years until three consecutive smears are negative; return to regular Pap smear testing routine at that point; if the repeated smears show abnormalities, colposcopy is indicated
- For high-risk poorly compliant patient, a colposcopy should be done without further Pap testing

---

    F.   Pap smear report of low-grade squamous intraepithelial lesion (LSIL); Manage as above under WHEN ASCUS IS QUALIFIED AS FAVORING A NEOPLASTIC PROCESS

    G.   Pap smear report of high-grade squamous intraepithelial lesion (HSIL); Endocervical curettage, colposcopy, and directed biopsy are required in patients with these high-grade lesions

H. Pap smear report of endometrial cells; endometrial cells found in a cytologically benign smear of a post-menopausal female not on estrogen replacement therapy are an indication for an endometrial biopsy

I. Pap smear report of atypical glandular cells of undetermined significance (AGUS); the diagnosis should include origin--endometrial or endocervical--of the atypical glandular cells
   1. Endometrial origin of the atypical cells requires an evaluation that includes endometrial biopsy, fractional dilation, and curettage, or hysteroscopy
   2. Endocervical origin of the atypical cells is an indication for colposcopy and endocervical curettage (ECC)

J. Pap smear report of squamous cell carcinoma or adenocarcinoma requires a prompt referral to an expert in the management of gynecologic cancers

K. Pap smear report of other malignant neoplasms: Females with abnormalities in this section should be referred immediately for evaluation

L. Hormonal evaluation
   1. Hormonal evaluation should be consistent with clinical picture of the patient
   2. Evidence of an estrogenic effect in a 75 year old not on HRT is an example of abnormal findings in this area

M. Follow Up: Variable depending on cytopathology report (see appropriate sections above)

ABNORMAL VAGINAL BLEEDING

I. Definition: Vaginal bleeding not associated with normal menses. Important terms:

A. Normal menstrual bleeding can be described as follows
   1. Duration of flow is 2-8 days
   2. Cycle length is 21-40 days
   3. Blood loss on average is 35-50 mL

B. Menorrhagia/hypermenorrhea: Menstrual bleeding of greater than 80 mL or greater than 7 days in duration

C. Polymenorrhea: Menstrual interval < 21 days (regular interval)

D. Metrorrhagia: Irregular menstrual bleeding with frequent intervals

E. Menometrorrhagia: Irregular, heavy or prolonged menstrual bleeding

F. Oligomenorrhea: Bleeding that occurs in intervals greater than 5 weeks (35 days)

II. Pathogenesis

A. Among adolescents, 90% of all cases of abnormal uterine bleeding is caused by dysfunctional uterine bleeding (DUB)
   1. The vast majority of cases of DUB in adolescents are due to anovulatory cycles resulting from an immature hypothalamic-pituitary-ovarian axis
   2. DUB results from persistent stimulation of the endometrium by estrogen which is unopposed by the periodic influence of progesterone
   3. The mechanism of DUB is as follows

MECHANISM OF OCCURRENCE OF DUB IN ANOVULATORY CYCLES

* At menarche, rising levels of follicle-stimulating hormone (FSH) cause follicular maturation in the ovaries and elevations in estrogen levels

* Rising estrogen levels stimulate the formation of a proliferative endometrium in the uterus and the growth of endometrial glands

* During ovulatory cycles, progesterone interrupts endometrial growth and stabilizes the endometrium

* With anovulatory cycles, however, progesterone is not produced and a secretory endometrium does not develop

* Unopposed estrogen during anovulatory cycles can produce the following

   * Estrogen breakthrough bleeding: Bleeding occurs (1) when estrogen levels fall or are too low to support the thickened endometrium, and (2) because unopposed estrogen does not supply the necessary structural support for the developing endometrium (stroma, glands, and blood vessels) thereby contributing to spontaneous superficial hemorrhages which occur randomly

   * Heavy, prolonged menses: Low levels of progesterone interfere with local uterine prostaglandin production; the resultant deficit in prostaglandins leads to weak myometrial and vascular contractions that are ineffective in halting blood loss

    B.   Pregnancy related cause of abnormal uterine bleeding
        1.   Ectopic pregnancy
        2.   Gestational trophoblastic neoplasm (Hydatid mole)
        3.   Threatened, incomplete, or missed abortion
        4.   Placenta previa or low lying placenta

    C.   Trauma resulting from sexual abuse, tampon use, IUD use, or foreign body can produce bleeding

    D.   Medications such as oral contraceptives, steroids, anticoagulants, neuroleptics, major tranquilizers can also cause bleeding

    E.   Organic gynecologic pathology such as benign polyps, myomas, endometrial hyperplasia, and malignancy (cervical, endocervical, ovarian, tubal) are also occasional causes of bleeding

    F.   Systemic diseases such as coagulation disorders, thyroid disorders, adrenal disorders, liver disease, and renal disease can cause uterine bleeding

III.   Clinical Presentation

    A.   DUB is the most frequent cause of abnormal uterine bleeding in adolescents, accounting for about 90% of cases
        1.   Well over half of cycles are anovulatory from menarche to 2 years after menarche
        2.   About 30% are anovulatory from 2-4 years after menarche
        3.   Up to one fifth are anovulatory for 4-5 years after menarche
        4.   Most anovulatory menstrual cycles are not associated with bleeding or cycle length that is substantially different from ovulatory cycles

    B.   Pattern of bleeding and associated signs and symptoms provide additional clues to possible causes
        1.   DUB results in irregularity of menstrual interval, episodes of amenorrhea, and periods of heavy, prolonged bleeding; **bleeding is painless**
        2.   Adolescents with coagulation disorders may have signs of petechia, ecchymoses, or epistaxis
        3.   Ectopic pregnancy has variable spotting due to hemorrhage, usually with cramping and possibly signs and symptoms of pregnancy
        4.   Infection is usually associated with vaginal discharge, lower abdominal pain, and pain on intercourse

5. Leiomyomas are a common cause of bleeding and result in uterine enlargement; abdominal exam may be positive for a large mass if the leiomyoma has grown larger than a 12 week pregnant uterus

6. In cervical carcinoma, bleeding is frequently postcoital, intermenstrual, and described as slight spotting

7. Endometrial carcinoma begins with intermenstrual discharge which is watery with small amounts of blood and then progresses to heavier bleeding

IV. Diagnosis/Evaluation

A. History
1. **Data relating to LMP**: Inquire about timing and duration of last normal menses and ask female if she has kept a menstrual calendar
2. **Timing and amount of abnormal bleeding**: Ask when bleeding begins, whether it is spotting or heavy, how long bleeding lasts, whether it is daily spotting, and how heavy the heavy days (**Note**: Daily spotting is suggestive of a polyp or infectious cause; heavy flow tapering to spotting, with no bleeding for several days, then returning to heavy flow again is characteristic of anovulatory bleeding)
3. **Associated signs and symptoms**: Ask about presence of abdominal pain, vaginal discharge, pain on intercourse, pain with urination, defecation, or pelvic heaviness (**Note**: Pelvic pain/heaviness may indicate a persistent corpus luteum cyst, endometriosis, or myomas)
4. **Contraceptive use and sexual practices/history**: Obtain this essential information
5. **Drugs and medications**: Ask about medications, including oral contraceptives
6. **Past medical history**: Inquire about past/present problems including endocrine, hematological, and gynecological problems (**Note**: Ask: "Are you seeing or have you recently seen a health care provider for any other problem?")
7. **Gynecologic/obstetric history**: Obtain complete history in these areas
8. **Behavior/lifestyle**: Ask about recent changes in weight, life, activity, exercise patterns

B. Physical Examination
1. Determine whether blood loss is significant by obtaining orthostatic B/P and pulse readings
2. Inspect skin for bruising, petechia, or purpura
3. Always do pelvic and speculum examinations
   a. Insure that bleeding is uterine and not from urethra or rectum
   b. Assess for foreign body in vault, examine cervical os for erosion, polyps, and mucopurulent discharge
   c. Evaluate the uterus for tenderness, size, and shape
   d. Carefully assess the adnexa
4. Assess for signs of hypothyroidism such as skin thickening and abnormal deep tendon reflexes
5. Assess thyroid and check for abdominal masses

C. Differential Diagnosis: Rule out all conditions noted under Pathogenesis

D. Diagnostic Tests
1. Order urine or serum pregnancy test (**Note**: May be the most important test!)
2. CBC, and platelet count
3. If anovulation is suspected, a prolactin, thyroid panel, TSH
4. Obtain Pap smear
5. Test for *N. gonorrhoae* and *C. trachomatis*
6. Coagulation studies are useful in adolescents and in females with bruising or history of bleeding diathesis
7. Another diagnostic test for abnormal bleeding is endovaginal ultrasound which can be used to rule out ectopic pregnancy, to assess myomas and abnormal uterine size, and to measure endometrial thickness

V.   Plan/Management

A.   Refer patient to an expert if bleeding is severe (HCT <25) or if patient is unstable (orthostatic hypotension); also refer patients with suspected malignancy or serious systemic disease

B.   Treat all known causes of vaginal bleeding such as the following
1.   Removal of foreign body from the vagina (most often impacted tampon)
    a.   Under good visualization, and with the patient in the lithotomy position, grasp the tampon with a pair of sponge holding forceps
    b.   Place a basin of water as close to the introitus as possible (to minimize malodor)
    c.   Quickly immerse the tampon under water without releasing the forceps
    d.   Flush the tampon and water down toilet
    e.   **Note**: The unpleasant odor that envelopes the room is the most problematic; immersing the removed tampon into water the instant it is removed from the vagina reduces the malodor and the embarrassment to the patient
2.   Prescribe antibiotics for infections that are diagnosed
3.   For breakthrough bleeding from oral contraceptives
    a.   Counsel that breakthrough bleeding decreases dramatically after first 3 months of pills
    b.   Instruct to take pills at same time each day
    c.   Last, change oral contraceptive to one with a higher progestational activity (usually effective regardless of when bleeding occurs in the cycle) such as Desogen, Ortho-Cept, or Demulen 1/35

C.   If bleeding is light, patient has normal hemoglobin level (>12 g/dL) and DUB is suspected
1.   Ask patient to maintain menstrual calendar
2.   Reevaluate in 3-6 months
3.   Prescribe mefenamic acid (Ponstel) 500 mg orally TID for 3 days starting with menses to correct relative prostaglandin overproduction

D.   If bleeding is moderate, hemoglobin is 10-12 g/dL, and DUB is suspected based on an absence of systemic disease or uterine disorder, a number of options are available and are outlined in the following table

TREATMENT FOR MODERATE DUB	
Goal of Treatment: Convert proliferative endometrium into secretory endometrium, thereby resulting in predictable uterine withdrawal bleeding	
Many different treatment regimens have been suggested; only 3 are considered here, but consult the literature for other options	
Select One of the Following Therapies	
Drug	**Dosage**
Medroxyprogesterone acetate (Provera)	5-10 mg QD for 12-14 days in the second half of the month
Any combination oral contraceptive with one not being preferred over another	One pill taken daily as directed and continued so long as the patient tolerates well and desires to continue (This regimen is recommended by Beckmann et al., 1998, pp. 379-380)
An oral contraceptive containing 50 mcg of estrogen such as Ovral	One pill QID x 5-7 days, then one pill QD for 21 days, followed by 7 pill-free days; repeat this regimen for several months (This particular regimen is recommended by Hatcher et al., 1998, pp. 435-436)

E.   If bleeding persists in females treated with hormonal therapies, endometrial sampling is indicated

F.   After successful hormonal therapy, a long-term plan should be established
1.   For females with first episode of bleeding, a 3 month treatment with an oral contraceptive unless contraindicated is usually sufficient (**Note:** DUB may return after therapy is discontinued)
2.   Patients with a second or third episode (and no etiology has been found) may need to be treated with the **addition** of NSAIDs to correct relative prostaglandin overproduction
a.   Mefenamic acid (Ponstel) 500 mg initially, then 250 mg TID for 3 days starting with menses OR
b.   Naproxen (Naprosyn) 500 mg BID for 3 days starting with menses

3.   Follow-up with patients on a regular schedule depending on the clinical situation

AMENORRHEA

I.   Definition: Absence of menses at any age when menstrual function should be present

II.   Pathogenesis

A.   The hypothalamic-pituitary-ovarian-uterine axis needs to function in a coordinated manner for menstruation to occur

B.   If any part of the system functions incorrectly, withdrawal menses do not occur and amenorrhea is the symptom

III.   Clinical Presentation

A.   Diagnostic Criteria: Primary Amenorrhea
1.   No bleeding by age 14 in the absence of growth and development of secondary sexual characteristics
2.   Failure to have menses by age 16, regardless of presence of normal growth and development with the appearance of secondary sexual characteristics

B.   Diagnostic Criteria: Secondary Amenorrhea
1.   Female must have had at least one spontaneous menstrual period
2.   Six months of amenorrhea (this is controversial, some say 3, others 12)

C.   Common causes of primary amenorrhea along with usual presenting signs are the following
1.   Gonadal dysgenesis -- there is a lack of mature (stages 4 or 5) breast/pubic hair development, but small amounts of development (stages 2 or 3) may be present secondary to only adrenal hormone secretion
2.   Müllerion (uterovaginal) anomalies -- normal breast/pubic hair development occurs
3.   Hypothalamic/pituitary disorders -- normal breast/pubic hair development does not occur
4.   Constitutional delay secondary to an immature hypothalamic-pituitary axis -- short stature (under 5 feet at age 14) is found

D.   Common causes of secondary amenorrhea
1.   Pregnancy
2.   Prolactin-secreting pituitary adenomas
3.   Hypothalamic amenorrhea secondary to excessive stress, weight loss, and/or exercise (As many as half of all competitive female athletes may experience some menstrual abnormality, with luteal phase deficiency, anovulation, and amenorrhea the three most common)
4.   Polycystic ovarian disease (PCOD)
5.   Androgen excess, endocrine disorders such as thyroid disease and diabetes mellitus

E.	There are numerous uncommon causes of amenorrhea including onset of systemic debilitating diseases such as Crohn's disease and lupus erythematosus

IV.	Diagnosis/Evaluation

A.	History: Primary Amenorrhea
1.	Question about growth and development; occurrence of growth spurt (Ask: "Was there a period of 6 months - 1 year when you grew out of all your clothes, shoes?")
2.	Ask questions about puberty (breast and pubic hair -- when development began and how far it has advanced)

B.	Physical Examination: Primary Amenorrhea
1.	Height, weight
2.	Observe for common anomalies associated with gonadal dysgenesis
a.	Neck folds, setting of ears
b.	Chest configuration, whether 4th metacarpal is short, cubitus, valgus
3.	Assess breast and pubic hair development using Tanner stages
4.	Speculum exam for imperforate hymen, presence of vagina and uterus, and bimanual exam for adnexal masses
a.	Estrogen exposed vaginal mucosa is thick, with rugae
b.	Presence of cervix at end of canal is sufficient evidence that uterus is present
c.	Clear cervical mucus in os is good indication that estrogen is present
d.	Bimanual exam to confirm presence, size of uterus, and any masses

C.	Differential Diagnosis: Primary amenorrhea is a symptom. There are numerous etiologies for this symptom

D.	Diagnostic Tests: Primary Amenorrhea
1.	Refer patient to specialist for management
2.	Initial tests are usually HCG, TSH, prolactin, and progesterone challenge tests

E.	History: Secondary Amenorrhea
1.	Question patient regarding the following
a.	Age at menarche, cycle regularity, duration of menstrual flow (was it fairly constant month to month?) (**Note**: The presence of cycle regularity leads to a strong presumption of ovulation)
b.	Presence of symptoms suggesting ovulation -- mittelschmerz, bloating, breast tenderness
c.	When and how deviation from prior menstrual cyclicity occurred
d.	Number and outcomes of pregnancies, postpartal course
e.	Type of contraception and possibility of pregnancy
2.	Obtain past medical history, medications currently taking
3.	Question regarding growth of excess hair on face, chest, abdomen, upper back; ask about presence of acne
4.	Ask about galactorrhea (breast milk). Persistent galactorrhea, even slight and unilateral, is significant
5.	Question regarding weight changes, skin texture, energy level, bowel habits, and temperature tolerance
6.	Take social history including exercise, eating habits and patterns, and stress at home, school, and work
7.	If female is competitive athlete, obtain information about intensity and duration of training (**Note**: A triad of disordered eating, amenorrhea, and osteoporosis occurs in the elite athlete)

F.	Physical Examination: Secondary Amenorrhea
1.	Vital signs, height and weight, and calculate BMI (see OBESITY section for how to calculate and interpret BMI)
2.	Examine skin for signs of androgen excess--acne and hirsutism
3.	Examine thyroid for size, presence of nodularity
4.	Assess breast development for Tanner staging and presence of galactorrhea

5. Pelvic and speculum exam for pubic hair distribution (Tanner staging), degree of vaginal rugation, type of cervical mucus (amount, stretchability, ferning pattern when dried on glass slide)

6. Bimanual exam for masses; for example, a unilateral ovarian enlargement can mean a steroid-producing tumor. Assess deep tendon reflexes as index of thyroid status

G. Differential Diagnosis: Secondary amenorrhea is a symptom. There are numerous etiologies for this symptom

H. Diagnostic Tests: Secondary Amenorrhea
1. Focused diagnostic tests are useful to isolate the underlying cause to the hypothalamic/pituitary, ovarian, or uterine/vaginal compartments, or to other organ systems
2. HCG to rule out pregnancy, TSH, LH, FSH, prolactin, and progesterone challenge test are usually the initial tests

V. Plan/Management

A. Primary Amenorrhea: Refer all patients with primary amenorrhea to specialist for further evaluation and management

B. Secondary Amenorrhea: Consult with specialist regarding management based on history, physical exam, and diagnostic test results

BARTHOLIN GLAND CYSTS AND ABSCESSES

I. Definition: An occlusion and/or infection of the Bartholin gland or its ducts

II. Pathogenesis:

A. Bartholin's glands are bilateral vulvovaginal structures located at about the 4 and 8 o'clock positions on the posteriolateral aspect of the vestibule (area enclosed by the labia at the mouth of the vagina) (see Figure 14.1)

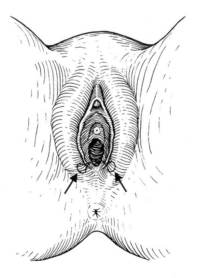

Figure 14.1. Bartholin's Glands.

465

B.   These vestibular glands are normally about the size of a pea and are made up of mucin-producing and excreting acini that drain into a transitional and squamous epithelium-lined ducts about 2.5 cm long; the ducts exit into a fold between the hymen and labium

C.   Obstruction of a Bartholin's duct occurs most commonly near the orifice
1.   The exact etiology is usually unknown although infection with inflammation probably plays a major role
2.   The duct becomes closed, while the mucus-secreting gland continues to produce fluid

D.   An enlargement in the absence of inflammation is a cyst

E.   With acute inflammation, an abscess develops
1.   Bartholin's duct abscesses may be caused from gonoccoccal or chlamydial infections
2.   However, other organisms such as *Staphylococcus aureus*, *Streptococcus fecalis*, and *Escherichia coli* also commonly cause the infection

III.   Clinical Presentation

A.   Dilatation of the Bartholin gland's duct due to obstruction is probably the most common finding in females complaining of vulvar masses and tends to be recurrent in some females

B.   A normal Bartholin's gland and duct are nonpalpable, and any cystic swelling in the labia minora on the posteriolateral aspect of the vestibule usually represents a cyst or abscess

C.   Cysts are generally 1 to 3 cm in size and are usually asymptomatic
1.   The patient may notice a bulge in the labia or mass may be found during routine clinical exam
2.   Cysts tend to grow slowly and noninfected cysts are nomally sterile (see Figure 14.2)

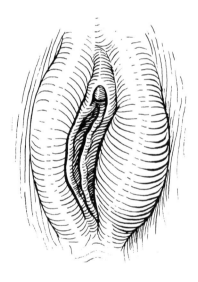

Figure 14.2. Bartholin's Gland Cyst.

D.   With acute inflammation, an abscess develops with symptoms of swelling, tenderness, and erythema; patient may be unable to engage in sex or sports due to pain

IV.   Diagnosis/Evaluation

A.   History
1.   Ask about onset, duration of cyst/abscess
2.   Ask about presence of associated symptoms such as pain, swelling, erythema and ask if presence of cyst/abscess has limited normal activities

3. Determine if there are any symptoms present that might indicate presence of a sexually transmitted disease--discharge, irregular bleeding, dyspareunia
4. Ask about trauma to the site
5. Ask about history of recurrent cysts/abscesses

B. Physical Examintion
1. Inspect external genitalia for presence of lesions and masses, other abnormalities
2. Carefully palpate the vaginal introitus with the thumb and forefinger for presence of swelling/masses, presence of fluctuance, areas of tenderness
3. Palpate inguinal nodes for enlargement

C. Differential Diagnosis
1. Sebaceous cyst
2. Vaginnal inclusion cyst
3. Fibromas
4. Lipomas
5. Hematoma

D. Diagnostic Tests: None indicated unless abscess is recurrent; then culture and sensitivity testing of discharge from the abscess should be performed

V. Plan/Treatment

A. Asymptomatic Bartholin's gland cysts in patients under age 40 may not require treatment
1. Many small ductal cysts do not interfere with intercourse, or cause discomfort with walking, sitting, or other activities, and usually wax and wane in size. Treatment consists of daily sitz baths or warm compresses applied to area and spontaneous resolution of the cyst usually occurs
2. Others eventually become symptomatic and require treatment
3. Referral to a specialist for drainage of the cyst and placement of a Word catheter in the cyst cavity is recommended
4. Word catheter is left in place for up to 4 weeks to allow drainage and formation of an epithelized outflow tract

B. Asymptomatic Bartholin's gland cysts in patients over 40 are usually excised because of concern about Bartholin's gland carcinoma (rare)

C. Most ductal abscesses will eventually "point" and spontaneously rupture resulting in immediate relief; the process will be hastened with frequent sitz baths
1. Because of the polymicrobial nature of most abscesses, broad-spectrum antibiotic coverage is recommended (erythromycin, 250 mg QID x 10 days)
2. Advise patient to continue with frequent sitz baths to provide relief and facilitate healing
3. Abscess may recur and definitive treatment with placement of a Word catheter may be necessary

D. Early abscesses (that have not ruptured) should be treated with sitz baths until the abscess points which makes incision and definitive treatment easier; broad spectrum antibiotics should also be prescribed
1. Refer the patient for incision, drainage, and placement of a Word catheter for up to 4 weeks to facilitate drainage and formation of an epithelized outflow tract
2. This procedure usually results in complete resolution of the condition

E. Follow Up: None indicated unless cyst/abscess fails to resolve

BREAST MASS

I. Definition: Benign and malignant lesions of the breast

II. Pathogenesis

    A. Common benign lesions
        1. Fibrocystic changes of the breast (FCB)
            a. Abnormal restructuring in the layering of the parenchyma most likely related to estrogen/progestin imbalance resulting in excessive ductal stimulation and proliferation
            b. Result of restructuring is atrophic epithelial segments and fibrous replacement
        2. Fibroadenoma
            a. Originates from the terminal duct -- lobular unit, and believed to be hormonally induced
            b. Composed of fibrous and epithelial elements
        3. Intraductal papilloma
            a. Arises from dilated ductules in unfolding lobules
            b. Found in both small and large ducts

    B. Breast cancer
        1. Arises from transformed epithelium that originates within ducts or lobules
        2. For a period of time, these transformed cells are non-invasive; if undisturbed, eventually there is local, lymphatic and hematogenous spread

III. Clinical Presentation

    A. The existence of a "dominant" area (lump, nodule, mass, or thickening) that is different from surrounding tissue or asymmetric compared to the opposite breast constitutes an abnormal finding
        1. The basic question is whether a dominant area exists; issues of smoothness, hardness, distinctness from surrounding tissue are secondary
        2. Causes of a specific dominant area must be determined by means other than physical examination

    B. Benign lesions
        1. Fibrocystic changes of the breast (FBC)
            a. Most common of all benign breast conditions
            b. Occurs in about 50% of females with highest incidence among females aged 20-50 who are in reproductive, premenopausal years; symptoms cease with menopause (unless hormone replacement is begun)
            c. Risk factors include nulliparity, late age of natural menopause, middle class, and Caucasian race
            d. Condition is characterized by cyclic bilateral breast pain (mastalgia), which usually worsens premenstrually and resolves after onset of menses
            e. Multiple small cysts are usually palpable, particularly prior to menses as the internal fibroglandular tissue changes in consistency based on hormonal effects
        2. Fibroadenoma
            a. The second-most common form of benign breast disease occurring in about 10% of females, most often in 20-30 year age group, and decreasing in incidence with advancing age
            b. May be stimulated by pregnancy and regress with menopause
            c. Usually presents as single, smooth, round, mobile lumps which are usually painless (**Note**: Can feel firm or "rubbery")
            d. In about 15%-20% of patients, multiple, often bilateral fibroadenomas are involved

3. Intraductal papilloma
   a. Tend to occur perimenopausally (median age of occurrence is 40)
   b. Usually presents as a spontaneous bloody or serous nipple discharge from a single duct
   c. Can cause a breast mass and nipple retraction, but often there is no associated palpable mass

C. Breast cancer
   1. Lifetime risk is 1 in 8 for US females (estimated lifetime risk of dying from breast cancer is 3.6%)
   2. Rare in females under 25; 48% of new breast cancer cases and 56% of breast cancer deaths occur in females age 65 and over
   3. Approximately 32% of all newly diagnosed cancers in females are cancers of the breast
   4. Risk factors include the following:
      a. Female gender, residence in North America or northern Europe and older age
      b. Family history of breast cancer in first degree relative, especially if bilateral and/or premenopausal in onset
      c. Menarche occurrence before age 11 or after age 14
      d. Onset of menopause after age 55 or more than 35 years duration of menses
   5. Usually presents as a painless, firm, fixed mass that does not change with menstruation; most common in upper, outer-quadrant though may occur in other areas
   6. Spontaneous nipple discharge that is most often clear may be associated with malignancy

D. Age is an important factor with most females <25 with masses having benign conditions and 75% of females >70 with palpable masses having cancer

IV. Diagnosis/Evaluation

A. History
   1. Question regarding presence/location of mass, characteristics of mass -- tenderness, mobility, size, single or multiple. Ask if any lymph nodes have seemed enlarged
   2. If presenting complaint is mastalgia, ask regarding frequency, severity, duration, location (localized, diffuse, or bilateral). Ask if the pain is cyclic occurring during the premenstrual phase or noncyclic. Determine if the pain is due to **trauma**
   3. Inquire about changes of breast mass with menstruation (if not postmenopausal), presence of nipple discharge (spontaneous rather than elicited), type of discharge (bloody, serous, clear, milky), and laterality (one or both nipples)
   4. Obtain detailed menstrual history including age at menarche, dates of last period, and age at menopause (if appropriate). Determine in which phase of menstrual cycle the patient is in at presentation (**Note**: Clinical breast exam is best performed a week or so after onset of menses when tissue is least congested)
   5. Question about medication history, including current and past use of oral contraceptives and hormone replacement therapy
   6. Obtain history of risk factors for breast cancer (see above), as well as information relating to previous breast masses, biopsies, and breast surgery
   7. Determine and document in chart time since last clinical breast exam, when last mammogram was done and the results, and breast self-examination practices

B. Physical Examination
   1. With patient sitting on table
      a. Inspect for symmetry, contour, and vascular pattern variation
      b. Inspect skin, noting discoloration, retraction, dimpling, edema
   2. Have patient raise arms above head and place hands on hip
   3. Palpate the axillary, supraclavicular, and infraclavicular nodes for adenopathy
   4. With patient supine and arm extended and slightly bent on side being examined
      a. Inspect breast and skin as in the upright position
      b. Palpate the breast tissue, supraclavicular region, and chest wall following a vertical strip pattern
      c. Gently palpate the entire nipple-areolar complex; do not squeeze the nipple unless the patient has complained of nipple discharge

5. Teach BSE during exam
6. If a dominant area (i.e., lump, mass, nodule, or thickening different from surrounding tissue or asymmetric compared to the opposite breast) is found, the area should be assessed and then described
    a. Use tip of forefinger as a ruler
    b. Do simultaneous mirror image palpation bilaterally
    c. Description of dominant area should be noted on a drawing in the chart and labeled appropriately

C. Differential Diagnosis: Benign versus malignant tumor

D. Diagnostic Tests: When a dominant mass is encountered, patients under age 30 may be rescheduled after their next menstrual period for re-evaluation of the mass, to assess whether it has gotten smaller or gone away, before proceeding with diagnostic tests
    1. Mammogram is the initial test ordered to evaluate a breast mass
    2. Alternative: Fine needle aspiration (FNA) biopsy may be performed in office procedure when mass is easily palpable and cyst-like
    3. Alternative: Ultrasound may also be used to differentiate a fluid-filled cyst from a solid tumor, but aspiration has the advantage of also treating the cyst; ultrasound may be more useful than mammogram in young females with dense breast tissue
    4. Open biopsy is the definitive step in determining if a breast mass is malignant

V. Plan/Management

A. If mammographic abnormalities are found, refer patient for open biopsy

B. If fibrocystic breast changes are diagnosed via FNA, the aspiration itself may be therapeutic for benign cysts and may relieve localized pain. Patient may be managed as follows to control symptoms
    1. Counsel patient that no cure exists for FBC but symptomatic therapy will control symptoms in most cases
    2. Wear support bra to stabilize the breasts
    3. Dietary modifications are controversial but reduction in caffeine intake and salt intake may help some patients
    4. If there are no contraindications, prescribe oral contraceptives that are low dose estrogen (20 mcg) and relatively high dose progesterone (1 mg) [product example is Loestrin 1/20]; patient usually has reduction in pain after a few months of therapy
    5. Low-dose danazol (Danocrine), a synthetic androgen, is the first-line treatment for severe mastalgia (works by blocking midcycle surges of LH and FSH; also reduces estrogen effects)
        a. Dosing: 50-200 mg BID x 4-6 months (**Note**: Begin therapy during menses or perform appropriate tests to ensure patient is not pregnant)
        b. Available as 50, 100, 200 mg caps
        c. Several months of use may be needed before drug becomes effective
        d. **Note**: Drug can cause alterations in the lipid profile and hepatic dysfunction
    6. Premenstrual use of diuretics, NSAIDs and vitamin E may be helpful in some patients
        a. Hydrochlorothiazide 25-50 mg/day for 7-10 days before menses
        b. Ibuprofen, 400 mg tabs, Q 4-6 hours for 2-3 days at time of maximal engorgement
    7. Vitamin E (150-600 IU/day) taken daily
    8. Patients whose breast pain does not resolve with above measures should be referred to a specialist for management

C. If fibroadenoma is diagnosed via FNA or ultrasound, refer for surgical excision (**Note**: If cytologic assessment of the aspirate from FNA provides a clear diagnosis of fibroadenoma, the mass can be left in place and followed with monthly self-exam, annual clinical breast exam, and annual mammogram)

D. If intraductal papilloma is diagnosed via excisional biopsy, the biopsy itself provides both diagnosis and treatment

E. Follow Up: None indicated unless condition does not improve

CONTRACEPTION

I.   Definition: Prevention of pregnancy by reversible or irreversible methods used by either or both sexual partners

II.   Pathogenesis: Not applicable

III. Clinical Presentation

   A.   Requests for contraceptives and contraceptive counseling are among the most frequent reasons females visit a health care provider

   B.   The proportion of never-married females currently in a sexual relationship has increased for all age categories over the past decade

   C.   Pregnancy rates among teens are greater in the US than in any other developed country with a least 1 in 5 sexually active teens not using contraception

   D.   Half of all pregnancies are unintended with 3.2 million unintended pregnancies in 1994, the last year for which data are available

   E.   Female sterilization, oral contraceptives, male condoms, and male sterilization are the dominant contraceptive methods in the US today

IV.   Diagnosis/Evaluation

   A.   History
      1.   **Obtain a menstrual history** including age at menarche, duration, frequency of, interval between menstrual periods, the last menstrual period (LMP, which is dated from the first day of the last normal menses), any intermenstrual bleeding, pain with menses, and perimenstrual symptoms
      2.   **Obtain an obstetric history**, including number of pregnancies and outcome of each
      3.   **Obtain a gynecologic history** including breast history, previous gynecologic surgery, infectious diseases involving the reproductive tract, any history of infertility, use of douching/feminine hygiene products, and diethylstilbestrol (DES) exposure in utero
      4.   **Obtain a sexual history** eliciting age at first intercourse; present sexual partner(s) and their gender; number of lifetime partners; types of sexual practices; level of satisfaction with sex lives
      5.   **Obtain a contraceptive history** including contraceptive method currently used and reason for its choice; when begun, any problems, and satisfaction with method; inquire about previous methods used and why discontinued
      6.   **Inquire about** past or present **sexual abuse** or assault
      7.   **Obtain a complete medical and surgical history**, including information about cardiovascular disease, thromboembolic disease, liver problems, diabetes mellitus and blood transfusions
      8.   **Inquire about substance use** including tobacco, alcohol, and drug use; ask what medications are currently being taken
      9.   **Question about allergies** and any history of adverse drug reactions
      10. **Determine childhood diseases**, especially rubella, and immunization status
      11. **Obtain family history**, asking about stroke, CVD, cancer, DM in first degree relative

   B.   Physical Examination
      1.   **General Principles**: Have patient empty bladder, get completely undressed, and don the gown provided
      2.   Obtain height, weight, temperature, pulse, respirations, and blood pressure

3. Complete physical exam, including funduscopic exam, palpation of thyroid gland for irregularities, abdominal exam for organomegaly, examination of extremities for evidence of varicose veins, edema, arterial competency (peripheral pulses)
4. Pelvic exam must include the following
   a. Inspection and examination of external genitalia
   b. Speculum examination of the internal structures
   c. Pap smear and specimens as appropriate
   d. Bimanual examination of the pelvic organs
   e. Rectovaginal exam of posterior aspect of pelvic organs (if indicated)
5. Breast exam and instruction in breast self exam (BSE)

C. Differential Diagnosis: Not applicable

D. Diagnostic Tests
   1. Variable depending on history and physical
   2. Screening tests commonly ordered are the following
      a. CBC
      b. VDRL or RPR
      c. Urine dipstick
      d. Pregnancy test
      e. Pap smear
      f. DNA probe for gonorrhea and chlamydia
      g. Wet prep of vaginal secretions to evaluate for vaginitis

V. Plan/Treatment

A. All patients should be counseled regarding the following and the counseling must be documented in the chart
   1. Anatomy and physiology of reproduction
   2. Contraceptive methods, including how they work, effectiveness, advantages, and disadvantages
   3. The need to use condoms to prevent STDs, regardless of contraceptive method selected
   4. Risks and benefits of all methods, as well as informed consent that is signed by patient and placed in chart when IUD, implants, injections, or oral contraceptives are chosen by patient
   5. Techniques of breast self exam (BSE)

B. Assist patient to select one of the methods contained in the following overview of commonly used contraceptive methods, and provide counseling appropriate to the method selected

VI. Brief Overview of Commonly Used Contraceptive Methods

A. **Spermicides** contain nonoxynol-9 (in the US) which disrupts the integrity of the sperm membrane. Spermicides are available as creams, gels, foams, film, tablets, and suppositories and should be placed deep in vagina near cervix prior to intercourse
   1. Effectiveness: About 5-50% of females experience an unintended pregnancy during a year of typical use; there is no significant difference among various forms
   2. Advantages: Inexpensive, easily available, convenient with infrequent intercourse, few side effects or user risk; provides some protection against some STDs
   3. Disadvantages: May cause local irritation

B. **Male condoms** are more commonly used today to prevent transmission of STDs than for pregnancy prevention. They are thin sheaths made from latex or polyurethane. The condom acts as a physical barrier
   1. Effectiveness: There is a 3% probability of pregnancy during a year of perfect use; causes of failure include slippage and breakage during intercourse and improper application
   2. Advantages: Inexpensive, easy to use, easily available, reduce risk of STDs

3.   Disadvantages: May decrease tactile sensation; condoms made of polyurethane are compatible with oil-based lubricants, but those made from latex are not
4.   Application of condoms

> Roll condom to base of erect penis
>
> Pinch tip of condom as it is unrolled and leave ½" of empty space at tip

C.   **Female condoms (Reality)** have been in use since 1992 and are the first barrier contraceptive for females offering some protection against STDs. Composed of a thin polyurethane sheath that is 7.8 cm in diameter and 17 cm in length, the sheath has two polyurethane rings. The inner ring is at the closed end of the sheath that is placed inside the vagina and a larger ring remains outside the vagina providing some protection to the labia and the base of the penis. The inner ring provides stability for the condom which is prelubricated with a dry silicone-based lubricant. The condom can be inserted up to 8 hours prior to intercourse and is intended for one-time use
   1.   Effectiveness: About 5% of females experience an unintended pregnancy during a year of perfect use
   2.   Advantages: Controlled by female and provides some STD protection
   3.   Disadvantages: Anatomy of females may make stable placement difficult

> **Patient Education Relating to Use of Spermicides and Condoms**
> ✔ The correct way to used spermicides and condoms including appropriate lubricants to use with condoms, and how to put on and remove both male and female condoms should be included
> ✔ Follow Up: In 1 year for annual exam

D.   **Diaphragms** are dome-shaped rubber caps with a flexible rim that fits over the cervix and blocks the passage of sperm; spermicides are applied to the inner aspect of the dome which is placed against the cervix
   1.   Effectiveness: Approximately 6% of females experience an unintended pregnancy during a year of perfect use
   2.   **Types**: Three types are commonly used
      a.   Flat spring rim: A thin rim with gentle spring strength, appropriate for use in females with normal vaginal size, contour, a shallow arch behind the symphysis pubis and normal vulvar tone
      b.   Arching spring rim: A sturdy rim with considerable strength, used in females with less than optimal vaginal support (indicated for females who have had a vaginal delivery which usually causes some amount of first degree cystocele) [**Note:** This type is the most commonly used]
      c.   Coil spring rim: A thin but sturdy rim useful in females with normal vaginal size, contour, and with an average or deep arch behind the symphysis pubis
   3.   **Goal** for fitting is to find the largest size that remains comfortable for the patient; most common problem in diaphragm fitting is selecting a size that is too small
      a.   Generally, a nulliparous female will be fitted with sizes 65, 70, or 75
      b.   A multiparous female, with sizes 75, 80, or 85
      c.   A grand multiparous female, with size 85 or larger
   4.   **Procedure** for fitting with diaphragm
      a.   May use fitting rings or sets of various sizes of diaphragms (for the purpose of this explanation, a diaphragm will be used)
      b.   Begin with a size in the middle of the probable range or estimate diaphragm size by using technique described below

> **DIAPHRAGM FITTING**
>
> ★ Insert your index and middle fingers into vagina until middle finger reaches vaginal posterior wall
> ★ With tip of your thumb, mark the place where your index finger touches the pubic bone.
> ★ Remove your fingers
> ★ Diaphragm is sized appropriately if it fits between mark on index finger and tip of middle finger

      c.   After selecting the size believed to be appropriate, introduce the diaphragm into the vagina (first, lubricate the rim of the diaphragm; then compress the sides with fingers and thumbs of one hand, and place in vagina as one would place a speculum--inserting downward and inward)

      d.   Check placement to make certain that the lower rim is in the posterior fornix, the circumference is against the lateral vaginal walls, and the upper rim is secured behind the symphysis pubis

      e.   Determine if the size is right by referring to the table below

---

IS THE DIAPHRAGM TOO SMALL, TOO LARGE, OR JUST RIGHT?

It's Too Small if
- it moves around in the vagina
- can't be stabilized behind the symphysis pubis
- it is loose
- comes out when female coughs/bears down
- there is more than enough space to place your fingertips between rim and symphysis pubis

It's Too Large if
- rim buckles forward against the vaginal walls
- female feels discomfort when the diaphragm is in place
- there is not enough space to place your fingertips between rim and symphysis pubis

It's Just Right if
- it fits snugly in the vagina without buckling forward
- it covers the cervix
- it fits both into posterior fornix and up behind symphysis pubis
- female cannot feel the diaphragm and it does not cause discomfort
- there is just enough space to place your fingertips between rim and symphysis pubis

---

      f.   Teach the female how to insert, place, check, and remove the diaphragm; give female detailed instructions on how to use and care for diaphragm

5.   Advantages: May be inserted up to 6 hours prior to intercourse; reduced risk of STDs and a reduced risk of cervical cancer; works well with infrequent intercourse

6.   Disadvantages: UTIs are more common; some females are sensitive to contraceptive jelly; use has been associated with toxic shock syndrome, so should be avoided during menses and left in place no longer than 24 hours

E.   **Cervical caps** are soft rubber cups with a firm, round rim (Prentif Cavity Rim Cervical Cap) that fit snugly around the base of the cervex. Spermicide is placed inside the cap prior to insertion

1.   Effectiveness: About 9-26% of females experience an unintended pregnancy during a year of perfect use (nulliparous females are less likely than parous females to become pregnant)

2.   Advantages: Provides continuous contraception protection for 48 hours with no need to remove for additional spermicide

3.   Disadvantages: Must be removed after 48 hours because of possible risk of TSS; some females experience odor problems with use for more than a few hours. Device must be fitted by a health care provider and thus requires a visit and replacement every year

---

Patient Education Relating to Use of Diaphragm and Cervical Cap
- ★ Provide patient with insertion and removal instructions and how to care for devices
- ★ Include information on application of spermicidal jelly or cream when using the devices and when to remove
- ★ Follow up: In 1 year for annual exam

F.   **Intrauterine devices (IUDs)** are inserted into the uterus and their mechanisms of action is believed to be via preventing sperm from fertilizing ova

1.   Effectiveness: About 0.6 to 1.5% of females experience unintended pregnancy in first year of use with perfect use

2.   Types: Presently there are two intrauterine contraceptive devices marketed in the US: the Copper T-380A (ParaGard) and the intrauterine progesterone contraceptive system (Progestasert)

a. The ParaGard is a T-shaped polyethylene device whose stem is wrapped with copper wire, and whose cross-arms are partly covered by copper tubing; fertilization is prevented primarily through creation of an intrauterine environment that is spermicidal; it is approved for 10 years of use

b. The Progestasert is a plastic T-shaped device, whose stem contains a reservoir of 38 mg progesterone, along with barium sulfate; 65 mcg of progesterone per day is released for at least one year

c. IUDs are not abortafacients

3. Contraindications to IUD use outlined in following table

CONTRAINDICATION TO IUD USE

Absolute Contraindications
- PID within the past 3 months, or current PID
- Known or suspected pregnancy

Strong Relative Contraindications
- History of ectopic pregnancy
- Abnormal vaginal bleeding whose cause remains unknown
- Risk factors for PID which includes multiple sexual partners
- Past history of infection with gonorrhea or chlamydia, or with mucopurulent cervicitis
- History of postpartum endometritis or
- infection following abortion in past 3 months
- Abnormal Pap smear which is unresolved
- Poor access to health care
- Impaired ability to check for IUD string
- Known or suspected bleeding disorder
- Valvular heart disease
- Anatomic variations that make inserting difficult
- Severe dysmenorrhea, heavy menses, endometriosis, anemia
- History of fainting or vasovagal response
- Allergy to copper (ParaGard only)
- History of impaired fertility in patient desiring future pregnancy

---

4. Timing of insertion: Usually recommended during menses to avoid pregnancy

5. Advantages: High efficacy, which is sustained over 10 years for the ParaGard but only 1 year for the Progestasert; absence of systemic metabolic effects; method is not related to coitus; immediately reversible

6. Disadvantages: Risk of uterine perforation, increase in spontaneous abortion, ectopic pregnancy, uterine bleeding and pain, pelvic infection; need to return for annual replacement (Progestasert only)

Patient Education Relating to Use of IUDs
★ Instruct on how to check for strings, especially during first few months when expulsion is more likely
★ Instruct on signs of infection to be alert for (fever, chills, pelvic pain, severe cramping, unusual bleeding)
★ Instruct to contact health care provider immediately if period is missed
★ Provide a copy of the FDA-approved and manufacturer-supplied leaflet or pamphlet to each IUD user; consent forms can be written to include a statement such as "I have been given a copy of (title) and have been encouraged to read it carefully"
★ Follow up after female's next menses (3-6 weeks after insertion) to make certain IUD is in place and that there are no signs of infection; further routine visits are not required. Schedule annual exam

---

G. **Combination oral contraceptives** prevent pregnancy by a number of effects of estrogen and progestin: they inhibit ovulation, presumably as a result of gonadotropin suppression induced by the estrogen and progestin effects on the hypothalamic/pituitary axis; they act directly on the cervical mucus, making it thicker which inhibits sperm penetration, and; they act directly on the endometrium, inhibiting its development into a state favorable for implantation

1. Effectiveness: About 0.1% of females experience an unintended pregnancy within the first year of use with perfect use (combined pills); the figure is 0.5% with progestin-only pills

2. Advantages: Easy to use convenient, rapidly reversible, use controlled by female, many noncontraceptive benefits such as prevention of gynecologic malignancies (endocervical and ovarian), prevention of benign conditions such as fibrocystic breast changes

3.   Disadvantages: Dependent on user adherence to daily use, provides no protection against STDs, expensive, prescription needed, many possible side effects

4.   Absolute contraindications to the use of oral contraceptives are the following

---

ABSOLUTE CONTRAINDICATIONS TO USE OF ORAL CONTRACEPTIVES

- Thrombophlebitis, thromboembolic disorders
- Past history of deep vein thrombophlebitis or thromboembolic disorder
- Cerebral vascular or coronary artery disease
- Known or suspected carcinoma of the breast
- Known or suspected carcinoma of the endometrium and known or suspected estrogen-dependent neoplasia
- Undiagnosed abnormal genital bleeding
- Cholestatic jaundice of pregnancy or jaundice with prior pill use
- Hepatic adenomas, carcinomas, or benign liver tumors
- Known or suspected pregnancy
- Marked impaired liver function
- Benign or malignant liver tumor that developed during prior use of OCs or other estrogen-containing products
- Leiden factor V mutation
- Type II hyperlipidemia (hypercholesterolemia)

Adapted from Dickey, R.P. (1998). Managing contraceptive pill patients. Durant, OK: EMIS, Inc.

---

5.   Strong relative contraindications are the following

STRONG RELATIVE CONTRAINDICATIONS TO USE OF ORAL CONTRACEPTIVES

- Severe headaches, particularly vascular or migraine headaches which begin after institution of oral contraceptives
- Diastolic blood pressure of 90 mm Hg or greater or hypertension by any other criteria
- Cardiac or renal dysfunction
- Impaired glucose tolerance or history of gestational diabetes
- Psychic depression
- Varicose veins
- Age ≥35 for smokers (considered absolute contraindication by some)
- Sickle-cell or sickle cell-hemoglobin C disease
- Cholestatic jaundice during pregnancy
- Worsening of any chronic condition during pregnancy
- Hepatitis or mononucleosis during past year
- Breast feeding
- Asthma
- First degree family histories of nonrheumatic cardiovascular disease or diabetes before age 50
- Use of drugs know to interact with OCs
- Ulcerative colitis

Adapted from Dickey, R.P. (1998). Managing contraceptive pill patients. Durant, OK: EMIS, Inc.

---

6.   Most females (those without absolute contraindications and strong relative contraindications) can be prescribed any sub-50 mcg OC based on its cost, availability, or the female's prior experience
   a.   No single OC in the sub-50 mcg category is clearly superior to another
   b.   One approach is to prescribe the lowest dose
   c.   OCs such as Alesse provide one-third less ethinyl estradiol (EE) than is present in a 30 mcg OC such as Nordette
   d.   Ovcon-35 has a total of 8.4 mg norethindrone per cycle compared with Tri-Norinyl which has 15 mg
   e.   Tri-Levlen has a total of 1.925 mg of levonorgestrel per cycle which is over one-third less than in Nordette
   f.   OCs containing more than 35 mcg of estrogen should rarely be used (clinical situations such as dysfunctional uterine bleeding [DUB] may be an indication for short-term use of higher estrogen dose in some females)

7.   Females who are not candidates for estrogen-containing OCs should be considered for progestin-only pills such as Micronor or others listed in table of contraceptives categorized according to composition

8.   Clinical considerations that might be a factor in OC choice are summarized in the following table

CHOICE OF ORAL CONTRACEPTIVE BASED ON PATIENT CHARACTERISTICS

Characteristics	Type of OC Indicated	Product Examples
Risk for thrombosis which includes females 40-50 years of age, young females who are heavy smokers, females with diabetes, and those who are very overweight*	Lowest estrogen	Loestrin 1/20 Alesse
Females who complain of nausea, breast tenderness, who have vascular headaches and other estrogen-related side effects	Low estrogen	Loestrin 1/20 Alesse Estrostep
Females who have spotting or break through bleeding (BTB)	Intermediate estrogenic or progestogenic activity (can either alter progestin dose or increase the estrogen dose)	Lo-Ovral Estrostep (increases the amount of EE from 20 mcg to 35 mcg during cycle)
Females with androgenic effects such as acne, hirsuitism, oily skin, or weight gain	Low dose norethindrone or a new progestin OC**to decrease androgen effects	Ovcon 35 Desogen
Females in whom lipid changes are a concern	New progestin OCs tend to increase HDL cholesterol and decrease LDL cholesterol***	Ortho-Cyclen, Desogen, Ortho-Cept

* For complete listing of absolute contraindications as well as relative contraindications, always consult the product information inserts and the PDR

**New progestin refers to the fourth generation progestins--desogenstrel, norgestimate, and gestodene

***Oral contraceptives containing a new progestin (gestoden, desogestrel, or norgestimate) were associated with increased risk for DVT in females based on findings from several epidemiologic studies conducted in England and transnationally; however, these findings have been questioned due to poor research design, methodolgical weaknesses, and failure to replicate the data in subsequent studies. The FDA concluded that the additional risk of DVT due to use of oral contraceptives containing these new progestins is not great enough to justify switching to other products

Adapted from Hatcher et al. (1998). Contraceptive technology. New York: Ardent Media, Inc.

9. The following table lists oral contraceptives categorized according to composition:

ORAL CONTRACEPTIVE CATEGORIZED BY COMPOSITION

Type	Preparation	Estrogen (mcg)	Progestin (mg)	Color of active tablets
COMBINATION ESTROPHASIC *Ethinyl estradiol/ norethindrone acetate*	Estrostep 21	(5 tabs)20 (7 tabs) 30 (9 tabs) 35	1 1 1	white (triangle) white (square) white (round)
	Estrostep Fe	(5 tabs) 20 (7 tabs) 30 (9 tabs) 35	1 1 1	white (triangle) white (square) white (round)
COMBINATION TRIPHASIC Ethinyl estradiol/ norethindrone	Ortho-Novum 7/7/7	(7 tabs) 35 (7 tabs) 35 (7 tabs) 35	0.5 0.75 1	white light peach peach
	Tri-Norinyl	(7 tabs) 35 (9 tabs) 35 (5 tabs) 35	0.5 1 0.5	blue yellow-green blue
Ethinyl estradiol/ norgestimate	Ortho Tri-cyclen	(7 tabs) 35 (7 tabs) 35 (7 tabs) 35	0.18 0.215 0.25	white light blue blue
Ethinyl estradiol/ levonorgestrel	Tri-Levlen	(6 tabs) 30 (5 tabs) 40 (10 tabs) 30	0.05 0.075 0.125	brown white light yellow
	Triphasil	(6 tabs) 30 (5 tabs) 40 (10 tabs) 30	0.05 0.075 0.125	brown white light yellow (continued)

Type	Preparation	Estrogen (mcg)	Progestin (mg)	Color of active tablets
COMBINATION BIPHASIC Ethinyl estradiol/ norethindrone	Ortho-Novum 10/11	(10 tabs) 35 (11 tabs) 35	0.5 1	white peach
	Jenest-28	(7 tabs) 35 (14 tabs) 35	0.5 1	white peach
COMBINATION MONOPHASIC Ethinyl estradiol/ norethindrone	Loestrin 1/20	20	1	white
	Loestrin (Fe) 1/20	20	1	white
	Loestrin 1.5/30	30	1.5	green
	Loestrin (Fe) 1.5/30	30	1.5	green
	Brevicon	35	0.5	blue
	Modicon	35	0.5	white
	Norethin 1/35E	35	1	white
	Norinyl 1+35	35	1	yellow-green
	Ortho-Novum 1/35	35	1	peach
	Ovcon-35	35	0.4	peach
	Ovcon-50	50	1	yellow
Ethinyl estradiol/ levonorgestrel	Alesse	20	0.10	Pink
	Levlen	30	0.15	light orange
	Nordette	30	0.15	light orange
Ethinyl estradiol/ norgestiel	Lo/Ovral	30	0.3	white
	Ovral	50	0.5	white
Ethinyl/estradiol/ ethynodiol diacetate	Demulen 1/35	35	1	white
	Demulen 1/50	50	1	white
Mestranol/ norethindrone	Norethin 1/50 m	50	1	white
	Norinyl 1+ 50	50	1	white
	Ortho-Novum 1/50	50	1	yellow
Ethinyl estradiol/ desogestrel	Desogen	30	0.15	White
	Ortho-Cept	30	0.15	orange
Ethinyl estradiol/ norgestimate	Ortho-Cyclen	35	0.25	blue
PROGESTIN-ONLY Norethindrone	Micronor	-	0.35	lime
	Nor-QD	-	0.35	yellow
Norgestrel	Ovrette	-	0.075	yellow

Adapted from Murphy, J.L. (1998, May). Tables: Oral contraceptives. Monthly Prescribing Reference.

Patient Education Relating to Use of Oral Contraceptives

★ Instruct to use a backup method of birth control during first pack of pills

★ Provide instructions on when to start the pills based on information in the following table

★ Instruct patient to contact you if she does not have a menstrual period when expected while taking OCs

★ Teach the patient the OC danger sign and symptoms which signal that the OC should be discontinued immediately. Use the acronym ACHES (Abdominal pain, Chest pain, Headaches, Eye problems, Severe leg pain) and also include teaching on unilateral numbness, weakness, or tingling, slurring of speech (possible stroke), hemoptysis (pulmonary embolism)

★ Provide a copy of the FDA-approved and manufacturer-supplied leaflet or pamphlet to each oral contraceptive OCs user; consent forms can be written to include a statement such as "I have been given a copy of (title) and have been encouraged to read it carefully"

★ When starting a female on the OCs for the first time, give her a 3 month supply and have her return to the clinic for a BP check and for evaluation on how she is doing on the OCs; then give her enough OCs to last for the remainder of the year

★ Follow Up: In 1 year for annual exam

INSTRUCTIONS FOR STARTING ORAL CONTRACEPTIVES

- Advise female to start the OCs on the first day of her menstrual cycle or on a the first Sunday after her period begins (if period begins Sunday, she should take the first pill on that day)
- Instruct patient to take 1 pill a day until pack is finished, then
- If on 28-day pack, begin a new pack immediately; skip no days
- If using 21-day pack, stop for 7 days, and then restart (Note: Caution patient to not wait until period starts, but to wait 7 days after completing pack, and then start next pack)
- Instruct to take at the same time each day and to associate with something that is done regularly at same time of day (going to bed, brushing teeth, etc.)
- Explain that a backup method such as condoms or foam should be used for first seven days during the first few cycles

Adapted from Dickey, R.P. (1998). Managing contraceptive pill patients. Durant, OK: EMIS, Inc.

INSTRUCTIONS ABOUT EARLY SIDE EFFECTS

- Advise that some side effects are common during the first few cycles of use, but that they should disappear after that time
- Side effects to expect include the following
  - ❖ Breakthrough bleeding (BTB) and spotting
  - ❖ Symptoms associated with early pregnancy, especially nausea
- Encourage patient to not make a decision about discontinuing the pill until after the 3rd cycle so that side effects will have had a chance to resolve

Adapted from Dickey, R.P. (1998). Managing contraceptive pill patients. Durant, OK: EMIS, Inc.

INSTRUCTIONS FOR DEALING WITH MISSED PILLS

First, explain to patients the difference between the 21-pill pack and the 28-pill pack (first 21 pills in 28-pill pack contain hormones and the last 7 contain no hormones)

Patients who are taking the 28-pill pack and miss any of the last 7 pills can discard the missed pill(s), take the remaining pills as scheduled to finish the pack
They should then start the next pack on usual schedule

Patients who are taking either the 21-pill or the 28-pill pack, and miss any of the 21 hormonal pills must do the following

Use back-up contraception even if one pill was missed, or even if a pill was taken as much as 12 hours late (if only 1 pill was missed or taken late, back-up contraception such as condoms should be used for 7 days or patient should abstain from sex for 7 days)

Advise Patient to Get Back on Schedule by Following These Guidelines

If patient is <24 hours late in taking a pill	Take the missed pill immediately and return to the daily pill-taking routine making sure to take the next pill at the regular time
If patient is 24 hours late in taking a pill	Take both the missed pill and today's pill at the same time
If patient is >24 hours late in taking one pill, and is late for or completely missed a second pill as well	Take the last pill that was missed immediately; take the next pill on time; throw out the other missed pills, and take the rest of the pills in pack right on schedule

If a pill was completely missed during the third week of pills (pills 15-21), advise the patient to do the following
- ✦ Finish the remainder of the hormonal pills in pack (take through pill 21 if using a 28-pill pack)
- ✦ Do not take a week off pills if using a 21-day pill pack OR do not take the last 7 pills (the nonhormonal pills) in the 28-pill pack
- ✦ Begin taking a new pack of pills as soon as the hormonal pills in the current pack have been taken
- ✦ Advise patient that she might not have a period until the end of the second pack of pills, but missing a period is not harmful
- ✦ In all cases, back-up contraception for at least 7 days must be used

Adapted from Hatcher et al. (1998). Contraceptive technology. New York: Ardent Media, Inc.

H.   **Norplant** is a long-acting subdermal contraceptive implant of the progestin levonorgestrel that suppresses ovulation in at least half the cycles; each set of implants contains 36 mg of progestin which is released at a slow, steady rate
   1.   Effectiveness: About 0.05% of females experience an unintended pregnancy within the first year of use with perfect use; rates are highest for females weighing 70 kg or more, but then is only 2.4% over 5 years

2. Advantages: Highly effective contraception; need little motivation on patient's part; rapid reversibility; avoids risks of estrogen
3. Disadvantages: Disruption of menstrual bleeding pattern and difficult removal
4. Indication: Sexually active females who
   a. Desire long-term contraception that is highly effective
   b. Have experienced estrogen-related side-effects with OCs
   c. Have difficulty taking OCs correctly
   d. Have completed childbearing but do not wish permanent sterilization
   e. Have a history of anemia with heavy menstrual bleeding.
5. Contraindications are generally the same as with oral contraceptives; consult the package insert and PDR for more detail
6. Relative contraindications are generally the same as with oral contraceptives; consult the package insert and PDR for more detail
7. Overview of insertion
   a. Should be done during the first 7 days after the onset of menstruation; pregnancy should be ruled out
   b. Insertion is through a 3-5 mm incision in the skin located on the medial aspect of the upper inner arm
   c. Implants are placed beneath skin in fan distribution with ends nearly touching to facilitate removal
   d. Insertion is through a specially designed trocar sleeve in a largely painless procedure requiring 5-10 minutes
   e. A pressure bandage is applied post-insertion to reduce bruising
8. Generally, it is recommended that the implants be removed at the end of the fifth year

---

Patient Education Relating to Use of Norplant

★ Advise to use a backup form of contraception for first 7 days after the implant placement
★ Explain that Norplant will change pattern of menses with periods usually becoming less regular, and sometimes stopping altogether
★ Review "red flags" with patient--purulent discharge at implant site, expulsion of an implant, severe headaches, blurred vision, heavy vaginal bleeding, delayed menses after long interval of regular periods
★ If breast tenderness is a problem, she should contact provider (treatment with vitamin E 600 U/day may be helpful)
★ Encourage patient to call with questions

I. **Depo-Provera** is an injectable form of long-acting progestins with a mechanism of action similar to that of other progestin-only contraceptives; a good choice for females in whom estrogen-containing OCs are contraindicated, barrier methods are inadvisable because of compliance problems, and in females older than age 35 who smoke
1. Effectiveness: About 0.3% of females experience an unintended pregnancy within the first year of use with perfect use
2. Advantages: Easy to use, decreased menstrual flow and avoidance of the rare but serious complications attributable to estrogen use
3. Disadvantages: Unpredictable vaginal bleeding, adverse changes in lipids
4. How Administered: Usual dose is 150 mg, given IM every 12 weeks
   a. Initial dose should be administered by the 5th day of menses in nonpostpartum females
   b. In non-nursing postpartum females, initial dose should be given 5 days postpartum and at 6 weeks postpartum for breast feeding mothers (breast feeding must be well established)
   c. Approximately half of females using this method experience amenorrhea after a year of injections

J.   **Emergency postcoital contraception** using emergency contraceptive pills (ECPs) has recently been approved by the FDA

1.   ECPs are birth control pills containing ethinyl estradiol and norgestrel or levongestrel

2.   These hormones are found in seven brands of combined oral contraceptives available in the US

3.   The following table presents regimens for administering these drugs for emergency contraception

REGIMENS FOR ORAL EMERGENCY CONTRACEPTIVE USE IN THE UNITED STATES*			
Brand	Pills per dose	Ethynyl estradiol per dose (μg)	Levonorgestrel per dose (mg)[a]
Ovral	2 white pills[b]	100	0.50
Alesse	5 pink pills[b]	100	0.50
Nordette	4 light-orange pills[b]	120	0.60
Levlen	4 light-orange pills[b]	120	0.60
Lo/Ovral	4 white pills[b]	120	0.60
Triphasil	4 yellow pills[b]	120	0.50
Tri-Levlen	4 yellow pills[b]	120	0.50
Ovrette	20 yellow pills[c]	0	0.75

*Ovral, Alesse, Nordette, Levlen, Lo/Ovral, Triphasil, and Tri-Levlen have been declared safe and effective for use as emergency contraceptives by the FDA

[a]The progestin in Ovral, Lo/Ovral, and Ovrette is norgestrel, which contains two isomers, only one of which (levonorgestrel) is bioactive; the amount of norgestrel in each tablet is twice the amount of levonorgestrel

[b]The treatment schedule is one dose within 72 hours after unprotected intercourse, and another dose 12 hours later

[c]Treatment schedule using levonorgestrel only was tested in a clinical trial in which 0.75 mg was given within 48 hours after unprotected intercourse followed by 0.75 mg 12 hours later. The WHO has completed a study indicating that this same regimen is effective when initiated up to 72 hours after unprotected intercourse

Adapted from Hatcher, R.A. et al. (1998). Contraceptive technology. New York: Ardent Media.

4.   Preven Emergency Contraceptive Kit was recently approved by the FDA

    a.   Kit is composed of 4 tabs containing both ethinyl estradiol 50 mcg and levonorgestrel 250 mcg

    b.   Dosing: 2 tabs within 72 hours of unprotected intercourse or a contraceptive failure and 2 tabs 12 hours later

    c.   **Note**: Kit also contains a urine pregnancy test

5.   Effectiveness: Reduces the risk of pregnancy by about 75% (**Note**: Risk of becoming pregnant during unprotected intercourse during 2nd or 3rd week of cycle is about 8 of every 100 females; with ECPs, this is reduced to about 2 out of every 100 females, which represents a 75% reduction)

6.   Side effects: Almost half of females who take ECPs have nausea and about a fourth have vomiting; if vomiting occurs within 2 hours after taking a dose, some authorities recommend repeating that dose

      a.   Antiemetics such as trimethobenzamide hydrochloride (Tigan) 250 mg caps or 200 mg suppositories may be administered 1 hour prior to the first dose, and then as needed every 6-8 hours x 24 hours

      b.   Recommend that the medication be taken with food to reduce nausea

   7.   Safety: Almost all females can safely use ECPs

      a.   The only absolute contraindication is confirmed pregnancy

      b.   Treatment may not be appropriate in females with active migraine or marked neurologic symptoms

      c.   In females with a history of stroke or blood clots in the lungs or legs, treatment with progestin-only pills may be preferable (consult table above)

K.   The Copper-T IUD has also been approved for emergency contraception and can be inserted up to five days after unprotected intercourse; reduce the risk of pregnancy following unprotected intercourse by more than 99%

DYSMENORRHEA

I.   Definition: Painful menstrual cramps

II.   Pathogenesis

    A.   Primary dysmenorrhea is painful uterine contractions associated with increased production and release of prostaglandins in the absence of pelvic pathology; a role may also be played by increased production of leukotrienes and vasopressin

    B.   Secondary dysmenorrhea is painful uterine contractions due to a clinically identifiable cause, and may be classified as follows:

      1.   External to the uterus (examples are endometriosis, tumors, adhesions, and nongynecologic causes)

      2.   Within the wall of the uterus (examples are adenomyosis, leiomyomas)

      3.   Within the cavity of the uterus (examples are polyps and infection)

III.   Clinical Presentation

    A.   Approximately half of all postpubescent females have some degree of dysmenorrhea, with about 10% having levels of discomfort that cause absence from school or work

    B.   Pattern of primary dysmenorrhea is as follows

      1.   Usually begins 6-12 months after menarche

      2.   Most commonly begins between the ages of 14-16 years

      3.   Peaks around 17-18 years of age; usually decreases in 20s and 30s

    C.   Secondary dysmenorrhea increases in incidence as females grow older due to the increased prevalence of processes that cause the condition among older females

    D.   Pain of primary dysmenorrhea is characterized by the following

      1.   Occurs first day or two of menstruation

      2.   Located in suprapubic area and radiates to back, upper thighs

      3.   Associated with diarrhea, nausea, vomiting, fatigue, and backache

    E.   Females with secondary dysmenorrhea usually experience pain consistent with the underlying pathology such as the following

      1.   GI symptoms, UTI symptoms, and so on suggest nongynecologic causes

      2.   Dyspareunia and pelvic pain unrelated to menses (but also occurring with menses) suggest causes such as endometriosis, infection (PID), adenomyosis, and leiomyomas

IV.   Diagnosis/Evaluation

    A.   History
        1.   Obtain a complete menstrual history and contraceptive history (including use of IUD)
        2.   Question patient about location of pain, when it begins, if it radiates, if there are associated symptoms of nausea, vomiting, and diarrhea
        3.   Inquire if pain occurs independently of menses in addition to occurring with menses Ask if there is dyspareunia
        4.   Ask if there are urinary tract symptoms, if there is any vaginal discharge
        5.   Question patient about treatments tried and results

    B.   Physical Examination
        1.   Measure blood pressure (in 2 positions if blood loss is suspected), pulse rate, temperature
        2.   Evaluate heart and lungs
        3.   Perform abdominal exam, evaluating for bowel sounds, tenderness, masses, rigidity, guarding, rebound tenderness
        4.   Do pelvic exam; inspect cervix for mucopurulent discharge draining from the endocervix. Gently scape cervix to test for friability
        5.   Perform bimanual exam to check for adnexal tenderness, uterine tenderness, and cervical motion tenderness

    C.   Differential Diagnosis
        1.   For primary dysmenorrhea, the most important differential diagnosis to consider is that of secondary dysmenorrhea
        2.   For secondary dysmenorrhea, must consider the following
            a.   Intrauterine causes such as adenomyosis, myomas, polyps, IUDs, infection
            b.   Extrauterine causes such as endometriosis, tumors, inflammation, adhesions, and nongynecologic causes

    D.   Diagnostic Tests
        1.   For primary dysmenorrhea, none indicated
        2.   For secondary dysmenorrhea, H & P should guide test selection

V.   Plan/Management

    A.   For secondary dysmenorrhea, treatment of the underlying cause is indicated; if no obvious cause is uncovered, refer to expert for management

    B.   For primary dysmenorrhea, drugs that suppress the production of prostaglandins are indicated; best accomplished by using nonsteroidal anti-inflammatory drugs (NSAIDs)

    C.   NSAIDs inhibit prostaglandin synthesis and exhibit antiinflammatory and analgesic activity
        1.   The most commonly used NSAIDs for dysmenorrhea come from two classes: propionic acids and fenamates
        2.   Propionic Acids
            a.   Ibuprofen (Motrin) 400 mg Q 6 H, OR
            b.   Naproxen (Naprosyn) 500 mg initial dose, then 250 mg Q 6-8 H, OR
            c.   Naproxen sodium (Anaprox) 550 mg initial dose, then 275 mg Q 6-8 H, OR
        3.   Fenamates
            a.   Mefenamic acid (Ponstel) 500 mg initial dose, then 250 mg Q 4-6 H, OR
            b.   Meclofenamate (Meclomen) 100 mg initial dose, then 50-100 mg Q 6 H
        4.   Drug that is selected for treatment should be tried over the course of 2-4 cycles before success or failure is judged
        5.   If treatment failure occurs with one class, the second trial should utilize the other class
        6.   Patients should be reminded to take drug at the onset of menstruation or symptoms, and continue taking for as long as symptoms would normally last if medication were not being taken

D. Oral contaceptives are also highly effective and may be used in addition to (reduce dose of NSAID) or instead of NSAIDs
   1. Oral contraceptives are first-line therapy for patients who also desire contraception
   2. Almost all patients with primary dysmenorrhea achieve good pain relief with use of OCs
   3. Low dose combination oral contraceptives should be prescribed if there are no contraindications

E. Nonpharmacologic management
   1. **Education:** Menstrual physiology and the relationship of changing hormones to symptoms should be briefly reviewed
   2. **Exercise:** A regular aerobic exercise program may be helpful and should be recommended
   3. **Alternative therapies:** Use of acupuncture and acupressure on a weekly basis may also be helpful
   4. **Stress reduction:** Refer for techniques for stress reduction including biofeedback and relaxation techniques
   5. **Other therapies:** Use of a transcutaneous electrical nerve stimulation (TENS) unit is effective in some patients

F. Follow Up: In 6 months to evaluate treatment efficacy

PREMENSTRUAL SYNDROME

I. Definition: A cyclical symptom complex that occurs with greatest frequency and severity in the late luteal phase (5-11 days prior to onset of menses) and abates within 1-2 days of the onset of menses

II. Pathogenesis

A. No single etiology has been identified and several mechanisms for pathogenesis have been described

B. Mechanisms such as reductions in endorphin and serotonin levels, underproduction and excess production of prostaglandins, nutritional imbalance, endocrine and neuroendocrine alterations have been studied in relation to possible etiology of PMS, but findings have been inconclusive

III. Clinical Presentation

A. Incidence of PMS is reported to be between 20-90% of females, with only about 20% having symptoms severe enough to limit daily functioning

B. Disorder is more prevalent in females from 30-40 years of age, and is more frequent in females with history of postpartum depression or affective illness

C. PMS presents as irritability, depression, crying spells, mood swings, sleep disturbance, appetite changes, and changes in libido; this presentation is similar to those seen in mood disorders and anxiety

D. Patients with true PMS will have symptoms in the luteal phase only

E. Diagnosis is made on the basis of history of a symptom-free follicular phase in contrast to emotional and physical disturbances that characterize the luteal phase

F. Diagnostic critera for premenstrual dysphoric disorder (PMDD) are contained in the table on page 662, and are adapted from the fourth edition of the Diagnostic and Statistical Manual of Mental Disorders (1994); focus is on psychological symptoms rather than on physical symptoms

G. Clinically, the two conditions--PMS and PMDD--overlap
  1. Many females with PMS meet the diagnostic criteria for PMDD
  2. PMDD is a much more narrowly defined disorder than PMS
  3. Presently, PMS and PMDD appear to be two points on a continuum, but further research is needed

---

DIAGNOSTIC CRITERIA FOR PREMENSTRUAL DYSPHORIC DISORDER

- The female must have **five or more** of the following 11 symptoms, including at least one of the first four for most of the time during the last week of the luteal phase in most menstrual cycles over the past 12 month period
    Depressed mood, feelings of hopelessness, or self-deprecating thoughts
    Marked anxiety or tension; feeling "keyed up"
    Significant mood lability
    Persistent anger or irritability
    Decreased interest in usual activities
    Difficulty concentrating
    Lethargy, or marked lack of energy
    Changes in appetite
    Hypersonmia or insomnia
    Feeling of being overwhelmed
    Physical symptoms such as breast tenderness, headache, joint/muscle pain, bloating, or weight gain
- Symptoms must start or resolve within a few days of onset of menses and be absent in week after menstruation ceases
- Additionally, symptoms must markedly impair patient's ability to work/attend school, or conduct usual social activities
- The diagnosis must be confirmed by prospective daily ratings for at least two consecutive symptomatic menstrual cycles

Adapted from American Psychiatric Association. (1994). Diagnostic and statistical manual of mental disorders (4th ed.). Washington, DC: Author.

IV. Diagnosis/Evaluation

  A. History: (**Note**: Be cautious in accepting patient's self-diagnosis of PMS)
    1. Ask about age at onset of symptomatology; when in cycle symptoms are experienced; most significant symptoms; degree of severity
    2. Inquire about variations from cycle to cycle
    3. Using the diagnostic criteria for PMDD, ask patient if the 11 symptoms listed are present during last week of luteal phase during menstrual cycles (**Note**: This is the best approach to the patient who reports significant impairment)
    4. Inquire about previous history of depression; previous treatment for PMS and results
    5. Determine if patient is experiencing dysmenorrhea (many females confuse PMS with dysmenorrhea), situational depression, or eating disorders
    6. Obtain data regarding drug and alchol use
    7. Use the SAFE Questions to screen for spousal abuse (see DOMESTIC VIOLENCE: PARTNER ABUSE section)

  B. Physical Examination: No specific physical findings aid in diagnosis; physical and pelvic exams as part of a general health survey may be completed, however

  C. Differential Diagnosis
    1. Depression
    2. Anxiety disorder
    3. Relationship discord/domestic violence
    4. Drug/alcohol abuse
    5. Eating disorder
    6. Dysmenorrhea

  D. Diagnostic Tests: None indicated (**Note**: Make certain patient understands that laboratory testing is not helpful)

V. Plan/Management

  A. Prospective data collection by the patient for at least 2 menstrual cycles must be done to establish pattern of symptoms and establish diagnosis

B. Several commercially available checklists can be used by the patient to record occurrence and severity of symptoms on a daily basis throughout entire cycle. Available forms are the Menstrual Distress Questionnaire (Moos, 1969) and the Premenstrual Syndrome Symptomatology Questionnaire (Vargyas, 1986) [see reference list]

C. After 2 months of data collection related to occurrence and severity of symptoms, interpretation of data can be made
    1. The suspected diagnosis of PMS is confirmed if other disorders (see differential diagnosis) are ruled out, and patient's symptomatology is limited to luteal phase
    2. Patients who report a high degree of symptomatology throughout menstrual cycle should be referred for further evaluation, as PMS is unlikely

D. Treatment must be individualized based on symptoms

E. Conservative measures such as the following should be instituted first
    1. **Support and reassurance**: Patient should know that her problems are not uncommon
    2. **Stress reduction**: Many patients benefit from formal instruction in stress management techniques such as relaxation exercises, biofeedback, and reflexology
    3. **Education**: Monitoring daily symptoms will help patient obtain a degree of control in life and will allow her to avoid making major decisions when symptoms are worse
    4. **Diet**: Advise to eat a well-balanced diet (see NUTRITION IN CHILDHOOD AND ADOLESCENCE); according to some sources, carboyhdrate-rich, low-protein foods, especially when eaten during the luteal phase may improve mood symptoms
    5. **Caffeine**: Sugggest that patient attempt a trial of caffeine elimiation to determine if this alleviates her symptoms (**Note**: Suggest that use be tapered to avoid caffeine-withdrawal headaches)
    6. **Exercise**: Personal preferences should be taken into account, but some type of regular daily activity should be undertaken (**Note**: Exercise is a great stress-reducer)
    7. **Vitamin Supplementation**: Studies to date suggest that vitamin B_6 supplementation may be helpful (<200 mg/day)
    8. **Herbal and other therapies**: Patients should not be discouraged from trying therapies such as teas and herbs so long as ingredients are clearly identified, the products are safe, and the patient's symptoms are not severe; ask patient to bring in product for you to evaluate the ingredients

F. Pharmacologic therapies may also be used in conjunction with the conservative measures listed above
    1. NSAIDs can be prescribed for those patients with premenstrual and menstrual pain including headache, cramping, low back pain, breast tenderness. See section on DYSMENORRHEA for appropriate NSAIDs and dosages
    2. Selective serotonin reuptake inhibitors are sometimes used in selected adolescents with severe symptoms unresponsive to other treatments. **NOTE:** Not recommended for routine use in adolescents!
        a. Fluoxetine (Prozac) 10-20 mg PO QD in AM OR
        b. Paroxetine (Paxil) 10 mg PO QD at bedtime
        c. Advise patient about common side effects, be aware of drug interactions and monitor response at 3 months
    3. Oral contraceptives work well for some patients; this method is most appropriate in patients needing contraception and who have also failed other treatments

G. Follow Up
    1. In 2 months to review diary
    2. Every 3-6 months until symptoms controlled

LABIAL ADHESIONS IN CHILDREN

I. Definition: Flap of skin formed by the adherence of the labia minora that completely or partially covers the vaginal opening

II. Pathogenesis: Condition is caused by a combination of inflammation and hypoestrogenization of the labia minora

III. Clinical Presentation

    A. Occurs primarily in girls between the age of 3 months and 6 years (due to hypoestrogenization of the labia minora) but may occur at any age until the time of puberty

    B. Parents are often concerned that child does not have a vagina

    C. Commonly, there are only small adhesions at the posterior fourchette which spontaneously separate with estrogenization at puberty

    D. Occasionally, the vaginal orifice is completely covered, resulting in poor drainage of vaginal secretions; urine flow may be partially impeded, resulting in pooling behind the fusion resulting in further irritation and adhesion

IV. Diagnosis/Evaluation

    A. History
        1. In children who are able to respond, inquire about dysuria and difficulty voiding
        2. Ask parent about amount, color, and odor of any vaginal discharge noted on child's underwear
        3. In children who are able to respond, ask about discomfort and pain
        4. Cautiously explore whether there is a history of trauma or injury (sexual abuse has been theorized to relate to labial adhesions)
        5. Explore hygiene practices such as whether child takes a shower or bath

    B. Physician Examination
        1. Visually inspect the vulva
        2. Check for signs of physical and sexual abuse
        3. If the vaginal introitus is obscured, insert a small probe through the anterior opening and direct it posteriorly beneath the membrane to determine degree of adhesion

    C. Differential Diagnosis: Imperforate hymen (hymen is apparent within the vaginal introitus and the labia are normal)

    D. Diagnostic Tests: None are indicated

V. Plan/Management

    A. If the opening in the adhesion is sufficient for good vaginal and urinary drainage, teach the parents to lubricate the labia with a bland ointment such as A and D ointment or vaseline ointment and apply gentle traction to the labia laterally for several weeks

    B. For adhesions that prevent vaginal and urinary drainage, use topical application of estrogen cream (0.1% or 0.01% diestrol) BID for 2 weeks followed by once daily application at bedtime for another 2 weeks. Must show parents to apply a thin layer of cream directly to the line of the labial adhesion rather than over the entire vulva and to apply gentle traction on the labia laterally at the time of application (**Note**: The older child can be taught to apply the cream herself with supervision)

C.   After separation, labia can be maintained apart by daily baths, good hygiene, and application of bland ointment at bedtime for 6-12 months (**Note:** The older child should be taught how do do this)

D.   Forceful separation is contraindicated because it may cause adhesions to form again and is traumatic for the child

E.   Occasionally a second course of treatment is needed

F.   Follow Up: None indicated

VULVOVAGINAL CANDIDIASIS

I.   Definition: Infection of the vulvar area and vagina by *Candida albicans* and other candida species

II.   Pathogenesis

A.   Little is known about factors that contribute to the overgrowth of normal flora in the vagina

B.   When the complex balance of microorganisms changes, however, potentially pathogenic endogenous microorganisms that are part of the normal flora such as *Candida albicans* proliferate to numbers that cause symptoms

C.   *C. albicans* causes 80% to 90% of vaginal fungal infections and other *Candida* species and *Torulopsis* sp., or other yeasts cause the remainder

III. Clinical Presentation

A.   Approximately 25% of all vaginal infections are due to vulvovaginal candidiasis (VVC); this condition is not transmitted sexually but is often diagnosed in females being evauated for STDs

B.   An estimated 75% of females will have at least one episode of VVC, and approximately 40% will have two or more episodes; a small percentage, less that 5% experience recurrent VVC

C.   Primarily a disease of the childbearing years; the majority of premenarcheal and postmenopausal females who develop the disease have recently taken antibiotics, estrogen, or will be found to have diabetes

D.   Pregnancy is the most common predisposing factor

E.   Depressed cell-mediated immunity (such as with HIV+ status) also is risk factor

F.   Vulvar pruritus is the cardinal symptom and a white dischage may also be present; vulvar erythema is the most often observed sign, with edema and excoriation of the vulva also often observed; vaginal secretions have a normal pH (≤ 4.5)

G.   Diagnosis can be made in a female with typical signs and symptoms and when either a) wet preparation or Gram stain of vaginal discharge demonstrates yeasts or pseudohyphae or b) culture yields a positive result for a yeast species

IV.   Diagnosis/Evaluation

A.   History
      1.   Question about vulvar itching, discharge, odor, dysuria, dyspareunia
      2.   Ask about previous occurrences of yeast infections

3. Ask about predisposing factors such as pregnancy, recent antibiotic or estrogen therapy, history of diabetes, HIV+ status
4. Ask about douching and use of feminine hygiene products

B. Physical Examination
    1. Examine vulva for erythema, edema, and excoriation
    2. Perform pelvic exam and examine vagina for erythema, white patches/plaques; note odor of secretions (should not be malodorous)

C. Diagnostic Tests
    1. Obtain sample of vaginal secretions from anterior or lateral vaginal walls on a dry swab and apply to pH paper. In candidiasis, pH of vaginal secretions is ≤4.5 (normal pH of vagina is 3.5-4.5)
    2. Microscopic examination of slide containing vaginal secretions mixed with 10% potassium hydroxide (KOH) shows typical hyphae and budding yeast (see Figure 14.1)

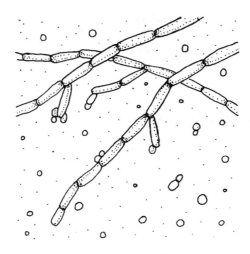

Figure 14.1. Hyphae and Yeast Buds.

D. Differential Diagnosis
    1. Other common causes of vaginitis -- bacterial vaginosis and trichomoniasis
    2. Common causes of cervicitis -- chlamydia and gonorrhea which can sometimes cause a vaginal discharge

V. Plan/Management

    A.   Recommended regimens for the treatment of VVC are contained in the following table

RECOMMENDED REGIMENS FOR TREATMENT OF VULVOVAGINAL CANDIDIASIS		
Medication	**Dose**	**Application**
Intravaginal agents		
Butoconazole OR	2% cream	5 g intravaginally for 3 days*[†]
Clotrimazole OR	1% cream	5 g intravaginally for 7-14 days*[†]
Clotrimazole OR	100 mg vaginal tablet	for 7 days*
Clotrimazole OR	100 mg vaginal tablet	2 tablets for 3 days*
Clotrimazole OR	500 mg vaginal tablet,	1 tablet single application*
Miconazole OR	2% cream	5 g intravaginally for 7 days*[†]
Miconazole OR	200 mg vaginal suppository	1 suppository for 3 days*[†]
Miconazole OR	100 mg vaginal suppository	1 suppository for 7 days*[†]
Tioconazole OR	6.5% ointment	5 g intravaginally in a single application*[†]
Terconazole OR	0.4% cream	5 g intravaginally for 7 days*
Terconazole OR	0.8% cream	5 g intravaginally for 3 days*
Terconazole	80 mg suppository	1 suppository for 3 days*
Oral agent		
Fluconazole	150 mg oral tablet	1 tablet in single dose

*These creams and suppositories are oil-based and may weaken latex condoms and diaphragms. Refer to product labeling for further information
[†]Over-the-counter (OTC) preparations
Source: US Department of Health and Human Services, Centers for Disease Control and Prevention. (1998). 1998 guidelines for treatment of sexually transmitted diseases. Morbidity and Mortality Weekly Report, 47(RR-1), 76.

    B.   Treatment of pregnant females: Only topical azole therapies should be used for the treatment of pregnant females
        1.   Most effective treatments that have been studied for pregnant females are clotrimazole, miconazole, butoconazole, and terconazole
        2.   Many experts recommend 7 days of therapy during pregnancy

    C.   Treatment of sexual partners is not necessary unless candidal balanitis is present

    D.   Treatment considerations in patients with recurrent VVC (RVVC) [defined as *four* or more episodes of symptomatic VVC in a 12 month period]
        1.   Pathogenesis of RVVC is poorly understood but risk factors include uncontrolled diabetes, immunosuppression, corticosteriod use, and repeated use of topical or systemic antibacterials (**Note**: The majority of females with RVVC have no apparent predisposing conditions)
        2.   Use of either topical or oral azoles for a period of 10-14 days is recommended

3. After the 10-14 days of initial therapy, maintenance therapy should be initiated for at least 6 months with ketoconazole 100 mg orally once daily for ≤ 6 months

4. **Note:** All cases of recurrent VVC should be confirmed by culture before maintenance therapy is initiated

E. Follow Up: None indicated

REFERENCES

American Psychiatric Association. (1994). Diagnostic and statistical manual of mental disorders (4th ed.). Washington, DC: Author.

Baker, S. (1998). Menstruation and related problems and concerns. In E.Q. Youngkin & M.S. Davis (Eds.), Women's health: A primary care clinical guide. Stamford,CN: Appleton & Lange.

Bayer, S.R., & DeCherney, A.H. (1993). Clinical manifestations and treatment of dysfunctional uterine bleeding. Journal of American Medical Association, 269, 1823-1828.

Beckman, C.R., Ling, F.W., Herbert, W.N., Laube, D.W., Smith, R.P., & Barzansky, B.M. (1998). Obstetrics and gynecology. Baltimore: Williams & Wilkins.

Caufield, K.A. (1998). Controlling fertility. In E.Q. Youngkin & M.S. Davis (Eds.), Women's health: A primary care clinical guide. Stamford,CN: Appleton & Lange.

Dickey, R.P. (1998). Managing contraceptive pill patients. Durant, OK: Emis Medical Publishers.

Endicott, J., Feemna, E.W. Kielich, A.M., & Sondeimer, S.J. (1996, April). PMS: New treatments that really work. Patient Care, 88-120.

Ettinger, B., Friedman, G. D., Bush, T., & Quesenberry, C. P. (1996). Reduced mortality associated with long-term postmenopausal estrogen therapy. Obstetrics & Gynecology, 87, 6-12.

Fiorica, J.V., Schorr, s.J., & Sickles, E.A. (1997, Apr). Benign breast disorders. Patient Care, 140-154.

Glasier, A. 91997). Emergency postcoital contraception. The New England Journal of Medicine, 337, 1058-1064.

Hatcher, R.A., Trussell, J., Stewart, F., Cates, W., Stewart, G., Guest, F., & Kowal, D. (1998). Contraceptive technology. New York: Adrent Media.

Hill, D.A., & Lense, J.S. (1998). Office management of Bartholin gland cysts and abscesses. American Family Physicain 57(7), 1611-1616.

Hindle, W.H., & Ling, F.W. (1992). Diseases of the breast. In T.G. Stovall, R.L. Summitt, Jr., C.R. Beckmann, & F.W. Ling (Eds.), Clinical manual of gynecology. New York: McGraw-Hill.

Moe, R.E. (1996). Clinical approach to breast disease. In M.A. Stenchever (Ed.), Office gynecology. St. Louis: Mosby.

Hindle, W.H. (1998, March). Palpable breast mass: The physical examination. Hospital Practice, 42-45.

Moos, R.H. (1969). The development of a premenstrual distress questionnaire. Psychosomatic Medicine, 30, 850-855.

Morgan, K.W., & Deneris, A. (1997). Emergency contraception: Preventing unintended pregnancy. Nurse Practitioner, 22(11), 34-48.

Mou, S.M. (1995). Gynecologic infections. In V.L. Seltzer & W.H. Pearse (Eds.), Women's primary heath care. New York: McGraw-Hill.

Murphy, E.J. (1998, May). Oral contraceptives: Classification of oral contraceptives. Monthly Prescribing Reference, 209.

Nand, S.L., Webster, M.A., Baber, R., & O'Connor, V. (1998). Bleeding pattern and endometrial changes during continuous combined hormone replacement therapy. Obstetrics and Gynecology, 91, 678-684.

Nelson, A.L. (1997). A practical approach to dysfunctional uterine bleeding. Family Practice Recertification, 19(8), 14-40.

Nesse, R.E. (1997). Menometrorrhagia and causes of abnormal premenopausal vaginal bleeding. In J.A. Rosenfeld (Ed.). Women's health in primary care. Baltimore: Williams & Wilkins.

Shy, K.K. (1996). Contraception. In M.A. Stenchever (Ed.), Office gynecology. St. Louis: Mosby.

Steege, J.F. (1996). Subjective disorders: Dysmenorrhea, chronic pelvic pain, and premenstrual syndrome. In M.A. Stenchever (Ed.). Office gynecology. St. Louis: Mosby.

Tamimi, H.K. (1996). Management of the abnormal or atypical papanicolaou smear. In M.A. Stenchever (Ed.), Office gynecology. St. Louis: Mosby.

Trussell, J., Ellerston, C., Stewart, F., Koenig, J., & Raymond, E.G. (1998). Emergency contraception. Women's Health in Primary Care, 1(1), 52-69.

US Preventive Services Task Force. (1996). Guide to clinical preventive services. Baltimore: Williams & Wilkins.

US Department of Health and Human Services, Centers for Disease Control. (1998). 1998 guidelines for treatment of sexually transmitted diseases. Morbidity and Mortality Weekly Report, 47(RR-1).

Uy, S., & McNicoll, K. (1998). Are you up-to-date on Pap smears? Family Practice Recertification, 20(1), 53-84.

Vargyas, J.M., & Ling, F.W. (1992). Premenstrual syndrome. In T.G. Stovall, R.L. Summitt, Jr., C.R. Beckmann, & F.W. Ling (Eds.), Clinical manual of gynecology. New York: McGraw-Hill.

Vargyas, J.M. (1986). Premenstrual syndrome. In D.R. Mishell, & V. Davajan (Eds.), Infertility, Contraception, and reproductive endocrinology. Cambridge, MA: Blackwell Scientific Publications.

Webb, T.S. (1996, Jan.). Common menstrual disorders: Primary care management. Advance for Nurse Practitioners, 20-23.

CHAPTER 15

Sexually Transmitted Disease

BACTERIAL VAGINOSIS

I.   Definition: Clinical syndrome resulting from replacement of the normal H_2O_2-producing *Lactobacillus sp.* in the vagina with high concentrations of anaerobic bacteria (e.g., *Prevotella* sp. and *Mobiluncus* sp.), *Garderella vaginalis*, and *Mycoplasma hominis*

II.   Pathogenesis

    A.   Causes of the microbial alteration are not fully understood

    B.   Bacterial vaginosis (BV) is associated with having multiple sex partners, but it remains unclear whether BV results from acquisition of a sexually transmitted pathogen

    C.   Females who have never been sexually active are rarely affected

III. Clinical Presentation

    A.   BV is the most prevalent cause of vaginal discharge and malodor in females

    B.   Approximately half of the females whose illness meet the clinical criteria for BV are asymptomatic

    C.   BV may be diagnosed by use of clinical or Gram stain criteria

    D.   Clinical criteria require three of the following signs or symptoms
       1.   A grayish-white, homogenous, malodorous discharge that may be scant or profuse, which adheres to the vaginal walls
       2.   The presence of clue cells on microscopic exam
       3.   pH of vaginal fluid >4.5
       4.   A fishy odor of vaginal discharge before or after addition of 10% KOH (whiff test)

    E.   When Gram stain is used, determining the relative concentration of the bacterial morphotypes characteristic of the altered flora of BV is an acceptable laboratory method for diagnosing BV

    F.   Because organisms do not invade vaginal wall, gross vulvitis and vaginitis do not occur; thus, few females experience irritative symptoms such as pruritus and burning

IV.   Diagnosis/Evaluation

    A.   History
       1.   Question about onset of symptoms, description of discharge (whether malodorous and appearance and amount)
       2.   Ask if other signs and symptoms are present
       3.   Ask if female uses frequent douching, feminine hygiene products to control odor
       4.   Obtain complete menstrual history and history of contraceptive use including condom use

    B.   Physical Examination
       1.   Examine introitus for homogenous discharge
       2.   Do speculum exam and look for homogenous discharge coating vaginal walls; note odor for characteristic foul, fishy odor
       3.   Inspect cervix (should be normal) and complete bimanual exam

    C.   Differential Diagnosis
       1.   Other common cause of vaginitis -- trichomoniasis and vulvovaginal candidiasis
       2.   Common causes of cervicitis -- chlamydia and gonorrhea

D.   Diagnostic Tests
1.   Obtain sample of vaginal secretions from anterior or lateral wall on a dry swab and apply to pH paper. In bacterial vaginosis, pH of vaginal secretions is >4.5 (normal pH of vagina is 3.5-4.5)
2.   Microscopic examination of slide containing vaginal secretions mixed with saline shows clue cells. Secretions have a fishy odor before or after being mixed with a drop of 10% KOH (positive whiff test)
3.   Figure 15.1 depicts a clue cell, an epithelial cell to which many bacteria are attached

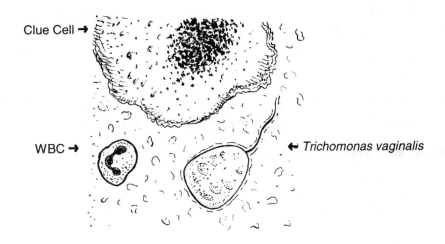

Clue Cell →

WBC →   ← *Trichomonas vaginalis*

Figure 15.1. Clue Cell, WBC, & *Trichomonas vaginalis*

V.   Plan/Management

A.   The principal goal of therapy is to relieve signs and symptoms

B.   All females with symptomatic disease require treatment, regardless of pregnancy status
1.   BV during pregnancy is associated with adverse outcomes
2.   Treatment of pregnant females who have BV and who are at high risk for preterm delivery might reduce risk for prematurity
3.   High-risk pregnant females who do not have symptoms of BV may be evaluated for treatment
a.   Presently, treatment for high-risk pregnant females who have asymptomatic BV remains controversial
b.   A large clinical trial is underway to assess benefits and risks of treatment for asymptomatic high-risk pregnant females
4.   Consideration should be given to treatment of females who have symptomatic or asymptomatic BV before invasive or surgical procedures such as endometrial biopsy, hysterectomy, cesarean section, and abortion are performed

C.   Treatment of choice for nonpregnant females
1.   Metronidazole (Flagyl) 500 mg orally BID x 7 days, OR
2.   Metronidazole gel 0.75%, one full applicator (5 g) intravaginally BID x 5 days, OR
3.   Clindamycin cream, 2%, one full applicator (5 g) intravaginally at bedtime x 7 days

D.   Alternative regimens for nonpregnant females
1.   Metronidazole (Flagyl) 2 g orally in a single dose, OR
2.   Clindamycin 300 mg orally BID x 7 days

E.   Treatment during pregnancy
1.   High-risk pregnant females may be screened and treated for BV at the earliest part of the second trimester of pregnancy

2. Low-risk pregnant females who have symptomatic BV should be treated to relieve symptoms
   a. Recommended regimen is metronidazole 250 mg orally TID x 7 days
   b. Alternative regimens: Metronidazole 2 g orally in a single dose OR clindamycin 300 mg orally BID x 7 days
3. Use of clindamycin vaginal cream during pregnancy is not recommended

F. Routine treatment of sex partners in **not** recommended

G. Follow Up
   1. None indicated except in high-risk pregnant females who should receive follow-up 1 month after completion of therapy to evaluate efficacy of treatment
   2. Recurrence of BV is common but no long-term maintenance regimen is recommended
   3. Use alternative treatment regimens for treatment of recurrent disease

TRICHOMONIASIS

I. Definition: Infection of the vagina by *Trichomonas vaginalis*. May also involve Skene's ducts and lower urinary tract in females, and the lower genitourinary tract in males

II. Pathogenesis

A. *Trichomonas vaginalis*, a unicellular flagellated protozoan, causes this primarily sexually transmitted disease

B. Incubation period is 4-20 days with the average being 1 week

III. Clinical Presentation

A. Trichomoniasis comprises about 10% of all vaginal infections and is observed primarily in females with normal estrogen levels

B. Infection is frequently asymptomatic. If symptomatic, symptoms are usually worse immediately after menstruation and during pregnancy

C. Cardinal symptom is a diffuse, malodorous, yellow-green discharge

D. Diffuse edema and redness is usually apparent in vulvar and vaginal tissue; the cervix may be inflamed and friable. Rarely, punctate lesions on the cervix give a "strawberry" appearance

E. Flagellated protozoa are seen in wet prep of vaginal secretions. Vaginal secretions have a pH of >4.5

F. Urethritis and prostatitis may be seen in the male; almost 80% of males harboring the organism are asymptomatic

IV. Diagnosis/Evaluation

A. History
   1. Question about presence of discharge, its odor, color and if dysuria, dyspareunia are present
   2. Obtain menstrual history and ask if menstruation makes symptoms worse
   3. In males, question about dysuria
   4. Obtain history of previous STDs; ask about condom use

B. Physical Examination
1. Examine external genitalia for discharge pooling at introitus or posterior fourchette
2. Do pelvic exam to determine if vagina has erythema, edema; note type, color, and amount of discharge; examine cervix for erythema, friability, discharge

C. Differential Diagnosis
1. Other common causes of vaginitis -- bacterial vaginosis and vulvovaginal candidiasis.
2. Common causes of cervicitis -- chlamydia and gonorrhea

D. Diagnostic Tests
1. Obtain sample of vaginal secretions from anterior or lateral wall on a dry swab and apply to pH paper. In trichomoniasis, pH of vaginal secretions is >4.5 (normal pH of the vagina is 3.5-4.5)
2. Microscopic examination of slide containing vaginal secretions mixed with saline solution shows organisms with whip-like flagellae that are motile and slightly larger than WBCs (see Figure 15.1 of trichomonad, WBC, and clue cell)
3. In males, collect the first 5-30 mL of an early morning specimen of urine. Examine under microscope for trichomonads

V. Plan/Management

A. Treatment of choice is metronidazole (Flagyl) 2 g orally in a single dose

B. Alternative: Metronidazole (Flagyl) 500 mg twice daily for 7 days

C. FDA has recently approved Flagyl 375 mg BID x 7 days

D. Management of treatment failure
1. If treatment failure occurs with either regimen, retreat with metronidazole (Flagyl) 500 mg twice daily for 7 days
2. If treatment failure occurs frequently, patient should be treated with a 2 g dose of metronidazole QD x 3-5 days

E. Sex partners should be treated and patients should be instructed to avoid sex until they have been cured (after therapy has been completed and patient and partner are asymptomatic)

F. Treatment during pregnancy: Patients should be treated with 2 g of metronidazole in a single dose

G. Follow Up: None indicated for males and females who become asymptomatic after treatment (or who are initially asymptomatic)

CHLAMYDIAL INFECTION

I. Definition: A sexually transmitted disease caused by *Chlamydia trachomatis*

II. Pathogenesis

A. *C. trachomatis,* a bacterial agent with at least 15 serologic variants (serovars) divided between the following two biologic variants: oculogenital (serovars A-K) and LVG (serovars L1-L3); genital infections are caused by serovars B and D-K

B. Infects the genital tract of females most commonly at the transition zone of the endocervix and infects the urethra in males

C. Incubation period is variable but is usually at least 1 week

III. Clinical Presentation

    A. One of the two most frequent causes of cervicitis in females and urethritis in males; *Neisseria gonorrhoeae* is the other

    B. Over 4 million new cases of chlamydial infection occur annually; presently the most common STD in the US

    C. Screening sexually active adolescent females for chlamydial infection is recommended as a routine screening test because of the high prevalence of this infection among females in this age group

    D. In females, several important sequelae can result from infection including PID, ectopic pregnancy, and infertility

    E. In females, chlamydial infection can cause mucopurulent cervicitis, urethritis, salpingitis, and proctitis

    F. In males, chlamydial infection can cause nongonococcal urethritis (NGU) and acute epididymitis (see NGU and EPIDIDYMITIS)

    G. Females may complain of vaginal discharge, dysuria, abnormal vaginal bleeding, and pelvic pain

    H. Males may complain of discharge of mucopurulent or purulent material from the urethra and burning during urination

    I. Asymptomatic infection is common among both males and females

IV. Diagnosis/Evaluation

    A. History
        1. In females, ask about presence of vaginal discharge, dysuria, abnormal bleeding, pelvic pain, and dyspareunia
        2. In females, obtain menstrual history and contraceptive history
        3. In males, ask about presence of mucopurulent/purulent discharge from urethra, presence of burning on urination
        4. Inquire about sexual history including age at first intercourse, number of partners in past year, types of sexual practices, use of condoms
        5. Ask about past history of STDs including types, frequency, and treatment

    B. Physical Examination
        1. In females, perform speculum exam to inspect cervix for mucopurulent discharge from the endocervix. Gently scrape cervix to test for friability
        2. Bimanual exam to check for adnexal tenderness, uterine tenderness, and cervical motion tenderness
        3. In males, examine the urethra for mucopurulent/purulent discharge
        4. In females, obtain specimen of vaginal secretions for wet-prep or Gram stain

    C. Differential Diagnosis
        1. PID in females
        2. Gonorrhea

    D. Diagnostic Tests
        1. Chlamydia culture is most definitive test but is expensive and takes 2-6 days to obtain results
        2. Currently available tests for detection without cell culture include
            a. Direct fluorescent antibody (DFA) staining for elementary bodies in clinical specimens using monoclonal antibody
            b. Enzyme immunoassay (EIA)

         c.   DNA probe

         d.   Nucleic acid amplification (PCR and LCR) [in males, perform test on first-void urine]

    3.   Always test for *N. gonorrhoeae* and also perform microscopic analysis of vaginal secretions (wet-prep or Gram stain)

V. Plan/Treatment

A. Treatment of choice is azithromycin (Zithromax) 1 g orally in a single dose OR doxycycline 100 mg orally BID x 7 days

B. Alternative regimens: Erythromycin base 500 mg orally QID x 7 day; OR erythromycin ethylsuccinate 800 mg orally QID x 7 days OR ofloxacin 300 mg orally BID x 7 days

C. Selecting a treatment
1. Doxycycline has the advantage of low cost and a long history of safety and efficacy
2. Azithromycin has the advantage of single-dose administration and may be more cost effective in patients in whom compliance is an issue (single-dose, directly observed therapy in the clinical setting is possible)
3. Ofloxacin is similar in efficacy to doxycycline and azithromycin, but it is more expensive than doxycycline and offers no advantage in dosing
4. Erythromycin is less efficacious than either azithromycin and doxycycline and gastrointestinal side effects are common and reduce patient compliance
5. Pregnant females should **not** be treated with doxycycline or ofloxacin

D. Treatment of sex partners: Patients should be instructed to refer their sex partners for evaluation and treatment
1. Sex partners should be evaluated and treated if they had sexual contact with the patient during the 60 days preceding onset of symptoms in the patient or diagnosis of chlamydia
2. The most recent sex partner should be treated even if the time of the last sexual contact was >60 days before symptom onset or diagnosis
3. Patients should be instructed to abstain from sexual intercourse until they and their sex partners have completed treatment (i.e., 7 days after a single-dose regimen or after completion of a 7-day regimen)

E. Treatment during pregnancy: Erythromycin base 500 mg orally QID x 7 days OR amoxicillin 500 mg orally TID for 7 days

F. Alternative regimens for pregnant females
1. Erythromycin base 250 mg orally QID x 14 days OR
2. Azithromycin 1 g orally in a single dose

G. Follow Up: None indicated when treated with doxycycline, azithromycin, or ofloxacin; retesting may be considered 3 weeks after completion of treatment with erythromycin

GONORRHEA

I. Definition: A sexually transmitted disease caused by *Neisseria gonorrhoeae,* a Gram-negative diplococcus that prefers columnar and pseudo-stratified epithelium

II. Pathogenesis

A. *N. gonorrhoeae* organisms are Gram-negative diplococci present in exudate and secretions of infected mucous surfaces

B. Transmission results from intimate contact, such as sexual acts and parturition

C. Incubation period is usually 2-7 days

D. Gonococcal infections occur only in humans

III. Clinical Presentation

A. An estimated one million new infections with *N. gonorrhoeae* occur in the US each year

B. Rate of infection is highest in sexually active young adolescents

C. Transmission risk from an infected male to a female is 70% after one exposure; from infected female to male is as low as 20% with one exposure but rises to 60-90% with four exposures

D. At least 20% of neonates of infected females delivered vaginally acquire the disease

E. Most infections among males produce symptoms that cause the person to seek treatment before serious sequelae develop

F. Many infections among females, on the other hand, do not produce symptoms until complications have occurred

G. In females, common sites of infection are the urethra, endocervix, upper genital tract, pharynx, and rectum
   1. Presenting symptoms include increased vaginal discharge, abnormal uterine bleeding, and dysuria
   2. Twenty to forty percent of pelvic inflammatory disease (PID) is caused by gonorrhea
   3. Disseminated disease occurs most often when gonorrhea is acquired during menses or pregnancy; common features of disseminated disease include tenosynovitis, skin lesions, fever, and polyarthralgias
   4. A primary measure for controlling gonorrhea is the screening of high-risk females

H. In males, common sites of infection are the urethra, epididymis, prostate, rectum, and pharynx; disseminated disease may also occur

IV. Diagnosis/Evaluation

A. History
   1. Inquire about onset and duration of symptoms
   2. In females, ask about presence of vaginal discharge, dysuria, abnormal bleeding, abdominal/pelvic pain, and dyspareunia
   3. In females, obtain menstrual history and contraceptive history
   4. In males, ask about dysuria, urethral discharge, rectal pain or discharge
   5. Inquire about sexual history including age at first intercourse, number of partners in past year, types of sexual practices, and use of condoms
   6. Ask about past history of STDs, including types, frequency, treatments

B. Physical Examination
   1. Take temperature to determine if febrile
   2. In females, perform pelvic exam; inspect Bartholin's and Skene's glands for tenderness and enlargement and the urethra for discharge; inspect cervix for mucopurulent discharge; gently scrape cervix to test for friability
   3. In females, perform a bimanual exam to check for adnexal tenderness and masses, for uterine tenderness, and cervical motion tenderness
   4. In males, examine for urethral discharge; if anal sex practiced, perform rectal exam for tenderness and discharge

C. Differential Diagnosis
   1. Pelvic inflammatory disease in females
   2. Chlamydia

D.   Diagnostic Tests
1.   Microscopic examinations of Gram-stained smears (for Gram-negative intracellular diplococci) of exudate from the endocervix in females and the urethra in males are helpful in the initial evaluation
2.   Cervical or urethral culture for *N. gonorrhoeae* using modified Thayer-Martin media
3.   In males, nucleic acid amplification tests on first-void urine
4.   DNA probe can also be used for both males and females to diagnose gonorrhea and chlamydia

V.   Plan/Treatment

A.   Treatment of adolescents with uncomplicated gonococcal infections of the cervix, urethra, and rectum (**Note**: Routine dual therapy for gonococcal and chlamydial infections is necessary)

> Ceftriaxone (Rocephin) 125 mg IM in a single dose
> OR
> Cefixime 400 mg orally in a single dose
> OR
> Ciprofloxacin 500 mg orally in a single dose
> OR
> Ofloxacin 400 mg orally in a single dose
> **PLUS**
> A regimen effective against possible coinfection with C. trachomatis--azithromycin 1 g orally in a single dose OR doxycycline 100 mg orally BID x 7 days

B.   Alternative Regimens: Spectinomycin 2 g IM in a single dose OR ceftizoxime 500 mg IM in a single dose

C.   Many other antimicrobials are active against *N. gonorrhoeae*. See 1998 Guidelines for Treatment of Sexually Transmitted Diseases available from US Department of Health and Human Services, Centers for Disease Control and Prevention (CDC), Atlanta, GA 30333 for additional drugs that can be used

D.   Pregnant females should be treated with a recommended or alternative cephalosporin as listed above. Either erythromycin or amoxicillin should also be used for presumptive or diagnosed chlamydia infection (see CHLAMYDIAL INFECTIONS section above for treatment of pregnant females) [**Note: Pregnant females should not be treated with quinolones or tetracyclines**]

E.   Patients should be instructed to refer sex partners for evaluation and treatment
1.   All sex partners of patients who have *N. Gonorhoeae* should be evaluated and treated for both *N. Gonorhoeae* and *C. Trachomatis* infections if their last sexual contact with the patient was within 60 days before onset of symptoms or diagnosis of infection in the patient
2.   If the patient's most recent sexual encounter was >60 days before onset of symptoms or diagnosis, the patient's most recent sex partner should be treated

F.   Patients should be instructed to avoid sexual intercourse until therapy is completed and symptoms are no longer present

G.   Persons with disseminated gonococcal infection (bacteremia) should be hospitalized for initial parenteral antibiotic therapy

H.   Follow Up
1.   Patients with uncomplicated gonorrhea and who are treated with any of the recommended regimens need not return for a test of cure
2.   Patients with persistent symptoms after treatment need to be re-evaluated for antimicrobial susceptibility
3.   Persistence of symptoms usually results from reinfection rather than treatment failure

MUCOPURULENT CERVICITIS

I. Definition: A sexually transmitted syndrome in which there is purulent or mucopurulent endocervical exudate visible in the endocervical canal or in an endocervical swab specimen

II. Pathogenesis

  A. Mucopurulent cervicitis (MPC) can be caused by *Chlamydia trachomatis* and *Neisseria gonorrhoeae*, but in **most cases** neither organism can be isolated
  B. Other non-microbiologic determinants (e.g., inflammation in an ectropion) could be involved

III. Clinical Presentation

  A. MPC is often asymptomatic, but some females have an abnormal vaginal discharge and vaginal bleeding (e.g., after sexual intercourse)

  B. MPC can persist despite repeated courses of antimicrobial therapy

  C. Some experts consider an increased number of polymorphonuclear leukocytes on Gram stain of endocervical secretions as being helpful in the diagnosis of MPC; however, this criterion has not been standardized and is not available in some settings

  D. Important to keep in mind that most females who have *C. trachomatis* or *N. gonorrhoeae* do not have MPC

IV. Diagnosis/Evaluation

  A. History
    1. Inquire about the onset and duration of symptoms, if present
    2. Ask about presence of vaginal discharge, dysuria, abnormal bleeding particularly after sexual intercourse
    3. Obtain menstrual history and contraceptive history
    4. Inquire about sexual history including age at first intercourse, present partner(s), types of sexual practices, and use of condoms
    5. Inquire about past history of STDs, including types, frequency, treatments

  B. Physical Examination
    1. Determine if febrile
    2. Perform speculum exam to inspect cervix and sample secretions for purulent or mucopurulent discharge; gently scrape cervix to determine friability
    3. Perform bimanual exam, checking for adnexal tenderness, masses

  C. Differential Diagnosis
    1. Urinary tract infection
    2. Chlamydia
    3. Gonorrhea
    4. Trichomonal vaginitis

  D. Diagnostic Tests
    1. Gram stain of endocervical secretions looking for PMNs and intracellular Gram-negative diplococci
    2. DNA probe to test for *C. trachomatis* and *N. gonhrrhoeae*
    3. Wet mount exam for trichomonas
    4. Urine for culture and sensitivity (if symptomatic)

V.   Plan/Management

   A.   Results of tests for *C. trachomatis* and *N. gonorrhoeae* should determine the need for treatment

   B.   Empiric treatment should be considered for patients in whom gonorrhea and/or chlamydia is SUSPECTED if the patient might be difficult to locate for treatment (see GONORRHEA and CHLAMYDIA sections for treatment recommendations)

   C.   Sex partners of females with MPC should be notified, examined, and treated for the STD identified or suspected in the index case

   D.   Follow Up
      1.   Should be as recommended for the infections for which the female is being treated
      2.   If symptoms persist, female should be instructed to return for reevaluation and to abstain from sexual intercourse even if the course of prescribed therapy has been completed

NONGONOCOCCOL URETHRITIS (NGU)

I.   Definition: Inflammation of the urethra not caused by gonococcal infection and characterized by a mucoid or purulent urethral discharge

II.   Pathogenesis

   A.   *Chlamydia trachomatis* is the most frequent cause of NGU (23%-55% of cases)

   B.   Etiology of most cases of nonchlaymdial NGU is unknown; *Ureaplasma urealyticum*, and possibly *Mycoplasma genitalium* are implicated in about one third of cases

   C.   *Trichomonas vaginalis* and HSV sometimes cause NGU

   D.   Complications of NGU among males infected with *C. Trachomatis* include epididymitis and Reiter's syndrome

III.   Clinical Presentation

   A.   Most common STD syndrome in males living in industrialized countries

   B.   NGU is substantially more common than gonococcal urethritis in most areas of US

   C.   Many males are entirely asymptomatic

   D.   In symptomatic males, primary complaints are urethral discharge (yellow, white, or cloudy), dysuria, or urethral itching

   E.   Urethritis can be documented by the presence of **any** of the following signs:
      1.   Mucopurulent or purulent discharge
      2.   Gram stain of urethral secretions demonstrating ≥5 WBCs per oil immersion field
      3.   Positive leukocyte esterase test on first-void urine, or microscopic examination of first-void urine demonstrating ≥10 WBCs per high power field

IV.   Diagnosis/Evaluation

   A.   History
      1.   Ask about onset, duration of symptoms
      2.   Inquire about presence and color of discharge, presence of dysuria, and urethral itching

3. Inquire about sexual history including age at first intercourse, number of partners in the past year, types of sexual practices, use of condoms
4. Inquire about past history of STDs, including types, frequency, and treatments

B. Physical Examination: Examine urethra for mucopurulent discharge

C. Differential Diagnosis: Gonorrhea

D. Diagnostic Tests
1. Gram-stain urethral smear (>5 WBCs per oil immersion field PLUS no intracellular Gram-negative diplococci are expected findings)
2. Positive leukocyte esterase test on first void urine, or microscopic examination of first-void urine demonstrating ≥10 WBCs per high power field
3. Test for *N. gonorrhoeae* and *C. trachomatis* using DNA probe

V. Plan/Treatment

A. If none of the criteria for confirming urethritis are met (see III. E. above), treatment should be deferred until the test results for *N. gonorrhoeae* and *C. trachomatis* tests are obtained
1. If the results are positive for either infection, the appropriate treatment should be given and sex partners referred for evaluation and treatment
2. Empiric treatment of symptoms without documentation of urethritis is recommended only for patients at high risk for infection who are unlikely to return for follow-up (such patients should be treated for both gonorrhea and chlamydia) [see GONORRHEA and CHLAMYDIA for treatment recommendations]

B. Management of sex partners: Should be evaluated and treated appropriately based on evaluation (see exposure intervals to base treatment on under section on CHLAMYDIA)

C. Recurrent NGU may be due to a lack of compliance, or more often, reinfection by untreated sex partner
1. Males with persistent or recurrent urethritis should be re-treated with the initial regimen if they failed to comply with the treatment regimen or if they were re-exposed to an untreated sex partner
2. Otherwise, a wet mount exam and culture of an intraurethral swab specimen for *T. vaginalis* should be performed;
3. If negative, the man should be retreated with an alternative regimen extended to 14 days (e.g., erythromycin base 500 mg orally 4 times a day for 14 days)
4. Refer for evaluation by an expert if objective signs of urethritis continue after adequate treatment

D. Follow Up: None required unless patient remains symptomatic

PELVIC INFLAMMATORY DISEASE (PID)

I. Definition: A spectrum of inflammatory disorders of the upper female genital tract, including any combination of endometritis, salpingitis, tubo-ovarian abscess, and pelvic abscess, and pelvic peritonitis

II. Pathogenesis

A. Sexually transmitted organisms, especially *Neisseria gonorrhoeae* and *Chlamydia trachomatis*, are implicated in most cases

B. Microorganisms that can be part of the vaginal flora (e.g., anaerobes, *G. vaginalis*, *H. influenzae*, enteric Gram-negative rods, and *Streptococcus agalactiae*) also can cause PID

C. In addition, *M. hominis* and *U. urealyticum* might be etiologic agents of PID

III.   Clinical Presentation

   A.   Incidence of PID is highest among sexually active adolescents

   B.   Variables that **increase** risk of PID include adolescence, multiple sex partners, previous episode of STD, use of an intrauterine device, and douching

   C.   Variables that **decrease** risk include use of oral contraceptives, barrier contraceptives, and spermicide use

   D.   Most typical presentation is continuous bilateral lower abdominal or pelvic pain that may be accompanied by fever, nausea, and vomiting

   E.   In many patients the infection is asymptomatic (silent PID) or symptoms are vague and mild with abnormal vaginal bleeding, dyspareunia, or change in vaginal discharge as the only signs and symptoms (atypical PID)

   F.   PID symptoms most often begin within one week of onset of menses

   G.   The diagnosis of PID usually is based on clinical findings; no single historical, physical, or laboratory finding is both sensitive and specific for the diagnosis

   H.   The following recommendations for diagnosing PID are made by the CDC to help health-care providers recognize when PID should be suspected and when there is a need to obtain additional information to increase diagnostic certainty

DIAGNOSTIC CRITERIA FOR PID
Minimum Criteria
Empiric treatment of PID should be instituted in sexually active young females and others at risk for STDs if all the following **minimum criteria** are present and no other cause(s) for the illness can be identified ✤ Lower abdominal tenderness ✤ Adnexal tenderness, and ✤ Cervical motion tenderness
Additional Criteria
For females with severe clinical signs, more elaborate diagnostic evaluation is warranted because incorrect diagnosis and management may cause unnecessary morbidity. These additional criteria may be used to increase the specificity of the minimum criteria listed above Listed below are the **additional criteria** that support a diagnosis of PID ✤ Oral temperature >101°F (>38.3°C) ✤ Abnormal cervical or vaginal discharge ✤ Elevated erythrocyte sedimentation rate ✤ Elevated C-reactive protein ✤ Laboratory documentation of cervical infection with *N. gonorrhoeae* or *C. trachomatis*
Definitive Criteria
The **definitive criteria** for diagnosing PID include the following ✤ Histopathologic evidence of endometritis on endometrial biopsy ✤ Transvaginal sonography or other imaging techniques showing thickened fluid-filled tubes with or without free pelvic fluid or tubo-ovarian complex, and ✤ Laparoscopic abnormalities consistent with PID

Source: Centers for Disease Control and Prevention. (1998). 1998 guidelines for treatment of sexually transmitted diseases. MMWR, 47(No.RR-1), 80.

IV.   Diagnosis/Evaluation

    A.   History
        1.   Ask about presence of lower abdominal/pelvic pain, including onset, duration, location, and character or pain
        2.   Ask the patient if she has had fever
        3.   Inquire about presence of vaginal discharge, postcoital bleeding, spotting between menstrual periods, fever, and gastrointestinal symptoms
        4.   Obtain sexual history including age at first intercourse, number of partners in past year, types of sexual practices, and contraceptive history (ask if IUD is used)
        5.   Inquire about past history of STDs, including type, frequency, treatments; ask about HIV+ status.
        6.   Obtain complete menstrual history including pattern of recent menstrual cycles and a description of the last menses (Ask: "Did onset of pain coincide with LMP?")

    B.   Physical Examination
        1.   Determine if febrile
        2.   Examine abdomen for tenderness, masses, signs of peritonitis
        3.   On speculum exam, inspect cervix for inflammation; insert a cotton swab into cervix to sample mucus and examine its gross appearance. (A thick transparent discharge similar to styling gel is normal; secretions that appear yellow on a cotton-tipped swab are not normal)
        4.   Perform bimanual exam to check for adnexal masses, uterine tenderness, and for cervical motion tenderness (pain that occurs when cervix is moved from side to side)

    C.   Differential Diagnosis
        1.   Appendicitis
        2.   Ectopic pregnancy
        3.   Tubo-ovarian abscess
        4.   Ovarian cyst
        5.   Pyelonephritis

    D.   Diagnostic Tests
        1.   Pregnancy Test
        2.   Endocervical and rectal cultures for *N. gonorrhoeae* and an endocervical test for *C. trachomatis* should be obtained before treatment
        3.   CBC with differential and sedimentation rate
        4.   Wet prep or Gram stain of endocervical secretions
            a.   If number of epithelial cells > than number of WBCs per high-powered field, then patient almost certainly does not have PID
            b.   If number of WBCs > epithelial cells per high powered field, patient may have PID
        5.   VDRL or RPR

V.   Plan/Management

    A.   Inpatient therapy for every case of PID is unrealistic. The CDC has made recommendations for when to select inpatient therapy and these recommendations are contained in the following table

---

SITUATIONS WHEN HOSPITALIZATION OF PATIENTS WITH ACUTE PID IS INDICATED

✓ Diagnosis is uncertain, and surgical emergencies such as appendicitis and ectopic pregnancy cannot be excluded

✓ Patient has a tubo-ovarian abscess

✓ Patient is pregnant

✓ Patient has severe illness, nausea and vomiting, or high fever

✓ Patient is immunodeficient

✓ Patient fails to respond clinically to oral antimicrobial therapy

✓ Patients is unable to follow or tolerate an outpatient oral regimen

---

B.   Outpatient therapy for PID is described in the table below

RECOMMENDED REGIMENS FOR AMBULATORY TREATMENT OF ACUTE PID
Regimen A
Ofloxacin 400 mg orally BID for 14 days **PLUS** Metronidazole 500 mg orally BID for 14 days
Regimen B
Cefoxitin 2 g IM <u>plus</u> Probenecid 1 g orally in a single dose concurrently, **OR** ceftriaxone 250 mg IM in a single dose, **OR** other parenteral equivalent third-generation cephalosporin **PLUS** Doxycycline 100 mg orally BID for 14 days

C.   Management of sex partners:
　　1.   Sex partners of patients with PID should be examined and treated if they had sexual contact with patient during the 60 day period preceding onset of symptoms in patient
　　2.   Evaluation and treatment of sex partners of females with PID is imperative because of the risk of reinfection
　　3.   Sex partners should be treated empirically with regimens effective against both *C. trachomatis* and *N. gonorrhoeae* regardless of the apparent etiology of PID

D.   Counsel female about importance of using condoms to prevent STDs and also importance of partner treatment

E.   Follow Up
　　1.   Patients treated on an ambulatory basis need to be monitored closely and reevaluated in 72 hours for clinical improvement (**Note**: Clinical improvement is defined as defervescence; reduction in direct or rebound abdominal tenderness; reduction in uterine, adnexal, and cervical motion tenderness within 3 days after initiation of therapy)
　　2.   Patients who do not demonstrate improvement within this time require additional diagnostic test, surgical intervention, or both
　　3.   Some experts recommend rescreening for *C. trachomatis* and *N. gonorrhoeae* 4-6 weeks after therapy is completed

SYPHILIS

I.   Definition: A systemic sexually transmitted disease involving multiple organ systems and caused by *Treponema pallidum*, a spirochete

II.   Pathogenesis

A.   *T. pallidum* is a thin, delicate organism with humans as the sole host

B.   Organism penetrates intact skin or mucous membrane during sexual contact, multiplies, and rapidly spreads to regional lymph nodes

C.   Spirochetes enter the blood stream within hours and are transported to other tissues

D.   Congenital syphilis results from transplacental passage of the organism

E.   Incubation period for acquired primary syphilis is about 3 weeks, but ranges from 10-90 days after exposure

III. Clinical Presentation

    A.   Since the end of the nationwide syphilis epidemic between 1986 and 1990, the syphilis rate has never been lower in the US, having declined by 84% between 1990 and 1997

        1.   The syphilis rate has declined 95% in the Northeast, 91% in the West, 80% in the South, and 73% in the Midwest

        2.   Despite declines in the South, that region has the highest syphilis rate in the nation

    B.   To guide therapeutic decisions and disease intervention strategies, acquired syphilis has been divided into the following clinical stages: Primary, secondary, latent, and tertiary

    C.   Primary syphilis: Characterized by appearance of ulcer or chancre at site of inoculation, usually on genitals 3-4 weeks after exposure

        1.   Genital lesions are usually indurated and painless

        2.   Extragenital lesions (e.g., lips, breast) are often painful

        3.   Regional lymphadenopathy usually present

        4.   Chancre persists for 1-5 weeks and heals spontaneously

    D.   Secondary syphilis: Occurs about 6-8 weeks later and is characterized by flu-like symptoms -- headache, generalized arthralgia, malaise, fever, and lymphadenopathy, followed by a generalized rash

        1.   Rash is macular, papular, annular, or follicular; often involves the palms and soles

        2.   Rash persists for 2-6 weeks then spontaneously heals

        3.   Mucous patches often occur in mouth, throat, on cervix; flat, papular lesions (condylomata lata) occur in intertriginous areas

        4.   About 25% of infected persons have at least one cutaneous relapse

        5.   Secondary syphilis is the most contagious state of the disease

        6.   Even without treatment, signs of first 2 stages resolve spontaneously, and persons enter the next state: the latent state

    E.   Latent syphilis: Arbitrarily divided into early and late latent stages

        1.   Infection of <1 year is defined as early latent (infectious)

        2.   Infections of >1 year is late latent or syphilis of unknown duration (non-infectious)

        3.   Difficult to make this distinction in practice, because exact date of infection is usually difficult to establish

        4.   Latent syphilis begins with the healing of the lesions in the secondary stage and may last a few years or a lifetime

        5.   About 1/3 of persons with latent syphilis are little inconvenienced by the disease

        6.   After a variable period of latency, about 1/3 of untreated cases go on to develop tertiary syphilis, and about 28% of these will die because of the disease

    F.   Tertiary syphilis: May take the form of gummatous, cardiovascular (both rare forms), or neurosyphilis

    G.   Congenital syphilis involves multiple organ systems with the stage of syphilis in the mother determining the effects on the fetus

        1.   Early congenital syphilis occurs from birth to age 2 and is characterized by mucocutaneous lesions, rhinitis, and other symptoms

        2.   Congenital syphilis can be asymptomatic, especially in the first weeks of life

        3.   Late congenital syphilis is characterized by bone and joint disorders, cranial neuropathies, and interstitial keratitis which causes blindness if untreated

IV. Diagnosis/Evaluation

    A.   History

        1.   Question about onset, duration of symptoms

        2.   Ask about presence or history of chancre (when it appeared, where located, if symptomatic, when healed)

        3.   Ask about presence (or history of) rash, mucous patches, condylomata lata

        4.   Ask about sexual behavior, use of condoms

5. Ask if sex partner has had similar symptoms
6. Ask about past history of STDs, including types, frequency, duration, treatment
7. Ask about HIV status
8. Obtain past medical history, medication history, drug and alcohol use, allergies

B. Physical Examination
1. Examine genital area and other skin surfaces (breast, buttocks) for characteristic chancre (primary syphilis)
2. Look for mucocutaneous lesions of secondary syphilis

C. Differential Diagnosis
1. Primary syphilis: Syphilis can mimic all lesions that appear to be genital ulcers: genital herpes, chancroid, lymphogranuloma venereum, scabies, balanitis should all be suspect
2. Secondary syphilis: Syphilis can mimic many skin disorders: all undiagnosed mucous or cutaneous eruptions should be suspect

D. Diagnostic Tests
1. Darkfield microscopy and direct fluorescent antibody tests of lesion exudate or tissue are the definitive methods for diagnosing early syphilis
2. A presumptive diagnosis is possible with the use of two types of serologic tests for syphilis
   a. Nontreponeal-specific tests: rapid plasma reagin (RPR) test and Venereal Disease Research Laboratory (VDRL) test
   b. Treponemal-specific tests: Fluorescent Treponemal antibody absorbed (FTA-ABS) and microhemagglutination assay for antibody to *T. Pallidum* (MHA-TP)
3. VDRL and RPR are used for initial screening and titers; fall in titer correlates with response to therapy; RPR is test most often used today, but the tests are comparable
4. For sequential serologic tests, the same test (VDRL or RPR) should be used
5. Treponemal tests are used to confirm diagnosis of syphilis in persons with positive VDRL or RPR
   a. Usually remains positive for life regardless of treatment or disease activity
   b. Reported as positive or negative

V. Plan/Treatment

A. Treatment is based on clinical and serologic staging of the disease and is summarized in the following table

RECOMMENDED TREATMENT OF SYPHILIS IN ADOLESCENTS	
Stage	**Treatment**
Primary, secondary, and early latent disease	Benzathine penicillin G 2.4 million units IM in a single dose. For patients allergic to penicillin: doxycycline 100 mg orally BID x 14 days, or tetracycline 500 mg orally QID x 14 days
Late latent syphilis or syphilis of unknown duration	Benzathine penicillin G 7.2 million units total, given as three doses of 2.4 million units IM each at 1-week intervals. For patients allergic to penicillin: doxycycline 100 mg orally BID for 4 weeks, or tetracycline 500 mg orally QID x 4 weeks
Tertiary disease, excluding neurosyphilis	As for late latent disease, with appropriate management of complications
Neurosyphilis	Aqueous crystalline penicillin G, 18-24 million units/day given as 3-4 million units IV every 4 hours for 10-14 days, or procaine penicillin 2-4 million units IM a day PLUS Probenecid 500 mg orally QID both for 10-14 days
Exposure: Sexual contacts of persons with infectious syphilis	Refer to MANAGEMENT OF SEX PARTNERS table below

B.   Management of sex partners should be guided by the following recommendations

MANAGEMENT OF SEX PARTNERS
Patients exposed sexually to a patient who has syphilis in any stage should be evaluated both clinically and serologically as follows:
Persons exposed within the 90 days preceding the diagnosis of primary, secondary, or early latent syphilis in a sex partner might be infected even if seronegative--**Treat presumptively**
Persons exposed >90 days before the diagnosis of primary, secondary, or early latent syphilis in a sex partner and in whom serologic test results are not available immediately and the opportunity for follow-up is uncertain--**Treat presumptively**
For purposes of **partner notification and presumptive treatment of exposed sex partners,** patients with syphilis of unknown duration with high nontreponemal serologic test titers (defined as ≥1:32) may be considered as having early syphilis
Note: Serologic titers should not be used to differentiate early from late latent syphilis for the purpose of determining treatment for the index case

C.   Congenital syphilis
    1.   Infants born to seroreactive mothers should be evaluated with a quantitative nontreponemal serologic test (RPR or VDRL)
        a.   Test should be performed on infant serum
        b.   Umbilical cord blood may be contaminated with maternal blood and might yield a false-positive result
        c.   A treponemal test of a newborn's serum is not necessary
    2.   Evaluation of infant includes the following
        a.   Complete physical exam of neonate for evidence of congenital syphilis
        b.   Examination of the placenta or umbilical cord using specific fluorescent antitreponemal antibody staining
        c.   Darkfield microscopic examination or direct fluorescent antibody staining of any suspicious lesions or body fluids (example, nasal discharge)
    3.   Consult expert regarding therapy decisions and treatment guidelines for all infants born to seroreactive mothers

D.   Syphilis in HIV infected persons
    1.   Diagnostic considerations
        a.   Both treponemal and non-treponemal serologic tests for syphilis can be interpreted in usual manner for most patients who are coinfected with *T. pallidum* and HIV
        b.   When clinical findings suggest syphilis, but serologic tests are nonreactive or unclear, alternate tests such as biopsy of lesion, darkfield examination or direct fluorescent antibody staining of lesion material may be helpful
    2.   Treatment
        a.   Treatment the same as for HIV-negative patients is recommended
        b.   HIV-infected patients who have either late latent syphilis or syphilis of unknown duration should have a CSF examination before treatment

E.   Follow Up
    1.   Patients with primary and secondary syphilis should be examined clinically and serologically at 6 months and 12 months; more frequent evaluation may be prudent if follow-up is uncertain
    2.   If nontreponemal antibody titers (either VDRL or RPR) have not declined fourfold within 6 months after therapy for primary or secondary syphilis, person is at risk or treatment failure
    3.   Optimal management of such patients is unclear, but the following steps should be taken
        a.   First, reevaluate for HIV infection (if positive for HIV, see V.D. above)
        b.   Then, provide more frequent follow-up (every 3 months instead of 6)
        c.   If additional follow-up cannot be ensured, re-treatment is recommended
        d.   Note: Some experts recommend CSF examination in such situations
        e.   Retreatment (according to most experts): 3 weekly injections of benazthine penicillin G 2.4 million units IM [unless CSF examination indicates neurosyphilis is present]
    4.   Patients with latent syphilis should be followed up with non-treponemal serologic testing at 6, 12, and 24 months; patient should be evaluated for neurosyphilis and retreated appropriately if

       a.   Titers increase fourfold

       b.   An initially high titer ($\geq$ 1:32) fails to decline at least fourfold within 12-24 months

       c.   Signs or symptoms attributable to syphilis develop in the patient

F.   HIV infected persons should have more frequent follow up, including serologic testing at 3, 6, 9, 12, and 24 months after therapy

GENITAL HERPES SIMPLEX VIRUS INFECTION

I.   Definition: Infections with herpes simplex viruses, large DNA viruses. Two major types have genomic and antigenic differences--Type 1 (HSV-1) usually involves the face and skin above the waist, but an increasing number of genital herpes cases are attributable to HSV-1; Type 2 (HSV-2) usually involves the genitalia and skin below the waist in sexually active adolescents (see SKIN PROBLEMS IN CHILDREN AND ADOLESCENTS for Herpes Simplex infections of the skin and mucous membranes)

II.   Pathogenesis

    A.   HSV-1 and HSV-2 are epidermotropic viruses with infection occurring within keratinocytes

    B.   Transmission is only by direct contact with active lesions, or by virus-containing fluid such as saliva or cervical secretions in persons with no evidence of active disease

    C.   Inoculation of the virus into skin or mucosal surfaces produces infection, with an incubation period of 2-14 days

    D.   About 48 hours after entering the host, the virus transverses afferent nerves to find host ganglion
        1.   The trigeminal ganglia are the target of the oral virus -- primarily HSV-1
        2.   The sacral ganglia are the target of the genital virus -- most often HSV-2

    E.   Upon reactivation, the virus retraces its route, causing recurrence in the cutaneous area affected by the same nerve root, but not necessarily in the original site

    F.   Generally HSV-1 is associated with infection of the lips, face, buccal mucosa, and throat; HSV-2, with the genitalia

    G.   In spite of the distinctive sites of herpetic lesions with each serotype, there is overlap in site of infection in approximately 25% of individuals who are infected
        1.   Type 1 strains can be recovered from the genital tract
        2.   Type 2 strains probably can be recovered from the pharynx as a result of oral-genital activity
        3.   Whereas type 1 HSV genital infections in children also can result from autoinoculation of virus from the mouth, sexual abuse must always be considered in prepubertal children with genital herpes

III.   Clinical Presentation

    A.   Based on serologic studies, approximately 45 million persons in the US have been diagnosed with genital HSV-2

    B.   Most HSV-2 infected persons have not received a diagnosis of genital herpes
        1.   Infections in these persons are either mild or unrecognized with the virus shed intermittently in the genital tract
        2.   Many cases are transmitted by persons unaware that they are infected or asymptomatic when transmission occurs

    C.   A small minority of first-episode genital herpes cases are manifest by severe disease that requires hospitalization

    D.   The usual sequence of disease in which signs/symptoms occur is painful papules followed by vesicles, ulceration, crusting, and healing

E. First clinical episode of genital herpes
   1. Symptoms of primary infection that is symptomatic often consists of hyperesthesia, burning, itching, dysuria, pain, and tenderness in the genital area
   2. Fever and lymphadenopathy are frequently present
   3. More systemic manifestations are present than with recurrent episodes
   4. Viral shedding is prolonged (average 12 days) and healing of lesions takes 21 days on average
   5. Persons with genital infection with HSV-1 (about 20-30% of patients with first episode herpes) have a much lower risk of symptomatic recurrent outbreaks

F. Recurrent episodes of HSV infection
   1. Most patients (about 50%) with symptomatic first episode HSV-2 infection will have recurrent episodes within 6 months after the first clinical episode
   2. Frequently have prodrome with recurrence
   3. Lesions often localized in recurrent episodes
   4. Length of viral shedding reduced compared to primary episode (average 7 days)
   5. Healing of lesions is also faster (5 days on average)

IV. Diagnosis/Evaluation

A. History
   1. Question regarding location, onset, duration, and appearance of lesions; ask if pain, burning, or paresthesia present prior to eruption
   2. Ask about associated symptoms of fever, myalgia, malaise
   3. Ask regarding previous occurrence of similar lesions, symptoms
   4. Inquire about exposures to infected persons and use of condoms

B. Physical Examination
   1. Examine genital area for characteristic location, distribution, appearance of lesions
   2. Check for enlarged lymph nodes in inguinal area

C. Differential Diagnosis
   1. Syphilis
   2. Chancroid
   3. Folliculitis
   4. Molluscum contagiosum

D. Diagnostic Tests
   1. Viral culture is the most sensitive and commonly available test for confirming the diagnosis of genital herpes
      a. Unroof vesicle and scrape the material with Dacron-tipped swab
      b. Place swab in viral transport media
      c. Virus grows rapidly and cultures may be positive within 2-3 days (can take longer)
      d. Additional advantage of culture is that it permits viral typing which is useful prognostic information for patients with primary episodes (**Note**: Patients with genital infection with HSV-1 have a much lower risk of symptomatic recurrent outbreaks)
   2. Direct fluorescent antibody test is an alternative when viral culture is not possible
      a. Yield rapid results at a relatively low cost
      b. Most antigen tests do not differentiate HSV-1 from HSV-2
   3. The Tzanck test is not recommended by the CDC for diagnosing HSV infection

V. Plan/Management

    A.   Management of first clinical episode of genital herpes is outlined in the following table

---

RECOMMENDED REGIMENS: FIRST CLINICAL EPISODE

Select one of the following regimens

Acyclovir 400 mg orally TID x 7-10 days
Acyclovir 200 mg orally 5 times/day x 7-10 days

Famciclovir 250 mg orally TID x 7-10 days
Valacyclovir 1 g orally BID x 7-10 days

Note: Treatment may be extended if healing is incomplete after 10 days of therapy

---

COUNSELING FOR MANAGEMENT OF PATIENTS WITH GENITAL HERPES

Natural history of the disease with emphasis on recurrent episodes, asymptomatic viral shedding, and sexual transmission
    Sexual transmission can occur during asymptomatic periods
    Asymptomatic viral shedding occurs more frequently in persons with genital HSV-2 than
        HSV-1 and also occurs more frequently in those with infection <12 months

After first episode,
    Episodic antiviral therapy during recurrent episodes might shorten duration
    Suppressive antiviral therapy can modulate or prevent recurrences

There is a risk for neonatal infection in pregnant females

Importance of use of condoms during all sexual exposures

Need to abstain from all sexual activity when lesions or prodromal symptoms are present

---

    B.   Management of recurrent episodes of HSV infection is outlined in the following table

---

RECOMMENDED REGIMENS FOR EPISODIC RECURRENT INFECTION

Select one of the following regimens

Acyclovir 400 mg orally TID x 5 days
Acyclovir 200 mg orally 5 x/day x 5 days
Acyclovir 800 mg orally BID x 5 days

Famciclovir 125 mg orally BID x 5 days
Valacyclovir 500 mg orally BID x 5 days

Options for treatment of recurrent episodes should be discussed with all patients
Treatment is most efficacious when begun during the prodrome or within 1 day after onset of lesions

If treatment for recurrence is chosen, patient should be provided with antiviral therapy, or a prescription for the medication, so that treatment can be initiated at the first sign of prodrome or genital lesions

---

RECOMMENDED REGIMENS FOR DAILY SUPPRESSIVE THERAPY

Select one of the following regimens

Acyclovir 400 mg orally BID
Famciclovir 250 mg orally BID

Valacyclovir 500 mg orally QD*
Valacyclovir 1,000 mg orally QD

Daily suppressive therapy reduces the frequency of genital herpes recurrences by ≥75% among patients who have frequent recurrences (defined as 6 or more recurrences per year)

Suppressive therapy with acyclovir reduces but does not eliminate asymptomatic viral shedding

Suppressive therapy has not been associated with emergence of acyclovir resistance among immunocompetent patients

After 12 months of continuous suppressive therapy, discontinuation should be discussed with patient

Famciclovir and valacyclovir should **not be used for over 12 months**

Safety and efficacy have been documented among patients using daily acyclovir for as long as 6 years

---

*May be less effective than other dosing regimens of valacyclovir in patients with ≥10 outbreaks per year

C. Management of sex partners
   1. Can usually benefit from evaluation and counseling
   2. Symptomatic sex partners should be evaluated and treated

D. Lesions caused by HSV are common among HIV-infected patients and may be severe
   1. Whereas the dosage of antiviral drugs for HIV-infected persons is controversial, clinical experience suggests the need for increased doses of antiviral drugs
   2. For initial and recurrent episodes, acyclovir 400 mg PO 3-5x/day, continued until clinical resolution is obtained is recommended
   3. For suppressive therapy, famciclovir 500 mg PO BID has been shown to be effective in decreasing the recurrence rate
   4. For severe cases, patients should be referred for expert care

E. Consult a specialist for management of pregnant females with HSV infection (**Note**: The safety of acyclovir and valacyclovir therapy in pregnant females has not been established)

F. Infants exposed to HSV during birth, as proven by virus isolation or presumed by observation of lesions should be followed by a specialist

G. Follow Up: None indicated

HUMAN PAPILLOMAVIRUS INFECTION (GENITAL WARTS)

I. Definition: A sexually transmitted disease caused by certain types of the human papillomavirus (HPV) that produces epithelial tumors of the skin and mucous membranes

II. Pathogenesis

A. Of the more than 60 HPV types identified in humans, more than 20 infect the lower genital tract

B. The virus enters the body via an epithelial defect and infects the stratified squamous epithelium of the lower genital tract

C. Visible genital warts usually are caused by HPV types 6 or 11

D. Other HPV types in the anogenital region--types 16, 18, and 31--have been strongly associated with cervical dysplasia

III. Clinical Presentation

A. Most HPV infections are asymptomatic, subclinical, or unrecognized

B. Genital warts are generally benign growths that cause minor or no symptoms aside from their cosmetic appearance

C. HPV infections are very common and account for an increasing proportion of primary care gynecologic visits

D. Clinical HPV infections develop following an incubation period of unknown length but is estimated to range from 3 months to several years

E. Present as small flesh-colored warty lesions

F. In males, warts may be found on shaft of penis, penile meatus, scrotum, and perianal areas

G. In females, warts are seen on labia and perianal areas with asymptomatic nonverrucous infections occurring in the vagina and on the cervix

H. Most anogenital infections are asymptomatic but can sometimes cause itching, burning, local pain, or bleeding

I. Individual warts may become confluent and appear as a single, large fleshy lesion

J. Growth of warts may be stimulated by pregnancy, oral contraceptive use, immunosuppression, and local trauma

IV. Diagnosis/Evaluation

A. History
1. Question about location, onset, duration, and presence of any associated symptoms
2. Inquire about exposures to sexually transmitted diseases (unprotected intercourse)
3. Ask if partner has similar lesions
4. Inquire about past history of HPV
5. Question regarding pregnancy, use of oral contraceptives, and immune status

B. Physical Examination
1. Examine external genitalia and rectal areas for characteristic lesions
2. To assist in visualization of warts, apply 3-5% acetic acid to the vulva (females), penis (males) and perianal areas to reveal acetowhitening
3. Perform Pap smear in females to detect cervical dysplasia

C. Differential Diagnosis
1. Herpes simplex
2. Syphilis

D. Diagnostic Tests: Most anogenital warts are diagnosed by clinical inspection

V. Plan/Management

A. Primary goal of treating visible warts is the removal of symptomatic warts
1. Treatment can induce wart-free periods in most patients
2. Currently available treatments do not affect the natural history of HPV infection
3. Most genital warts are asymptomatic and many warts resolve on their own, when left untreated
4. There is no evidence that treatment of visible warts affects development of cervical cancer in females

---

OVERVIEW OF TREATMENT

Treatment of genital warts should be guided by
  Preference of the patients after they have been informed of the options
  Available resources
  Experience of health care provider

Most patients have 1-10 warts with a total wart area of 0.5-1.0 cm^2
Most warts are responsive to most treatment modalities

Factors that influence selection of treatment
  Wart size and number   Patient preference
  Anatomic site of wart   Convenience and cost of treatment
  Wart morphology   Provider experience

Treatment protocol is important because many patients require a course of therapy rather than a single treatment!
  Treatment modality should be changed if
    Patient has not improved substantially after 3 provider-administered treatments, OR
    Warts have not cleared after 6 treatments

Avoid overtreatment!

To increase efficiency and efficacy, providers should be knowledgeable about
  At least one patient-applied treatment
  At least one provider-administered treatment

Note: Most experts believe that combining modalities does not increase efficacy but may increase complications; therefore, it is best to not combine therapies (use two or more modalities on same wart at same time)

Because of the limitations of currently available treatments, some providers employ combination therapy

---

EXTERNAL GENITAL WARTS: RECOMMENDED TREATMENT

Patient-Applied (**Note**: for patient-applied treatments, patient must be able to identify and reach warts!)

Podofilox 0.5% solution or gel
Dosing: Apply BID x 3 days, followed by 4 days of no therapy
Repeat cycle as necessary for a total of 4 cycles
Instruction to patient:
Apply solution with cotton swab, gel with finger to visible genital warts
Total wart area treated should be ≤ 10 cm^2, and total volume of podofilox should be ≤ 0.5 mL per day
Most patients experience mild/moderate pain or local irritation after treatment
If possible, provider should apply initial treatment to demonstrate proper application technique and identify
    which warts should be treated
Not for use in pregnancy

Imiquimod 5% cream
Dosing: Apply QD at bedtime, 3 times/week for as long as 16 weeks
Instructions to patient:
Apply cream with a finger at bedtime and wash off with mild soap/water after 6-10 hours
Many patients may be clear of warts by 8-10 weeks
Not for use in pregnancy

Provider-Administered

Select **one** of the following
    Cryotherapy with liquid nitrogen or cryoprobe
    Repeat applications Q 1-2 weeks
    Pain after application followed by necrosis and sometimes blistering are common

Note: Major limitation of this modality is that proper use requires substantial training; most warts are overtreated or undertreated by providers who have not been trained resulting in poor efficacy or increased complications

Podophyllin resin 10%-25% in compound tincture of benzoin
Apply small amount to each wart and allow to air dry
Limit application to ≤ 0.5 mL of podophyllin or ≤ 10 cm^2 of warts per session
Instruct patient to thoroughly wash preparation off 1-4 hours after application
Repeat weekly if necessary
Not for use in pregnancy

TCA or BCA 80%-90%
Apply small amount to warts only
Allow to dry--a white "frosting" develops
Powder with talc or sodium bicarbonate to remove untreated acid (if excess amount was applied)
Repeat weekly if necessary

B.   For treatment of cervical and vaginal warts, referral to an expert is recommended

C.   For treatment of urethral meatus warts, referral to an expert is recommended

D.   For treatment of anal warts, use of cryotherapy with liquid nitrogen or TCA or BCA 80%-90%; apply as directed above under EXTERNAL GENITAL WARTS: RECOMMENDED TREATMENT

E.   Management of warts on rectal mucosa should be referred to an expert

F.   Subclinical genital HPV infection (without exophytic warts)
1.   Subclinical genital HPV infection occurs more frequently than visible warts in both males and females
2.   Infection is usually diagnosed via Pap smear, colposcopy, or biopsy of vulva in females, and via biopsy of penis in males. In both males and females, the use of acetic acid soaks and examination of genital skin with light and magnification may be helpful
3.   Screening for subclinical genital HPV infection using DNA or RNA tests or acetic acid is not recommended
4.   In the absence of coexistent dysplasia, treatment is not recommended for subclinical genital HPV infection diagnosed via Pap smear, colposcopy, biopsy, acetic acid soaking of genital skin/mucous membranes, or DNA/RNA methodologies

G. Management of pregnant females: Refer to specialist

H. Management of sexual partners
1. Examination of partners not necessary because most partners of infected patients probably are already infected subclinically with HPV
2. Partner should be cautioned that patient remains infectious even though warts are gone
3. Use of condoms reduces, but does not eliminate risk of transmission

I. Recommendations relating to cervical cancer screening for females who attend STD clinics or have a history of STDs
1. If female has not had a Pap smear during previous 12 months, a Pap smear should be obtained as part of the routine pelvic examination
2. Provide female with printed information about Pap smears and a report containing a statement that a Pap smear was obtained during her clinic visit
3. A copy of the Pap smear result should be provided to the patient for her records
4. **Note:** Females who have a history of STD are at increased risk for cervical cancer
5. Counsel female about need for an annual Pap smear, and provide her with names of local clinics/providers where Pap smears can be obtained on an annual basis

J. Follow Up
1. After visible warts have cleared (which may require several visits for provider-administered treatments), a follow-up evaluation is not necessary
2. Patient should be advised to watch for recurrences, which occur most often during first 3 months after treatment
3. Females should be reminded of the need for regular cytologic screening (Pap smear) as recommended for females without genital warts [annual screening]

REFERENCES

American Medical Association. (1997). Genital herpes: A clinician's guide to diagnosis and treatment, part I. Chicago: Author.

American Medical Association. (1997). Genital herpes: A clinician's guide to diagnosis and treatment, part II. Chicago: Author.

Baker, D.A. (1997). Diagnosis and treatment of viral STDs in women. International Journal of Fertility, 42 (2), 107-114.

Centers for Disease Control and Prevention. (1998). 1998 guidelines for treatment of sexually transmitted. Morbidity and Mortality Weekly Report, 47(No. RR-1)

Cox, J.T. (1998). HPV testing: Is it useful in triage of minor pap abnormalities? Journal of Family Practice, 46 (2), 121-132.

Dull, P., & Miller, K.E. (1997). STDs in women: An update. Family Practice Recertification, 19 (6), 13-30.

Eschenbach, D.A. (1996). Diagnosis and treatment of vaginitis. In M.A. Stenchever (Ed.). Office gynecology. St. Louis: Mosby.

Faro, S., Apuzzio, J., Bohannon, N., & Elliott, K. (1997). Treatment considertions in vulvovaginal candidiasis. The Female Patient, 22, 21-36.

Hook, E.W., & Marra, C.M. (1992). Acquired syphilis in adults. New England Journal of Medicine, 326(16), 1060-1067.

Mayeaus, E.J., & Spigener, S.S. (1997, Nov). Epidemiology of human papillomarirus infections. Hospital Practice, 39-41.

Mayeaus, E.J., & Spigener, S.S. (1997, Dec). Treatment of human papillomarirus infections. Hospital Practice, 87-90.

Moran, G. (1997, Jan). Diagnosing STDs: Ulcerating diseases. Emergency Medicine, 59-72.

Moran, G. (1997, Feb). Diagnosing and treating STDs: Lesionless disorders. Emergency Medicine, 20-31.

Slade, C.S. (1998, Mar). HPV and cervical cancer: Breaking the deadly link. Advance for Nurse Practitioners, 39-55.

Rosen, T., & Ablon, G. (1997, Aug). Cutaneous herpesvirus infections update. Consultant, 2021-2042.

Verdon, M.E. (1997). Issues in the management of human papillomavirus genital disease. <u>American Family Physician, 55</u> (5), 1813-1817.

Vincent, M.T., & Adeyele, E. (1998). Are you comfortable taking the sexual history? <u>Family Practice Recertification, 20</u> (1), 87-101.

Wolner-Hanssen, P. (1996). Acute pelvic inflammatory disease. In M.A. Stenchever (Ed.), <u>Office gynecology</u>. St. Louis: Mosby.

CHAPTER 16

Human Immunodeficiency Virus Infection and Acquired Immunodeficiency Syndrome

HUMAN IMMUNODEFICIENCY VIRUS INFECTION AND ACQUIRED IMMUNODEFICIENCY SYNDROME IN CHILDREN

I. Definition: Children under age 13 with Human Immunodeficiency Virus (HIV) infection and/or Acquired Immunodeficiency Syndrome (AIDS)

    A. HIV Infection: Infection with human retrovirus, Human Immunodeficiency Virus

    B. Acquired Immunodeficiency Syndrome: Definition of AIDS in children <13 years incorporates the age-dependent decline in CD4+ T-cells (see table on Immune Cateogies in IV.D.3.b.) and differentiates mild, moderate and severe degrees of clinical symptoms (see table on Clinical Categories in IV.D.3.b.)

II. Pathogenesis:

    A. Human immunodeficiency virus enters and destroys cells, predominantly CD4+ T-lymphocyte (CD4+ T-cells) cells which are involved in cell-mediated immunity; the progressive destruction of CD4+ T-cells results in increased susceptibility of the patient to infections by opportunistic organisms

    B. Transmission of HIV infection in children
        1. More than 90% of pediatric AIDS cases reported in 1994 occurred via maternal to infant transmission or vertical transmission
            a. The vertical transmission rate is about 20-30%, with the majority of children born to infected mothers being uninfected
            b. Transmission from mother to infant can occur during the following times:
                (1) Pregnancy or gestation (in uteru); accounts for about 25-30% of perinatal HIV transmission
                (2) Labor and delivery (intrapartum); accounts for about 70-75% of perinatal transmission
                    (a) Possible mechanisms for neonatal HIV acquisition include direct exposure to maternal blood and genital tract secretions and transplacental microtransfusions
                    (b) Cesarean delivery has a partially protective role against transmission
                (3) Postpartum period through breastfeeding; accounts for a small percentage of transmission
            c. The following factors increase the risk of vertical HIV transmission: Low maternal peripheral blood CD4+ T-cell counts, high maternal plasma HIV RNA levels, and prolonged rupture of amniotic membranes
            d. Zidovudine (AZT) therapy to mothers during the antepartum and intrapartum periods and to newborns for 6 weeks after birth, reduced perinatal transmission by 70% in the Pediatric AIDS Clinical Trials Group Protocol (PACTG) 076
        2. Other means of transmission in children include exposure to HIV-contaminated blood or blood products, sexual abuse, and sexual transmission during adolescence

III. Clinical Presentation

    A. Epidemiology
        1. The annual number of perinatally acquired AIDS cases in the U.S. has declined in recent years
        2. The AIDS epidemic continues to disproportionately affect African American and Hispanic females and children

B. Disease progression
1. Generally, HIV infection progresses to AIDS more rapidly in infants than in adults due to the immature immune systems of infants or exposures to increased viral loads relative to body masses
2. Approximately 20% of infants progress rapidly and are symptomatic during the first few months after birth; infants infected in utero are believed to be rapid progressors
3. Slower progression occurs in the majority of children who are probably infected during labor and delivery; these children typically become symptomatic within the first several years of life
4. A small percentage of children do not develop manifestations of disease progression until after 8-10 years of age

C. Usually, children have a triad of symptoms: failure to thrive, chronic interstitial pneumonitis, and hepatosplenomegaly

D. Other common clinical manifestations include lymphadenopathy, recurrent diarrhea, chronic parotid swelling, hepatitis, malignancies, recurrent infections, recurrent febrile episodes, skin rashes, cardiomyopathy, and dysmorphic syndrome

E. When a significant quantity of CD4+ T-cells have been destroyed by the virus, immunosuppression occurs and children develop opportunistic infections and other complications (also see section on HIV/AIDS in Adolescents for further discussion of common clinical presentations of opportunistic infections)
1. The lung is the most common site of infection with pneumocystis carinii pneumonia (PCP) the most common opportunistic infection
2. The gastrointestinal tract is the next most common site for opportunistic infections with candida esophagitis the most common GI infection
3. Central nervous system involvement is common in children; one of the earliest signs of CNS involvement is failure to achieve developmental milestones
4. Chronic otitis media and sinusitis are common
5. Endocrine and skeletal muscle manifestations are common and include short stature and delay of puberty

F. The clinical presentation of HIV infection is different in children and adults:
1. The following AIDS-related problems are more common in children than adults: hypergammaglobulinemia, lymphocytic interstitial pneumonia, bacterial sepsis, recurrent bacterial infections, failure to thrive and parotitis
2. Manifestations more common in adults than children: Kaposi's sarcoma, B-cell lymphoma, peripheral lymphopenia, acute mononucleosis-like presentations, opportunistic infections and tumors of the central nervous system

IV. Diagnosis/Evaluation

A. History
1. Determine if the child is at risk for HIV infection based on the HIV positive status of the mother
2. Gather a complete pregnancy history of the mother including drug use and labor and delivery information
3. Obtain a neonatal history including birth weight and complications
4. Carefully explore feeding behaviors and developmental milestones
5. Inquire about associated symptoms such as fevers, rashes, and diarrhea
6. Carefully explore frequency and duration of infections

B. Physical Examination
1. Measure and plot height and weight on growth chart; compare with previous measurements
2. Observe general appearance, noting alertness, responsiveness, and level of activity
3. A complete physical examination is required with focus on the skin, lymph nodes, mouth, lungs, heart, abdomen, and neuromuscular systems
4. Perform a Denver II to assess development

C. Differential Diagnosis
   1. Failure to thrive
   2. Recent therapy with an immunosuppressive agent
   3. Lymphoproliferative disease
   4. Congenital immunological states
   5. Congenital cytomegalovirus infection
   6. Congenital toxoplasmosis

D. Diagnostic Tests
   1. Early identification of HIV-infected females is essential for the health of such females and for the care of HIV-exposed and HIV-infected children
      a. Universal counseling and voluntary testing with HIV tests are recommended as the standard of care for all pregnant females
      b. Positive diagnosis of HIV infection requires both of the following tests which detect antibodies to HIV: A positive enzyme-linked immunosorbent assay (ELISA) as a screening test and a positive Western blot for confirmation
   2. Diagnosis of HIV infection in infants
      a. Diagnosis of HIV infection in neonates is difficult because most children born to HIV-infected mothers are initially HIV positive because of placental transfer of maternal antibodies
      b. However, HIV infection can be definitively diagnosed in most infected infants by age 1 month and in virtually all infected infants by age 6 months by using viral diagnostic assays
         (1) HIV DNA polymerase chain reaction (PCR) is the preferred method, but HIV RNA assays and HIV culture are acceptable alternative tests
         (2) Perform testing 48 hours after birth, at age 1-2 months, and at age 3-6 months (testing at age 14 days is also recommended by some experts)
         (3) Positive tests indicate possible HIV infection and should be confirmed by a repeat virologic test on a separate occasion
         (4) HIV can be reasonably excluded among children with the following:
            (a) Two or more negative virologic tests, two or which are performed at age ≥1 month and one of those being performed at age ≥4 months
            (b) Two of more negative HIV immunoglobulin G (IgG) antibody tests performed at age >6 months with an interval of at least 1 month between tests
            (c) HIV IgG antibody which is negative in the absence of hypogammaglobulinemia at age 18 months
      c. Testing for HIV infection in children who are over 18 months of age is similar to testing of adults with a positive ELISA and positive Western blot tests for confirmation
   3. Monitoring immunologic parameters in children with CD4+ T-cell counts is used in conjunction with other measurements to guide antiretroviral treatment decisions and primary prophylaxis of PCP after age 1 year
      a. Obtain CD4+ T-cell counts as soon as possible after child has a positive virologic test for HIV and every 3 months thereafter
      b. The following two tables on CD4+ T-cells and clinical categories present a pediatric clinical and immunologic staging system for HIV infection

1994 REVISED HIV PEDIATRIC CLASSIFICATION SYSTEM: IMMUNE CATEGORIES BASED ON AGE-SPECIFIC CD4+ T-LYMPHOCYTE COUNT AND PERCENTAGE					
	<12 mos		1-5 yrs		6-12 yrs	
Immune category	No./μL	(%)	No./μL	(%)	No./μL	(%)
Category 1-- no suppression	≥1,500	(≥25%)	≥1,000	(≥25%)	≥500	(≥25%)
Category 2-- moderate suppression	750-1,499	(15%-24%)	500-999	(15%-24%)	200-499	(15%-24%)
Category 3-- severe suppression	<750	(<15%)	<500	(<15%)	<200	(<15%)

Source: Centers for Disease Control. (1998). Guidelines for the use of antiretroviral agents in pediatric HIV infection. MMWR, 47 (RR-4), 1-47

1994 Revised HIV Pediatric Classification System: Clinical Categories

Category N: Not Symptomatic

Children who have no signs or symptoms considered to be the result of HIV infection or who have only **one** of the conditions listed in category A

Category A: Mildly Symptomatic

Children with **two** or more of the following conditions but none of the conditions listed in categories B and C:
- Lymphadenopathy ($\geq$0.5 cm at more than two sites; bilateral = one site)
- Hepatomegaly
- Splenomegaly
- Dermatitis
- Parotitis
- Recurrent or persistent upper respiratory infection, sinusitis, or otitis media

Category B: Moderately Symptomatic

Children who have symptomatic conditions other than those listed for category A or category C that are attributed to HIV infection. Examples of conditions in clinical category B include but are not limited to the following:
- Anemia (<8 gm/dL), neutropenia (<1,000/mm^3), or thrombocytopenia (<100,000/mm^3) persisting $\geq$30 days
- Bacterial meningitis, pneumonia, or sepsis (single episode)
- Candidiasis, oropharyngeal (i.e., thrush) persisting (>2 mo) in children >6 mo of age
- Cardiomyopathy
- Cytomegalovirus infection with onset before age 1 month
- Diarrhea, recurrent or chronic
- Hepatitis
- Herpes simplex virus (HSV) stomatitis, recurrent (i.e., more than two episodes within 1 year)
- HSV bronchitis, pneumonitis, or esophagitis with onset before age 1 month
- Herpes zoster (i.e., shingles) involving at least two distinct episodes or more than one dermatome
- Leiomyosarcoma
- Lymphoid interstitial pneumonia (LIP) or pulmonary lymphoid hyperplasia complex
- Nephropathy
- Nocardiosis
- Fever lasting >1 month
- Toxoplasmosis with onset before age 1 month
- Varicella, disseminated (i.e., complicated chickenpox)

Category C: Severely Symptomatic

Children who have any condition listed in the 1987 surveillance case definition for acquired immunodeficiency syndrome (see AIDS Surveillance Case Definition in section on HIV INFECTION IN ADOLESCENTS), with the exception of LIP (which is a category B condition)

Source: Centers for Disease Control. (1998). Guidelines for the use of antiretroviral agents in pediatric HIV infection. MMWR, 47 (RR-4), 1-47

    4.   The viral load (burden) can be determined by using quantitative HIV RNA assays; viral load is essential in deciding when to initiate and change antiretroviral therapy in adults and adolescents, and probably helpful in perinatally infected children aged >3 years but HIV RNA levels are difficult to interpret in young children

V.   Plan/Management

    A.   To reduce perinatal transmission the following guidelines are recommended:
        1.   Care of HIV-infected pregnant females and newborn should be coordinated with an HIV-specialist, obstetrician, and primary health care provider
        2.   Assessment of the pregnant female should include evaluation of existing immunodeficiency (CD4+ T-cell count), risk of disease progression (level of plasma HIV RNA), history of prior or current antiretroviral therapy, gestational age of the baby, and supportive care needs
        3.   Recommendations for females currently taking antiretrovirals should involve the same parameters as those for females who are not pregnant
        4.   Additionally, all infected pregnant females should be offered the following three-part zidovudine (ZDV) chemoprophylaxis regimen, alone or in combination with other antiretrovirals:
            a.   In antepartum, prescribe ZDV 200 mg TID or ZDV 300 mg BID (may consider delaying ZDV until 10-12 weeks gestation)
            b.   During labor, order intravenous administration of ZDV in 1-hour-initial dose of 2 mg/kg followed by continuous infusion of 1 mg/kg/hour until delivery

      c.   ZDV should be administered orally to the newborn for first 6 weeks of life
          (1)   For infants in first two weeks, give ZDV 1.5 mg/kg PO or IV every 12 hours
          (2)   For infants 2-6 weeks old, give ZDV 2 mg/kg PO every 8 hours
   5.   Provide primary pneumocystis carinii pneumonia prophylaxis to the pregnant female when CD4+ T-cells fall below 200/mm^3: Prescribe trimethoprim/sulfamethoxazole (Bactrim) one DS tablet QD on Monday, Wednesday, Friday or aerosolized pentamidine once a month if unable to tolerate Bactrim
   6.   General counseling should be provided about risk factors for transmission including the need to refrain from breastfeeding

B.   Additional recommendations for caring for the newborn of the HIV-infected mother
   1.   Order CBC and differential at birth and at 6 weeks of age
   2.   Monitor for adverse reactions from zidovudine such as anemia, neutropenia, myositis, elevated transaminases; mild, transient anemia is common and resolves when therapy is discontinued
   3.   More intensive monitoring of hematologic and serum chemistry measurements is needed for infants whose mothers received combination antiretroviral therapy

C.   Follow-up care of child at risk for HIV infection from birth until HIV status is determined must be aggressive until it is assured that the child is not HIV infected
   1.   Prophylaxis for PCP should begin at 6 weeks following completion of ZDV prophylaxis regardless of the results of testing because of the difficulty in making an accurate diagnosis of HIV infection in infancy
   2.   PCP prophylaxis is continued until the child's HIV status is definitely determined
   3.   If the child is determined to have HIV infection then PCP prophylaxis is based on the guidelines related to the age adjusted CD4+ T-cell counts (See V.D.9)

D.   Care of the child with confirmed HIV infection
   1.   CD4+ T-cell counts should be performed regularly (every 3 months)
   2.   Neurodevelopmental assessments should be completed every 6 months
   3.   Tuberculosis should be screened for annually with skin tests (PPDs)
   4.   Pulmonary status should be evaluated regularly
   5.   Growth and development should be evaluated at least every 6 months
   6.   Nutritional assessments should be periodically performed
      a.   Encourage a high calorie, high protein diet
      b.   Recommend daily vitamin supplements
      c.   Eliminate irritating foods such as lactose and caffeine
      d.   Oral supplements such as Pediasure and Ensure may be helpful
      e.   Cyproheptadine HCl (Periactin) 2-4 mg BID or TID may be used in children >2 years to increase appetite
   7.   Provide routine immunizations EXCEPT:
      a.   The inactivated polio vaccine (IPV) should be given in place of the oral polio vaccine (OPV)
      b.   <u>Do not</u> administer varicella vaccine
      c.   Pneumococcal vaccination is recommended at 2 years of age
      d.   Annual influenza vaccinations are recommended beginning at 6 months
   8.   Prophylaxis for herpes simplex, mycobacterium avium complex, and chronic candidiasis is controversial in children (consult specialist); see section on HIV/AIDS IN ADOLESCENTS for further information on patient education to prevent opportunistic infections
   9.   Initiation of PCP prophylaxis should follow the guidelines listed in the following table: trimethoprim-sulfamethoxazole (TMP/SMX) is the most effective choice with dapsone, pentamidine aerosol and intravenous pentamidine as alternatives

PCP PROPHYLAXIS AND CD4+ T-CELL MONITORING FOR HIV-EXPOSED INFANTS AND HIV-INFECTED CHILDREN BY AGE AND HIV INFECTION STATUS

Age and HIV Infection Status	PCP Prophylaxis	CD4+ Monitoring
Birth to 4-6 wk, HIV-exposed	No prophylaxis	1 mo of age
4-6 wk to 4 mo, HIV-exposed	Prophylaxis	3 mo of age
4-12 mo, HIV-infected or indeterminate HIV infection reasonably excluded	Prophylaxis	6,9, and 12 mo of age
1-2 y, HIV-infected	No prophylaxis	None
	Prophylaxis if CD4+ count <750 cells/μL in first 12 mo or <500 cells/μL at 12-24 mo, or CD4+ percentage <15	Every 3-4 mo
2-5 y, HIV-infected	Prophylaxis if CD4+ count <500 cells /μL or CD4+ percentage <15	Every 3-4 mo
6-12 y, HIV-infected	Prophylaxis if CD4+ count <200 cells/μL or CD4+ percentage <15	Every 3-4 mo
All ages, HIV-infected, prior PCP infection	Prophylaxis	Every 3-4 mo

Adapted from American Academy of Pediatrics Committee on Pediatric AIDS. (1997). Evaluation and medical treatment of the HIV-exposed infant. Pediatrics, 99, 909-917.

E. Antiretroviral therapy for children
1. Adolescents in early puberty (Tanner Stages I and II) should be given pediatric dosing schedules; adolescents in late puberty (Tanner Stage V) should follow adult dosing schedules; closely monitor adolescents who are in their growth spurt (females in Tanner Stage III and males in Tanner Stage IV)
2. An infectious disease specialist should be consulted for recommendations on initiating and changing antiretroviral therapy in children
3. The following table provides guidelines on when to initiate therapy

INDICATIONS FOR INITIATION OF ANTIRETROVIRAL THERAPY

- Clinical symptoms associated with HIV infection (i.e., clinical categories A, B, or C [Table: Classification System: Clinical categories])
- Evidence of immune suppression, indicated by CD4+ T-lymphocyte absolute number or percentage (immune category 2 or 3 [Table: Classification System: Immune categories])
- Age <12 months–regardless of clinical, immunologic, or virologic status
- For asymptomatic children aged ≥1 year with normal immune status, two options can be considered:
  –Preferred Approach
    Initiate therapy–regardless of age or symptom status
  –Alternative Approach
    Defer treatment in situations in which the risk for clinical disease progression is low and other factors (e.g., concern for the durability of response, safety, and adherence) favor postponing treatment. In such cases, the health-care provider should regularly monitor virologic, immunologic, and clinical status. Factors to be considered in deciding to initiate therapy include the following:
    –High or increasing HIV RNA copy number
    –Rapidly declining CD4+ T-lymphocyte number or percentage to values approaching those indicative of moderate immune suppression (i.e., immune category 2)
    –Development of clinical symptoms

Source: Centers for Disease Control. (1998). Guidelines for the use of antiretroviral agents in pediatric HIV infection. MMWR, 47 (RR-4), 1-47

4. Combination antiretroviral therapy is recommended for all infants, children and adolescents; monotherapy is appropriate only when used in infants of indeterminate HIV status during the first 6 weeks of life to prevent perinatal HIV transmission; see table that follows

RECOMMENDED ANTIRETROVIRAL REGIMENS FOR INITIAL THERAPY

Preferred Regimen

Evidence of clinical benefit and sustained suppression of HIV RNA in clinical trials in HIV-infected adults; clinical trials in HIV-infected children are ongoing

- One highly active protease inhibitor plus two nucleoside analogue reverse transcriptase inhibitors (NRTIs)
  - Preferred protease inhibitor for infants and children who cannot swallow pills or capsules: nelfinavir or ritonavir. Alternative for children who can swallow pills or capsules: indinavir
  - Recommended dual NRTI combinations: the most data on use in children are available for the combinations of zidovudine (ZDV) and dideoxyinosine (ddI) and for ZDV and lamivudine (3TC). More limited data are available for the combinations of stavudine (d4T) and ddI, d4T and 3TC, and ZDV and zalcitabine (ddC)*

Alternative Regimen

- Nevirapine[†] and two NRTIs

Secondary Alternative Regimen

- Two NRTIs

Not Recommended

Evidence against use because of overlapping toxicity and/or because use may be virologically undesirable

- Any monotheraphy
- d4T and ZDV
- ddC and ddI
- ddC and d4T
- ddC and 3TC

*ddC is not available in a liquid preparation commercially, although a liquid formulation is available through a compassionate use program of the manufacturer (Hoffman-LaRoche Inc., Nutley, New Jersey). ZDV and ddC is a less preferred choice for use in combination with a protease inhibitor

[†]A liquid preparation of nevirapine is not available commercially but is available through a compassionate use program of the manufacturer (Boehringer Ingelheim Pharmaceuticals, Inc., Ridgefield, Connecticut)

Source: Centers for Disease Control. (1998). Guidelines for the use of antiretroviral agents in pediatric HIV infection. MMWR, 47 (RR-4), 1-47

---

5.   See following table for when to change antiretroviral therapy

---

CONSIDERATIONS FOR CHANGING ANTIRETROVIRAL THERAPY

Virologic Considerations*

- Less than a minimally acceptable virologic response after 8-12 weeks of therapy. For children receiving antiretroviral therapy with two nucleoside analogue reverse transcriptase inhibitors (NRTIs) and a protease inhibitor, such a response is defined as a <10-fold ($1.0 \log_{10}$) decrease from baseline HIV RNA levels. For children who are receiving less potent antiretroviral therapy (i.e., dual NRTI combinations), an insufficient response is defined as a less than fivefold ($0.7 \log_{10}$) decrease in HIV RNA levels from baseline
- HIV RNA not suppressed to undetectable levels after 4-6 months of antiretroviral therapy[†]
- Repeated detection of HIV RNA in children who initially responded to antiretroviral therapy with undetectable levels
- A reproducible increase in HIV RNA copy number among children who have had a substantial HIV RNA response but still have low levels of detectable HIV RNA. Such an increase would warrant change in therapy if, after initiation of the therapeutic regimen, a greater than threefold ($0.5 \log_{10}$) increase in copy number for children aged ≥2 years and a greater than fivefold ($0.7 \log_{10}$) increase is observed for children aged <2 years

Immunologic Considerations*

- Change in immunologic classification
- For children with CD4+ T-lymphocyte percentages of <15% (i.e., those in immune category 3), a persistent decline of five percentiles or more in CD4+ cell percentage (e.g., from 15% to 10%)
- A rapid and substantial decrease in absolute CD4+ T-lymphocyte count (e.g., a >30% decline in <6 months)

Clinical Considerations

- Progressive neurodevelopmental deterioration[‡]
- Growth failure defined as persistent decline in weight-growth velocity despite adequate nutritional support and without other explanation
- Disease progression defined as advancement from one pediatric clinical category to another (e.g., from clinical category A to clinical category B)

*At least two measurements (taken 1 week apart) should be performed before considering a change in therapy

[†]The initial HIV RNA level of the child at the start of therapy and the level achieved with therapy should be considered when contemplating potential drug changes.

[‡]New treatment for children with neurodevelopmental deterioration should include one antiviral drug with substantial CNS penetration such as zidovudine or nevirapine.

Source: Centers for Disease Control. (1998). Guidelines for the use of antiretroviral agents in pediatric HIV infection. MMWR, 47 (RR-4), 1-47

6. See following table for dosing of nucleoside analogue reverse transcriptase inhibitors

DOSAGE SCHEDULE OF NUCLEOSIDE ANALOGUE REVERSE TRANSCRIPTASE INHIBITORS				
Drug	**Preparation**	**Neonatal Dose**	**Pediatric Dose**	**Adolescent Dose**
Didanosine (dideoxyinosine) (ddI), VIDEX	Powder for oral solution; Chewable tabs 25, 50, 100, 150 mg	Infants <90 days: 50 mg per m^2 of body surface area every 12 hours	90 mg per m^2 of body surface area every 12 hours	Body weight ≥60 kg: 200 mg BID; body weight <60 kg: 125 mg BID
Lamivudine (3TC), EPIVIR	Solution: 10 mg/mL; Tablets: 150 mg	Infants aged <30 days: 2 mg per kg of body weight BID	4 mg per kg of body weight BID	Body weight ≥50 kg: 150 mg BID. Body weight <50 kg: 2 mg per kg body weight BID
Stavudine (d4T), ZERIT	Solution: 1 mg/mL; Capsules: 15, 20, 30, 40 mg	Under evaluation in Pediatric AIDS Clinical Trial Group protocol 332	1 mg per kg of body weight every 12 hours (up to weight of 30 kg)	Body weight ≥60 kg: 40 mg BID. Body weight <60 kg: 30 mg BID
Zalcitabine (ddC), HIVID	Syrup: 0.1 mg/mL (investigational); Tablets: 0.375 and 0.75 mg	Unknown	0.01 mg per kg of body weight every 8 hours	0.75 mg TID
Zidovudine (ZDV, AZT), RETROVIR	Syrup: 10 mg/mL; Caps: 100mg; Tabs: 300 mg; concentrate for injection or IV infusion: 10mg/mL	Premature infant: 1.5 mg/kg q 12 hours from birth to 2 weeks Neonate: 2 mg/kg q 6-8 hours PO; IV 1.5 mg/kg q 6-8 hours	160 mg m^2 of body surface every 8 hours PO; IV intermittent infusion: 120 mg per m^2 of body surface q 6 hours	200 mg TID or 300 mg BID

Adapted from Centers for Disease Control. (1998). Guidelines for the use of antiretroviral agents in pediatric HIV infection. <u>MMWR</u>, <u>47</u> (RR-4), 1-47

7. See table for doses of non-nucleoside analogue reverse transcriptase inhibitors

DOSAGE SCHEDULE OF NON-NUCLEOSIDE ANALOGUE REVERSE TRANSCRIPTASE INHIBITORS				
Drug	**Preparation**	**Neonatal Dose**	**Pediatric Dose**	**Adolescent Dose**
Delavirdine (DLV), RESCRIPTOR	Tablets: 100 mg	Unknown	Unknown	400 mg TID
Nevirapine (NVP), VIRAMUNE	Suspension: 10 mg/mL - investigational; Tablets: 200 mg	5 mg/kg QD for 14 days, then 120 mg per m^2 of body surface area q 12 hours for 14 days; then 200 mg of m^2 of body surface q 12 hours	120-200 mg per m^2 of body surface every 12 hours; initiate therapy with 120 mg per m^2 of body surface QD for 14 days, then increase to full dose	200 mg every 12 hours; initiate therapy at 100 mg for first 14 days, then increase to full dose

Adapted from Centers for Disease Control. (1998). Guidelines for the use of antiretroviral agents in pediatric HIV infection. <u>MMWR</u>, <u>47</u> (RR-4), 1-47

8.   See the following table for dosing protease inhibitors

DOSAGE SCHEDULE OF PROTEASE INHIBITORS				
Drug	Preparation	Neonatal Dose	Pediatric Dose	Adolescent Dose
Indinavir, CRIXIVAN	Capsules: 200 and 400 mg	Unknown. Due to side effect of hyperbilirubinemia, should not be given to neonates	Under study: 500 mg per m^2 of body surface	800 mg every 8 hrs
Nelfinavir, VIRACEPT	Powder for oral suspension: 50 mg per 1 level gram scoopful; Tablets: 250 mg	(Investigational) 10 mg per kg of body weight TID	20 to 30 mg per kg of body weight TID	750 mg TID
Ritonavir, NORVIR	Oral solution: 80 mg/mL	Unknown	400 mg per m^2 per body surface area q 12 hours; start at 250 mg per m^2 and increase to full dose over 5 days	600 mg BID; initiate at 300 mg BID and increase to full dose over 5 days
Saquinavir, FORTOVASE (soft gel capsule)	200 mg soft gel capsule	Unknown	Unknown	1200 mg TID

Adapted from Centers for Disease Control. (1998). Guidelines for the use of antiretroviral agents in pediatric HIV infection. MMWR, 47 (RR-4), 1-47

9.   CD4+ T-cell counts and HIV viral loads should be monitored regularly to determine the effectiveness of therapy
10.   In children, clinical parameters such as growth failure, abnormal neurodevelopmental function, and frequency and severity of infections are also helpful in evaluating drug efficacy

F.   New drugs will be available soon (see section V.N. in section on HIV INFECTION IN ADOLESCENTS)

G.   Adherence is a major issue
   1.   Patient education, cues or reminders to administer drugs, and individualized treatment plans are helpful
   2.   Teach strategies to make drugs more palatable to increase adherence such as mixing liquid formulations with chocolate milk, pudding or ice cream; dulling senses prior to drug administration with popsicles, iced drinks, ice cream, or ice; coating mouth with peanut butter before drug administration; ingesting strong-tasting foods after drugs

H.   Treatment of opportunistic infections in children: typically a specialist in infectious disease will manage the care of children who develop opportunistic infections (see section on HIV/AIDS IN ADOLESCENTS for additional information)

I.   Nutritional, psychiatric, behavioral and neuropsychological problems are important clinical issues and should be evaluated and addressed at each visit

J.   Patient education and counseling is extremely important and is best managed with an interdisciplinary team of professionals who are specialists in the care of children

K.   Follow up is individualized based on immune status and clinical parameters

HUMAN IMMUNODEFICIENCY VIRUS (HIV) INFECTION AND ACQUIRED IMMUNODEFICIENCY SYNDROME (AIDS) IN POST PUBERTAL ADOLESCENTS

I. Definitions:

    A. HIV infection: Infection with human retrovirus, Human Immunodeficiency Virus (HIV)

    B. AIDS: Disease characterized by opportunistic infections (see following table for case definition of AIDS)

CONDITIONS INCLUDED IN THE 1993 AIDS SURVEILLANCE CASE DEFINITION
• HIV+ persons with CD4 cells counts <200/μL or a CD4 percent <14%*
• Candidiasis of bronchi, trachea, or lungs
• Candidiasis, esophageal
• Cervical cancer, invasive*
• Coccidioidomycosis, disseminated or extrapulmonary
• Cryptococcosis, extrapulmonary
• Cryptosporidiosis, chronic intestinal (>1 mo duration)
• Cytomegalovirus disease (other than liver, spleen, or nodes)
• Encephalopathy, HIV-related
• Herpes simplex: Chronic ulcer(s) (>1 mo duration); or bronchitis, pneumonitis, or esophagitis
• Histoplasmosis, disseminated or extrapulmonary
• Isosporiasis, chronic intestinal (>1 mo duration)
• Kaposi's sarcoma
• Lymphoma, Burkitt's (or equivalent term)
• Lymphoma, immunoblastic (or equivalent term)
• Lymphoma, primary, of brain
• *Mycobacterium avium* complex or *M. kansasii*, disseminated or extrapulmonary
• *Mycobacterium tuberculosis*, any site (pulmonary* or extrapulmonary)
• *Mycobacterium*, other species or unidentified species, disseminated or extrapulmonary
• *Pneumocystis carinii* pneumonia
• Pneumonia, recurrent*
• Progressive multifocal leukoencephalopathy
• *Salmonella* septicemia, recurrent
• Toxoplasmosis of brain
• Wasting syndrome due to HIV

*Added January 1993

Source: Center for Communicable Diseases. 1992. 1993 revised classification system for HIV infection and expanded surveillance case definition of AIDS among adolescents and adults. MMWR, 41 (RR-17).

II. Pathogenesis

    A. HIV invades the body and may enter any cell, but it has a propensity to infect and kill cells of the immune system, particularly the CD4+ T-cells (T-lymphocytes)

B.   HIV actively replicates which leads to immune system damage and results in susceptibility to opportunistic infections (OIs), cancer, neurologic diseases, wasting, and death

C.   Transmission occurs by direct contact of a person's blood or body secretions with the blood or body secretions of a person infected with HIV virus
1.   Body fluids considered to be infectious include blood, tissues, cerebrospinal fluid, synovial fluid, peritoneal fluid, pleural fluid, pericardial fluid, amniotic fluid, semen and vaginal secretions
2.   Body fluids that are **not** considered infectious include feces, nasal secretions, sputum, sweat, tears, urine, vomitus and saliva (unless contaminated with blood)
3.   Certain activities are associated with high risk of infection such as unprotected anal, oral, or vaginal sex with multiple partners; unprotected sex with an HIV positive person; IV drug abuse; blood transfusions outside the U.S. or during 1977-1985; unprotected sex with a person who has recent or past history of sexually transmitted diseases
4.   Highest percentage of HIV transmissions occurs during sex acts where body fluids are exchanged
5.   IV drug use is the second most frequent route of transmission

D.   Most adolescents have been infected in teen-age years either sexually or via intravenous drug use and are in early stages of disease; a limited but growing number of adolescents are long-term survivors and became infected perinatally or via blood products

III.   Clinical Presentation

A.   Epidemiology
1.   The first AIDS cases were reported in 1981
2.   Seroprevalence of HIV in U.S. is 0.3%
3.   Highly active antiretroviral therapy (HAART) has revolutionized HIV care
   a.   In late 1995 and early 1996, introduction of 3TC, non-nucleoside reverse transcriptase inhibitors and protease inhibitors brought a new wave of hope that there would be chronic nonprogressors
      (1)   To date, however, there are no cures
      (2)   Studies show that these new drugs (i.e., protease inhibitors) have potent activity in most recipients for up to 1-2 years, but there are few studies to confirm long-term benefits
   b.   During transition period from late 1995 through 1997, there has been a 60-80% decline in AIDS-defining complications, a 60-80% decrease in the number of hospitalizations, and a 44% decrease in mortality rate
4.   White males who had sex with males had the largest proportional decline in AIDS incidence
5.   Incidence of AIDS has proportionately increased among black males, Hispanic males, and black females with heterosexual exposures
6.   In U.S., there is growing incidence of AIDS in persons older than 50 years; older persons are often diagnosed late in the course of their disease and progress more rapidly
7.   HIV infection is no longer the leading cause of death in individuals between the ages of 25 and 44 in U.S.

B.   Viral load and CD4+ T-cell counts help to assess the prognosis of HIV-infected patients
1.   Viral load measures the level of circulating plasma HIV-RNA
   a.   Viral load is the most powerful predictor of progression to AIDS and death
   b.   The greater the number of virus, the more active the infection and the worse the prognosis
2.   CD4+ T-cell counts are obtained to assess the general level of immunity or the extent of HIV-induced immune damage already suffered; the lower the CD4+ T-count the greater the risk for opportunistic infections
3.   A decrease in viral load of one log is associated with an average increase in CD4+ T-cells of about 85/mm^3

C. The natural history of HIV infection encompasses a wide spectrum of disease
  1. There is great variability in the progression of the disease among individuals
  2. Infection with HIV is always harmful; true long-term survival free of major immune damage is uncommon

D. The acute retroviral syndrome develops after HIV exposure and a 1-3 week incubation period
  1. Symptoms resemble those of infectious mononucleosis or influenza and are usually self-limited
    a. Fever, fatigue, lymphadenopathy, pharyngitis, and arthralgias are typical
    b. Rash, diarrhea, nausea, vomiting, hepatosplenomegaly, thrush, weight loss, and neurological are less common problems
  2. Syndrome is accompanied with rapid HIV replication or high viral load
  3. Recovery is usually in 1-3 weeks
  4. There is a sharp decrease in viral replication after recovery; however, replication is probably continuing in various tissues such as the lymphatic tissue and the central nervous system even though it can no longer be detected by blood tests

E. Early HIV disease: period between seroconversion to 4 months following HIV transmission
  1. Approximately at 4 months, the plasma levels of HIV RNA reach a set point that shows a very gradual increase averaging 7% a year over several years in the absence of antigenic stimuli such as intercurrent illness or immunizations or antiretroviral therapy
  2. This set point predicts the subsequent rate of progression
    a. High concentrations (>100,000 copies/mL) are associated with median survival of 4.4 years
    b. Low concentrations (<5,000 copies/mL) are associated with median survival exceeding 10 years
  3. Symptoms occurring early in the course of disease include the following:
    a. Lymphadenopathy and dermatologic abnormalities (seborrheic dermatitis, psoriasis, eosinophilic folliculitis)
    b. Oral lesions such as aphthous ulcers, herpes simplex labialis, and oral hairy leukoplakia usually occur later but may present
  4. As the disease progresses, patients have more frequent skin disorders, oral lesions, and infections as well as the following symptoms: recurrent diarrhea, intermittent fevers, night sweats, chills, unexplained weight loss, myalgias, arthralgia, headache and fatigue

F. Symptomatic HIV disease: complications are due to direct effects of the virus or to immunosuppression which occurs after a significant quantity of CD4+ T-cells has been destroyed
  1. Direct effect of HIV: persistent generalized lymphadenopathy, HIV-associated dementia, lymphocytic interstitial pneumonia, HIV-associated nephropathy, and progressive immunosuppression; other possible consequences are anemia, neutropenia, thrombocytopenia, cardiomyopathy, myopathy, peripheral neuropathy, chronic meningitis, polymyositis, and Guillain-Barré syndrome
  2. Immunosuppression results in opportunistic infections and tumors, primarily from compromised cell-mediated immunity (see tables in V.E.1.2.3.4.5.6. for further clinical presentation of opportunistic infections)
  3. Only about 2% or less of HIV-infected patients can maintain CD4+ T-cell counts in the normal range for lengthy periods of time (>12 years) without antiretroviral therapy
  4. In untreated patients, CD4+ T-cells average a 40-60/mm^3 decrease per year
  5. Opportunistic infections, particularly pneumocystic pneumonia, may occur when CD4+ T-cell counts fall below 200/mm^3
  6. Risk for opportunistic infections increases dramatically as CD4+ T-cell counts drop below 50/mm^3 (see tables in V.E.1.2.3.4.5.6. for further clinical presentation of opportunistic infections)

IV. Diagnosis/Evaluation

  A. History
    1. Determine risk factors for HIV; because a recent study found that many primary health care providers are missing opportunities to identify and test persons at high risk for HIV infection, the following questions may be helpful (see following table)

2. History at initial visit after the diagnosis is confirmed; at this initial visit the patient's health status may range from asymptomatic to advanced immunodeficiency; this first encounter sets the stage for a partnership with the patient that may last for years
   a. Explore the duration of HIV positivity as well as when and how the patient was infected
   b. Document when the patient was first diagnosed with HIV infection
   c. Inquire about testing (when and where was it done?; what led to testing?)
   d. Ask about results of prior diagnostic tests
   e. Inquire about prior treatments and responses to treatment
   f. Obtain past risk history (see preceding table) including a detailed sexual history such as number of partners within last year, use of condoms, and history of other sexually transmitted diseases
   g. Determine immunization status (pneumovax, flu vaccine, tetanus, hepatitis B, varicella)
   h. Document significant past medical history (opportunistic infections, hospitalizations, chicken pox, and other chronic diseases, particularly tuberculosis, hepatitis, shingles)
   i. In females, obtain a gynecological history including current menstrual pattern, date of last pelvic exam and pap smear, history of abnormal pap smear, and history of vaginal bleeding
   j. Inquire about travel to Ohio and Mississippi River Valleys (risk of histoplasmosis) and to Southwestern desert (risk of coccidioidomycosis)
   k. Assess patient's and family's knowledge about HIV
   l. Obtain a detailed social and mental health history to determine psychosocial assets and needs
   m. Screen for domestic violence
   n. Perform an HIV-related review of systems (ROS) directed toward uncovering symptoms of infection (fevers, night sweats, weight change, lymphadenopathy, skin changes, new headaches, memory problems, mouth lesions, difficulty swallowing, cough/chest pain, diarrhea, nausea, vomiting, vaginitis, peripheral neuropathy)
3. History on subsequent visits
   a. Document most recent CD4+ T-cell count and HIV viral load
   b. Document medications used for treating HIV infection
      (1) Inquire about adverse effects from medications
      (2) Always ask about adherence; a simple, direct question such as "How many doses have you missed in the past 24 hours?" may be nonthreatening
   c. Inquire about new or worsening symptoms
   d. Perform an HIV-related ROS (see IV.A.2.n.)

B. Physical Examination
   1. Vital signs (fever is a sign of opportunistic infections and neoplasms)
   2. Measure weight (important in detecting "wasting syndrome" and determining the type of dietary intervention that is needed)
   3. Observe general appearance, noting signs of distress and depression
   4. Examine skin for lesions, ecchymosis, and signs of dehydration
   5. Perform ophthalmological exam including a fundoscopic exam for retinopathy
   6. Examine mouth, noting thrush, hairy oral leukoplakia, herpes simplex, peridontal problems, ulcerations

7. Palpate lymph nodes as generalized lymphadenopathy is frequently present; localized lymphadenopathy may indicate carcinoma
8. Perform pulmonary and cardiac exam for pneumonia and cardiomyopathy
9. Perform examination of abdomen, noting organomegaly
10. Examine anal area for detection of sexually transmitted diseases, ulcerations, and fissures
11. Perform pelvic and speculum exam on females for cervical dysplasia, vaginal candidiasis, and sexually transmitted diseases; perform a complete genitourinary examination on males
12. Perform complete neurologic exam, including testing of cranial nerves, cerebellar function, reflexes, sensory function, and mental status for dementia and neuropathy
13. Perform a psychiatric examination

C. Diagnostic tests
1. Methods to **determine the diagnosis of HIV**
   a. Typically, the diagnosis is made with antibody testing using enzyme-linked immunoabsorbent assay (ELISA) and a Western blot (both tests must be positive to confirm the diagnosis)
      (1) ELISA is the initial test; it is sensitive but not highly specific (may have false positives)
      (2) Either a Western blot (WB) or an immunofluorescence assay (IFA) is used for confirmation of positive ELISA tests; WB and IFA are specific but labor intensive
      (3) Testing should be preceded by pretest counseling
      (4) Test results are usually available in 1-3 weeks and should be given in person with posttest counseling
   b. Other tests for detection of antibodies
      (1) FDA approved HIV ELISA and Western Blot urine tests are available but they are less accurate and cause more false positive results than serum tests
      (2) Orasure HIV-1 can detect antibodies from a sample of oral mucosal transudate
      (3) Home Access is an anonymous, finger-stick blood test for antibodies which can be done by an individual at home and purchased over-the-counter
   c. Rapid tests
      (1) Three FDA approved rapid tests are SUDS, Recombigen latex agglutination assay, Genie HIV-1
      (2) Results are available within 10 minutes
      (3) Advantageous in settings in which there are occupational exposures to health care workers and where reliable follow-up is unlikely such as in emergency rooms and STD clinics
   d. Persons with positive antibody tests are considered HIV seropositive; however, a negative antibody test does not guarantee that an individual is seronegative
      (1) A window period exists: it may take 1-3 months after HIV exposure for antibodies to form in sufficient amounts to be detectable by antibody tests
      (2) Because of this window period, it is recommended that persons with initial negative antibody tests and low risks have retesting at 6 months and high risk persons have repeat testing at 6 months and 1 year
2. **Antigen tests** are expensive, but can directly detect the virus
   a. Nucleic acid testing can detect the presence of HIV and is used for patients suspected of having acute retroviral syndrome which occurs before antibody tests become positive
   b. HIV blood culture is labor intensive and reliability is low
   c. p24 antigen can identify the presence of the HIV protein, but cannot quantify the amount of HIV
   d. RNA polymerase chain reaction (PCR) and branched DNA (bDNA) assay can measure the amount of HIV RNA in the plasma of infected persons

3.   **Tests to monitor disease progress**
   a.   RNA PCR or bDNA assay (viral load) is the most important test to order when making decisions to initiate and change antiretroviral drug therapy; order at the following times:
      (1)   At time of diagnosis and then every 3-4 months in untreated patients
      (2)   Immediately prior to and again at 4-8 weeks after initiating or changing antiretroviral drug therapy (ideally viral loads should be ordered on two occasions before beginning or altering drugs)
      (3)   Once patient is stable, order every 3-4 months
      (4)   Do not measure viral load during or within 4 weeks after successful treatment of any intercurrent infection, resolution or symptomatic illness, or immunization because of the immune activation of virus associated with these events
      (5)   "Third generation" assays or ultra sensitive RNA PCR will detect HIV RNA at a threshold of 20-50 copies/mL
   b.   Measurement of CD4+ T-cell counts, CD8 and CD4/CD8 ratio are the primary tests for monitoring immune function
      (1)   Determine stage of HIV infection, prognosis of disease, and need for prophylaxis of opportunistic infections; these tests play a secondary role in helping providers determine when to initiate and change drug therapy (viral loads are the essential test in decisions concerning drug therapy)
      (2)   Changes >50% (0.3 log) are considered significant
      (3)   Order at time of diagnosis and generally every 3-6 months thereafter
4.   **Tests to screen for concomitant diseases, immunity status and as a base-line before drugs are administered;** ordered at first visit after diagnosis is confirmed
   a.   Mantoux method using the purified protein derivative (PPD) to screen for tuberculosis (anergy testing is no longer recommended); positive PPD for person with HIV is >5 mm of induration
   b.   Rapid plasma reagin (RPR) or the Venereal Disease Laboratories (VDRL) to screen for syphilis which occurs in approximately 20% of patients with HIV infection; for patients with high-risk of developing STDs order annually
   c.   Pap smear for females to screen for cervical dysplasia; perform every 6-12 months
   d.   Typically the following additional tests are recommended:
      (1)   Chemistry panel including liver function tests and renal profile: useful as a baseline since patient may be receiving drugs with potential hepatic or renal toxicity
      (2)   Hepatitis B serology (HbsAg) to determine hepatitis immunity and need for vaccination as well as to detect hepatitis B infection which is common in HIV infected patients
      (3)   Hepatitis C serology to detect infection, particularly important in patients who are/were IV drug users and those with liver function abnormalities
      (4)   Toxoplasmosis serology (anti-toxoplasma antibody or IgG titer)
         (a)   Patient is at risk for reactivation toxoplasmosis when CD4+ T-cells drop below 100/mm^3
         (b)   Consider repeating in seronegative patients when their CD4+ T-cell is <100/mm^3
      (5)   Cytomegalovirus (CMV) IgG; CMV retinitis is a common complication and develops in seropositive patients when CD4+ T-cell drops below 50-75/mm^3
      (6)   Glucose-6-phosphate dehydrogenase deficiency (G-6-PD): If test is positive, patient has a deficiency and should not be prescribed dapsone and possibly should not be given a sulfonamide
      (7)   Varicella IgG to determine need for post-exposure prophylaxis with varicella zoster immune globulin
      (8)   CBC with differential and platelet count; anemia, leukopenia, or thrombocytopenia are common in HIV infection and can also result from drug therapy
      (9)   Chest x-ray to screen for latent TB and as a baseline

5. **New monitoring tests** that are being developed
   a. Resistance testing
   b. CD4+ cell subset determinations to enumerate memory and naive cells are used in clinical trials to help define the degree of immune reconstitution
   c. Therapeutic drug level monitoring is available

V. Plan/Management (care should be supervised by infectious disease specialist); because treatment of HIV infection changes rapidly consult following websites for updated information: CDC Clearinghouse (http://www.cdc.org) and the HIV Information Network (http://www.hivatis.org)

   A. Provide **patient education and counseling** at each visit; adjust amount and complexity of teaching and counseling based on patient's degree of stress, prior knowledge, readiness to learn, and cognitive abilities
      1. Provide information about transmission and how to prevent spread of infection such as not sharing razors or toothbrushes, carefully cleaning up blood spills, disposing of used feminine sanitary products
      2. Discuss ways to handle notification of partners and others; the local health department can assist with anonymous partner notification/elicitation
      3. Discuss lifestyle choices and safe sex practices such as latex barriers including condoms and female vaginal pouches
         a. Even patients with undetectable viral loads should be considered infectious and should practice safe sex
         b. HIV infected males should wear condoms even when engaging in sexual activity with other HIV infected individuals to prevent transmission of drug-resistant strains of HIV and other sexually transmitted diseases
      4. Discuss healthy diet; referral to nutritionist is beneficial
         a. Recommend eating a variety of foods from different food groups
         b. Encourage nutrient density or making every bite of food count; avoid foods with little protein, vitamins, and minerals
         c. Choose foods that are close to their natural states as possible; use whole wheat instead of white bread or brown rice instead of white
         d. Use olive and canola oils instead of margarine and vegetable oils which are rich in polyunsaturated fatty acids and may suppress the immune system
         e. One or two daily multivitamin/mineral supplement(s) is(are) recommended
      5. Encourage smoking cessation and decreasing or eliminating other types of substance abuse (alcohol, recreational drugs)
      6. Teach about food safety
         a. Foods should be well done and thoroughly cooked; avoid raw/rare meat, fish and poultry, raw eggs, or unpasteurized dairy products
         b. Wash hands after contact with raw meat
         c. Wash fruits and vegetables before eating
         d. Consider using filtered or bottled water
      7. Recommend that patient wash hands after gardening or other contact with soil; avoid changing cat liter box due to risk of toxoplasmosis; avoid rough play with kittens due to risk of cat scratch disease
      8. Reinforce the importance of good oral hygiene
      9. Discuss susceptibility to contagious disease and how to protect self
      10. Discuss ways to improve sleep habits and receive sufficient rest
      11. Explore stress levels, and recommend stress reduction interventions such as exercise, relaxation techniques, and guided imagery; massage therapy and referral to a psychologist may be beneficial
      12. Provide information on available community services
      13. Listen to fears and concerns and provide social support
      14. Provide information on prognosis and future therapy plans
      15. Discuss what to do if an emergency arises and which symptoms require immediate attention
      16. Help empower patients to become actively involved in their care through support groups, learning about the disease and treatments, and developing a partnership with the health care provider
      17. For patients in the late stage of disease offer information on advance directives; discuss living wills, health care surrogates; consider referral for home care or hospice care

B. **Immunization** recommendations
1. Administer annual influenza vaccine to all patients with CD4+ T-cell counts >100/mm³ who are on effective antiretrovirals
2. Administer pneumococcal (Pneumovax) vaccine, 05 mL IM X 1
3. *Haemophilus influenzae* type B vaccine is no longer recommended as most infections in HIV-infected persons involve nontypable strains
4. Consider Hepatitis B vaccine (series of 3) in all susceptible persons (anti-HB$_c$-negative), if they have not been previously immunized
5. Tetanus-diphtheria, mumps, rubella, measles identical to patients without HIV
6. If polio vaccine is needed, use enhanced inactivated polio vaccine (eIPV)
7. Do **not** use any of the following vaccines: Live polio, varicella zoster, BCG, or any live or attenuated vaccine except measles, mumps, and rubella

C. **Health maintenance referrals**
1. Schedule twice-yearly dental examinations
2. Periodic ophthalmology examinations are recommended; screening for CMV retinitis by a trained ophthalmologist or optometrist is recommended every 4-6 months once the patient's CD4+ T-cell count falls below 75/mm³

D. Medications should be given to **prevent opportunistic infections** when a person's CD4+ T-cell counts fall to certain levels or after exposure to certain pathogens (see following table)

PREVENTION OF OPPORTUNISTIC DISEASE IN HIV-INFECTED ADULTS AND ADOLESCENTS

Pathogen	Indication	Preventive regimens	
		First Choice	Alternatives
I. Strongly recommended as standard of care			
Pneumocystis carinii	CD4+ count <200/μL or prior PCP or oropharyngeal candidiasis or unexplained fever ≥2 weeks	Trimethoprim-sulfamethoxazole (TMP-SMZ), 1 DS PO QD; TMP-SMZ, 1 SS PO Q.D.	TMP-SMV, DS PO three times a week; dapsone, 50 mg PO BID or 100 mg PO QD or aerosolized pentamidine, 300 mg every month via Respirgard II™ nebulizer
Mycobacterium tuberculosis	PPD reaction ≥5 mm or prior positive PPD result without treatment or contact with case of active tuberculosis	Isoniazid, 300 mg PO plus pyridoxine, 50 mg PO QD x 12 mo or isoniazid, 900 mg PO plus pyridoxine, 50 mg PO twice a week x 12 mo	Rifampin, 600 mg PO QD x 12 mo
Toxoplasma gondii	IgG antibody to *Toxoplasma* and CD4+ count <100/μL	TMP-SMZ, 1 DS PO QD	TMP-SMZ, 1 SS PO QD; dapsone, 50 mg PO QD plus pyrimethamine, 50 mg PO QW plus leucovorin, 25 mg PO QW
Mycobacterium avium complex	CD4+ count <50μL	Clarithromycin, 500 mg PO BID or azithromycin, 1,200 mg PO QW	Rifabutin, 300 mg PO QD
Varicella zoster virus (VZV)	Significant exposure to chickenpox or shingles for patients who have no history of either condition or, if available, negative antibody to VZV	Varicella zoster immune globulin (VZIG), 5 vials (1.25 mL each) IM administered ≤96 h after exposure, ideally within 48 h	Acyclovir, 800 mg PO 5 times/d for 3 weeks
II. Not recommended for most patients; indicated for use only in unusual circumstances			
Candida species	CD4+ count <50/μL	Fluconazole, 100-200 mg PO QD	
Cryptococcus neoformans	CD4+ count <50/μL	Fluconazole, 100-200 mg PO QD	Itraconazole, 200 mg PO QD
Cytomegalovirus (CMV)	CD4+ count <50/μL and CMV antibody positivity	Oral ganciclovir, 1 g po TID	None

Adapted from U.S. Department of Health and Human Services. (1997). 1997 USPHS/IDSA guidelines for the prevention of opportunistic infections in persons infected with human immunodeficiency virus. MMWR, 46(RR-12), 1-46

E. It is important to recognize the signs and symptoms of **opportunistic diseases** and to diagnose and treat appropriately and then provide prophylaxis to prevent recurrences (see V.F. for prevention of recurrences)

    1. Dosages for antiretrovirals and drugs to treat opportunistic infections should be prescribed according to Tanner staging of puberty

        a. Adolescents in early puberty (Tanner stages I and II) should be given doses using pediatric schedule

        b. Adolescents in late puberty (Tanner stage V) should follow adult schedule

        c. Youth in midst of growth spurt (Females in Tanner III and males in Tanner IV) should be closely monitored for medication efficacy and toxicity

    2. See following table for diagnosis and treatment of bacterial infections

ASSESSMENT, DIAGNOSIS, AND TREATMENT OF COMMON BACTERIAL OPPORTUNISTIC INFECTIONS			
Transmission	**Clinical Characteristics**	**Diagnosis**	**Treatment**
Mycobacterium Avium Intracellulare (MAI) or M. Avium Complex Infections			
Widely dispersed in environment and found in most water supplies	Diarrhea, abdominal pain, organomegaly, high fevers, weight loss, fatigue, enlarged nodes, elevated alkaline phosphatase	Cultures of blood, stool, or bone marrow; Lymph node and liver biopsy	Clarithromycin 500 mg BID **plus** ethambutol 15-25 mg/kg/day ± rifabutin 300 mg/day or ciprofloxacin 500-750 mg BID; Alternatively, substitute azithromycin 500 mg QD for clarithromycin
Mycobacterium Tuberculosis			
Spread through droplet nuclei coughed up by persons with untreated TB	Productive, prolonged cough; fever, chills, night sweats, fatigue, weight loss, hemoptysis, lymphadenopathy	PPD skin test, chest x-ray, sputum smear and culture	**PPD but no active disease:** Isoniazid (INH)* 300 mg QD x 12 months **Active disease: 12 months treatment;** INH*, Rifampin, Pyrazinamide, & Ethambutol for 8 weeks; then INH & Rifampin
Syphilis			
Caused by *Treponema pallidium*; Sexually transmitted disease	Primary: chancre Secondary: Rash on palms and soles Tertiary: No outward signs Neurosyphilis: CNS problems	RPR or VDRL and then FTA-ABS and a lumbar puncture	If VDRL is ≥1:32 **and** CSF VDRL is negative: 2.4 million units Bicillin q week x 3 weeks; If VDRL is ≥1:32 and CSF VDRL is positive: 3.5 million units Penicillin G IV q 4 hrs. x 10 days followed by 2.4 million units of Bicillin q week x 3 weeks

*If on INH, give pyridoxine 50 mg/day

3. See following table for diagnosis and treatment of fungal infections

ASSESSMENT, DIAGNOSIS, AND TREATMENT OF COMMON FUNGAL OPPORTUNISTIC INFECTIONS			
Transmission	**Clinical Characteristics**	**Diagnosis**	**Treatment**
Candidiasis			
Caused by *candida albicans* when CD4+ T-cells drop below 500/mm^3	Oral: White plaques anywhere in oral cavity, burning sensation, absence of taste, pain when swallowing	Swab lesion: KOH prep	Clotrimazole 10 mg troches; dissolve in saliva, 1 troche 5 times daily for 14 days; Fluconazole 100 mg PO QD for 7-14 days
	Vaginal: Thick white vaginal discharge; itching, burning, redness in vaginal area	Swab vagina: KOH prep	Terconazole vaginal suppositories: 1 suppository HS X 3 nights; Fluconazole 150 mg tab. PO single dose
Cryptococcal Meningitis			
Yeast-like fungus found widely in environment, especially in soil contaminated with bird excrement	Fever, headache, fatigue, nausea, memory loss, confusion, problems with coordination	Cryptococcal serum antigen; Lumbar puncture: India ink, cryptococcal antigen, culture	Amphotericin B 0.7 mg/kg/day IV X 10-14 days or Fluconazole 400 mg/day for 8-10 weeks; Lifelong suppressive therapy with 200 mg/day

4. See following table for diagnosis and treatment of protozoal infections:

ASSESSMENT, DIAGNOSIS, AND TREATMENT OF COMMON PROTOZOAL OPPORTUNISTIC INFECTIONS			
Transmission	**Clinical Characteristics**	**Diagnosis**	**Treatment**
Pneumocystis Carinii Pneumonia (PCP)			
Believed to infect most humans during childhood, and then remains dormant	Dry, non-productive cough; shortness of breath, fever, fatigue, weight loss	Chest X-ray; Induced sputum; Broncho-alveolar lavage	Mild-Moderate Disease TMP/SMX* PO 15 mg/kg, TMP equivalent in 4 divided doses PO or IV for 21 days; TMP 5 mg/kg PO q 6 hours plus Dapsone 100 mg/day times 21 days for sulfa allergy Severe Disease:TMP/SMX 15 mg/kg TMP equivalent/day in 4 divided doses for 21 days with prednisone
Toxoplasmic Encephalitis			
30% U.S. adults infected with parasite which remains dormant until immune system is damaged	Fever, headache, neurological problems such as seizures, changes in mental status, coma	CT scan or MRI of brain for ring enhancing lesions; Positive toxoplasma IgG in serum	Pyrimethamine 100-200 mg QD PO then 50-75 mg QD with sulfadiazine 4-8 g PO QD plus folinic acid 10-20 mg PO QD for 6 weeks
Cryptosporidiosis			
Transmitted to humans via contact with feces, contaminated water or food	Chronic watery diarrhea, abdominal cramps, nausea, fever, weight loss, headache	Modified acid fast stain of stool; endoscopy with biopsy or bowel biopsy	Treatment is difficult - refer to specialist; sometimes Paromomycin 500 mg PO QID with food X 14-28 days then 500 mg BID may be effective

*Trimethoprim/sulfamethoxazole

5. See following table for diagnosis and treatment of viral infections:

ASSESSMENT, DIAGNOSIS, AND TREATMENT OF COMMON VIRAL OPPORTUNISTIC INFECTIONS			
Transmission	**Clinical Characteristics**	**Diagnosis**	**Treatment**
Cytomegalovirus Retinitis			
High percentage of US adults are infected with virus which remains dormant until immune system is damaged	Cytomegalovirus may infect GI tract, brain, and other organs but common site is the eye with blurred vision, floaters, flashing lights, loss of peripheral vision, area of vision that is missing	Diagnosis made with indirect fundoscopy by a trained ophthalmologist	Need chronic IV therapy or ocular implant plus oral therapy with ganciclovir or foscarnet (refer to specialist)
Oral Hairy Leukoplakia			
Caused by Epstein-Barr virus	White, non-removable lesion with a corrugated surface on lateral margins of tongue	Clinical presentation	None usually needed; may treat with acyclovir 400 mg PO QID
Progressive Multifocal Leukoencephalopathy (PML)			
Caused by J. C. virus; most people are infected by 2 years of age, but virus remains latent in brain until immune system is sufficiently damaged	Insidious onset with rapid progression; confusion, lack of energy, loss of balance, memory and speech problems, blurred or double vision, hallucinations, seizures, paralysis and eventual death	CT scan or MRI which may reveal focal brain lesions which do not enhance or cause surrounding edema	Refer to specialist; no universally accepted treatment
Herpes Simplex, Herpes Zoster, and Molluscum Contagiosum (see Chapter 7, SKIN PROBLEMS)			

6. See following table for diagnosis and treatment of cancers:

ASSESSMENT, DIAGNOSIS, AND TREATMENT OF CANCERS ASSOCIATED WITH HIV INFECTION			
Transmission	**Clinical Characteristics**	**Diagnosis**	**Treatment**
Kaposi's Sarcoma			
May be sexually transmitted and is caused by herpes virus, HHV-8	Red, brown or pink blotches on skin which change to hard, raised purplish-red lesions; can be on internal organs as well as common places of arms, legs, and chest	Visual examination or skin biopsy	Referral to specialist, sometimes left untreated or can remove with alpha interferon, radiation, chemotherapy
Lymphomas			
Cancers of lymphoid cells; B-cell non-Hodgkin's lymphoma is most common	Spreads quickly, occurs in brain and outside of the lymph nodes	Depending on site; biopsy or CT/MRI	Refer to specialist

F. Patients who have a history of opportunistic diseases should be administered chemoprophylaxis to prevent recurrence (see following table)

PROPHYLAXIS FOR RECURRENCE OF OPPORTUNISTIC DISEASE (AFTER CHEMOTHERAPY FOR ACUTE DISEASE) IN HIV-INFECTED ADULTS AND ADOLESCENTS			
		Preventive regimens	
Pathogen	**Indication**	**First choice**	**Alternatives**
I. Recommended for life as standard of care			
Pneumocystis carinii	Prior *P. carinii* pneumonia	Trimethoprim-sulfamethoxazole (TMP-SMZ), 1 DS PO QD TMP-SMZ 1 SS PO QD	TMP-SMZ DS PO three times a week; dapsone, 50 mg PO BID or 100 mg PO QD; aerosolized pentamidine, 300 mg QM via Respirgard II™ nebulizer
Toxoplasma gondii	Prior toxoplasmic encephalitis	Sulfadiazine 500-1000 mg PO QID plus pyrimethamine 25-75 mg PO QD plus leucovorin 10 mg PO QD	Clindamycin, 300-450 mg PO Q 6-8 h plus pyrimethamine, 25-75 mg PO QD plus leucovorin, 10-25 mg PO QD-QID
Mycobacterium avium complex	Documented disseminated disease	Clarithromycin, 500 mg PO BID plus one or more of the following: ethambutol, 15 mg/kg PO QD; rifabutin, 300 mg PO QD	Azithromycin, 500 mg PO QD plus one or more of the following: ethambutol, 15 mg/kg PO QD; rifabutin, 300 mg PO QD
Cytomegalovirus	Prior end-organ disease	Ganciclovir, 5-6 mg/kg IV 5-7 days/wk or 1,000 mg PO TID or foscarnet, 90-120 mg/kg IV QD; or cidofovir 5 mg/kg every other week; or (for retinitis) ganciclovir sustaned-release implant every 6-9 months	
Cryptococcus neoformans	Documented disease	Fluconazole, 200 mg PO QD	Amphotericin B, 0.6-1.0 mg/kg IV QW-TIW; itraconazole, 200 mg PO QD
II. Recommended only if subsequent episodes are frequent or severe			
Herpes simplex virus	Frequent/severe recurrences	Acyclovir, 200 mg PO TID or 400 mg PO BID	
Candida (oral, vaginal, or esophageal)	Frequent/severe recurrences	Fluconazole, 100-200 mg PO QD	Ketoconazole, 200 mg PO QD; itraconazole, 200 mg PO QD

Adapted from Center for Disease Control. (1997). 1997 USPHS/IDSA guidelines for the prevention of opportunistic infections in persons infected with Human Immunodeficiency Virus. MMWR, 46, 1-46.

G.	Summary of the **principles of antiretroviral drug therapy** of HIV infection (see following table)

PRINCIPLES OF THERAPY

1. Because rates of disease progression vary among patients, treatment decisions must be individualized by level of risk indicated by viral loads and CD4+ T-cell levels

2. Maximum achievable suppression of HIV replication is the goal of drug therapy

3. Simultaneous initiation of combinations of effective anti-HIV drugs that the patient has not previously received and that are not cross-resistant with antiretroviral agents that the patient has previously received is the most effective method to achieve durable suppression of HIV replication

4. Drug monotherapy is **NOT** a recommended option as it presents risk for development of drug resistance and potential development of cross-resistance to related drugs

5. Each antiretroviral drug should be used according to optimum schedules and dosages

6. Any change in antiretroviral therapy increases future therapeutic constraints

7. Females need optimal antiretroviral therapy regardless of pregnancy status

8. Patient adherence is extremely important as intermittent use leads to resistance; emphasize that patient should not stop any medications without consulting health care provider

Adapted from NIH Panel To Define Principles of Therapy of HIV Infection. (1998). Report of the NIH Panel To Define Principles of Therapy of HIV Infection. Annals of Internal Medicine, 128, 1057-1078

H.	**Initiating antiretroviral therapy** (see V.H 2. & 4. for discussion of combination therapies; see K.L. & M. for discussion of specific drug classifications and agents)
1.	Criteria of when to offer antiretroviral therapy to patients
a.	In asymptomatic patients begin therapy when CD4+ T-cell counts are <500/mm^3 or plasma HIV RNA levels are > 5,000-10,000 copies/mL (bDNA) or >10,000-20,000 copies/mL (RT-PCR)
(1)	Some experts recommend treating all patients who have a detectable viral loads, particularly if the patient has a concomitant pattern of declining CD4+ T-cells
(2)	Treatment decisions for asymptomatic patients should also be based on patient's willingness to begin a complicated regimen, likelihood of adherence, and benefits/risks of early initiation (see following table)
b.	Symptomatic patients should be treated regardless of laboratory values

BENEFITS AND RISKS OF EARLY INITIATION OF ANTIRETROVIRAL THERAPY

Potential Benefits:	Control of viral replication and mutation Prevention of progression of immunodeficiency Delayed progression to AIDS	Decreased risk for selection of resistant virus Decreased risk for drug toxicity
Potential Risks:	Reduction in quality of life from adverse drug effects Inconvenience of drug administration Earlier development of drug resistance Limitation of future choices of antiretroviral agents Unknown long-term toxicity of drugs Unknown duration of effectiveness of current antiretroviral agents	

Adapted from NIH Panel to Define Principles of Therapy of HIV Infection. (1998). Guidelines for the use of antiretroviral agents in HIV-infected adults and adolescents. Annals of Internal Medicine, 128, 1079-1100

2.	Initiating therapy with a naive patient (patient who has never been on antiretroviral medications):
a.	Begin with 2 nucleoside reverse transcriptase inhibitors (NRTIs) and 1 protease inhibitor (PI)
b.	Alternative regime: Ritonavir and saquinavir (soft-gel capsule) plus one or two NRTI(s) or nevirapine as a substitute for PI
c.	When initiating therapy, start all drugs simultaneously and at a full dose with following exceptions: Dose escalation needed with ritonavir, nevirapine, and in some cases ritonavir plus saquinavir

3. Patients on monotherapy and dual therapy regimes should be offered triple combination therapy; even if these patients have no detectable virus in the plasma, triple combination therapy is more effective in preventing virologic failure than regimens with one or two drugs

4. See following table for acceptable antiretroviral combinations

ANTIRETROVIRAL COMBINATIONS*
Acceptable combinations include the following:
Zidovudine (AZT) and lamivudine (3TC) plus a protease inhibitor (PI)
Lamivudine (3TC) and stavudine (d4T) plus PI
Zidovudine (AZT) and didanosine (ddI) plus PI
Didanosine (ddI) and stavudine (d4T) plus PI
Zidovudine (AZT) and zalcitabine (ddC) plus PI
Saquinavir-SGC (Fortovase) and ritonavir (Norvir) plus a NRTI
Alternative therapy which is less likely to provide sustained virus suppression
1 non-nucleoside reverse transcriptase inhibitor (NNRTI) plus 2 NRTI (listed above)
The following are generally not recommended:
Saquinavir-HGC (Invirase) with any combination
Two NRTIs
Unacceptable combinations of NRTI used in triple therapy include the following:
Didanosine (ddI) and zalcitabine (ddC)
Stavudine (d4T) and zidovudine (AZT)
Zalcitabine (ddC) and stavudine (d4T)
Lamivudine (3TC) and didanosine (ddI)

*Some authorities recommend PI-sparing regimens (see V.H.7.)

5. If possible, nevirapine should not be combined with a PI, because dose of PI must be increased if combined with nevirapine

6. If only one NRTI is used in a triple combination use zidovudine, stavudine, or didanosine; never use lamivudine as high-level resistance develops within 2-4 weeks in partially suppressive regimens

7. PI-sparing regimens: Because of fears of treatment failures leading to cross-resistance to all PIs and serious side effects, some experts recommend that patients with modest degrees of immunocompromise and no treatment experience should defer exposure to PIs and instead should be prescribed combinations of NRTIs and a NNRTI

I. Interruption of antiretroviral therapy: stop all antiretroviral agents simultaneously

J. Considerations for **changing an antiretroviral regimen**
1. If change is due to drug toxicity, substitute one or more alternative drugs of same potency from the same class of agents as causing suspected toxicity
2. Criteria to use when deciding whether or not to change regimens (see following table)

CRITERIA THAT SHOULD PROMPT CONSIDERATION OF CHANGING THERAPY
1. < a 0.5- to 0.75-log reduction in plasma HIV RNA by 4 weeks after initiation of therapy or < a 1-log reduction by 8 weeks
2. Failure to suppress plasma HIV RNA to undetectable levels within 4-6 months after initiation of therapy*
3. Repeated detection of virus in plasma after initial suppression of undetectable levels which suggests development of resistance
4. Any reproducible significant increase (defined as threefold or greater) from nadir of plasma HIV RNA levels not attributable to intercurrent infection, vaccination, or test methods
5. Patients on monotherapy and dual therapy regimens should be considered for triple combination therapy, regardless of viral load
6. Persistently declining CD4+ T-cell counts (measured on two separate occasions)
7. Clinical deterioration**

*Before changing therapies, consider the degree of initial decrease in plasma HIV RNA and the overall trend in decreasing viremia (patients with high initial viral loads may have slower rates of declining plasma HIV RNA)
**Professional judgement is needed; a new opportunistic infection may not suggest failure of drug therapy if there has been a sufficient decline in viremia

Adapted from NIH Panel to Define Principles of Therapy of HIV Infection. (1998). Guidelines for the use of antiretroviral agents in HIV-infected adults and adolescents. Annals of Internal Medicine, 128, 1079-1100.

3. With drug failure, best approach is to change to all new drugs, not previously taken
4. Limited information is available on restarting a drug that the patient has previously received; avoid if possible
5. Because of the likelihood of high-level cross resistance avoid the following:
    a. Changing from ritonavir to indinavir or vice versa
    b. Changing from nevirapine to delavirdine or vice versa
6. See the following table for possible regimens for patients in whom antiretroviral therapy has failed

TREATMENT OPTIONS WHEN CHANGING ANTIRETROVIRAL REGIMENS	
Prior Regimen	**New Regimen (Not listed in priority order)**

2 NRTIs +
    Nelfinavir
	2 new NRTIs +
	    RTV; or IDV; or SQV + RTV; or NNRTI# + RTV; or NNRTI + IDV*

Ritonavir	SQV + RTV*; NFV + NNRTI; or NFV + SQV
Indinavir	SQV + RTV; NFV + NNRTI; or NFV + SQV
Saquinavir	RTV + SQV; or NNRTI + IDV
2 NRTIs + NNRTI	2 new NRTIs + a protease inhibitor
2 NRTIs	2 new NRTIs + a protease inhibitor 2 new NRTIs + RTV + SQV 1 new NRTI + 1 NNRTI + a protease inhibitor 2 protease inhibitors + NNRTI
1 NRTI	2 new NRTIs + a protease inhibitor 2 new NRTIs + NNRTI 1 new NRTI + 1 NNRTI + a protease inhibitor

#Of the two available NNRTIs, clinical trials support a preference for nevirapine over delavirdine based on results of viral load assays. These two agents have opposite effects on the CYP450 pathway and this must be considered in combining these drugs with other agents
*There are some clinical tests with viral burden data to support this recommendation

Adapted from NIH Panel to Define Principles of Therapy of HIV Infection. (1998). Guidelines for the use of antiretroviral agents in HIV-infected adults and adolescents. Annals of Internal Medicine, 128, 1079-1100.

K. Nucleoside reverse transcriptase inhibitors (NRTIs)
    1. Mechanism of action: Blocks the conversion of virus RNA into viral DNA through inhibition of reverse transcriptase; inhibits viral spread to uninfected cells rather than eradicating the virus
    2. Factors to consider when selecting a NRTI: advantages and disadvantages

SELECTION OF NUCLEOSIDE REVERSE TRANSCRIPTASE INHIBITORS		
Drug	**Advantages**	**Disadvantages**
Zidovudine (Retrovir, AZT, ZDV, Azidothymidine)	✓ Superior CNS penetration compared to other NRTIs ✓ Twice daily dosing ✓ Can be combined with lamivudine in one tablet (Combivir)	✓ Numerous nuisance adverse effects ✓ Major objective adverse effect: bone marrow suppression with anemia and/or granulocytopenia ✓ May not be given with stavudine
Didanosine (ddl, dideoxyinosine, Videx)	✓ Efficacious ✓ Twice daily dosing	✓ Must be taken on empty stomach ✓ Only available in chewable tablets, powder or liquid ✓ Decreases absorption of other drugs when taken simultaneously ✓ Adverse effect of pancreatitis which can be fatal
Zalcitabine (ddC, dideoxycytidine, Hivid)	✓ None	✓ Efficacy is less than other NRTIs ✓ TID dosing ✓ Adverse effect of peripheral neuropathy is common

(continued)

SELECTION OF NUCLEOSIDE REVERSE TRANSCRIPTASE INHIBITORS (CONTINUED)

Drug	Advantages	Disadvantages
Stavudine (d4T, Zerit)	✓ Twice daily dosing	✓ Adverse effect of peripheral neuropathy is common ✓ May <u>not</u> be given with zidovudine
Lamivudine (3TC, Epivir)	✓ Twice daily dosing ✓ Few adverse effects ✓ Can be combined with zidovudine in one tablet (Combivir) ✓ Has activity against Hepatitis B	✓ Resistence develops rapidly if not given with another antiretroviral
Abacavir (Ziagen, 1592)	✓ Good bioavailability ✓ Penetrates CNS ✓ Well Tolerated	✓ Serious hypersensitivity reaction mandates stopping drug permanently

NUCLEOSIDE REVERSE TRANSCRIPTASE INHIBITORS

Dosing	Adverse Effects	Contraindications/ Precautions	Comments
Zidovudine: 600 mg/day in 2-3 divided doses; Available 100 mg and 300 mg caps **or** with lamivudine as **Combivir** 1 tab BID	✓ Major: bone marrow suppression with anemia and/or neutropenia ✓ Common subjective: nausea, headaches, insomnia, fatigue, malaise, vomiting, GI pain ✓ Less common: myopathy and muscle pain ✓ Long term: nail pigmentation	✓ Consider dose adjustment in patients with liver dysfunction	✓ Do **not** use with ganciclovir or other marrow-suppressing drugs ✓ Do **not** use with stavudine ✓ Discontinue if hemoglobin falls below 7.5 g/dL ✓ Monitor CBC 2-4 weeks after initiating and then periodically
Didanosine: <60 kg: 125 mg q 12 hours; ≥60 kg: 200 mg q 12 hours; Available 25, 50, 100, 150 mg chewable tablets and 100,167, 250 mg packets of buffered powder; must take on empty stomach	✓ Pancreatitis (potentially fatal) ✓ Peripheral neuropathy ✓ Diarrhea and GI problems	✓ Consider dose adjustment in patients with renal and liver dysfunction; do not prescribe to alcoholics, patients with history of pancreatitis, and those with poor seizure control	✓ Do not give within two hours following drugs requiring an acid environment: ketoconazole, dapsone, tetracyclines, quinolones, cimetidine, indinavir, delavirdine ✓ Monitor amylase levels and assess for abdominal pain, nausea, and vomiting ✓ Contains 8.6 mEq of magnesium hydroxide ✓ Must chew tabs
Zalcitabine: <45 kg: 0.375 mg q 8 hours; ≥45 kg 0.75 mg q 8 hours; Available 0.375, 0.75 tabs	✓ Peripheral neuropathy ✓ Aphthous ulcers ✓ Pancreatitis (less frequently than with didanosine)	✓ Extreme caution when given to patients with Hepatitis B; consider dose adjustment in patients with renal disease	✓ Used infrequently today because it is less efficacious than other NRTIs
Stavudine: <60 kg: 30 mg BID; ≥60 kg 40 BID; Available 15, 20, 30, 40 caps	✓ Peripheral neuropathy	✓ Consider dose adjustment in patients with renal and liver dysfunction	✓ Use cautiously with other drugs that cause peripheral neuropathy
Lamivudine: 150 mg BID; Available 150 mg tabs **or** with zidovudine as **Combivir** 1 tab BID	✓ Minimal toxicity but may have headache, nausea, diarrhea, abdominal pain, insomnia	✓ Consider dose adjustment in patients with renal dysfunction	✓ Increased drug absorption when given with trimethoprim/sulfamethoxazole ✓ Delays or reverses resistance of zidovudine ✓ Best to always administer concurrently with a protease inhibitor ✓ Not recommended with ddC and ddI
Abacavir 300 mg every 12 hours	✓ Usually well tolerated; may have mild nausea, headache, malaise, abdominal pain, and diarrhea ✓ Serious hypersensitivity reaction with flu-like symptoms, fever, nausea, vomiting, malaise, and rash		✓ May be combined with any PI and with zidovudine and lamivudine (no known clinically significant drug interactions with other antiretroviral agents)

L.   Protease inhibitors (PI)
   1.   Mechanism of action: Inhibit HIV replication in cells that are chronically infected with HIV; competitively inhibit the HIV protease enzyme, a necessary enzyme for formation of the protein capsule surrounding the viral RNA in mature virions
   2.   Factors to consider when selecting a PI
       a.   Saquinavir (Invirase) hard-gel formulation has decreased bioavailability; use Fortovase, soft-gel formulation
       b.   Saquinavir and nelfinavir have less cross-resistance than other PIs
       c.   Ritonavir is the most potent PI but has many drug interactions and adverse effects
       d.   Indinavir is the least expensive PI, but is difficult for patient to take because it must be taken on an empty stomach and patient must drink >48 ounces of fluids
   3.   Toxicities of PIs sometimes limit their use
       a.   Elevated glucose, serum triglycerides, and cholesterol are often reported
           (1)   Monitor these levels every 3 months
           (2)   Teach patients to maintain a healthy diet by reducing intake of saturated fatty acids, cholesterol and simple sugars
           (3)   Consider prescribing gemfibrozil (Lopid) 1.2 g/day in 2 divided doses 30 minutes before morning and evening meals if trigylceride levels are >1000
       b.   Changes in body habitus: peripheral lipodystrophy (fat wasting of face and limbs with central obesity), posterior cervical fat pads ("buffalo hump"), and breast enlargement in females
   4.   Patient adherence is a major consideration; to enhance adherence
       a.   Use combination medications if possible such as combivir
       b.   Simplify medication regimen
       c.   Individualize therapy and seek patients' input on their preferences for drug regimens
   5.   See following tables for selecting PIs, drug interactions and other drugs requiring dose modifications

CHARACTERISTICS OF PROTEASE INHIBITORS

Characteristic	Indinavir (Crixivan)§	Ritonavir (Norvir)*	Saquinavir-SGC* (Fortovase)	Nelfinavir (Viracept)§
Form	200-,400-mg caplets	600 mg/7.5 mL po solution	200-mg soft gel caps	250-mg tablets 50-mg/g oral powder
Dosing recommendations	800 mg q8h Take 1 h before or 2 h after meals; may take with skim milk or low-fat meal Reduce dose to 600 mg q 8 hours with ketoconazole or itraconazole	600 mg q 12h*† Take with food if possible	1,200 mg TID* Take with large meal	750 mg TID Take with food (meal or light snack)
Patient Teaching	Drink >48 ounces of fluid to reduce risk of nephrolithiasis Grapefruit juice decreases levels Separate by 2 hrs. from ddI Can use with oral contraceptives	Liquid contains alcohol; caution about driving and working with machinery; avoid in patients with alcohol abuse problems Reduces effectiveness of oral contraceptives Tobacco decreases levels	Not bioequivalent to Invirase or hard gel formulation Grapefruit juice increases levels	Do not take with carbonated beverages due to high phosphorus content Reduces effectiveness of oral contraceptives
Adverse effects	Nephrolithiasis GI intolerance, nausea Laboratory: increased indirect bilirubinemia (inconsequential) Miscellaneous: headache, asthenia, blurred vision, dizziness, rash, metallic taste, thrombocytopenia Hyperglycemia ↑Cholesterol ↑Trigylcerides	GI intolerance, nausea, vomiting, diarrhea Paresthesias– circumoral and extremities Hepatitis Asthenia Taste perversion Laboratory: ↑ triglycerides, ↑ aminotransferase, ↑ creatine phosphokinase and uric acid, ↑glucose	GI intolerance, nausea, diarrhea, abdominal pain, and dyspepsia Headache Elevated aminotransferase enzymes Hypergylcemia	Diarrhea Hyperglycemia

*Combination of ritonavir 400 mg BID and saquinavir-SGC 400 mg BID
†Dose escalation of ritonavir: days 1-2, 300 mg BID; days 3-5, 400 BID; days 6-13, 500 mg BID; day 14, 600 mg BID.
§Twice-daily regimens of indinavir 1200 mg BID (three 400 mg caps BID) and nelfinavir 1000 mg. in am (four 250 mg tabs) and 1250 mg in pm (five 250 mg tabs) in combination with zidovudine and lamivudine is not recommended in 1998

Adapted from NIH Panel to Define Principles of Therapy of HIV Infection. (1998). Guidelines for the use of antiretroviral agents in HIV-infected adults and adolescents. Annals of Internal Medicine, 128, 1079-1100.

DRUG INTERACTIONS: PROTEASE INHIBITORS

Indinavir *(Crixivan)*	Ritonavir *(Norvir)*	Saquinavir-SGC *(Fortovase)*	Nelfinavir *(Viracept)*
Inhibits cytochrome p450 (less than ritonavir) Do not use with rifampin Contraindicated for concurrent use: terfenadine, astemizole, cisapride, triazolam, midazolam, and ergot alkaloids Indinavir increased by ketoconazole*, delavirdine, and nelfinivir Indinavir reduced by rifampin, rifabutin, grapefruit juice, and nevirapine Didanosine reduces indinavir absorption unless taken >2 h apart	Inhibits cytochrome p450 (potent inhibitor) Ritonavir increases levels of multiple drugs that are not recommended for concurrent uses§ Didanosine may reduce absorption of both drugs; should be taken ≥2 h apart Ritonavir decreases ethinyl estradiol, theophylline, sulfamethoxazole, and zidovudine Ritonavir increases clarithromycin and desipramine	Inhibits cytochrome p450 Saquinavir increased by ritonavir, ketoconazole, grapefruit juice, nelfinavir, and delavirdine Saquinavir reduced by rifampin, rifabutin, and possibly phenobarbital, phenytoin, dexamethasone, carbamazepine, and nevirapine Contraindicated for concurrent use: rifampin, rifabutin, terfenadine, astemizole, cisapride, ergot alkaloids, triazolam, and midazolam	Inhibits cytochome p450 (less than ritonavir) Nelfinavir reduced by rifampin and rifabutin Contraindicated for concurrent use: triazolam, midazolam, ergot alkaloids, terfenadine, astemizole, and cisapride Nelfinavir decreases ethinyl estradiol and norethindrone Nelfinavir increases rifabutin, saquinavir, and indinavir Not recommended for concurrent use: rifampin

§Drugs contraindicated for concurrent use with ritonavir: amiodarone (Cordarone), astemizole (Hismanal), bepridil (Vascar), bupropion (Wellbutin), cisapride (Propulsid), clorazepate (Tranxene), clozapine (Clozaril), diazepam (Valium), encainide (Enkaid), estazolam (ProSom), flecainide (Tambocor), flurazepam (Dalmane), meperidine (Demerol), midazolam (Versed), piroxicam (Feldene), propoxyphene (Darvon), propafenone (Rythmol), quinidine, rifabutin, terfenadine (Seldane), triazolam (Halcion), zolpidem (Ambien), and ergot alkaloids

*Decrease indinavir to 600 mg every 8 hours

Adapted from NIH Panel to Define Principles of Therapy of HIV Infection. (1998). Guidelines for the use of antiretroviral agents in HIV-infected adults and adolescents. Annals of Internal Medicine, 128, 1079-1100.

DRUG INTERACTIONS BETWEEN PROTEASE INHIBITORS AND OTHER DRUGS REQUIRING DOSE MODIFICATIONS

Drug	Indinavir	Ritonavir	Saquinavir*	Nelfinavir
Fluconazole Ketoconazole and Itraconazole	No dose change Decrease dose to 600 mg q8h	No dose change Increases ketoconazole >3-fold; dose adjustment required	No data Increases saquinavir levels 3-fold; no dose change†	No dose change No dose change
Rifabutin	Reduce rifabutin to half dose: 150 mg qd	Consider alternative drug or reduce rifabutin dose to one quarter	Not recommended with either Invirase or Fortovase	Reduce rifabutin to half dose: 150 mg qd
Rifampin	Contraindicated	Unknown‡	Not recommended with either Invirase or Fortovase	Contraindicated
Oral contraceptives	Modest increase in Ortho-Novum levels; no dose change	Ethinyl estradiol levels decreased; use alternative or additional contraceptive method	No data	Ethinyl estradiol and norethindrone levels decreased; use alternative or additional contraceptive method
Miscellaneous	Grapefruit juice reduces indinavir levels by 26%	Desipramine levels increased by 145%: reduce dose Theophylline levels decreased; increase dose	Grapefruit juice increases saquinavir levels†	

*Several drug interaction studies have been completed with saquinavir given as Invirase or Fortovase. Results from studies conducted with Invirase may not be applicable to Fortovase.

†With Invirase.

‡Rifampin reduces ritonavir levels by 35%. Increased ritonavir dose or use of ritonavir in combination therapy is strongly recommended. The effect of ritonavir on rifampin is unknown. Concurrent use may increase liver toxicity. Therefore, patients on ritonavir and rifampin should be monitored closely.

Adapted from NIH Panel to Define Principles of Therapy of HIV Infection. (1998). Guidelines for the use of antiretroviral agents in HIV-infected adults and adolescents. Annals of Internal Medicine, 128, 1079-1100.

M. Non-nucleoside reverse transcriptase inhibitors (NNRTI)
    1. Mechanism of action: Act on a nonsubstrate binding site of the enzyme which alters the shape of the active site
    2. Drugs in this class should be used only in regimens designed to be maximally suppressive because of the potential for high-level resistance
    3. See following table for characteristics of NNRTIs

NON-NUCLEOSIDE REVERSE TRANSCRIPTASE INHIBITORS			
Variable	Nevirapine (Viramune)	Delavirdine (Rescriptor)	Efavirenz (Sustiva)*
Form Dosing recom- mendations	200-mg tablets 200 mg po QD x 14 days, then 200 mg po BID	100-mg tablets 400 mg po TID (four 100-mg tabs in ≥3 oz of water to produce slurry) Decrease dose to 600 mg TID with indinavir	200-mg tablets 600 mg HS
Drug interactions	Induces cytochrome p450 enzymes The following drugs have suspected interactions that require careful moni-toring if coadminis-tered with nevirapine: rifampin, rifabutin, oral contraceptives, protease inhibitors, triazolam, and midazolam	Inhibits cytochrome p450 enzymes Not recommended for concurrent use: terfenadine, astemizole, alprazolam, midazolam, cisapride, rifabutin, rifampin, triazolam, ergot derivatives, amphetamines, nifedipine, and anticonvulsants (phenytoin, carbamazepine, phenobarbitol) Delavirdine increases levels of clarithromycin, dapsone, quinidine, warfarin, indinavir, and saquinavir Antacids or didanosine: separate delavirdine administration by ≥1 hr	Metabolized by cytochrome P450 Induces metabolism of indinavir (increase indinavir dose to 1000 mg every 8 hours)
Adverse events	Rash Increased aminotrans-ferase levels Hepatitis Reduces effectiveness of oral contraceptives	Rash Headaches	Central nervous system symp-toms (dizziness, light-headedness, nightmares, drowsiness, insomnia, impaired concentration) Rash Birth defects (use with caution in females of reproductive age)

*May be given with indinavir, zidovudine, lamivudine
Adapted from NIH Panel to Define Principles of Therapy of HIV Infection. (1998). Guidelines for the use of antiretroviral agents in HIV-infected adults and adolescents. Annals of Internal Medicine, 128, 1079-1100.

N. Investigational therapies
    1. Several investigational drugs are in the advanced stages of clinical evaluation:
        a. Amprenavir (141W94) is a new PI
            (1) Dosage is 800 mg TID or 1200 mg BID
            (2) Available in 150 mg tablets
            (3) Can be taken with or without food
            (4) May be given with other PIs or NRTIs; metabolized by cytochrome P450 so drug interactions with other PIs may prove to be important
            (5) Does not have high-level cross-resistance to other PIs which suggests it may be good first-line option
            (6) Usually well tolerated, but may have gastrointestinal symptoms and rash
        b. Adefovir dipivoxil (bis-POM, Preveon) is in a different category than any of other currently approved antiretrovirals; it is a nucleotide analogue
            (1) It has activity against herpes simplex virus; may have activity against hepatitis B and CMV
            (2) Does not appear to be as potent as the other new agents, but it has limited cross-resistance to other currently available antiretroviral agents
            (3) Once daily dosing; 60-120 mg QD
            (4) No drug interactions with other antiretroviral agents
            (5) Usually well tolerated but may have mild nausea, vomiting, malaise, and diarrhea

    (6) Most common adverse effects are abnormal levels of creatinine and proteinuria (monitor renal function routinely)

    (7) It can cause lowered L-carnitine levels, so L-carnitine should be administered with adefovir

  2. Hydroxyurea (Hydrea) in combination with other antiretrovirals therapies is being investigated

    a. Best to prescribe hydroxyurea with didanosine (ddI) plus a protease inhibitor and a NRTI (stavudine is often recommended)

    b. Dosages are 1.0 gram daily in single dose; 500 mg BID; or 300 mg TID

    c. May cause leukopenia

  3. HIV vaccine is in the exploratory stage

O. Treatment regimen for primary HIV infection (acute retroviral syndrome)

  1. Prescribe a combination of two NRTIs and one potent PI (see V.H.4)

  2. Testing for plasma HIV RNA levels and CD4+ T-cells counts should be performed on initiation of therapy, after 4 weeks, and every 3-4 months thereafter

  3. The optimal duration and composition of therapy is unknown; some experts recommend that treatment should be indefinite whereas others treat for 1 year and then re-evaluate the patient with HIV RNA measurements and CD4+ T-cell counts

P. Symptom management

  1. Wasting syndrome defined as otherwise unexplained loss of 10% of body weight

    a. Causative factors include;

      (1) Decreased food intake due to mouth or esophageal ulcers, anorexia (often related to depression), early satiety, or nausea

      (2) Decreased absorption from loss of enzymes causing lactose intolerance; to avoid this problem teach patient to avoid all milk products by reading labels

      (3) Increased metabolic demand from infection and fever

      (4) Malabsorption due to infections and bacterial overgrowth

    b. Order following diagnostic tests to rule-out infection and treat as needed: stool culture, blood culture, cryptococcal serum antigen and other tests based on patient's clinical presentation

    c. Recommend daily multivitamin

    d. Consider prescribing one of the following appetite stimulants

      (1) Megestrol acetate (Megace) 40 mg/ml susp.; 800 mg/day; adverse effects include impotence, decreased libido, hypertension

      (2) Dronabinol (Marinol)

        (a) 2.5 mg BID before lunch and supper, may gradually increase to maximum of 20 mg/day

        (b) Adverse effects include abuse potential, euphoria, psychomimetic reactions, altered mental status

    e. Recommend nutritional supplements (10 cans per day are needed for total daily caloric needs)

      (1) If patient needs to gain weight and can tolerate milk use Carnation Instant Breakfast or SportsShake

      (2) If the patient needs to gain weight but cannot tolerate milk give Ensure, Sustacal, Scandishake

      (3) If patient has constant diarrhea give a low or special fat supplement such as Lipisorb or a supplement with special dietary fiber such as Ensure with Fiber

      (4) For patients with severe diarrhea an elemental diet (with easily absorbed nutrients) is needed such as Criticare HN or Peptamen

      (5) Advera and Hi-Cal VM are specifically formulated for persons with HIV/AIDS

      (6) Elemental formulas: Vivonex TEN

    f. Consider other beneficial therapies such as serostim (growth hormone) 6 mg SC QD X 12 weeks, recombinant growth hormone, thalidomide 100 mg PO/day, anabolic steroids (oxandrolone 20 mg/day PO)

  2. Testosterone failure may cause a decrease in energy levels and muscle mass

    a. To diagnose, order serum testosterone level

    b. Treatment is testosterone injections 200 mg IM every 2 weeks or testosterone patch (Testoderm TTS), apply 5 mg patch every 22-24 hours to arm, back or upper buttocks (application site rotation is not necessary)

3. Diarrhea
   a. Order following diagnostic tests to rule-out parasites or infection: Stool for ova and parasites, bacterial stool culture, *C-difficile* toxin, acid-fast bacterial smear of stool can sometimes detect *Myobacterium avium* and cryptosporidiosis
   b. If infection is ruled-out, prescribe one of following
      (1) Imodium (Loperamide) 2 mg. caps, two in am and one after each BM up to maximum of 8 caps
      (2) Alternative: Lomotil (diphenoxylate) 2.5 mg; 2 tabs or 10 ml four times a day
   c. Patient education
      (1) Increase fluids
      (2) Follow a low lactose, low fat, high fiber diet
      (3) Use LactAid instead of milk
      (4) Avoid caffeine, fried foods, carbonated beverages, cabbage, broccoli
4. Nausea and vomiting
   a. Rule out infections
   b. Symptomatically treat with metroclopramide (Reglan) 10 mg PO QID, or prochlorperazine (Compazine) 5-10 mg QID, or ondansetron (Zofran) 4-10 mg QID
5. Pain is a common symptom (see section on PAIN)
6. Fever
   a. Common causes are *Mycobacterium avium complex*, tuberculosis, lymphoma, cytomegalovirus infection, secondary syphilis
   b. Following diagnostic tests should be obtained: blood culture for acid-fast bacteria, cryptococcal serum antigen, CBC; consider PPD, RPR, chest x-ray
   c. Symptomatic treatment (see section on FEVERS)
7. Anemia may develop due to drugs such as zidovudine or may result from the HIV infection
   a. Order the following diagnostic tests
      (1) Iron profile, reticulocyte count, erythropoietin levels, B_{12}, folate
      (2) If patient has normal WBCs but decreased RBCs consider infection with parvovirus
   b. If patient is on zidovudine, consider switching to another NRTI
   c. For severe anemia (<7.5 hemoglobin), prescribe erythropoietin (Epogen, Procrit)
      (1) Need to determine endogenous levels of erythropoietin; if >500 units of endogenous erythropoietin, patient won't respond to this drug
      (2) Measure ferritin levels, patient must have adequate iron stores to respond to drug
      (3) Administer 100-250 U/kg, 3 subcutaneous injections every week
   d. Neutropenia may be due to drugs (zidovudine, ganciclovir) or HIV infection: give G-CSF, filgrastim (Neupogen) 5-10 micrograms/kg 2-4 times a week; available 300 micrograms/ml
8. Mouth ulcers are common, particularly if patient is on zalcitabine (See sections on APHTHOUS ULCERS, HERPES SIMPLEX, CANDIDIASIS)
9. Dermatological problems
   a. Eosinophilic folliculitis or red, itchy bumps: prescribe astemizole (Hismanal) 10 mg QD and one of following:
      (1) Camphor 0.5/Menthol 0.5 lotion (sarna)
      (2) Topical steroids
   b. See treatment of other dermatological conditions in SKIN chapter
10. Peripheral neuropathy: treat with one of following:
    a. Nortriptyline (Pamelor) 10 mg HS; increase dose by 10 mg q 5 days to maximum of 50 mg HS or 10-20 mg TID
    b. Ibuprofen 600-800 mg TID
    c. Capsaicin-containing ointments (Zostrix) for topical application
11. Mental health problems are common (see sections on DEPRESSION, INSOMNIA, and ANXIETY)

Q. Ethical issues
   1. Disclosure of HIV status to sexual partners
      a. Recent study found that 40% of HIV infected patients failed to tell their sexual partners that they were HIV positive; 43% of those who did not disclose failed to used condoms all the time

549

   b. Persons sometimes fail to disclose due to fear of abuse and abandonment

   c. Assist patients to safely and readily disclose; state health departments can help with confidential partner notification

  2. Needle exchange programs have been developed to reduce the spread of HIV infection; research results have been inconclusive

  3. The need for post-sexual exposure prophylaxis programs is being debated; programs typically offer the following:

   a. Assess sexually exposed persons risk of HIV infection

   b. Provide HIV testing and STD evaluation

   c. If risks are evident, prescribe postexposure prophylaxis regimen (PEP) within 72 hours after sexual exposure; delaying treatment more than 24 to 36 hours dramatically decreases the likelihood of effectiveness

R. Follow Up; adjust followup to clinical condition of patient

  1. Patients who are asymptomatic and not on antiretroviral therapy should be seen every 3-6 months

  2. Patients who begin antiretroviral therapy or begin a new antiretroviral regimen should be reevaluated in one month

  3. Patients who are stable and on antiretroviral therapy should be seen every 1-3 months depending on their clinical situation

REFERENCES

American Academy of Pediatrics Committee on Pediatric AIDS. (1997). Evaluation and medical treatment of the HIV-exposed infant. Pediatrics, 99, 909-917.

American Academy of Pediatrics Committee on Pediatric AIDS. (1998). Surveillance of pediatric HIV infection. Pediatrics, 101, 315-319.

Association of Nurses in AIDS Care. (1996). In K.M. Casey, F. Cohen, & A.M. Hughes. (Eds.). ANAC's core curriculum for HIV/AIDS nursing. Nursecom: Philadelphia.

Barnhart, H.X., Caldwell, M.B., Thomas, P., Mascola, L., Ortiz, I., Hsu, H., Schulte, J., Parrott, R., Maldonado, Y., Byers, R. & the Pediatric Spectrum of Disease Clinical Consortium. (1996). Natural history of human immunodeficiency virus disease in perinatally infected children: An analysis from the Pediatric Spectrum of Disease Project. Pediatrics, 97, 710-716.

Barrett, Douglas J. & Sleasman, John W. (1997). Pediatric AIDS: So now what do we do? Contemporary Pediatrics, 14, 111-124.

Bartlett, J.G. (1997). The John's Hopkins Hospital 1997 guide to medical care of patients with HIV infection (7th ed.). Baltimore: Williams & Wilkins

Burman, W.J., Reves, R.R. & Cohn, D.L. (1998). The case for conservative management of early HIV disease. JAMA, 280, 93-95.

Carpenter, C.C. J., Fischl, M.A., Hammer, S.M., Hirsch, M.S., Jacobsen, D.M., Katzenstein, D.A., Montaner, J.S.G., Richman, D.D., Saag, M.S., Schooley, R.T., Thompson, M.A., Vella, S., Yeni, P.G. & Volberding, P.A. (1998). Antiretriviral therapy for HIV infection in 1998. JAMA, 280, 78-86.

Center for Communicable Diseases. (1992). 1993 revised classification system for HIV infection and expanded surveillance case definition of AIDS among adolescents and adults. MMWR, 41 (RR-17).

Center for Disease Control. (1997). 1997 USPHS/IDSA guidelines for the prevention of opportunistic infections in persons infected with Human Immunodeficiency Virus. MMWR, 46, 1-46.

Center for Disease Control. (1998). Guidelines for the use of antiretroviral agents in pediatric HIV infection. MMWR, 47 (RR-4), 1-45.

Flexner, C. (1998). HIV-protease inhibitors. The New England Journal of Medicine, 338, 1281-1292.

Klaus, B.D., & Grodesky, M. J. (1998). Drug interactions and protease inhibitor therapy in the treatment of HIV/AIDS. The Nurse Practitioner, 23 (2), 102-106.

Klaus, B.D., & Grodesky, M.J. (1998). News from the 5th Conference on Retroviruses and Opportunistic Infections. The Nurse Practitioner, 23, 117-127.

Luzuriaga, K., & Sullivan, J.L. (1998). Prevention and treatment of pediatric HIV infection. JAMA, 280, 17-18.

Maenza, J., Flexner, C. (1998). Combination antiretroviral therapy for HIV infection. The American Family Physician, 57, 2789-2798.

NIH Panel To Define Principles of Therapy of HIV Infection. (1998). Report of the NIH Panel To Define Principles of Therapy of HIV Infection. Annals of Internal Medicine, 128, 1057-1078.

NIH Panel to Define Principles of Therapy of HIV Infection. (1998). Guidelines for the use of antiretroviral agents in HIV-infected adults and adolescents. Annals of Internal Medicine, 128, 1079-1100.

Provisional Committee on Pediatric AIDS. (1995). Perinatal Human Immunodeficiency Virus testing. Pediatrics, 95, 303-307.

Rodriguez, E.M., Diaz, C. & Fowler, M.G. (1997). The clinical management of children perinatally exposed to HIV. HIV/AIDS Management In Office Practice, 24, 643- 666.

Rutstien, R.M., Feingold, A., Meislich, D., Word, B. & Rudy, B. (1997). Protease inhibitor therapy in children with perinatally acquired HIV infection. Fast Track, 11, f107-f111.

Shands, J.W., Jr. & Bentrup, K.L. (Eds.).(1998). HIV/AIDS primary care guide: For health care professionals providing HIV/AIDS care. Gainesville, Fl: University of Florida.

Stephenson, J. (1998). AIDS vaccine moves into phase 3 trials. JAMA, 280, 7-8.

Working Group on Antiretroviral Therapy and Medical Management of Infants, Children, and Adolescents with HIV Infection. (1998). Antiretroviral therapy and medical management of pediatric HIV infection. Pediatrics, 102, 1005-1058.

Musculoskeletal Problems

ANKLE SPRAIN

I.   Definition: Injury to the ligaments of the ankle

II.   Pathogenesis:

   A.   Due to sudden stress on one or more of the supporting ligaments of the ankle

   B.   Often occurs from stepping off a curb or into a hole

   C.   If injury is sports-related, it is often due to jumping or falling on outstretched ankle; basketball, football, and cross-country running are the sports in which sprains occur most frequently

   D.   Inversion injuries which involve the anterior talofibular or the calcaneofibular ligaments occur most frequently

   E.   Eversion injuries which usually involve the deltoid ligament are the second most common type

III.   Clinical Presentation

   A.   Although the percentage is lower in children, approximately 85% of all ankle injuries in adults are due to sprains

   B.   Classification of sprains
      1.   First-degree sprain occurs when the ligament is minimally torn and the joint is stable with minimal pain and swelling
      2.   Second-degree sprain is a more severe injury with the ligament appreciably torn but the joint remains stable; tends to have more swelling and ecchymosis than Grade I injury; usually patient has difficulty bearing weight
      3.   Third-degree sprain is a complete tear of the ligament with an unstable joint; usually there is marked swelling, ecchymosis, pain, and difficulty bearing weight

   C.   Immediate pain is noticed and swelling over the injured ligament often occurs within 1 hour of the injury

   D.   Persons with previous ankle injuries have increased risk of reinjuring the same ankle

   E.   Characteristics of severe ankle injuries
      1.   Eversion injury
      2.   Immediate diffuse swelling which may indicate bleeding
      3.   Inability to bear weight immediately
      4.   Sensation of a "pop", "snap", locking of joint, or kick into the heel
      5.   On physical exam, patient often has a positive drawer sign and a positive squeeze test

IV.   Diagnosis/Evaluation

   A.   History
      1.   Ask patient to precisely describe how the injury occurred
      2.   Ask patient to describe the foot position at the time of injury
      3.   Determine whether the patient was able to bear weight after injury
      4.   Determine whether the patient had a sensation of a "pop," a "snap," or had any locking of the joint which may indicate a partial- or full-tendon rupture
      5.   Question when and where the swelling and ecchymosis were first noticed
      6.   Ascertain whether there is any associated pain in the leg, knee or foot
      7.   Inquire about previous musculoskeletal injuries
      8.   Inquire about self-treatment

B.   Physical Examination
1.   Always compare injured side with unaffected side; examine most painful area last
2.   Observe ankle, concentrating on the lateral and medial aspects of the foot and ankle, for swelling, ecchymosis, and deformity
3.   Check neurovascular status of foot
4.   Palpation should be systematic (see Figure 17.1 of anatomical structures)
       a.   Start with bony structures: shaft of fibula, distal fibula over lateral malleolus, medial malleolus, base of the fifth metatarsal, all the tarsals, metatarsals, and phalanges
       b.   Next palpate the ligamentous structures
              (1)   Palpate the anterior tibiofibular ligament
              (2)   Palpate the anterior talofibular ligament
              (3)   Palpate the calcaneofibular ligament
              (4)   Palpate the medial compartment to determine deltoid ligament damage
       c.   Palpate tendons including the Achilles, the peroneal tendons, and the anterior tibial tendon

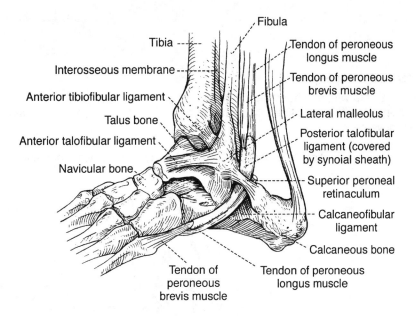

Figure 17.1. Anatomical Structures of the Ankle.

5.   Perform active range of motion and assess the limits of unassisted movement
6.   Perform passive range of motion and assess the limits of manipulation by the examiner without effort of the patient
7.   Perform resisted range of motion to determine muscular strength by measuring the patient's active movement against resistance
8.   Perform three special tests:
       a.   Anterior drawer test is used to assess the anterior talofibular and other ligaments of the lateral side of the ankle (see Figure 17.2)

555

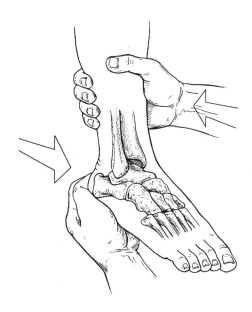

Figure 17.2. Anterior Drawer Sign.

Examiner grasps distal tibia with one hand and heel with other hand; Patient's foot is held firmly while backward force is applied to tibia; Positive test is graded 1+ for slight movement, 2+ for moderate movement, and 3+ for marked movement

          b.   Talar tilt test is used to assess stability of the calcaneofibular ligament (see Figure 17.3)

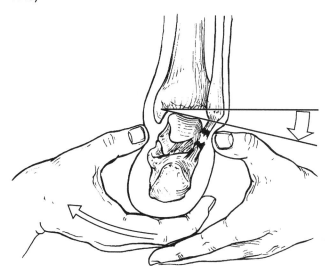

Figure 17.3. Talar Tilt Test.

Grasping the distal tibia and heel with other hand, apply gentle inversion force to affected ankle; ligaments are probably damaged if the talar tilt around the ankle is 5-10° greater around injured than around uninjured ankle

          c.   Squeeze test is not often performed but should be done if medial or severe lateral injury has taken place
              (1)   Examiner's hands are placed 6 inches inferior to the knee with thumbs on the fibula and fingers on the medial tibia
              (2)   Leg is squeezed as if to bring fibula and tibia together
              (3)   Pain with this test denotes syndesmotic injury which is a severe injury with a long rehabilitation time
    9.   Assess joints above and below injury

C. Differential Diagnosis
   1. Strains: Injuries to the tendons and muscles; usually have gradual onset of pain due to overuse rather than trauma
   2. Tenosynovitis usually occurs from a direct blow or overuse with repetitive overloads or faulty technique; Achilles tendonitis is an example and presents with pain on palpation of tendon and pain which is worse with active stretching and plantar flexion against resistance; tenderness is worse with hill running; treatment is rest, ice, and pain control
   3. Tendon ruptures such as Achilles
      a. While exercising, patient has a sudden onset of shooting pain in calf, followed by weakness in leg and inability to stand or walk on toes
      b. Signs include absence of normal plantar reflex and a positive Thompson test (with patient prone, flex the affected leg 90° at knee and squeeze calf; if foot doesn't move, the tendon is ruptured)
      c. Refer to orthopedist
   4. Fractures often occur in persons who engage in high velocity, high impact sports
      a. Salter type I and II fractures of the fibula are the most common ankle injuries in children
      b. Four basic injury mechanisms for fractures: lateral displacement of talus (most common), medial displacement of talus, axial compression of talus, and repetitive microtrauma
   5. Gout, arthritis, or infection may present with a painful ankle, but examination findings and history are inconsistent with trauma

D. Diagnostic Tests
   1. When to order x-rays is controversial; some authorities suggest x-rays should be routinely ordered to rule out bony involvement whereas the recently-developed Ottawa rules recommend the following:
      a. Order ankle series if there is pain near the malleoli and either inability to bear weight both immediately and in the emergency department or bone tenderness at the posterior edge or tip of either malleolus
      b. Order foot x-ray series if there is pain in the midfoot and either inability to bear weight both immediately and in emergency department or bone tenderness at the navicular or the base of the fifth metatarsal
   2. For children or adolescents with open growth plates, the chances of a growth plate fracture are higher and x-rays should be considered to rule out a Salter-Harris fracture
   3. Consider ordering of stress films when the ankle cannot be easily manipulated to test for stability or when the patient has chronically unstable ankles

V. Plan/Management

   A. Refer patient to orthopedist with Grade III sprain; consider orthopedist referral for eversion injury

   B. Patient education for the first 48 hours: follow RICE therapy (Rest, Ice, Compression, Elevation)
      1. Immediately after injury, stop all weight-bearing
      2. Apply ice to injury as many times as possible a day for 20 minutes
      3. Compression can be accomplished by using an ace wrap to hold ice in place and after ice application to prevent swelling (when wrapping ankle, make sure to include heel)
      4. Elevate ankle above the level of heart
      5. A posterior splint and crutches may also be needed

   C. Patient education after first 48 hours if patient's pain and swelling are resolving normally
      1. Use hot and cold contrast baths
         a. Submerge ankle in hot water (115°F) for 4 minutes then in cold water (50°F) for 1 minute
         b. Alternate between hot and cold water 4 times, ending with cold water
         c. Repeat procedure 4 times each day
      2. Begin exercising
         a. Toe alphabet in which entire foot and ankle traces letters of alphabet in air
         b. Isometrics in which side of injured foot/ankle is placed against an immovable object and pressed

c.   Toe raising in which patient raises up and down on toes while holding onto object to maintain balance

D.   Patient education 2 weeks post-injury for individuals who have no further problems:
1.   Resistive exercises with surgical or bicycle tubing (see Figure 17.4)
2.   Remind patient that once an injury has occurred, the joint will never be as strong which will increase likelihood of reinjury unless strengthening exercises are continued

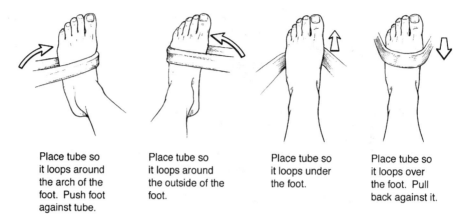

Place tube so it loops around the arch of the foot. Push foot against tube.

Place tube so it loops around the outside of the foot.

Place tube so it loops under the foot.

Place tube so it loops over the foot. Pull back against it.

Figure 17.4. Resistence Exercises.

E.   May order an air stirrup orthosis (e.g., Swede-O, Air Cast) to support ankle

F.   For pain, prescribe acetaminophen (Tylenol) 325 mg or 5-15 mg/kg/dose every 4 hours prn or ibuprofen (Motrin) 400 mg or 4-10 mg/kg per dose every 4-6 hours prn

G.   Prevention should include high-top lace-up shoes or a combination of proper shoes with a lace-up brace underneath (e.g., Swede-O)

H.   Follow Up
1.   Examine ankle in 7-10 days or sooner if pain and swelling do not decrease
2.   If there is little improvement or the condition has worsened in 2-3 weeks, consider referral to orthopedist or the ordering of additional films or bone scans

COMMON ORTHOPEDIC DEFORMITIES IN CHILDHOOD

I.   Definition: Orthopedic problems usually not related to trauma or other musculoskeletal disease

II.   Pathogenesis

A.   Developmental dysplasia of hip (formerly known as congenital dislocation of the hip)
1.   Results from partial or complete dislocation/subluxation of the femoral head out of the acetabulum
2.   Mechanical factors such as breech birth may have a role
3.   Hormonal factors may create increased ligamentous laxity
4.   Heredity seems to be a factor as 20% of affected children have a positive family history

B.   Increased femoral anteversion results when the femur is medially rotated on its long axis at birth and is usually idiopathic

C. Internal tibial torsion is due to a medially rotated tibia on its long axis at birth and is usually idiopathic

D. Pes planus (flat feet)
1. Longitudinal arch of the foot appears flat on the floor when child is bearing weight
2. Flexible or pseudo flat feet are familial in origin and due to increased laxity of the ligaments and joint capsules of the plantar aspect of the foot
3. Rigid flat feet are uncommon and considered a congenital deformity caused by a fibrous or bony connection between various bones

E. Metatarsus adductus
1. Results when the forefoot is turned in or adducted
2. Hypothesized to be caused by increased medially directed intrauterine pressure
3. Rigidity and tightness of muscles and ligaments of forefoot cause in-toeing

F. Talipes equinovarus (type of club foot) is characteristic of cerebral palsy, spina bifida, or muscular disease, but the majority of children with this condition are healthy and the cause is idiopathic

G. Genu varum (bowlegs)
1. Considered an angular variation which involves symmetrical bowing of the tibia and femur
2. Physiologic genu varum is often familial and a normal developmental variation
3. Pathologic genu varum is rare and due to rickets, dwarfing conditions, epiphyseal injury or Blount's disease

H. Genu valgum (knock-knees)
1. Considered an angular variation in which there is deviation of the axis of the thighs and calves
2. Frequently has a positive family history
3. Often a normal developmental variation
4. Associated with ligamentous relaxation, pronated feet, and overweight

III. Clinical Presentation

A. Developmental dysplasia of the hip (see table on SIGNS OF DEVELOPMENTAL DYSPLASIA OF HIP BY AGES)
1. Higher incidence in breech deliveries, first born children and females; left side is affected in 60% of cases (right 20%, bilateral 20%); less prevalent in African Americans
2. In the newborn period, there is ligamentous laxity resulting in hip instability without fixed deformity
3. About 60% of unstable hips in newborns spontaneously become normal within the first 2-4 weeks
4. In some children as they age, dislocation becomes more fixed and pathologic changes occur such as flattening of femoral head, excessive femoral anteversion, and valgus neck-shaft angle; these changes result in limitation of movements

SIGNS OF DEVELOPMENTAL DYSPLASIA OF HIP BY AGES		
Birth to 6 months	**Older Infant**	**Walking Child**
Barlow's maneuver causes hip to dislocate (see Figure 17.5 in physical examination)	Limited abduction of hip	Curvature of spine (scoliosis)
	Unequal leg lengths	Leg length discrepancy
Ortolani's maneuver reduces the joint and a click is felt (see illustration in physical examination)	Unequal knee heights when supine and knees are flexed (Galeazzi sign)	Occasional asymmetric intoeing or outtoeing
	Asymmetry of thigh folds	

5. In the ambulating child, the pelvis may tilt with weight-bearing and gait may be asymmetrical
6. Long-term complications include flexion contractures, osteoarthritis, pain, abnormal gait, and decreased agility; most serious complication is vascular necrosis of the hip

B. Increased femoral anteversion
1. Often familial and occurs more frequently in females
2. Typically presents between 3-10 years of age
3. Child often sits in "W" position and walks with in-toeing; often trips and falls
4. Patella and feet are rotated inwardly
5. Internal rotation of hip is greater than external rotation of hip in supine and prone lying positions
6. Usually is bilateral and symmetrical
7. Usually condition significantly improves by age 7-8 years
8. Resolution of intoeing secondary to femoral anteversion occurs in more than 80% of affected children without treatment

C. Internal tibial torsion (ITT)
1. Is the most common cause of in-toeing between the ages of 1 and 3 years; unusual in preterm infants
2. Often has a familial tendency
3. More common in precocious walkers and dark-skinned races
4. Often is accompanied with metatarsus adductus
5. May be associated with increased running speed; study found that sprinters where more internally rotated than a control group
6. Typically, the majority of affected children have spontaneous improvement by age 7

D. Pes planus
1. Feet have depression of the longitudinal arch; rigid flat foot may be associated with pathological conditions whereas flexible flat foot is common and not associated with problems
2. Plantar fat pad is normal until ages of 4-6; therefore, diagnosis is difficult before age 6
3. With flexible flat feet, the heel cord is flexible and the longitudinal arch is depressed during weight-bearing but reconstituted when non-weight-bearing
4. Patients may have pain, particularly in the calcaneus, on the plantar surface or on the lateral subtalar joint or the sinus tarsi
5. A history of difficulties during birth, delay in motor development, or recent onset of flat feet may suggest a neuromuscular problem
6. Fractures and tendon ruptures can result in flat foot

E. Metatarsus adductus
1. Occurs at birth to 6 months
2. Feet turn inward when child is both weight-bearing and non-weight-bearing
3. Approximately 85% of the cases of metatarsus adductus spontaneously correct
4. Usually the more flexible the foot, the more rapidly resolution takes place
5. Differential diagnosis
   a. Talipes equinovarus: forefoot is rigidly fixed in an inward position, the heel is turned inward and downward and ankle cannot be dorsiflexed
   b. Congenital metatarsus varus involves uncorrectable turning in of forefoot; heel is positioned outward and there is limitation of dorsiflexion of the ankle
6. Often associated with torticollis and developmental dysplasia of hip

F. Talipes equinovarus
1. Involved foot is usually smaller and shorter than uninvolved foot
2. Involves metatarsal adduction and stiffness
3. Hindfoot and ankle are plantar flexed
4. Heel is smaller or absent and is turned downward and inward while forefoot is curved inward
5. Ranges from mild and easily correctable to a severe and difficult-to-treat form

G. Genu varum
1. Genu varum up to 20° is normal in children until age of 18 months
2. By 24-35 months of age there should be spontaneous resolution and the knees should touch when the child is positioned supine; as growth occurs genu varum changes to genu valgum until age 7-9 years when there is normal straightening as child ages

H. Genu valgum
1. Considered normal from ages 2-6 years
2. Spontaneous resolution with growth is expected
3. Often associated with pronation of feet and more marked in child who is overweight

IV. Diagnosis/Evaluation

A. History
1. Specifically ask parents to discuss their concerns and to describe their child's musculoskeletal problem
2. If child is walking, inquire about gait and falling
3. Determine when child reached developmental milestones
4. Inquire about birth history, family history, nutritional problems, and incidents of trauma

B. Physical Examination
1. Measure height; short stature may indicate metabolic growth disturbance which is sometimes present with genu varum
2. Inspect skin; café-au-lait spots may indicate neurofibromatosis
3. Observation for alignment of bones, deformities, and muscle development in supine, prone, and standing positions
4. Observe gait if child is walking; scissor gait is suggestive of cerebral palsy; waddling with a wide stance suggests bilateral hip dysplasia
5. Observe for unequal leg length
6. Observe the shape of the bones such as lateral bowing of tibia in genu varum
7. Perform passive and active range of motion, noting limitations in movement
8. Assess motor strength

9. Perform special tests for each suspected problem.
    a. Congenital hip dysplasia: Barlow's and Ortolani's tests (see Figure 17.5)

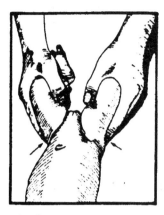
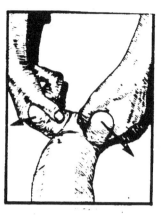
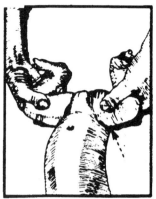

Ortolani's test (1): To be of any value the examination must be carried out on a relaxed child, preferably after feeding. Flex the knees and encircle them with the hands so that the thumbs lie along the medial sides of the thighs and the fingers over the trochanters.

Ortolani's test (2): Now flex the hips to a right angle, and starting from a position where the thumbs are touching, smoothly and gently abduct the hips.

Ortolani's test (3): If a hip is dislocated, as full abduction is approached the femoral head will be felt slipping in to the acetabulum. An audible click may accompany the displacement but in no way must this be considered an essential element of the test. Note that *restriction* of abduction may be pathological, and represent an irreducible dislocation (see also 11.71).

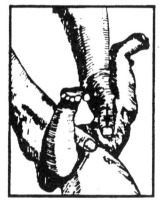
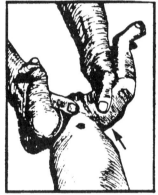

Barlow's provocative test (1): If the Ortolani test is negative the hip may nevertheless be unstable. Fix the pelvis between symphysis and sacrum with one hand. With the thumb of the other attempt to dislocate the hip by gentle but firm backward pressure. Check both sides.

Barlow's test (2): If the head of the femur is felt to sublux backwards, its reduction should be achieved by forward finger pressure or wider abduction. The movement of reduction should also be appreciated with the fingers. If either test is positive, treatment is essential.

Figure 17.5. Ortolani's Test and Barlow's Test.

Source: McRae, R. (1990). Clinical orthopaedic examination (p. 160). Edinburgh, Scotland: Churchill. Copyright 1990 by Longman Group UK Limited. Reprinted by permission.

b.   Increased femoral anteversion (see Figure 17.6)

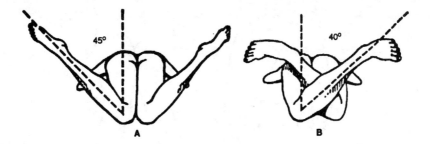

Figure 17.6. Evaluating Increased Femoral Anteversion.

With child lying prone and knees flexed to 90° measure ability to internally (A) and externally (B) rotate femur (make sure pelvis is level); in children with no problem, the external and internal measurements are similar; with increased femoral anteversion, internal rotation is increased (up to 90°) and external rotation is decreased (to as little as 20-30°)

Source: Killam, P.E. (1989). "Orthopedic assessment of young children: Developmental variations. <u>Nurse Practitioner, 14</u>, 32. Copyright 1989 by Vernon Publications. Reprinted by permission.

    c.   Internal tibial torsion
        (1)   Observe legs and feet while child walks; knee-caps will be positioned straight ahead or slightly outward with one or both feet pointing inward
        (2)   Observe legs and feet with patient sitting on examining table with thighs together and both knees bent over edge of table; feet will point inward toward each other
    d.   Pes planus
        (1)   Assess heel cord flexibility by passively dorsiflexing the ankle with the knee in extension and the foot inverted
        (2)   Assess also eversion and inversion of foot and abduction and adduction of the forefoot
        (3)   Heel cord and foot should be flexible; inflexibility suggests rigid flat feet
    e.   Metatarsus adductus
        (1)   Examiner should grasp heel with nondominant hand and gently push the inward-turning forefoot outward with the dominant hand, attempting to realign the foot in normal position; degree to which forefoot is passively correctable will allow classification as flexible, partially correctable or rigid
        (2)   Another way to determine foot flexibility is by scratching first the outside and then the inside of the lower border of the foot. With metatarsus adductus the foot will flex, but with metatarsus varus or talipes equinovarus the foot will straighten
    f.   Talipes equinovarus
        (1)   Examine dorsum of foot; heel cord will be inflexible
        (2)   Grasp the foot by the heel with sole lying in examiner's hand and dorsiflex (inflexible cords are present if dorsiflexion cannot be carried to about 20-30° beyond a right angle)
        (3)   Carefully, ascertain that the child with clubfoot does not have a generalized neuromuscular disorder such as spina bifida or cerebral palsy
    g.   Genu varum (see Figure 17.7)
        (1)   Position child supine with medial malleoli together and measure the distance between the knees (intercondylar distance)
        (2)   Normally, by 24-36 months the knees should be touching or have a only a small space between the medial surfaces of the knees
        (3)   Assess the child with genu varum every 4 months
    h.   Genu valgum (see Figure 17.7)
        (1)   Position child supine with knees touching and measure distance between the medial malleoli
        (2)   Genu valgum in children over age 6 should be assessed every 6 months

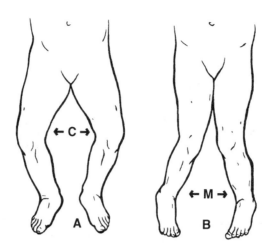

Figure 17.7. Measurement of Genu Varum and Genu Valgum.

For genu varum (bowing) (A) the intercondylar distance (C) is measured with ankles touching. In genu valgum (knock-knees) (B) the intermalleolar (M) is measured with the knees together. A measurement of more than 5 to 6 inches suggests a severe condition requiring further evaluation

    C.   Differential Diagnosis: See disorders under pathogenesis

    D.   Diagnostic Tests
        1.   If developmental dysplasia of hip is suspected:
            a.   In infant <3-4 months, order an ultrasound of the hip
            b.   In older infant, order x-ray (anteroposterior and frog lateral pelvis x-ray)
        2.   Computed tomogram is best for quantitating femoral anteversion, but is usually not needed
        3.   X-rays can be ordered to measure the degree of tibial torsion, but usually are not needed
        4.   Order x-rays if genu varum is extreme or unilateral to rule out rickets, osteogenesis imperfecta, Blount's disease or injury to the medial proximal epiphysis

V.   Plan/Management

    A.   Developmental dysplasia of hip: Refer to orthopedist
        1.   Infants <6 months are treated with a Pavlik harness
        2.   Infants 6-18 months usually need traction and closed reduction with cast immobilization
        3.   Older children usually need surgical reduction; beyond 4 years of age in bilateral cases and 8 years in unilateral cases, reduction is usually not attempted

    B.   Increased femoral anteversion
        1.   Teach child to avoid the prone, in-toed sleeping position and the "reverse tailor" sitting position (research to support this teaching is limited)
        2.   Reevaluate child every 6-12 months
        3.   Refer to orthopedist if there is no improvement in in-toeing on subsequent visits, if in-toeing causes child problems, or if in-toeing persists beyond 7 years of age (surgery is rarely indicated)

    C.   Internal tibial torsion
        1.   Teach child to avoid the prone, intoed sleeping position and the "reverse tailor" sitting position (limited research data to support this practice)
        2.   Reevaluate child every 4-12 months
        3.   Children who have a 20° internal rotation that persists past age 15 months should be referred to orthopedist and may be given braces or corrective shoes
        4.   Usually no treatment is needed until child is older than 36 months; although controversial, a Denis-Brown bar which positions the feet and lower legs in outward-turning position during night and naptime may be used
        5.   Surgical intervention is sometimes recommended by age 7 if condition has not resolved

D. Pes planus
1. Refer to orthopedist if no arch is visible when the child is non-weight-bearing, if there is heel cord tightness or foot rigidity, or if the child has marked foot or ankle pain
2. No treatment is needed for children who are asymptomatic; shoe modifications may be beneficial for children who experience rapid shoe wear because of excessive pronation or who experience discomfort
3. Child and parents should be told that shoe modifications will not change the foot structure and are used for comfort

E. Metatarsus adductus
1. For flexible metatarsus adductus, teach parents to do passive exercises several times a day to bring forefoot into a straight position
   a. Heel should be held firmly in palm while opposite hand pushes forefoot toward its outer side
   b. Stretch should be held for count of 3 seconds and repeated ten times
   c. Perform exercises 4 times a day
   d. Care should be taken to not twist forefoot on the heel as this may result in stretching of the longitudinal arch
2. If condition persists beyond 6 weeks with stretching, refer to orthopedist
3. Fixed metatarsus adductus should be referred to orthopedist
4. Ineffective strategies: reverse shoes, bars or shoe wedges

F. Talipes equinovarus: Refer immediately to orthopedist; often treated with abductor shoes, serial casting and surgery

G. Genu varum: Refer to orthopedist if condition persists past 2 years of age, if bowing is increasing rather than decreasing, if bowing is severe (>5-6 inches between knees or intercondylar distance) or if there is bowing of only one leg

H. Genu valgum: refer to orthopedist if condition persists beyond 8 years of age or if condition is severe or unilateral

I. Follow up is variable depending on condition

ELBOW PAIN

I. Definition: Acute or recurrent pain or discomfort of the elbow caused by selected common problems

II. Pathogenesis

A. Lateral epicondylitis or "tennis elbow"
1. Inflammation of the common tendinous origin of the extensor muscles of the forearm on the humeral lateral epicondyle
2. Exact mechanism of injury is uncertain but activities that combine excessive pronation and supination of the forearm with an extended wrist are probably responsible

B. Medial epicondylitis or "pitcher's elbow"
1. Inflammation of the common forearm flexor origin at the humeral medial epicondyle
2. Occurs in persons performing repetitive pronation activities

C. Sublaxation of the radial head or "nursemaid's elbow"
1. Sudden traction on the outstretched arm pulls the radius distally causing it to slip partially through the annular ligament and tearing it in the process (see Figure 17.8 of anatomical structures of the elbow)
2. When traction is released, the radial head recoils trapping the proximal portion of the ligament between it and the capitellum

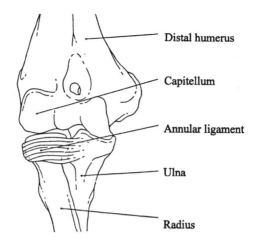

Distal humerus

Capitellum

Annular ligament

Ulna

Radius

Figure 17.8. Anatomical Structures of the Elbow.

III.   Clinical Presentation

A.   Lateral epicondylitis is one of the most common syndromes affecting the upper extremities
1.   Commonly occurs in patients who frequently play tennis, badminton, or bowl
2.   Also occurs in persons who engage in occupations that require using a wrench or screwdriver repetitively
3.   The commonality among these activities is use of a strong grasp during wrist extension
4.   Onset of symptoms is usually gradual with the patient complaining of tenderness on the lateral aspect of the elbow; swelling may occasionally be present

B.   Medial epicondylitis is similar in presentation to "tennis elbow" described above but occurs less commonly
1.   Occurs in baseball and softball pitchers during adolescence
2.   Clinical presentation is similar to that of lateral epicondylitis except that the pain is located in the area of the medial, rather than the lateral, epicondyle
3.   Inflammation can involve the ulnar nerve and compression of the nerve may cause numbness in the little and ring fingers on the affected side

C.   Nursemaid's elbow is the most common elbow injury in childhood occurring most commonly in children between the ages of 1 and 4 years
1.   Typical history involves an adult suddenly and vigorously pulling the child by the arm or of the child being swung by the arms (see Figure 17.9 for mechanism of injury)
2.   Pain in the involved arm may be immediately present causing the child to cry; the pain quickly subsides, but the child is unable to use the arm, which is held close to the body with the elbow flexed and the forearm pronated
3.   The child resists attempts to supinate the forearm and mild limitation of elbow flexion and extension may also be present
4.   Usually, there is no bony tenderness or evidence of swelling of the affected elbow

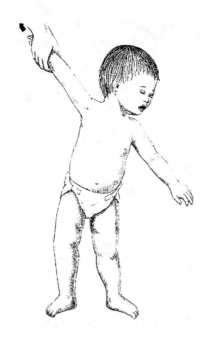

Figure 17.9. Mechanism of Injury: Nursemaid's Elbow.

IV.   Diagnosis/Evaluation

    A.   History
        1.   Inquire about onset, duration, and location of pain; if nursemaid's elbow suspected, ask about mechanism of injury
        2.   Determine if associated symptoms of swelling, numbness and tingling of hand/fingers, or loss of strength in arm or hand are present
        3.   If tennis or pitcher's elbow suspected, inquire about participation in activities, either occupational or recreational that require the following
            a.   Strong grasp during wrist extension (if lateral epicondylitis is suspected)
            b.   Repetitive pronation of the arm (if medial epicondylitis is suspected)
        4.   If nursemaid's elbow is suspected (but to rule out an infectious disease), ask if there is a history of fever, recent illness, or prior joint pain
        5.   Inquire about what makes the pain better or worse
        6.   Determine what treatments (either by the patient or another provider) have been tried and their result
        7.   Ask about past medical history and medication history

    B.   Physical Examination
        1.   If lateral epicondylitis is suspected, examine the elbow to determine the following
            a.   Assess for tenderness over the lateral epicondyle or over the radiohumeral joint
            b.   Assess range of motion (flexion and extension should be normal though extension may cause minimal pain)
            c.   Evaluate motor function of the hand by asking patient to abduct the thumb, index, and little fingers against resistance
            d.   Evaluate sensation at the dorsal web space between thumb and index finger (radial nerve), the tip of the long finger (median nerve), and the tip of the little finger (ulnar nerve)
            e.   Have the patient perform supination (palms up) and pronation (palms down) against resistance
            f.   To reproduce the patient's symptoms, perform the maneuver in Figure 17.10. Sharply localized tenderness in area of palpation or just distal is diagnostic of tennis elbow

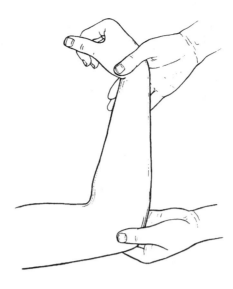

Figure 17.10. Palpation of the Lateral Epicondyle with the Thumb.

2.   If medial epicondylitis is suspected, examine the elbow to determine the following
   a.   Assess for point tenderness over the medial epicondyle
   b.   Assess range of motion (flexion and extension should be normal though extension may cause minimal pain)
   c.   Evaluate motor function of the hand by asking patient to abduct the thumb, index, and little fingers against resistance
   d.   Evaluate sensation at the dorsal web space between thumb and index finger (radial nerve), the tip of the long finger (median nerve), and the tip of the little finger (ulnar nerve)
   e.   To reproduce the patient's symptoms, perform the maneuver in the Figure 17.11. Tenderness on palpation occurs in pitcher's elbow, tears of the ulnar collateral ligament, and injuries to the medial epicondyle

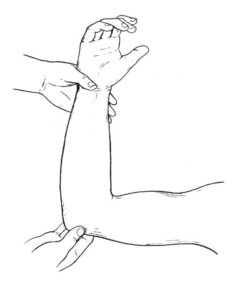

Figure 17.11. Palpation of the medial epicondyle.

3. If nursemaid's elbow is suspected, exam the elbow to determine the following
   a. Look for swelling, deformity, or point tenderness of the affected elbow (none of these features should be present)
   b. Examine the elbow joint for warmth and/or erythema (should be absent)
   c. Evaluate the fingers for neurovascular compromise (rare)
   d. Compare the affected and uninjured arms

C. Differential Diagnosis
   1. Nerve entrapment syndromes
   2. Arthritis
   3. Septic arthritis
   4. Fracture

D. Diagnostic Tests
   1. None indicated with history and physical examination that are consistent with the suspected diagnosis
   2. If atypical findings on history or physical examination, x-rays should be ordered

V. Plan/Management

A. Lateral epicondylitis
   1. Focus is on reduction of the inflammation, strengthening the involved muscle, and avoidance of further injury
   2. Rest (immobilization in a sling for several days), ice, and use of rapidly acting NSAIDs (such as naproxen or piroxicam) are helpful in reducing the inflammation
   3. Referral to physical therapy can reduce symptoms and strengthen the involved muscle groups in the forearm and wrist through an appropriate exercise program, possibly preventing recurrences
   4. Avoidance of the activity that caused the problem for several weeks or months is necessary
   5. Use of an elbow strap (available at sporting goods stores) in the area of the muscle mass of the proximal portion of the forearm can be helpful, but is usually of limited value
   6. Patients who fail to respond to conservative therapy should be referred to a specialist for management

B. Medial epicondylitis
   1. Treatment is the same as described under V.A. above
   2. If ulnar nerve involvement is suspected based on history and physical examination, prompt orthopedic referral is indicated

C. Nursemaid's elbow
   1. Apply pressure over the radial head, and at the same time, supinate the child's forearm with the elbow in a flexed position (see Figure 17.12 for reduction maneuver)
   2. Often, a click can be felt as the annular ligament is freed from the joint
   3. Symptoms resolve within 30 minutes, and immobilization after reduction is usually not required
   4. Acetaminophen may be prescribed for the aching discomfort in the arm that may persist for several hours after the reduction
   5. Parents should be cautioned to avoid pulling on the child's arms as there is a significant risk of recurrence

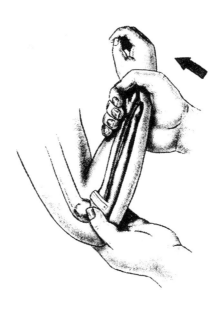

Figure 17.12. Nursemaid's Elbow: Reduction Maneuver Technique.

D. Follow Up
1. In lateral and medial epicondylitis, in one month to determine treatment effectiveness and to assess whether referral to a specialist is warranted
2. In nursemaid's elbow, no follow up is necessary unless the child fails to resume normal activities involving use of the arm in 1-2 days

EXTREMITY PAIN, LOWER

I. Definition: Acute or chronic discomfort or pain in a limb

II. Pathogenesis

A. Growing Pains
1. Etiology unknown
2. Possibly involves edema of muscle bodies within tight fascial sheaths during periods of activity or overuse

B. Shin splints: microtears and inflammation of the sites of origin of the muscles originating from the shaft of the tibia; often due to overactivity

C. Tibial and fibular stress fractures are due to repetitive forces being applied to the lower leg during strenuous activity; a malaligned lower leg may precipitate a stress fracture

D. Osgood-Schlatter disease
1. Degeneration of the tibial tubercle at the insertion site of the quadriceps ligament
2. Associated with overuse and rapid growth, particularly during adolescence
3. Result of repetitive, micro stress fractures

E. Patellofemoral pain syndrome (PFPS) is due to one or both of the following:
1. Mild malalignment of the extensor mechanism of the knee
2. Repetitive microtrauma from overuse

F. Chondromalacia patellae is due to degeneration of the cartilage on the articular surface of the patella; overuse and malalignment of the lower leg predispose individuals to this condition

G.   Patellar subluxation is associated with trauma and results in a lateral displacement of the patella

H.   Iliotibial band syndrome is caused by overuse and excessive friction between the iliotibial band and the lateral femoral condyle; related to change in footwear, increase in running schedule, or prolonged downhill running

I.   Legg-Calvé-Perthes disease results from compromise of the vascular supply to the femoral capital epiphysis which causes femoral head to become flattened; may be idiopathic or due to one of following:
1.   Slipped capital femoral epiphysis
2.   Trauma
3.   Steroid use
4.   Sickle cell crisis
5.   Congenital dislocation of the hip

J.   Slipped capital femoral epiphysis is a disorder of the growth and development of the upper femur due to a sudden or gradual dislocation of the head of the femur from its neck and shaft at the upper epiphyseal plate level; may be associated with endocrinopathies and heredity

K.   Toxic synovitis is an acute inflammatory reaction of the hip joint with unknown etiology

L.   Bursitis may be caused by acute trauma, contusion over bursae, overuse, or acute or chronic intra-articular inflammation (Baker's cyst)

M.   Plantar fascilitis results from small tears near the origin of the plantar fascia (the plantar fascia arises from the plantar aspect of the calcaneus and extends to proximal phalanges)

N.   Other important causes of lower extremity pain include osteomyelitis, neoplasms, fractures, sprains, sickle cell anemia, septic arthritis, thyroid disorders, and conditions with psychosocial origins

III.   Clinical Presentation

A.   Growing pains
1.   Most common in 3-5 year olds or 8-12 year olds with pain resolving in 12-24 months
2.   Usually bilateral and intermittent with deep, aching pain or restlessness that spares the joints
3.   Absent abnormal physical finding
4.   Commonly occurs at night with resolution by morning

B.   Shin splints
1.   Usually does not occur before age 10
2.   Most often develop in persons who undergo exercise and are not properly conditioned, do not warm up properly, run on hard or uneven surfaces, wear improper shoes, and/or have anatomical abnormalities
3.   Achy pain over the medial tibia that increases with exercise and improves with rest
4.   Tenderness over the medial tibia; may also have warmth

C.   Tibial and fibular stress fractures
1.   More common in adults than children; occur in athletes
2.   Pain at the start of running activity; pain reproduced by jumping on affected leg
3.   Diffuse tenderness over medial aspect of tibia or lateral aspect of fibula

D.   Osgood-Schlatter disease
1.   Most common in late childhood and adolescence
2.   Painful swelling and point tenderness of the anterior aspect of the tibial tubercle; resisting knee extension worsens pain
3.   Bilateral involvement occurs in 30% of cases
4.   Occurs with strenuous activity, particularly involving the quadriceps muscles

5. May have permanent prominence of the tibial tubercle
6. Reoccurrence rate is 60%

E. Patellofemoral pain syndrome (PFPS)
   1. Most common complaint in sports medicine clinics, particularly for the running athlete
   2. Females are affected more than males, probably due to females having increased width of the gynecoid pelvis which results in an exaggerated Q angle
   3. Patients often complain of dull, achy knee pain of insidious onset which may have associated clicking or popping of knee on movement; pain is often poorly localized and bilateral
   4. Pain is exacerbated with extended sitting, and activity involving knee flexion such as running and climbing and descending stairs
   5. Patient often has a positive patellar apprehension test: patient experiences pain when trying to contract the patella by tightening the quadriceps
   6. No history of swelling
   7. Tenderness is elicited by compression of patella in the femoral groove
   8. May have pain with movement of the patella laterally
   9. Often associated with malalignment such as femoral anteversion, external tibial torsion, ankle valgus and excessive foot pronation
   10. May lead to chondromalacia patellae and patellofemoral degenerative arthritis in adulthood

F. Chondromalacia patellae
   1. Occurs mainly in adolescents and adults; more in females than males
   2. Diffuse pain especially with climbing stairs or getting up from a squatting position
   3. Usually has a greater degree of malalignment than occurs with PFPS

G. Patellar subluxation
   1. Initial episode usually involves trauma
      a. Usually patient has severe knee pain and effusion
      b. Typically, patient can recall that knee "gave way"
   2. On pivoting and running, patients often complain of "locking" or "popping" of knee

H. Iliotibial band syndrome: typically involves mild pain over lateral side of knee

I. Legg-Calvé-Perthes Disease
   1. Most common in males, aged 4-8 years
   2. Limp may be presenting complaint
   3. Pain often is minimal, intermittent, and referred to medial aspect of knee
   4. Limitation of internal rotation and abduction of the femur is often present
   5. May have unequal iliac crest height and lower limb length discrepancy

J. Slipped capital femoral epiphysis
   1. Condition is a surgical emergency and requires immediate nonweight-bearing status to prevent further slippage
   2. Commonly affects sedentary, obese male adolescents
   3. Limp and varying degrees of ache and pain in the groin or referred pain in the knee are the common symptoms
   4. May have sudden dislocation of the head of the femur resulting in severe pain with associated inability to bear weight or gradual dislocation resulting in increasing dull pain
   5. Abduction, internal rotation, and flexion of the hip are the movements most limited
   6. Most cases are stable with a good prognosis if diagnosed early
   7. Unstable cases have a poorer prognosis because of high risk of avascular necrosis

K. Toxic synovitis is a diagnosis of exclusion and may resemble more serious conditions such as Legg-Calvé-Perthes, juvenile rheumatoid arthritis, or slipped capital femoral epiphysis
   1. Typically affects children 2-6 years old, but can occur to those as young as 12 months
   2. Most common cause of limping and hip pain in children
   3. Self-limited, unilateral hip or groin pain of insidious or acute onset
   4. Symptoms usually persist no longer than one week with bed rest and analgesics

5.   Hip is often held in flexion, abduction and external rotation positions

6.   Often follows a viral upper respiratory infection

L.   Bursitis: Typically has swelling and pain over respective bursae (prepatellar, infrapatellar, and anserine bursae); may be associated with a Baker's cyst

M.   Plantar fascilitis
1.   Patients have subcalcaneal pain which may radiate to arch of foot with walking or running
2.   Pain is typically present in morning and improves after taking a few steps
3.   Pain increases with forced dorsiflexion of toes
4.   Tenderness is present at medial plantar aspect of calcaneous

IV.   Diagnosis/Evaluation

A.   History
1.   Inquire about mode of onset, duration, frequency and location of pain
2.   Question about discomfort in areas above and below the stated location of pain
3.   Ask patient to describe pain
4.   Ask about joint pain, especially without a history of trauma, as joint pain is often related to rheumatologic diseases and needs to be ruled out
5.   Query patient about recent trauma involving the lower leg
    a.   Determine how injury occurred
    b.   Ask patient to specifically describe the position and movement of his/her leg during the trauma
6.   Question about history of fevers and joint/muscle swelling and redness
7.   Inquire about a history of a limp, stiffness, grinding, or any audible popping or snapping sound
8.   Inquire about exercise without pretraining, change in intensity or duration of exercise, recent viral infections, previous musculoskeletal problems, or repetitive activity
9.   Ask about medication use, particularly steroid use, and recent immunizations such as rubella
10.   Inquire about family history of musculoskeletal problems, autoimmune disease, sickle cell disease, and recent exposure to infectious disease
11.   Inquire about self-treatments and what aggravates and relieves pain
12.   Perform a review of systems to rule-out systemic disease

B.   Physical Examination
1.   Assess vital signs as increased temperature may point to a systemic disease
2.   Observe gait
3.   Observe for misalignment of bones such as femoral anteversion and external tibial torsion
4.   Observe for signs of trauma, development of muscles, deformities, swelling, and erythema
5.   May need to measure limb length
6.   Determine quadriceps angle (Q angle) if PFPS and chondromalacia patellae are suspected (see Figure 17.13)

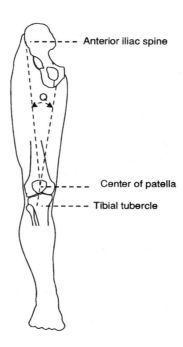

- - - - Anterior iliac spine

Q

- - - Center of patella
- - - Tibial tubercle

Figure 17.13. Measurement of Q-Angle or the Patellofemoral Angle.

Q angle is measured as the angle between a line drawn from the center of the patella to the anterior superior iliac spine and a line drawn from the center of the patella to the tibial tubercle. Average Q angle is 10-13° in males and 15-18° in females. Any angle less than or greater than average angles may be associated with PFPS.

7.   Palpate limb and joints for tenderness, swelling, deformity, and warmth
8.   Perform range of motion of affected joints, noting any limitation in movement, crepitus, and tenderness
9.   Assess peripheral vascular status by palpating pulses and determining capillary refill time distal to site of pain
10.   Assess sensation of affected extremity
11.   Assess muscle strength (distal weakness is often due to a neurological problem and proximal weakness is often due to a muscular problem)
12.   Evaluate joint stability
13.   Assess hamstring flexibility by having patient lie on back with hips flexed to 90° and then extend leg; failure to extend knee completely indicates hamstring tightness and may be a contributing factor in the extremity pain
14.   Compare opposite limb for swelling, muscle wasting, color, mobility, strength, pulses, and sensation
15.   A complete physical examination is often needed to rule out rheumatological diseases

C.   Differential Diagnosis:
1.   Septic arthritis often involves abrupt onset of fever, malaise, pain and a tense, hot joint effusion
2.   Inflammatory arthritis presents with warm, swollen, tender joints
3.   Osteomyelitis commonly has extremity pain along with systemic signs of infectious disease such as fever and a septic appearance

D.   Diagnostic Tests
1.   If there is suspicion of systemic or infectious disease, or if pain has a longer duration than expected, is not relieved by common therapies, or is more intense than usually expected, the following tests may be helpful

a. CBC
b. Erythrocyte sedimentation rate
c. Sickle cell preparation or hemoglobin electrophoresis
2. Consider rheumatologic studies for chronic pain
3. X-rays are usually ordered for the following:
    a. Pain due to trauma
    b. Suspected pathologic fractures, tumors or metabolic defects
    c. Pain lasting longer than 4-6 weeks
    d. Any history of swelling
4. Bone scan is often ordered if stress fractures or osteomyelitis is suspected.
5. Diagnostic tests are usually ordered for suspected common causes of extremity pain:
    a. Growing pains: None usually needed
    b. Shin splints: Order X-ray or bone scan if uncertain about diagnosis
    c. For suspected tibial and fibular stress fractures, x-rays (AP, lateral, and both oblique views of leg) are usually ordered; x-rays may be negative in early stages; technetium-99m bone scans and MRI are most helpful
    d. Osgood-Schlatter disease: None usually needed; may order x-ray to rule out other conditions or if diagnosis is uncertain; x-ray will reveal changes in tibial tuberosity
    e. PFPS: Order X-rays if pain lasts longer than 4-6 weeks
    f. Chondromalacia patellae: Order knee x-rays which include a tangential or sunrise view to look for lateral subluxation of the patella
    g. Patellar subluxation: Order knee x-rays; need a tangential or sunrise view
    h. Iliotibial band syndrome: none usually needed
    i. Legg-Calvé-Perthes disease: Order x-rays (anteroposterior and frog-leg lateral pelvis) or bone scan
    j. Slipped capital femoral epiphysis: Order x-rays
    k. Toxic synovitis: Consider ordering CBC, sedimentation rate, and x-rays
    l. Bursitis: Arthrography is ordered to definitively diagnose a Baker's cyst; otherwise none are needed

V. Plan/Management

A. Growing Pains
    1. Heat and Massage
    2. Acetaminophen (Tylenol) 5-10 mg/kg/dose every 4-6 hours

B. Shin Splints
    1. Rest: Unless the pain is severe, the athlete does not need to completely stop exercising but needs to reduce intensity and duration of exercise
    2. Ice should be applied to reduce swelling and inflammation
    3. Anti-inflammatory medication such as naproxen (Naprosyn) 250-500 mg every 6-8 hours
    4. May need to treat concomitant hyperpronation of foot with flexible orthotics or sturdy, well-fitting footwear
    5. Instruct patient to run on soft, flat surfaces; begin a program of preactivity conditioning exercises

C. Tibial and fibular stress fractures
    1. Initial treatment is rest, ice, and antiinflammatory medication
    2. Often fractures heal without casting or surgery
    3. Rest until there is no longer point tenderness on palpation or pain with running (usually takes 6-8 weeks to resolve)
    4. Can bike, swim or do other activities that do not produce pain

D. Osgood-Schlatter disease: Rest, ice, quadriceps strengthening exercise, hamstring stretching exercises, and limited use of antiinflammatory medication

E. PFPS
    1. Modify activities to avoid full flexion of the knee and stress on the patellofemoral joint
    2. Begin stretching and strengthening program for quadriceps muscles (perform three sets of 10 repetitions each day during the acute phase)

          a.   Quadriceps setting: Patient lies supine with affected knee fully extended, dorsiflexes foot, then tightens the thigh muscles or pushes the thigh into the floor

          b.   Straight leg raise: Patient sits on floor, leans back on elbows with one leg fully extended and the other leg flexed to 90 degrees; the extended leg is raised until it is parallel with the thigh of the flexed leg and held in this position for 5 seconds

          c.   Terminal-arc extension: Patient lies on floor with knees in about 20 degrees of flexion over a rolled towel of about 6 inches in diameter; patient then extends knee fully and holds for 5 seconds

          d.   After the acute phase, progressive resistance with ankle weights should be initiated

          e.   Encourage flexibility exercises as well

      3.   Consider flexible orthotics for malalignment of lower extremities

      4.   For exacerbations, use ice and antiinflammatory medication

      5.   Teach that pain tends to be chronic with exacerbations and remissions, but pain can be controlled; swimming or walking are better sports to participate in than running, basketball, and volleyball

F.   Chondromalacia patellae: Plan is similar to treatment for PFPS (see above)

G.   Recurrent patellar subluxation: Refer to orthopedist

H.   Iliotibial band syndrome: Rest for approximately 1-2 weeks (may take as long as 6 weeks), ice, limited use of NSAIDS, and gradual resumption of full activities with rehabilitation (quadriceps strengthening exercises); consider one-eighth-inch lateral heel wedge

I.   Legg-Calvé-Perthes disease: Refer to orthopedic surgeon

J.   Slipped Capital Femoral Epiphysis: Refer to orthopedic surgeon immediately

K.   Toxic Synovitis
      1.   May need to hospitalize if septic arthritis cannot be completely ruled out
      2.   Recommended treatment: bed rest and analgesics with frequent follow up

L.   Bursitis
      1.   Rest (couple days to weeks), ice for 24 hours, and limited use of NSAIDS
      2.   Aspirate tense, inflamed bursa and inject corticosteroid solution
      3.   Aspirate Baker's cyst to relieve pressure and pain

M.   Plantar fascilitis
      1.   Trial of heel lifts, padded heel cups or orthotic devices may be helpful
      2.   For acute treatment, rest, ice and NSAIDS are recommended
      3.   Local injection of steroids are used in more severe cases
      4.   Heel cord stretching exercises may prevent symptoms
      5.   A dorsal night splint is used for refractory cases

N.   Follow up for extremity pain is variable depending on patient's problem

FIBROMYALGIA

I.   Definition: Complex syndrome involving fatique and widespread, nonarticular musculoskeletal pain

II.   Pathogenesis

    A.   Etiology is unknown

    B.   The following mechanisms have been hypothesized to trigger fibromyalgia (FMS): metabolic processes, immunological abnormalities, sleep disturbances, stress and trauma from accidents or surgery and infection due to Epstein Barr virus, cytomegalovirus, human herpesvirus 6, enteroviruses, *B. burgdorferi*

III.   Clinical presentation

   A.   Age of onset is typically between 20-40 years; prevalence increases with age but can occur in childhood

   B.   Females are affected 8-10 times more than males

   C.   Most common symptoms are diffuse musculoskeletal pain, sleep disturbance, and persistent fatigue

   D.   Other symptoms include swelling of hands and feet, morning stiffness, headaches, paresthesias, sensitivity to cold and/or hot, dypsnea, chest pain, night sweats, visual problems, dizziness, painful menses, gastrointestinal complaints, memory impairment, anxiety and depression; children often have hypermobility

   E.   Patients may have associated conditions such as mitral valve prolapse, episodic hypoglycemia, Raynaud's disease, and irritable bowel syndrome

   F.   Symptoms can be severe and patients may become functionally disabled

   G.   Because patients have chronic, multiple, vague complaints and no outward signs, they are often misdiagnosed as hypochondriacs and relationships with family and friends may deteriorate

   H.   Patients often have disturbance of stage 4 of sleep; disturbance of this stage for 2-3 consecutive nights can produce physical symptoms of FMS even in normal controls

   I.   Tender points (localized areas of muscle tenderness that result in pain when pressure is applied) are essential to the diagnosis; trigger points (pain is elicited at initial site of palpation as well as in a linear or circumferential pattern surrounding the site or at a distant site) are also common

   J.   The American College of Rheumatology (ACR) established clinical criteria for diagnosing FMS (see table on ACR Criteria and Figure 17.14 on Tender Point Sites)

THE AMERICAN COLLEGE OF RHEUMATOLOGY 1990 CRITERIA
FOR CLASSIFICATION OF FIBROMYALGIA

*1. History of widespread pain

   Definition. Pain is considered widespread when all of the following are present: pain in the left side of the body, pain in the right side of the body, pain above the waist, and pain below the waist. In addition, axial skeletal pain (cervical spine or anterior chest or thoracic spine or low back) must be present. In this definition, shoulder and buttock pain is considered as pain for each involved side. "Low back" pain is considered lower segment pain.

2. Pain in 11 of 18 tender point sites on digital palpation.

   Definition. Pain, on digital palpation must be present in at least 11 of the following 18 tender point sites:
   Occiput: Bilateral, at the suboccipital muscle insertions
   Low cervical: Bilateral, at the anterior aspects of the intertransverse spaces at C5-C7
   Trapezius: Bilateral, at the midpoint of the upper border
   Supraspinatus: Bilateral, at origins, above the scapula spine near the medial border
   Second rib: Bilateral, at the second costochondral junctions, just lateral to the junctions on upper surfaces
   Lateral epicondyle: Bilateral, 2 cm distal to the epicondyles
   Gluteal: Bilateral, in upper outer quadrants of buttocks in anterior fold of muscle
   Greater trochanter: Bilateral, posterior to the trochanteric prominence
   Knee: Bilateral, at the medial fat pad proximal to the joint line

For a tender point to be considered "positive" the subject must state that the palpation was painful.

*For classification purposes, patients must satisfy both criteria. Widespread pain must have been present for at least 3 months.

Source: Wolfe, F., et al. (1990). The American College of Rheumatology 1990 criteria for the classification of fibromyalgia. Arthritis and Rheumatism, 33(2), 160-173.

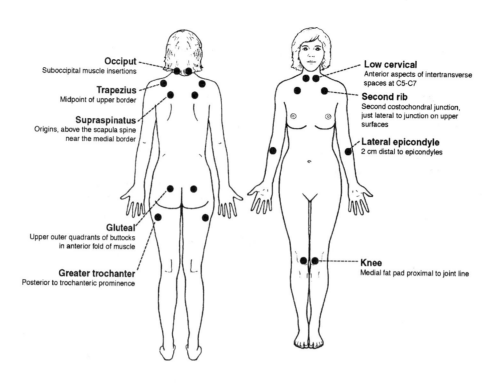

Figure 17.14. Tender Points Identified by American College of Rheumatology.

IV.   Diagnosis/Evaluation

    A.   History
        1.   Question about associated symptoms such as headaches, diarrhea, lack of concentration
        2.   Ask about factors that may precipitate symptoms
        3.   Explore how the disease has impacted on patient's family, interpersonal relationships, work, school, and activities of daily living

    B.   Physical Examination
        1.   Measure vital signs
        2.   Observe general appearance
        3.   Assess neck for thyromegaly
        4.   Perform bilateral digital palpation using a force of about 4 kg/cm$_2$ which is approximately equal to pressing finger on bathroom scale until it registers 10 pounds, or until the nail bed just begins to blanch; to meet criteria of a positive tender point, patient must label the palpation as "painful," not just tender
        5.   Perform a complete musculoskeletal, particularly assess each joint
        6.   Assess mental status and perform a mental health assessment

    C.   Differential Diagnosis
        1.   Patients with chronic fatigue syndrome have vague, systemic symptoms but do not usually complain of pain as is characteristic of FMS
        2.   Rheumatoid arthritis in contrast to FMS presents with warm, erythematous joints in addition to pain
        3.   Patients with FMS may have a mildly elevated ANA but other criteria of systemic lupus erythematosus (SLE) are not present (see section on RHEUMATOID ARTHRITIS for criteria for SLE)
        4.   Somatization and depression often accompany FMS but are not the primary diagnoses; patients with psychological problems do not have characteristic tender points
        5.   Myofascial pain syndrome presents with referred trigger points and occurs more frequently in males than females which is not characteristic of FMS

6. Polymyalgia rheumatica can be diagnosed by an elevated erythrocyte sedimentation rate (ESR)
7. Severe hypothyroidism can mimic FMS but usually patient has signs such as lid lag, dry skin, and an elevated thyroid stimulating hormone

D. Diagnostic Tests: no tests are available to detect FMS, consider the following tests to exclude other possible diagnoses
1. Complete blood count
2. Erythrocyte sedimentation rate (order in all persons >50 years who present with symptoms)
3. Measurement of muscle enzymes
4. Thyroid stimulating hormone
5. Rheumatoid factor

V. Plan/Management: a multifaceted approach with an interdisciplinary team is ideal

A. Patient Education
1. Provide reassurance that patient has a distinct, recognizable disease and that symptoms are real but can be managed
2. Help patient shift from a sense of helplessness and frustration to a sense of self-efficacy and hope
   a. Self-management courses to control symptoms and promote health are effective
   b. Social support interventions may be beneficial
   c. Cognitive behavioral therapy such as helping patients to prioritize their time and activities to include meaningful work, activities of daily living as well as leisure is helpful

B. Exercise: A program which includes pain reduction techniques of stretching, proper posture, body mechanics with careful and gentle exercise such as walking, bicycling, and swimming is helpful
1. Strenuous or excessive exercise should be avoided
2. Referral to a physical therapist can be beneficial

C. Pharmacological treatment
1. Medications to help the patient receive a restful sleep may be helpful
   a. Amitriptyline (Elavil) is commonly used and in the FMS patient this drug increases non-REM stage 4 sleep by increasing serotonin levels; prescribe amitriptyline 10 mg at HS and can increase to 50 mg over a few weeks
   b. Zolpidem (Ambien) 10 mg HS is an alternative drug to treat sleep problems; limit to 2-3 nights per week
   c. To help combat the concomitant fatigue and depression, a serotonin reuptake inhibitor like fluoxetine (Prozac) 20 mg can be given in the morning; a combination of amitriptyline and prozac was found to be more effective than either drug alone in a recent study
2. To treat muscle spasms, cyclobenzaprine (Flexeril) 10 mg TID can be prescribed; do not use more than three weeks
3. Tramadol (Ultram) 50-100 mg every 4-6 hours and topical anesthetics such as capsaicin (Zostrix) may be effective in relieving pain; because of chronic nature of FMS avoid narcotic agents; there are contradictory research findings concerning the benefits of nonsteroidal anti-inflammatory drugs

D. Massage therapy, acupuncture, local infiltration of trigger points with 1% solution of lidocaine, stress management, relaxation techniques, transcutaneous electrical nerve stimulation, visualization and meditation are additional effective therapies

E. Followup is variable and depends on the severity of symptoms as well as coping abilities and resources of the patients and their support systems

JOINT PAIN

I.   Definition: Discomfort or tenderness in one or more joints

II.   Pathogenesis: see clinical presentation for common causes

III.   Clinical presentation of common forms of joint pain

    A.   Pain involving multiple joints
        1.   Rheumatoid arthritis (RA): Chronic inflammatory polyarthritis with symmetric joint involvement and rheumatoid factor positivity (see section on RHEUMATOID ARTHRITIS)
        2.   Systemic lupus erythematosus (SLE): American Rheumatism Association Classification (1982) (see following table)

CLASSIFICATION OF SYSTEMIC LUPUS ERYTHEMATOSUS
• Malar rash: fixed, erythematous, flat, or raised rash over malar eminences
• Discoid rash: erythematous raised patches with scaling
• Photosensitivity
• Oral ulcers
• Arthritis involving 2 or more peripheral joints
• Serositis involving either pleuritis or pericarditis
• Renal disorder involving persistent proteinuria or cellular casts
• Neurologic disorder involving seizures or psychosis
• Hematologic disorders of hemolytic anemia, leukopenia, lymphopenia, or thrombocytopenia
• Immunologic disorder such as positive lupus erythematosus cell preparation or anti-DNA antibody to native DNA in abnormal titer or Anti-Sm or false positive serologic test for syphilis for at least 6 months
• Abnormal titer of antinuclear antibody

* A person is said to have SLE if 4 or more of 11 criteria are present

Adapted from Tan, E.M., Cohen, A.S., Fries, J.F., et al. (1982). The 1982 revised criteria for the classification of systemic lupus erythematosus. Arthritis Rheumatology, 25, 1275-1277.

        3.   Fibromyalgia is a poorly understood syndrome involving widespread musculoskeletal pain and accompanied by fatigue, nonrestorative sleep, reduced functional ability and sometimes accompanied with headaches, irritable bowel syndrome, paresthesias, restless leg syndrome, and cold sensitivity (see section on FIBROMYALGIA)
        4.   Reiter's syndrome involves classic triad of arthritis, urethritis, and conjunctivitis
        5.   Psoriatic arthritis often presents with asymmetric joint involvement and characteristic nail and skin lesions
        6.   Gonococcal arthritis presents as migratory polyarthritis, tendinitis and often has vesicular-pustular skin lesions
        7.   Lyme arthritis usually has classic history of tick bite and rash with arthritis in knees (see section on LYME DISEASE)
        8.   Rheumatic heart disease presents in a migratory pattern of joint involvement with evidence of antecedent streptococcal infection
        9.   Inflammatory bowel disease such as ulcerative colitis and Crohn's disease are associated with gastrointestinal complaints
        10.   Ankylosing spondylitis presents with back pain and stiffness
        11.   Infections such as influenza, rubella, mumps, chickenpox, infectious mononucleosis, hepatitis, Rocky Mountain-spotted fever, and rat-bite fever can also involve joints
        12.   Growing pains occur in about 18% of school-aged children and peak at age 11 (see section on EXTREMITY PAIN, LOWER)
        13.   Sickle cell disease causes pain, swelling, tenderness, and effusion in large joints
        14.   Malignancies such as leukemia and lymphoma; typically child has severe bone pain at night, fever, and weight loss

15. Vasculitic syndromes such as Henoch-Schönlein purpurea, Kawasaki disease, and polyarteritis nodosa usually have associated physical findings such as a purpuric rash

B. Pain involving single joint
1. Infection
   a. Septic arthritis due to disseminated gonorrhea or gram positive bacteria, especially *Staphylococcus aureus,* is a serious condition, presenting with fever, chills, skin lesion, joint pain, and swelling
   b. Gram-negative bacterial infections and infections due to anaerobes are increasingly frequent causes of monarthritis due to the rising number of persons who are parenteral drug users and immunosuppressed persons
   c. Tuberculous arthritis with subsequent periarticular bone lesions and synovial involvement may occur even if pulmonary tuberculosis is not present
   d. Monarthritis can herald the onset of HIV infection
2. One joint may be involved in crystal-induced arthritis such as gout and pseudogout which results from crystals of calcium pyrophosphate inducing joint inflammation and seems to be associated with hyperparathyroidism and hemochromatosis in the older patient
3. Trauma, and foreign-body reactions may present with sudden pain and swelling in one joint
4. Osteomyelitis involves localized swelling, limitation of joint mobility, erythema and tenderness over involved area, fever, and and/or an associated ulcer or skin lesion with possibly a sinus tract draining infected fluid; risk factors include history of bacteremia, peripheral vascular disease, diabetes mellitus, trauma, or surgery in the affected area
5. Toxic synovitis is seen in children < 10 years of age who have unilateral hip pain; typically occurs after an upper respiratory infection (see section on EXTREMITY PAIN, LOWER)
6. Localized tumors (e.g., osteogenic sarcoma) and metastatic processes (e.g., neuroblastoma) may cause solitary joint pain; usually accompanied with fever, weight loss, and lethargy

C. Other diseases such as rheumatoid arthritis, systemic lupus erythematosus, arthritis of inflammatory bowel disease, Lyme disease, psoriatic arthritis, Behcet's disease, Reiter's syndrome, and hemarthrosis (bleeding into a joint commonly due to a clotting abnormality) can result in pain in single or multiple joints

IV. Diagnosis/Evaluation

A. History
1. Ascertain pain characteristics, location, what aggravates pain, and what functional loss has occurred
2. Ask about distribution of involved joints (symmetric involvement of metacarpophalangeal joints (MCP) and wrists suggests rheumatoid arthritis (RA)
3. Determine severity of pain by asking if it awakens patient at night or hinders activities of daily living
4. Explore history of previous attacks; past episodes lend support for a crystalline or other noninfectious cause
5. Inquire about previous trauma to joint or surrounding tissues
6. Question about tick bites, fever, sexual risk factors, intravenous drug use, alcohol abuse, and travel in foreign countries -- all of which suggest an infectious cause
7. Inquire about rash, diarrhea, urethritis, or uveitis which supports a diagnosis of arthritides
8. Explore systemic symptoms such as fatigue, fever, sleep problems which suggest rheumatoid arthritis, SLE, fibromyalgia
9. Ask about history of gastrointestinal problems and determine whether there is a history of an ulcer, because this will affect choice of analgesic medication
10. A complete family history is important
11. Often a complete review of systems is needed to determine other involved organs

B. Physical Examination
1. Measure temperature and other vital signs (fever suggests infection such as septic arthritis)
2. Observe gait and general appearance

3. Examine joints for presence of tenderness, erythema, warmth, effusion, bony enlargement, and mechanical abnormalities
   a. Assessment must distinguish an arthritis, which involves the articular space, from conditions involving the periarticular area, such as bursitis, cellulitis, or tendinitis; painful limitation of motion probably indicates joint involvement
   b. Helpful to compare paired joints
   c. Remember to inspect, palpate, perform range of motion activities, and perform additional tests such as Tinel's sign [percuss over median nerve on palmar side or volar surface of wrist; shooting pain in the long or index finger is a positive sign] (see Figure 17.22)
4. Assess for muscle atrophy
5. Detailed physical examination often needed to detect extra-articular manifestations
   a. Observe eyes, nose, and mouth for dryness as occurs with sicca syndrome which suggests Sjögren's syndrome that often accompanies rheumatoid arthritis
   b. Palpate elbows, Achilles tendons, and pinnae for nodules (rheumatoid arthritis)
   c. Observe nails for pitting (psoriatic arthritis)
   d. Observe skin for malar and discoid lesions of SLE and exanthem of gonococcal arthritis
   e. Examine eyes for conjunctivitis of Reiter's syndrome
   f. Inspect mouth for ulcers in Behcet's syndrome, Reiter's syndrome, and SLE
   g. Auscultate heart and lungs noting pleural rubs and heart murmurs from RA and SLE
   h. Urethral or cervical discharge suggests gonococcal arthritis

C. Differential Diagnosis: Rule out all conditions listed in section III.

D. Diagnostic tests are useful in differentiating the specific type of arthritis present.
   1. Synovial fluid analysis is done to differentiate inflammatory from non-inflammatory joint disease and to determine whether a joint is infected
   2. Erythrocyte sedimentation rate (ESR) can be useful as a screen for inflammatory disease
   3. Rheumatoid factor may be helpful in confirming the diagnosis of RA, but is also often positive when the patient has other conditions
   4. Antinuclear antibody (ANA) is sensitive but not specific in diagnosing SLE
   5. X-rays are often ordered to obtain baseline data rather than to help determine diagnosis; best utilized in bone and joint evaluation
   6. Magnetic resonance imaging can sometimes localize an infectious or inflammatory process in a joint, tissue, or bone; best utilized in soft tissue evaluation
   7. Bone scans and bone marrow aspiration are useful in detecting tumors
   8. Tests for HIV antibodies should be ordered when risk factors for this disease are present
   9. Blood cultures are needed when sepsis is suspected
   10. Bone biopsy or culture are needed when osteomyelitis is suspected

V. Plan/Management

A. Determine severity of disease and the need for hospitalization; rapid onset on pain, heat, swelling, and erythema of joint should be evaluated immediately for septic arthritis or osteomyelitis

B. Treat known causes. For example, ceftriaxone (Rocephin) should be used to treat gonococcal arthritis

C. Symptomatic therapy often includes rest of involved joint, hot and/or cold therapy and pain relief with aspirin (not gout) or NSAIDs

D. Follow up is variable

KNEE INJURY, ACUTE

I. Definition: Injury to the knee from acute trauma

II. Pathogenesis

   A. Strains and sprains of the collateral and cruciate ligaments are caused by forces that create abduction of the leg at the knee, hyperextension of the knee, or a direct blow to the knee
       1. Strains involve stretching of the muscles or tendons
       2. Grade I sprains involve stretching fibers without significant structural damage
       3. Grade II sprains involve partial disruption of fibers with increased laxity
       4. Grade III sprains involve complete tearing of ligamentous tissues

   B. Tears of the medial and lateral meniscus are common and typically involve a simple twisting motion or a rotary force applied to a flexed knee joint; often caused by a noncontact injury

   C. Patellar subluxation or dislocation usually occurs with knee near extension and the tibia externally rotated or may result from a direct blow to knee; may accompany an anterior cruciate ligament (ACL) injury

   D. Fractures of the patellar result from fall or direct blow to knee; tibial tubercule avulsion fractures typically occur secondary to a fall or a jumping sport in children

   E. Hemarthrosis, or blood collecting in joint, is a serious injury and results from extensive trauma

   F. Excessive pronation of the foot or misalignment of an extremity can cause inappropriate stress on structures of the knee and result in injury

III. Clinical Presentation

   A. Musculoskeletal system of children differs from adults
       1. Children's bones are more porous and plastic than adults which creates a greater risk for unicortical or "greenstick" fractures
       2. Avulsion injuries in which a piece of bone is torn off at the point where a tendon or ligament attaches is common
       3. Meniscal injuries occur less frequently in children than adults

   B. Ligament injuries
       1. Most frequently injured ligament is the medial collateral ligament
       2. Patients have variable amounts of pain, stiffness, tenderness and swelling depending on severity of ligament damage
       3. Anterior cruciate ligament injury may involve an audible pop and "giving way" sensation (patient typically falls to ground and is unable to arise without assistance); involves a positive Lachman's test; large effusion develops within first few hours
       4. Posterior cruciate ligament injury has a positive posterior drawer test; observation of knee may reveal hyperflexion
       5. Collateral ligament injury involves local swelling, laxity, tenderness over the ligament and may or may not be painful; effusion is usually minimal

   C. Meniscus injury
       1. Medial meniscus injuries are more common than lateral meniscus injuries
       2. Patient often recalls a twisting flexion injury of the knee following by pain and difficulty flexing the knee and bearing weight
       3. May have clicking, locking, catching, or giving way of knee
       4. Knee joint effusion and tenderness over the joint line are often noted

D. Patellar subluxation or dislocation occurs more frequently in females and involves medial tenderness and effusion; often the dislocation reduces when the leg is completely extended

E. Fractures are difficult to differentiate from other injuries; may result in severe pain, inability to bear weight, swelling, limited range of motion, and unequal leg length
   1. Crepitus is palpable with patellar fractures
   2. Neurovascular compromise may occur with femoral condylar fractures
   3. Pain with compression of the side of joint may occur with tibial plateau fractures
   4. Injuries, particularly fractures, to growth plates can lead to deformity and growth irregularities
   5. The Salter-Harris classification system groups fractures into 5 categories ranging from Type I which is a separation of the growth plate which does not affect future bone growth to Type V which is a crush injury and has the worst prognosis for normal growth

IV. Diagnosis/Evaluation

A. History
   1. Ask patient to precisely describe circumstances surrounding injury and mechanism of the injury; particularly ask if injury involved hyperextension of the knee, a direct blow to knee, or a twisting injury
   2. Inquire about location of pain, tenderness, and swelling in knee as well as hip, thigh, shin, ankle and foot
   3. Inquire about sensations of locking, clicking, catching, giving way or buckling of the knee
   4. Ask patient to point to site of greatest pain
   5. Ask how quickly after the injury the swelling developed; swelling in the joint within 24 hours suggests hemarthrosis
   6. Ask about previous musculoskeletal injuries; important to determine if this is an acute problem or a preexisting condition which has been aggravated
   7. Inquire about systemic symptoms such as fever, chills, night sweats
   8. Determine patient's occupation and job requirements
   9. Determine whether patient is involved in leisure or competitive athletics which will affect decisions about management
   10. Inquire about self treatments

B. Physical Examination
   1. Always compare injured side with unaffected side during observation, palpation, range of motion, and special tests
   2. Observe gait and stance, noting lower extremity alignment
   3. Observe knee while standing for deformity, discoloration, and swelling
   4. With patient seated and knee flexed at 90°, look for bulge of fluid on either side of patellar ligament
   5. Palpate in a proximal to distal direction with patient sitting and supine (see Figure 17.15 for anatomical structures)
      a. Begin with distal thigh, palpating quadriceps, hamstrings, and articular surfaces of the femoral condyles; consider measuring thigh girth to detect disuse atrophy
      b. Palpate patella and all around the joint line (tenderness at joint line suggests meniscal tear, whereas tenderness slightly above or below suggests ligament damage)
      c. Palpate muscles around patella and collateral ligaments
      d. Palpate around each growth plate
      e. Palpate tibial plateau and tibial tuberosity

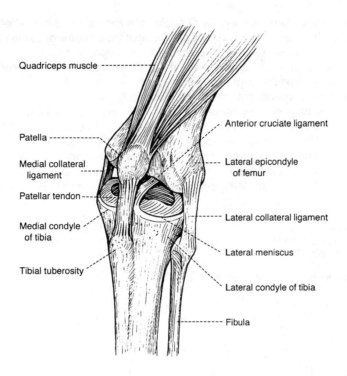

Figure 17.15. Anatomical Structures of the Knee.

6. Assess for effusion or fluid in knee joint (see Figure 17.16)

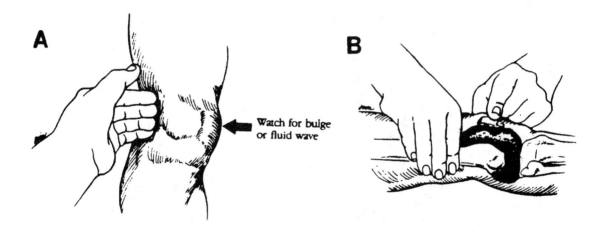

Figure 17.16. Testing for Fluid in the Knee Joint.

A. The bulge sign. B. The patellar tap will suggest fluid in the knee as the patella clicks against the femur. With greater amounts of knee fluid, the patella will be ballottable.

Source: Judge, R.D., Zuidema, G.D., & Fitzgerald, F.T. (Eds.), 1989. Clinical Diagnosis (p. 445). Boston: Little, Brown and Company. Copyright 1989 by A.C. Judge, P.C. Judge, S.M. Judge, N.C. Judge. Reprinted by permission.

7. Perform range of motion of knee
8. Assess mobility of patella by flexing knee 30° and applying medial and lateral pressure to determine amount of subluxation that is possible

9. Determine the quadriceps or Q angle (see Figure 17.13 in section on EXTREMITY PAIN)
    a. This angle is formed by lines drawn from center of patella to the tibial tubercle and from the center of patella to anterior superior spine
    b. When angle exceeds 15° it is abnormal and may be associated with patellar subluxation and dislocation
10. Determine ligament stability (see Figure 17.17)
    a. Apply valgus (medial) or varus (lateral) stress when knee is at full extension and then at 30° flexion to assess stability of medial and lateral collateral ligaments
        (1) In first-degree sprains, end point is solid
        (2) In second-degree sprains, laxity is evident at 30° flexion but not at full extension
        (3) In third-degree sprains, there are no solid end points at either 30° flexion or full extension

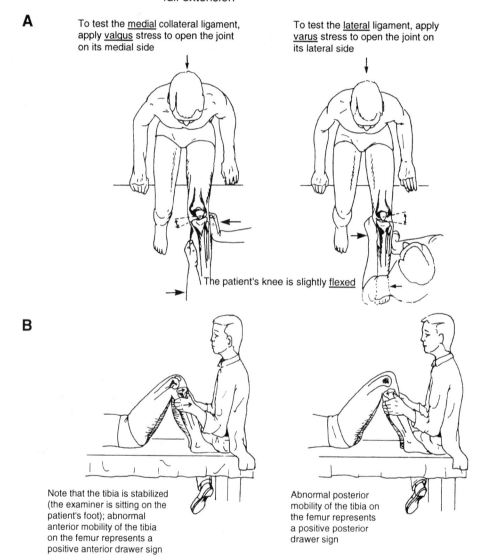

A

To test the medial collateral ligament, apply valgus stress to open the joint on its medial side

To test the lateral ligament, apply varus stress to open the joint on its lateral side

The patient's knee is slightly flexed

B

Note that the tibia is stabilized (the examiner is sitting on the patient's foot); abnormal anterior mobility of the tibia on the femur represents a positive anterior drawer sign

Abnormal posterior mobility of the tibia on the femur represents a positive posterior drawer sign

Figure 17.17. Collateral Ligament Testing.

A: Collateral ligament testing. B: The "drawer" sign for cruciate ligament testing.

Source: Reilly, B.M. (1991). Practical Strategies in Outpatient Medicine (p. 1193). Philadelphia: Saunders. Copyright 1991 by Saunders. Reprinted by permission.

        b. Assess stability of cruciate ligaments with the drawer test by applying anterior (see aforementioned illustration) and posterior forces to the proximal tibia when the knee is flexed and the foot is stabilized

c. Lachman's test can also test cruciate ligaments and is performed with knee flexed to 30°; anterior drawer force is applied to the proximal tibia with one hand while the other hand stabilizes the femur (see Figure 17.18)

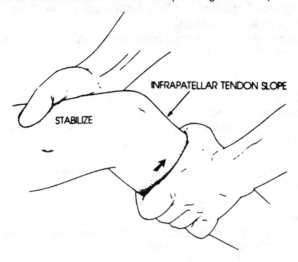

Figure 17.18. Lachman's Test.

Source: Magee, D.J. (1987). Orthopedic Physical Assessment (p. 284). Philadelphia: Saunders. Copyright 1987 by Uniform Copyright Convention. Reprinted by permission.

11. Assess meniscus
    a. Flex knee to 90° and palpate joint line
    b. Perform McMurray's test (see Figure 17.19)
        (1) Maximally flex knee, externally rotate tibia and apply varus stress as the knee is extended to test for lateral meniscus injury
        (2) Perform flexion, external rotation as above but then apply valgus stress to test medial meniscus injury
        (3) Pain and a palpable click at joint line are positive tests

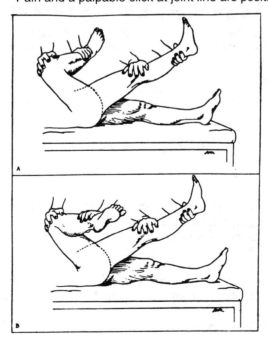

Figure 17.19. McMurray Maneuver.

A. Extension in internal rotation. A palpable or audible snap suggests a lesion in the lateral meniscus.
B. Extension in external rotation. A palpable or audible snap suggests a lesion in the medial meniscus.

Source: Judge, R.D., Zuidema, G.D., & Fitzgerald, F.T. (Eds.). (1989). Clinical Diagnosis (p. 448). Boston: Little, Brown and Company. Copyright 1989 by A.C. Judge, P.C. Judge, S.M. Judge, N.C. Judge. Reprinted by permission.

12. Assess hip and back whenever a history of knee pain is combined with normal findings on the knee exam

C. Differential Diagnosis: important to differentiate acute injuries from overuse injuries, inflammatory processes, infection, and neoplasms
   1. Overuse injuries have insidious onset and usually result from repetitive stress (see section on EXTREMITY PAIN, LOWER)
      a. Chondromalacia patellae
      b. Osgood-Schlatter disease
      c. Patellar tendinitis
      d. Stress fractures
   2. Inflammatory processes, infections, and neoplasms are typically associated with systemic symptoms
   3. Hip problems should be considered; referred pain from the hip occurs, especially in children and older patients who are at risk for metastatic disease, osteoarthritis, and fractures

D. Diagnostic Tests
   1. Consider ordering x-rays of the knee including anteroposterior, lateral and sunrise patella views; the Ottawa Knee Rule is helpful in deciding when to use radiography (see following table)

OTTAWA KNEE RULE
Order knee x-ray series for patients with the following findings:
1) Isolated tenderness of patella* Or
2) Tenderness at head of fibula Or
3) Inability to flex to 90° Or
4) Inability to bear weight immediately or walk more than four steps immediately after injury

*No bone tenderness of knee other than patella

Adapted from Stiell, I.G., Wells, G.A., Hoag, R.H., et al. (1997). Implementation of the Ottawa Knee Rule for the use of radiography in acute knee injuries. JAMA, 278, 2075-2079.

   2. Aspirate a large effusion and order cell count, gram stain, and culture
   3. Injuries which do not heal after 2 weeks of conservative treatment may require magnetic resonance imaging or in the case of a meniscus injury, an arthrogram which is less accurate
   4. An arteriogram is ordered for suspected knee dislocations

V. Plan/Management

A. The following are indications for immediate orthopedic referral; patient's knee should be immobilized in a splint or rigid knee immobilizer
   1. Neurovascular compromise
   2. Suspected fracture or dislocated tibia or femur
   3. Suspected growth plate injury
   4. Torn ligaments (Grade II and III sprains)
   5. Locked knee which is unable to be manipulated into place
   6. Large meniscus tear or hemarthrosis
   7. Suspected infection or tumor

B. For other, less extensive knee injuries teach patient the following:
1. Rest depending on extent of injury; minor injuries may need only 1-2 days of rest, whereas more extensive injuries may need 8-10 weeks
2. Apply ice (never directly to skin) 20 to 30 minutes with at least 10 minute breaks in application as often as possible during first 48 hours after injury
3. After first 48 hours, hot and cold applications can be used (see section on ANKLE INJURY)
4. Elevate extremity
5. Consider prescribing NSAIDs
   a. Prescribe ibuprofen (Motrin) 200-800 mg TID every 6 to 8 hours
   b. Children's Motrin is available 100 mg/5 mL; 24-35 lbs give 5 mL; 36-47 lbs. give 7.5 mL; 48-59 lbs give 10 mL; 60-71 lbs. give 12.5 mL; 72-95 lbs. give 15 mL every 6-8 hours
   c. Some clinicians believe that NSAIDs hamper early healing and should be used conservatively
6. Teach crutch walking and the need to avoid weight-bearing until acute inflammation subsides
7. For injuries with pronounced symptoms immobilize knee in brace for a minimal period of time
8. Exercise is important
   a. For minor injuries, exercise can be permitted within 1-2 days, but patient should be cautioned to gradually increase activity
   b. For more extensive injuries, activity should initially consist of isometric quadriceps tensing exercises
   c. Begin isotonic quadriceps exercises and range of motion exercises after acute inflammation subsides
9. Incision and drainage of large and fluctuant hematomas may be needed

C. Surgery is needed for more extensive knee injuries; a promising new method of repairing damaged knees is extraction of autologous chondrocytes from patient's cartilage which are grown in vitro and then reimplanted

D. Follow Up
1. For extensive injuries, schedule return visit in 24 hours
2. For less extensive injuries, return visits should be scheduled in two weeks or sooner if problems occur
3. Consult specialist for patients with ligament and meniscus injuries which have had only minimal improvement after 2 weeks of conservative treatment; patient with meniscus injury may need magnetic resonance imaging and/or an arthrogram before orthopedic visit
4. At the return visit, all patients should be taught ways to prevent further injuries to their knees particularly by proper exercising and conditioning and possibly the use of prophylactic braces

LOW BACK PROBLEMS, ACUTE

I. Definition: Activity intolerance due to lower back or back-related leg symptoms of less than 3 months duration

II. Pathogenesis: In preadolescents isolated back pain is uncommon and often indicates an underlying pathology that needs increased attention; from early adolescence into adulthood, back pain is frequent and usually is a benign problem due to mechanical stress or trauma

A. Spondylolysis and spondylolisthesis are most common cause of low back pain in children
1. Spondylolysis is a break of the pars interarticularis; usual site is L4 or L5
2. Spondylolisthesis is a slip of the vertebrae (after spondylolysis) which allows one vertebrae body to slide forward on its neighbor; usual site is L5 or S1

589

B. Discitis occurs primarily in preschool-age children and is a bacterial infection
    1. Probably due to vascular disruption in hyaline epiphyseal endplates of vertebrae distal to T12 which results in vascular necrotic changes to disc
    2. Disc becomes permanently deformed and narrowed

C. Lumbosacral strain
    1. Etiology is often unclear but results from stretching or tearing of muscles, tendons, ligaments or fascia of back secondary to trauma or chronic mechanical stress
    2. Predisposing factors include chronic occupational strain, obesity, exaggerated lumbar lordosis, abnormal forward tipped-pelvis, weak paraspinal and/or abdominal muscles, leg length discrepancy, chronic poor posture, inadequate/inappropriate conditioning and sub-optimal lifting habits

D. Herniated intervertebral discs are uncommon in children
    1. Intervertebral discs are composed of collagenous annulus fibrosis and gelatinous nucleus pulposus
    2. Herniation occurs with tears in annulus fibrosis which allows contents of nucleus pulposus to protrude
    3. When nerve roots are compressed by these contents, pain and other neurological signs and symptoms develop

E. Scoliosis is rarely painful but in some children may cause back discomfort

F. Tumors, juvenile ankylosing spondylitis, infections such as spinal tuberculosis and nontuberculosis vertebral osteomyelitis are less common causes of back pain in children

III. Clinical Presentation of common syndromes of acute low back problems; 90% of patients with acute low back problems will recover spontaneously in 4 weeks

A. Spondylolysis and spondylolisthesis
    1. Often occurs from a stress fracture of the posterior vertebral elements or from hyperextension sports such as gymnastics, diving, or weight lifting
    2. Family history for spondylolysis is often positive
    3. Neurologic examination is usually normal, but patients may have tight hamstrings, and hyperextension (back bending) often reproduces pain at L5 or just below the iliac crests
    4. If spondylolysis is suspected x-rays are ordered; if x-rays are negative and suspicion is still high, a bone scan is ordered

B. Discitis: Patients' main complaints are related to their ages
    1. Children <3 years refuse to walk
    2. Children >3 years complain of abdominal pain and tenderness of hamstrings
    3. Most children have no systemic illness signs but have irritability which is relieved by lying in a prone, lumbar lordotic position

C. Lumbosacral strain
    1. Typically, patient experiences minimal discomfort during or immediately after injury or activity with stiffness and pain occurring 12-36 hours later as soft tissue swells
    2. Pain is located in back, buttocks or in one or both thighs
    3. Pain is aggravated by standing, flexion and is relieved with rest and reclining

D. Herniated intervertebral disc
    1. Characterized by radicular pain which is described as shooting, sharp, electric-type pain, associated with foot and leg pain and worsened with valsalva maneuvers
    2. Paresthesia or numbness may occur in sensory distribution of nerve root
    3. Deep tendon reflexes are absent or depressed in distribution of nerve root
    4. Muscular weakness and atrophy may result
    5. Most common disc ruptures affect L-5 or S-1 nerve roots

6. Cauda equina involvement (compression of the lower portion of the nerve roots inferior to spinal cord proper) may occur secondary to central disc herniation and presents as insidiously worsening rectal and/or perineal pain with decreased perineal sensation, loss of sphincter control, and disturbances in bowel and bladder functions

7. Signs and symptoms depend on level of herniation (see Figure 17.20 on Common Disc Syndromes)

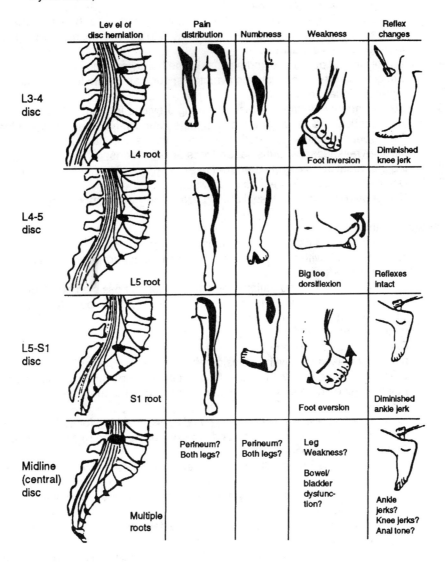

Figure 17.20. Common Disc Syndromes: Neurologic Findings.

Source: Reilly, B.M. (1991). Practical Strategies in Outpatient Medicine (p. 915). Philadelphia: Saunders. Copyright 1991 by Saunders. Reprinted by permission.

E. Scoliosis (see section on SCOLIOSIS)

F. Worrisome findings include constant pain in child <11 years that lasts for several weeks or occurs spontaneously at night, interferes with school or play or is associated with marked stiffness, limitation of motion, fever, or neurologic abnormalities

IV. Diagnosis/Evaluation

A. History
   1. Ask patient to point with one finger where he/she feels pain and then to describe pain and/or radiation of pain
   2. Determine onset because acute onset without trauma may signal serious conditions such as dissecting aortic aneurysm
   3. Differentiate whether pain is mechanical and worsens after bending or lifting or is nonmechanical, occurring at rest, and related to extraspinal disorders such as pelvic or intra-abdominal conditions
   4. Inquire about pattern of symptoms; ask whether symptoms are constant or intermittent
   5. Explore occurrence of systemic symptoms, such as weight loss, and fever, which could signal malignant disease
   6. Obtain careful past medical history, noting previous trauma, TB, cancer, immunosuppression, urinary infection, osteoporosis, previous back problems and surgery
   7. Ask about possible associated symptoms such as dysuria, bowel or bladder incontinence, muscle weakness, paresthesia, and loss of sensations
   8. Inquire about steroid and other drug use
   9. Determine patient's limitations in activities
   10. Use of pain drawings or visual analog scales may augment history

B. Physical Examination
   1. Observe gait and general appearance
       a. Patients with herniated disc usually are uncomfortable sitting and gait is cautious and awkward
       b. Limping or coordination problems suggest a possible neurological problem
       c. Severe guarding of lumbar motion may indicate spinal infection, tumor, or fracture
   2. Observe spine for alignment and abnormalities; observe skin overlying spine for signs of trauma or infection
   3. Perform range of motion.
       a. Increased pain with extension often indicates osteoarthritis.
       b. Increased pain with flexion most often indicates strain or injured or herniated disc
   4. Palpate spine and paraspinal structures noting point tenderness and paravertebral muscle spasm
       a. If fell on tailbone, need to do rectal exam checking for stability of coccyx
       b. Palpate ischial tuberosity and greater trochanter to rule out bursitis
   5. Perform traction maneuvers
       a. Straight leg raise (SLR): Elevate each leg passively with flexion at hip and extension of knee; positive SLR is radicular pain when leg is raised between 30-60°
       b. Crossed leg raise is very diagnostic for disc injury; positive when patient complains of radicular pain in the leg that is not raised
       c. Yeoman maneuver: Unilateral hyperextension in prone position (checking for lumbosacral mechanical disorders)
       d. Patrick's test in which heel is placed on opposite knee and lateral force is exerted on knee (check for hip or sacroiliac disease)
   6. Check for malingering
       a. Observe for overreaction
       b. Apply slight pressure to top of head (should not produce pain)
       c. Perform distracted straight leg raise
       d. Observe for nonanatomical motor or sensory regional disturbances
   7. Perform complete neurological examination
       a. Determine pain and sensation distribution; pain and diminished or absent sensation should follow nerve root distribution (see Figure 7.1 Dermatomes in HERPES ZOSTER in SKIN chapter)
       b. Do complete motor strength assessment, including dorsiflexion of great toe (only abnormality of the common L4-5 disc protrusion may be great toe weakness)
           (1) Ask patient to toe walk which tests calf muscles and mostly S1 nerve root
           (2) Ask patient to heel walk which tests ankle and toe dorsiflexor muscles, L5 and some L4 nerve roots

        (3)   Ask patient to perform a single squat and rise which tests quadriceps muscles, mostly L4 nerve root

    c.   Circumferential measurements of calf and thigh bilaterally can detect muscle atrophy; differences of greater than 2 cm in measurements of the two limbs often indicate an abnormality

    d.   Deep tendon reflex testing
        (1)   Ankle jerk tests mostly the S1 nerve root
        (2)   Knee jerk tests mostly the L4 nerve root
        (3)   Up-going toes in response to stroking the plantar footpad (Babinski or plantar response) may indicate motor-neuron abnormalities such a myelopathy or demyelinating disease

8.   Check sensation of perineum to rule out cauda equina syndrome (compression of the lower portion of the nerve roots inferior to the spinal cord proper)

9.   Examine abdomen (masses or bruits)

10.   Consider pelvic and rectal examinations

11.   Palpate peripheral pulses

C.   Differential Diagnosis
    1.   Important to rule out red flags for potentially serious conditions (see following table)

RED FLAGS FOR POTENTIALLY SERIOUS CONDITIONS		
Possible Fracture	**Possible Tumor or Infection**	**Possible Cauda Equina Syndrome**
Major trauma such as vehicle accident or fall from a high place Minor trauma or even strenuous lifting (in older or potentially osteoporotic patient)	Age <20 years	Saddle anesthesia
	History of cancer	Recent onset of bladder dysfunction such as urinary retention, increased frequency, or overflow incontinence
	Constitutional symptoms such as fever, chills, or unexplained weight loss	Severe or progressive neurologic deficit in legs
	Risk factors for infection: recent bacterial infection, IV drug abuse, or immunosuppression	Unexpected laxity of anal sphincter Perianal/perineal sensory loss
	Pain that worsens when supine; severe nighttime pain	Major motor weakness such as knee extension weakness or foot drop

Adapted from Bigos, S., Bowyer, O., Braen, G., et al. (1994). Acute low back problems in adults. Clinical practice guideline No. 14. AHCPR Publication No. 95-0642. Rockville, MD: Agency for Health Care Policy and Research, Public Health Service, U.S. Department of Health and Human Services.

    2.   Pseudosciatica with a normal neurologic exam includes simple mechanical back pain, disorders of hip, thigh, pelvis, rectum, and vascular claudication

    3.   True radicular pain (sciatica or shooting, sharp pain down to the lower leg and foot) includes herniated intervertebral disc, spondylolisthesis, compression fracture, degenerative spondylosis, herpes zoster, and neoplasm

    4.   Extreme, tearing pain with syncope and diaphoresis may indicate an aneurysm

    5.   Fever or meningeal symptoms may suggest vertebral osteomyelitis

    6.   Other less common ominous causes: metabolic bone disease, inflammatory disease, spinal cord disease, unstable spine, pyelonephritis

    7.   Other diseases may or may not be accompanied with back pain: peripheral neuropathy, depression, hysteria, cystitis, prostatitis, endometriosis, spinal stenosis, bursitis, osteoporosis

D.   Diagnostic Tests
    1.   In preadolescent children determine if history of trauma exists
        a.   If trauma occurred, order plain radiograph; if x-ray is normal, CT or MRI may be needed unless strain or sprain is most likely

        b.   Consider technetium T$_c$ 99m bone scan when there is no history of trauma
- (1) Discitis is diagnosed early by technetium T$_c$ 99m uptake
- (2) By 4 weeks, discitis can usually be detected on plain x-ray by disc space narrowing

2. For patients older than 13 years with low back pain less than 3 weeks and in the absence of signs and symptoms of dangerous conditions (see preceding table on RED FLAGS FOR POTENTIALLY SERIOUS CONDITIONS), usually no tests are needed
   a. If spinal fracture is a possibility, order plain x-ray of lumbosacral spine; if fracture still suspected after 10 days or there are multiple sites of pain, consider bone scan or consultation
   b. If cancer and/or infection is suspected, order CBC, erythrocyte sedimentation rate, urinalysis; if after these tests, there is still suspicion consider consultation or order bone scan, x-ray or other lab test

3. For patients older than 13 years whose back pain does not improve over 3 weeks:
   a. If symptoms are primarily in the low back consider ordering CBC, ESR, x-rays, or bone scan depending on symptomatology and risk factors
   b. If sciatica symptoms are present >3 weeks, consult surgeon about choice of imaging study (MRI, CT) to define nerve root compression **or** order electromyography (EMG) if the level of nerve root dysfunction is not obvious from the physical examination; sensory evoked potentials may be added if spinal stenosis or spinal cord myelopathy is suspected

V. Plan/Management

A. Consult specialist for patients with suspected discitis, herniated intervertebral disc, tumors, infections, and juvenile ankylosing spondylitis

B. Management of spondylolysis
   1. Begin with rest, analgesics and hamstring stretching exercises
   2. Back muscle strengthening exercises are recommended when the pain has subsided
   3. Immobilization with back braces may be needed to achieve healing of fractures or to relieve irritation if patient is not responding to analgesics and exercises
   4. Consult surgeon after trial of conservative therapy; spinal fusion is rarely required

C. Management of spondylolisthesis
   1. Children with minimal pain and less than 25% slip need the following: periodic assessment to detect possible increase in slip (repeat x-ray at 6 months, then in one year), an exercise program and possible lumbo-sacral corset and rest
   2. If slip percentage is between 25-50%, rest and conservative treatment are usually indicated
   3. Spinal fusion is usually needed if slip is ≥75%

D. Pharmacological therapy for lumbosacral strain; remember that back pain in preadolescents is uncommon and a diagnosis of exclusion
   1. Safest, effective medication is acetaminophen which may be used safely in combination with non-steroidal anti-inflammatory drugs (NSAIDs) or physical therapeutics
   2. NSAIDs including aspirin are also effective but can cause gastrointestinal problems, renal or allergic problems
      a. Do not use combination of NSAIDs
      b. Recommend Ibuprofen (Motrin) 400 mg or 4-10 mg/kg per dose every 4-6 hours
   3. Muscle relaxants are no more effective than NSAIDS in relieving low back symptoms and have adverse effects including drowsiness; they are seldom indicated in children and adolescents
   4. Opioids should be avoided if possible, and if selected, used only for a short time
   5. The following therapies are not recommended: oral steroids, colchicine, and antidepressants

E. Physical methods for lumbosacral strain
   1. Self application of heat and cold therapy may provide temporary symptom relief
      a. Cold therapy for 20-30 minutes several times a day for first 24 hours.
      b. Topical heat 20-30 minutes several times a day after first day
   2. The following have not been found effective: traction, massage, diathermy, ultrasound, biofeedback, transcutaneous electrical nerve stimulation, acupuncture, shoe lifts, back corsets, back belts

F. Activity for lumbosacral strain
   1. For most patients, no bed rest is needed; prolonged bed rest may have debilitating consequences
   2. For patients with severe limitations, 2-4 days of bed rest may be beneficial
   3. Teach patient to minimize stress to the back
      a. Avoid jerky, hurried movements when lifting
      b. Lift with legs by straddling the load; bend knees to pick up load; keep back straight (do not bend back)
      c. Keep objects close to the body at navel level when lifting
      d. Avoid twisting, bending, reaching while lifting
      e. Avoid prolonged sitting
      f. Change positions often while sitting
      g. A soft support at small of back, armrests to support some body weight, a slight recline in chair back may make sitting more comfortable
      h. Firm mattress/bed board, lying supine with hips and knees flexed on pillows is beneficial when sleeping
   4. Low-stress, aerobic exercise (walking, riding bike, swimming, and eventually jogging) can be gradually and incrementally started within the first 2 weeks of symptoms; conditioning exercises for trunk muscles are not recommended during the first few weeks of symptoms

G. Surgical consultation should be considered if patients have any of the following:
   1. Severe and disabling sciatica
   2. Symptoms of sciatica _____ ithout improvement for >3 weeks or with extreme progression
   3. Strong physiologic e_____ ction of a specific nerve root with intervertebral disc herniation is confir_____ ing level and side by imaging studies

H. Prevention of further back p_____
   1. Discuss that low back pain, like o_____ conditions, will get worse unless preventive measures are taken.
   2. Exercises to condition specific tr_____ ded a few weeks after acute symptoms; encourage p_____ s partial sit-ups or extension exercises such as lying_____ rso off floor for at least 5 minutes a day
   3. Instruct patient in proper lifting_____ mechanics (see V.F.3)

I. Follow Up
   1. For patients with s_____ eva
   2. If patient is in moderate_____
   3. In 4-6 weeks, schedule offic_____ cation
   4. Children with spondylol_____

RHEUMATOID ARTHRITIS, JUVENILE

I. Definition: A chronic inflammatory disease which primarily affects joints but may have generalized manifestations

II. Pathogenesis

    A. Autoimmune disorder of unknown etiology; immunologic changes due to multiple factors

    B. Inflammation of synovial membranes results in panus or thickened synovium which adheres to articular cartilage and later erodes cartilage and underlying bone

    C. Adhesions between opposing joint surfaces and/or cysts develop

III. Clinical Presentation

    A. Criteria for diagnosing juvenile rheumatoid arthritis (JRA) (see following table)

DIAGNOSTIC CRITERIA FOR CLASSIFICATION OF JUVENILE RHEUMATOID ARTHRITIS (JRA)
• Age of onset less than 16 years.
• Arthritis of one or more joints, defined as swelling or effusion or the presence of 2 or more of following signs: Limitation of range of motion, tenderness or pain in motion, increased heat.
• Duration of disease is 6 weeks to 3 months.
• Type of onset of disease during first 4-6 months classified as: ▲ Oligoarthritis or Pauciarthritis: 4 joints or fewer.   ▲ Polyarthritis: 5 or more joints.   ▲ Systemic disease: Arthritis with intermittent fever, rheumatoid rash or visceral disease.
• Exclusion of other forms of juvenile arthritis.

Adapted from Cassidy, J.T., et al. (1986). A study of classification criteria for diagnosing juvenile rheumatoid arthritis. Arthritis Rheumatology, 29, 274.

    B. Systemic JRA (approximately 10% of cases)
        1. Occurs equally in both sexes; no age predilection
        2. Associated symptoms may include fever, joint pain, and macular rash
        3. Some children have pericarditis, pleuritis, hepatomegaly, splenomegaly or lymphadenopathy
        4. Often remission within one year

    C. Pauciarticular JRA (approximately 40% of cases)
        1. Onset approximately 2 years; affects females more than males
        2. Involves four or fewer joints; typically affects large joints such as knees, wrists, ankles, elbows
        3. At risk for asymptomatic chronic iridocyclitis which can lead to visual loss if not treated

    D. Polyarticular JRA (approximately 50% of cases)
        1. Typically presents with multiple symmetric involvement of joints of hands, feet, cervical spine, temporomandibular joint, and sternoclavicular joint
        2. May have short duration of systemic symptoms
        3. Many children (approximately 50-60%) do **not** have permanent joint disability

IV. Diagnosis/Evaluation

    A. History
        1. Exactly determine duration, location and characteristics of pain, tenderness, inflammation and morning stiffness
        2. Question about systemic symptoms such as weight loss, fever, and fatigue
        3. Inquire about associated symptoms such as nodules, eye pain, or conjunctivitis
        4. Ask about past medical history and medication use
        5. Inquire about family medical history
        6. Specifically determine degree of limitation in patient's activities of daily living

    B. Physical Examination
        1. Measure vital signs
        2. Assess growth and development; plot height and weight
        3. Count number of swollen joints, noting bilateral symmetry of joint involvement
        4. Check for various deformities of the hand such as swan-neck deformity, mallet finger, boutonnière deformity
        5. Carefully palpate joints noting tenderness, temperature, and swelling
        6. Apply traction maneuvers to determine joint stability
        7. Assess muscular strength, particularly grip strength
        8. A complete physical examination is often needed because of systemic problems such as pleurisy, pericarditis, splenomegaly

    C. Differential Diagnosis (see section on JOINT PAIN)
        1. Reiter's syndrome
        2. Systemic lupus erythematosus
        3. Gouty arthritis, gonococcal arthritis, psoriatic arthritis
        4. Lyme disease
        5. Acute rheumatic fever
        6. Ulcerative colitis and Crohn's disease
        7. Lyme disease
        8. Leukemia

    D. Diagnostic Tests
        1. Baseline laboratory information in patient suspected of RA includes CBC with differential, erythrocyte sedimentation rate, urinalysis, rheumatoid factor titer; consider ANA
        2. Before initiating any drugs it is important to get the following: electrolytes, serum creatinine, liver function tests, hepatic panel, urinalysis, stool guiac
        3. In selected patients, consider ordering the following:
            a. Synovial fluid analysis to rule out other diseases; may need repeated during disease flares to rule-out septic arthritis
            b. X-rays of selected joints; limited diagnostic value early in disease, but helpful in establishing a baseline to periodically monitor progression and response to therapy
            c. Additional serological studies such as antinuclear antibodies (ANAs) and serum hemolytic complement (CH50) may be needed to rule-out other diseases

V. Plan/Management: Goals are to relieve pain, preserve joint function, and prevent further disease progression

    A. Initially, patients are treated by specialists; consultation is also needed when patients have exacerbations or flares of their symptoms

    B. In children, a referral to an ophthalmologist should be made at the time of diagnosis of JRA; frequency of subsequent ophthalmologic visits is presented in the table that follows

FREQUENCY OF OPHTHALMOLOGIC VISITS FOR CHILDREN WITH JUVENILE RHEUMATOID ARTHRITIS (JRA) AND WITHOUT KNOWN IRIDOCYCLITIS*		
	Age of Onset	
JRA Subtype at Onset	<7 years[†]	≥7 years[‡]
Pauciarticular		
+ ANA	H[§]	M
- ANA	M	M
Polyarticular		
+ ANA	H[§]	M
- ANA	M	M
Systemic	L	L

*High risk (H) indicates ophthalmologic examinations every 3 to 4 months. Medium risk (M) indicates ophthalmologic examinations every 6 months. Low risk (L) indicates ophthalmologic examinations every 12 months. ANA indicates antinuclear antibody test.
[†]All patients are considered at low risk 7 years after the onset of their arthritis and should have yearly ophthalmologic examinations indefinitely.
[‡]All patients are considered at low risk 4 years after the onset of their arthritis and should have yearly ophthalmologic examinations indefinitely.
[§]All high-risk patients are considered at medium risk 4 years after the onset of their arthritis.

Source: American Academy of Pediatrics section on Rheumatology and section on Ophthalmology. (1993). Guidelines for ophthalmologic examination in children with juvenile rheumatoid arthritis. Pediatrics, 92(2), 295-296.

C. Patient education includes discussion of chronicity of disease and ways to decrease exacerbations and prevent deformities
1. Maintain ideal body weight
2. Exercise with emphasis on joint extension (physical therapy is always helpful).
3. Receive adequate rest with naps
4. Perform correct body mechanics
5. Always use large joints, such as shoulders or hands, rather than fingers to carry pail of water, etc.
6. In younger children, management of behavior is important; parents should be encouraged to avoid overprotection

D. Prescribe splints and protheses to protect joints, to keep in functional position, and to reduce pain

E. Hot and cold therapy, ultrasound, electrical stimulation with transcutaneous nerve stimulator are often beneficial

F. Visual imagery, massage, acupuncture and hypnosis may be helpful

G. Drug therapy in children
1. Nonsteroidal anti-inflammatory drugs (NSAIDs) are used more frequently today because of the fears of Reye syndrome with aspirin. Prescribe one of the following:
a. Naproxen (Naprosyn) 10 mg/kg/day in 2 divided doses. Available in suspension 125 mg/5 mL
b. Ibuprofen (Children's Motrin): 5-10 mg/kg/dose every 6-8 hours; available 100 mg/5 mL suspension
2. Aspirin may be prescribed; therapeutic doses (80 to 100 mg/kg/day in four divided doses for children smaller than 25 kg; 2.4 to 4.8 g/day in larger children); enteric coated pills should be used in children who can swallow pills; stop medications if child is exposed to varicella or influenza
3. Disease-modifying antirheumatic drugs (DMARDs) (secialist consultation needed): If disease is rapidly progressing or if aspirin and NSAIDs are not sufficiently beneficial, rheumatologists often prescribe one of the following DMARDs
a. Methotrexate: Consult specialist for pediatric dosage
(1) Often drug of choice for those unresponsive to NSAIDs or aspirin
(2) Adolescents should be counseled about teratogenic effects of drug

b. Hydroxychloroquine (Plaquenil), Pediatric dosage: 5 mg/kg/day in divided doses

c. Sulfasalazine (Azulfidine): Pediatric dosage: Consult specialist

d. Gold sodium thiomalate: Consult rheumatologist concerning starting dosage and lengthening intervals

e. Oral gold: Consult specialist for pediatric dosage

f. Others: penicillamine, cyclophosphamide, and azathioprine

g. Common characteristic of all DMARDs is that they are slow acting; clinical response may not be evident for 1-6 months

h. DMARDs have potential to delay or prevent joint damage

i. DMARDs have adverse effects and many need frequent monitoring (see table below on RECOMMENDED MONITORING STRATEGIES)

RECOMMENDED MONITORING STRATEGIES FOR DMARDS

Drugs	Toxicities requiring monitoring	Baseline evaluation	Monitoring
Nonsteroidal antiinflammatory drugs	Gastrointestinal ulceration and bleeding	CBC, creatinine, AST, ALT	CBC yearly, LFTs, creatinine testing may be required
Hydroxychloroquine	Macular damage	None unless patient has previous eye disease	Funduscopic and visual fields every 6-12 months
Sulfasalazine	Myelosuppression	CBC, and AST or ALT in patients at risk, G6PD	CBC every 2-4 weeks for first 3 months, then every 3 months
Methotrexate	Myelosuppression, hepatic fibrosis, cirrhosis, pulmonary infiltrates or fibrosis	CBC, chest radiography, hepatitis B and C serology in high-risk patients, AST or ALT, albumin, alkaline phosphatase, and creatinine	CBC, platelet count, AST, albumin, creatinine every 4-8 weeks
Gold, intramuscular	Myelosuppression, proteinuria	CBC, platelet count, creatinine, urine dipstick for protein	CBC, platelet count, urine dipstick every 1-2 weeks for first 20 weeks, then at the time of each injection
Gold, oral	Myelosuppression, proteinuria	CBC, platelet count, urine dipstick for protein	CBC, platelet count, urine dipstick for protein every 4-12 weeks
D-penicillamine	Myelosuppression, proteinuria	CBC, platelet count, creatinine, urine dipstick for protein	CBC, urine dipstick for protein every 2 weeks until dosage stable, then every 1-3 months
Azathioprine	Myelosuppression, hepatotoxicity, lymphoproliferative disorders	CBC, platelet count, creatinine, AST or ALT	CBC and platelet count every 1-2 weeks with changes in dosage, and every 1-3 months thereafter
Cyclophosphamide	Myelosuppression, myeloproliferative disorders, malignancy, hemorrhagic cystitis	CBC, platelet count, urinalysis, creatinine, AST or ALT	CBC and platelet count every 1-2 weeks with changes in dosage, then every 1-3 months, urinalysis and urine cytology every 6-12 months
Corticosteroids (oral ≤10 mg of prednisone or equivalent)	Hypertension, hyperglycemia	BP, chemistry panel, bone densitometry in high-risk patients	Urinalysis for glucose yearly, BP at each visit

Adapted from American College of Rheumatology Ad Hoc Committee on Clinical Guidelines. (1996). Guidelines for monitoring drug therapy in rheumatoid arthritis. Arthritis and Rheumatism, 39, 723-731.

4. Oral corticosteroids are used only for severe systemic manifestations; topical corticosteroids may be beneficial in controlling eye problems; intra-articular corticosteroids can relieve pain from tender, swollen joints

H. Surgery is needed if there is marked structural damage on x-ray, lack of response to medical therapy, or significant pain and loss of function

I. Future antirheumatoid therapies: cytokine antagonist, an oral type II collagen derived from sternal cartilage of chicks, minocycline, recombinant human interleukin 1ra, antibodies to TNF-α

J. Follow Up
1. When initiating new drug therapies, patient should be seen every 1-2 weeks
2. Interval between follow up visits depends upon patient's condition and monitoring recommendations of medications (see preceding table on RECOMMENDED MONITORING STRATEGIES)

SCOLIOSIS

I. Definition: Lateral curvature of the spine; usually thoracic or lumbar spine but may involve cervical spine

II. Pathogenesis:

   A. Etiology is usually unknown or idiopathic; genetic factors are probably involved

   B. Scoliosis can be congenital and caused by anomalous bony development

   C. Scoliosis can be associated with neuromuscular diseases (cerebral palsy), genetic diseases (neurofibromatosis), metabolic diseases (juvenile osteoporosis), infections, trauma or tumors

III. Clinical presentation

   A. Present in approximately 3% of children; 10% of these children have scoliosis that requires treatment

   B. Idiopathic scoliosis (65-75% of all cases) can be divided into three types according to age when scoliosis was first noticed
      1. Infantile type occurs in children <3 years, predilection for males, and resolves without treatment
      2. Juvenile type occurs in ages 6-10 years; affects both genders equally, and tends to progress during growth spurts
      3. Adolescent type affects mainly girls and tends to rapidly progress during growth spurts

   C. Condition is usually painless and discovered on routine physical examination

   D. Scoliotic curves progress less rapidly after skeletal growth is completed

   E. Complications:
      1. If untreated, can result in severe deformity of the spinal column
      2. Spinal deformity can impair respiratory and cardiovascular functions as well as limit physical activity and cause pain

IV. Diagnosis/Evaluation
   A. History
      1. Determine onset and duration of any symptoms such as back pain
      2. Ask questions to rule out possible neurologic causes of scoliosis such as muscle weakness, incoordination, skin lesions
      3. Explore etiological factors such as family history and medical history of infection, trauma, congenital abnormalities
      4. Inquire about sexual development; onset of menses and end of puberty signals limited growth potential and less likelihood of curve progression

   B. Physical Examination
      1. Observe gait
      2. Observe posture; evaluate shoulder, scapular, rib, iliac crest, and breast symmetry
      3. Inspect skin for hairy patches, nevi, café au lait spots, dimples, and lipoma

4. Inspect back
   a. Curve may have one turn ("C curve") or two compensating curves ("S curve")
   b. Closely inspect spinal column as well as ribs to look for deviation and rotation of individual vertebra; increased or decreased thoracic kyphosis or lumbar lordosis may be associated with scoliosis
   c. Perform forward bend test (see Figure 17.21)

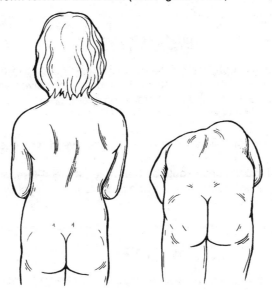

Figure 17.21. Bend Test.

Ask patient to bend forward at hips with both palms held at midline; a simple, level-like instrument, the scoliometer, can document the degree of symmetry of the trunk; Prominence of one scapula of one side of rib cage or of the lumbar paraspinous muscles indicates scoliosis

5. Observe thorax, noting unequal rib prominences and chest asymmetry
6. Measure leg lengths
7. Evaluate for secondary sex characteristics; determine Tanner stage (see section in PRECOCIOUS PUBERTY)
8. Perform complete neurological and musculoskeletal examinations

C. Differential diagnosis
   1. Important to differentiate functional scoliosis from structural or true scoliosis
      a. Functional or nonstructural scoliosis refers to the appearance of a lateral curve when there is no structural change in the vertebral column and may be due to unequal leg lengths, poor posture, muscle spasm, or herniated discs
      b. Functional scoliosis may eventually become structural if means to prevent progression are overlooked
   2. Important to rule-out systemic problems such as neurofibromatosis, cerebral palsy, multiple sclerosis, rickets, tuberculosis, and tumor
   3. If pain is presenting symptom, idiopathic scoliosis is unlikely and there is a need to search for another diagnosis

D. Diagnostic Tests
   1. Limit spinal x-rays to children in whom clinical findings are suggestive of scoliosis of at least 10 degrees
   2. X-rays determine degree of curvature and structure of vertebrae
   3. For children who present with pain, bone scans and/or MRIs may be needed

V. Management

A. Refer to orthopedist or subspecialist, any child who has congenital scoliosis or any child who has curvature on initial examination that is greater than 15°; any child who has progressive scoliosis as indicated by a change of at least 5°; any child who may have associated diseases such as neuromuscular, metabolic, infectious conditions

B. Typically, children with mild curves of less than 20° or 25° require no active intervention, but frequent reevaluations are important; exercises, physical therapy, and chiropractic manipulation are ineffective

C. Children with curves greater than 20° or 24° typically are given ambulatory brace treatments with rigid spinal instrumentation and an exercise program; braces prevent progression of curve in about 85% to 90% of cases

D. Surgery is indicated for children who have progressive curves despite brace treatment

E. Follow Up: serial evaluations should be performed every 4-6 months, and are especially important during rapid growth spurts when progression is most likely

SHOULDER PAIN

I. Definition: Pain in the shoulder that is either acute or chronic

II. Pathogenesis

A. Acute shoulder pain
    1. Fractures, dislocations, sprains and strains are the most common causes
    2. Trauma is usually responsible

B. Chronic shoulder pain
    1. The rotator cuff, the dynamic stabilizer of the glenohumeral joint, is composed of four muscles--the subscapularis, the supraspinatus, the infraspinatus, and the teres minor, along with their musculotendinous attachments
    2. Rotator cuff injury or dysfunction occurs in many circumstances in which the space between the undersurface of the acromion and the superior aspect of the humeral head becomes so narrowed that there is impingement of the acromion onto the rotator cuff tendons (this impingement occurs during forward shoulder elevation that takes place in many overhead activities relating to occupational and recreational pursuits)

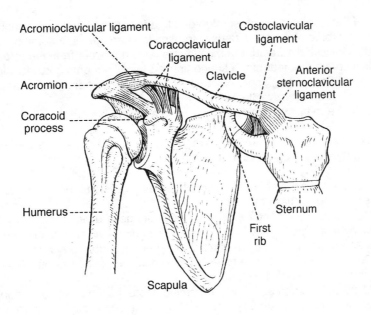

Figure 17.22. Shoulder Bones and Joints

III. Clinical Presentation

A. Shoulder problems are one of the most common orthopedic complaints in primary care

B. Most common fractures of the shoulder involve the proximal humerus and the clavicle (fractures of the scapula are infrequent and are usually associated with multiple fractures relating to severe trauma)

C. Fractures of the proximal humerus most often occur in older patients who fall on an outstretched hand
1. Incidence increases with age and females are twice as likely as males to sustain this type of fracture
2. Patient typically presents with complaints of pain, tenderness, and swelling in the shoulder region in the area of the greater tuberosity
3. Crepitus may or may not be present

D. Fractures of the clavicle are by far the most common fracture that occurs in childhood; in recent decades, this type fracture has become much more common in adults secondary to motor vehicle accidents and participation in contact sports
1. Mechanisms of injury are usually either a fall on outstretched hand or a direct blow to the shoulder
2. Considerable force is needed to crack the clavicle in an adult; therefore, if trauma is minor, look for an underlying cause (neoplastic disease, infection)
3. Patient usually presents with pain at the fracture site; a displaced fracture may be obvious
4. Patient may avoid moving the arm or may angle head toward the injured side to relax the pull of the trapezius to limit pain

E. Dislocations make up about 25% of all shoulder injuries, with about 95% being anterior glenohumeral dislocations
1. Anterior dislocations occur when the arm is forcefully elevated and pulled backwards
2. First-time dislocations are always the result of significant trauma; once glenohumeral instability is present, however, dislocations tend to recur
3. Patient usually presents with the affected arm in external rotation and abduction
4. Shoulder is painful, especially with passive range of motion; active range of motion may be very difficult due to muscle spasm

603

F. Sprains of the shoulder are most often due to a fall on the point of the shoulder
   1. Direct force of the fall is usually transmitted through the acromioclavicular (AC) joint into the clavicle; if a fracture of the clavicle does not occur from the force of the fall, the result is a sprain or a tear of the supporting AC joint ligaments and capsule
      a. Patients with sprains most often experience point tenderness directly over the joint; there is very little if any deformity
      b. Patients with tears usually have a noticeable bump at the AC joint

G. The diagnosis of shoulder strain is a diagnosis of exclusion and is reserved for a muscle injury, usually involving the large deltoid muscle

H. The most frequent cause of chronic shoulder pain is injury to the rotator cuff with pain, weakness, and loss of motion usually reported
   1. Most common among patients 40 years of age and older
   2. Many activities of daily living including combing hair, putting on a coat, reaching high shelves, and driving a car can place demands on the rotator cuff
   3. Occupations that require repetitive overhead work such as painting and carpentry place extra demands on the shoulder
   4. Many sports such as tennis, swimming, football, and basketball require constant overhead positioning of the arms and shoulders; sports such as golf require external rotation of the shoulders

I. Rotator cuff impingement syndrome (and associated tears of the rotator cuff) is usually classified into three stages (see following table)

STAGES OF ROTATOR CUFF IMPINGEMENT SYNDROME	
Stage I	❖ Usually involves patients <25 years of age ❖ Most often occurs in athletes, with pain developing after exercise ❖ Pain is dull, aching, and diffuse ❖ Rotator cuff edema and hemorrhage may by present ❖ Process is reversible at this point
Stage II	❖ Typically occurs in laborers aged 25-40 ❖ Work requires repeated and constant overhead reach for many hours during the day ❖ Pain occurs both during and after activity ❖ Pain frequently occurs at night, interfering with sleep ❖ Pathologic changes become evident and include fibrosis and irreversible tendon changes
Stage III	❖ Final stage usually occurs in patients >50 years of age ❖ Usually, person has been a laborer for many years ❖ In addition to the pain described under stage II, above, additional complaints of stiffness and weakness may be present ❖ Patients present with a long history of shoulder problems ❖ May also present with sudden, severe episode of pain with resultant shoulder disability from an apparently minor recent trauma ❖ Rotator cuff is either partially or completely torn ❖ Damage is irreversible at this stage

IV. Diagnosis/Evaluation

   A. History
      1. Acute shoulder pain
         a. Ask about the onset (sudden or gradual), duration, location, and intensity of pain (have patient rate on a scale of 1 to 10 with 1 being no pain at all and 10 being the worst pain the patient has ever experienced)
         b. Ask if the onset of pain is related to a single event (macrotrauma) or reinjury of a chronically symptomatic joint
         c. If macrotrauma involved, ask about the activity or sport being performed at the time of the injury and the exact mechanism of injury. Ask if there was a direct blow to the shoulder or an indirect injury such as falling on the elbow or arm
         d. If macrotrauma involved, determine if there was immediate pain, swelling, or deformity

e. If reinjury of a chronically symptomatic joint is suspected, ask what activities were being engaged in when pain started (was the patient lifting overhead, pulling, throwing, or was there no apparent cause for the reinjury?) [**Note**: If no apparent cause, consider systemic arthritis, neoplasm, infection, or cardiac disease]

f. Ask what reduces the pain and what makes it worse

g. Ask if the shoulder feels loose or unstable

h. Inquire about treatments that have been initiated by patient or another provider

i. Obtain past medical history (including past surgeries for orthopedic problems) and medication history; ask about allergies

j. Complete a ROS focusing on pathology in other body systems that could cause referred pain to the shoulder

2. Chronic shoulder pain

a. Ask about the onset (sudden or gradual) duration, location, and usual intensity of pain (have patient rate on a scale of 1 to 10 with 1 being no pain at all and 10 being the worst pain the patient has ever experienced) [**Note**: Gradual onset of pain is the hallmark of impingement syndrome]

b. Determine if pain awakens patient from sleep and if lying on the affected shoulder is avoided because of discomfort

c. Ask appropriate questions to grade the patient's overuse pain in terms of impact on function (from less to most impact)

(1) Grade 1: Pain occurs only after activity (implies early inflammatory activity)

(2) Grade 2: Pain during activity but not restricting performance

(3) Grade 3: Pain during activity and restricting performance

(4) Grade 4: Pain chronic and unremitting, even at rest

d. Ask if the shoulder feels loose or unstable; if there is shoulder weakness or stiffness; if there is swelling or deformity

e. Determine source of microtrauma or repetitive overload of shoulder joint: Is it related to patient's occupation or to leisure activities?

f. Ask about exacerbating and ameliorating factors

g. Ask about previous treatments (including diagnostic testing, hospitalizations, surgeries, and pain management)

h. Ask about problems with other joints, especially the neck and elbow

i. Obtain complete neurologic history for the upper extremity to include paresthesia, weakness, or radiating pain

j. Obtain a complete ROS to detect remote, nonshoulder sources of symptoms (with a focus on respiratory, cardiovascular, gastrointestinal systems); ask about systemic symptoms including fevers, night sweats, and weight loss

k. Obtain past medical history, social history, medication history, and allergies

B. Physical Examination

1. Acute shoulder pain

a. Inspect the affected shoulder from both front and back for swelling, discoloration, deformity, abrasions, and lacerations

b. Palpate the entire shoulder for point tenderness, subtle deformities, or bony crepitus; palpate the area distal and proximal to the pain location

c. Assess for nerve injury

(1) Sensation in the arm and hand on the affected side should be evaluated

(2) Muscles that are innervated by the major nerves of the extremity should be examined for motor function

d. Assess for arterial blood flow

(1) Assess for circulatory compromise on the affected side

(2) Color, warmth, and nail bed capillary refill time should be assessed in each finger

(3) Radial, ulnar, and brachial pulses should be evaluated

e. **Note**: Examination of the unaffected shoulder should be performed at each step of the exam for comparison with the involved shoulder

f. In the absence of trauma (i.e., patient denies a precipitating event for the acute onset of shoulder pain), it is important to carefully check the neck, chest, heart, and abdomen for sources of referred pain

2.   Chronic shoulder pain
  a.   Observe the height of the shoulders and scapulae, the symmetry of the contours, and muscle bulk (common for the dominant shoulder to be slightly lower). This is best done with patient standing, facing both toward and away from the examiner
  b.   Perform muscle strength testing as weakness is often both the underlying cause and the result of injury (on a standard scale of 0 to 5, results of muscle testing should be in 4 to 5 range)
  c.   Palpation should be done with patient at rest and with shoulder movement
      (1)   Bony structures and joints should be palpated with the patient at rest
      (2)   Palpation during active ROM may reveal grinding, popping, and snapping in the AC or glenohumeral joints
  d.   **Note**: Examination of the unaffected shoulder should be performed at each step of the exam in order to compare it with the involved shoulder
  e.   Perform maneuvers to screen for cervical spine pathology and to reproduce shoulder pain as described in the following table

MANEUVERS TO ASSESS SUBACUTE SHOULDER PAIN

Test	Description	Interpretation
Maneuver to Screen for Cervical Spine Pathology		
Head compression test	◆ With patient sitting on low stool, stand behind patient, lock hands together, and then apply gentle but firm downward pressure on head, using both hands locked together (see A below)	◆ Pain localized to neck suggests disk degeneration or facet joint arthritis ◆ Burning pain or pain radiating to involved shoulder suggests nerve root involvement ◆ If test is negative (shoulder pain is not reproduced), continue with exam
Maneuvers to Test Range of Motion		
Scratch test	◆ Evaluate adduction and internal rotation by having patient place arm and hand behind back and reach toward the opposite scapula with the thumb pointed up (see B below) ◆ Evaluate abduction and external rotation by having patient place the hand behind the neck and touch the border of the scapula on the opposite side (see C below)	◆ Repeat with the unaffected side and compare differences ◆ Adhesive capsulitis reduces range of motion on the affected side
Painful arc test	◆ Patient begins test with arm held at side, and then lifts arm to position over head. At 45 degrees of abduction, pain is felt when inflamed tissue is forced under the acromion; pain continues until the 120 degree point on the arc is reached; then, pain subsides as the inflamed tissue passes from beneath the acromion as the arm moves into full abduction (see D below)	◆ This pattern of pain strongly supports impingement

A

B

C

Pain decreases

Painful arc

Painless

D

C. Differential Diagnosis
   1. Acute shoulder pain: Necessary to differentiate among intrinsic causes (fracture, dislocation, strains and sprains) and to determine if pain is being referred from areas such as the chest, abdomen, or cervical spine
   2. Chronic shoulder pain: Many conditions can mimic impingement (examples are adhesive capsulitis, biceps tendon rupture, glenohumeral arthritis, septic arthritis, gout, rheumatoid arthritis, cervical radiculopathy, avascular necrosis, tumor)

D. Diagnostic Tests
1. All patients with acute shoulder pain should be evaluated via x-ray; for suspected proximal humeral and clavicle fractures, AP and lateral (Y view) x-rays made in the scapular plane are recommended; for suspected dislocations and shoulder sprains, an AP view is usually diagnostic, but in anterior dislocation, the axillary view is the test of choice (**Note**: If systemic disease is suspected, perform appropriate tests to detect abnormalities)
2. For patients with chronic shoulder pain, the following diagnostic testing is recommended
   a. The routine radiograph or x-ray film should be used first before consideration of more sophisticated and expensive studies
   b. The standard views include the anteroposterior and lateral views (can disclose basic bony structures but not helpful in viewing the coracoacromial arch or the glenohumeral joint)
   c. Scapular Y (outlet) view discloses the coracoacromial arch as well as the supraspinatus outlet
   d. West Point axillary view can be used to rule out dislocation and assess for avulsion fractures of the glenoid caused by dislocation
3. Further imaging studies such as MRI and arthrography should be done by the specialist to whom patients with Stages II and III impingement syndrome are referred

V. Plan/Management

A. All patients with acute shoulder pain should be referred to an orthopedist for management

B. Patients who are determined to have Stage I impingement (pain is Grade 1 or 2 which suggests mild to moderate inflammation) can be managed conservatively with the goal of decreasing the inflammation that is compressing the subacromial space before irreversible damage occurs

---

CONSERVATIVE TREATMENT FOR STAGE I SHOULDER IMPINGEMENT
ADVICE THAT SHOULD BE GIVEN TO PATIENT

✔ **Rest without** immobilization
✔ **Use** arm and shoulder in activities that do not require overhead motion
✔ **Refrain** from activities that precipitated the injury
✔ **Apply ice** as often as desired and as long as inflammation is present
  (**Note**: Ice is a potent anti-inflammatory agent that can both reduce pain and muscle spasm)
✔ **Use** nonsteroidal anti-inflammatory drugs (NSAIDs) for 2-4 weeks
✔ **Visit** physical therapist for therapeutic modalities such as high-voltage electrical stimulation and ultrasound, and training in stretching and strengthening exercises

---

C. Patients with Stage I impingement that does not respond to conservative therapy in 4 weeks should be referred for further evaluation and possible corticosteroid injections

D. Patients with Stages II and III impingement syndrome require referral to an orthopedist

E. Follow Up
1. For patients with acute shoulder pain, should be to specialist to whom patient was referred
2. For patients with Stage I impingement syndrome (chronic pain) follow up should be in 4 weeks to assess the efficacy of conservative management
3. For patients with Stages II and III impingement syndrome, follow up should be with specialist to whom patient was referred

REFERENCES

American Academy of Pediatrics, Section on Rheumatology and Section on Ophthalmology. (1993). Guidelines for ophthalmologic examinations in children with juvenile rheumatoid arthritis. Pediatrics, 92(2), 295-296.

American College of Rheumatology Ad Hoc Committee on Clinical Guidelines. (1996). Guidelines for management of rheumatoid arthritis. Arthritis and Rheumatism, 39, 713-722.

American College of Rheumatology Ad Hoc Committee on Clinical Guidelines. (1996). Guidelines for monitoring drug therapy in rheumatoid arthritis. Arthritis and Rheumatism, 39, 723-731.

Bach, B.R. (1997). Acute knee injuries: When to refer. The Physician and Sportsmedicine, 25, 39-50.

Baker, D.G. & Schumacher, H.R. Jr. (1993). Acute monarthritis. The New England Journal of Medicine, 329(14), 1013-1020.

Ballas, M.T., Tytko, J., & Cookson, D. (1997). Common overuse running injuries: Diagnosis and management. American Family Physician, 55, 2473-2480.

Ballas, M.T., Tytko, J., & Mannarino, F. (1998). Commonly missed orthopedic problems. American Family Physicians, 57, 267-274.

Ballinger, S.H., & Bowyer, S.L. (1997). Fibromyalgia: The latest "great imitator." Contemporary Pediatrics, 14, 140-154.

Ballock, R.T., & Richards, B.S. (1997). Hip dysplasia: Early diagnosis makes a difference. Contemporary Pediatrics, 14(7), 108-117.

Bergfeld, J., Ireland, M.L., Wojtys, E.M., & Glaser, V. (November 15, 1997). Pinpointing the cause of acute knee pain. Patient Care, 100-117.

Bigos, S., Bowyer, O., Braen, G., et al. (1994). Acute low back problems in adults. Clinical practice guideline No. 14. AHCPR Publication No. 95-0642. Rockville, MD: Agency for Health Care Policy and Research, Public Health Service, U.S. Department of Health and Human Services.

Branstetter, B. (1998). Practical solutions to the mystery of fibromyalgia. Journal of American Association of Physicians Assitants, 11, 27-37.

Brown, L.M. (1999). Injuries of the upper extremity. In R.A. Dershewitz (Ed.), Ambulatory pediatric care. Philadelphia: Lippincott.

Bruce, R.W. (1996). Torsional and angular deformities. Pediatric Clinics of North America, 43, 867-881.

Brunet, M.E., Norwood, L.A., & Sykes, T.F. (1997, January). What to do for the painful shoulder. Patient Care, 56-83.

Brunet, M.E., Norwood, L.A., & Sykes, T.F. (1997, November). A systematic approach to acute shoulder pain. Patient Care, 34-51.

Cassidy, J.T., Levinson, J.E., Bass, J.C., et al. (1986). A study of classification criteria for diagnosis of juvenile rheumatoid arthritis. Arthritis Rheumatology, 29, 274.

Davids, J.R. (1996). Pediatric knee: Clinical assessment and common disorders. Pediatric Clinics of North America, 43, 1067-1090.

Davidson, K. (1993). Patellofemoral pain syndrome. American Family Physician, 48(7), 1254-1262.

Fongemie, A.F., Buss, D.D., & Rolnick, S.J. (1998). Management of shoulder impingement syndrome and rotator cuff tears. American Family Physician, 57, 667-674.

Gillette, R.D. (1996). A practical approach to the patient with back pain. American Family Physician, 53, 670-676.

Goroll, A.H., May, L.A., & Mulley, Jr., A.G. (1995). Evaluation of acute monoarticular arthritis. In A.H.Goroll, L.A. May, A.G.Mulley, Jr., Primary care medicine, (3rd ed.). Lippincott: Philadelphia.

Goroll, A.H., May, L.A., & Mulley, Jr., A.G. (1995). Evaluation of polyarticular complaints. In A.H.Goroll, L.A. May, A.G.Mulley, Jr., Primary care medicine, (3rd ed.). Lippincott: Philadelphia.

Hoffinger, S.A. (1996). Evaluation and management of pediatric foot deformities. Pediatric Clinics of North America, 43, 1091-1111.

Howard, T.M., & O'Connor, F.G. (1997). The injured shoulder: Primary care assessment. Archives of Family Medicine, 6, 376-384.

Jones, A.K. (1997). Primary care management of acute low back pain. <u>Nurse Practitioner, 22</u>(7), 50-73.

Jupiter, J.B. (1995). Approach to minor orthopedic problems of the foot and ankle. In A.H. Goroll, L.A. May, & A.G. Mulley, Jr. (Eds). <u>Primary care medicine</u>, Philadelphia: Lippincott.

Karol, L.A. (1997). Rotational deformities in the lower extremities. <u>Current Opinion in Pediatrics, 9,</u> 77-80.

Koop, S., & Quanbeck, D. (1996). Three common causes of childhood hip pain. <u>Pediatric Clinics of North America, 43,</u> 1053-1066.

Loder, R. (1998). Slipped capital femoral epiphysis. <u>American Family Physician, 57,</u> 2135-2142.

Lyon, R.M., & Street, C.C. (1998). Pediatric sports injuries: When to refer or x-ray. <u>Pediatric Clinics of North America, 45,</u> 221-242.

Magee, D.J. (1992). <u>Orthopedic physical assessment</u>. Philadelphia: Saunders.

Malmivaara, A., et al. (1995). A treatment of acute low back pain--bed rest, exercises, or ordinary activity. <u>New England Journal of Medicine, 332,</u> 351-355.

Mankin, K.P., & Zimbler, S. (1997). Gait and leg alignment: What's normal and what's not. <u>Contemporary Pediatrics, 14</u>(11), 41,45-46, 51-58, 62-70.

Maurizio, S.J., & Rogers, J.L. (1997). Recognizing and treating fibromyalgia. <u>Nurse Practitioner, 22</u>(12), 18-31.

Morgan, D.L. (1998). Orthopedic emergencies. In S.H. Plantz & J.N. Adler (Eds), <u>Emergency medicine</u>. Baltimore: Williams & Wilkins.

Novacheck, T.F. (1996). Developmental dysplasia of the hip. <u>Pediatric Clinics of North America, 43,</u> 829-848.

Payne, W.K., & Ogilvie, J.W. (1996). Back pain in children and adolescents. <u>Pediatric Clinics of North America, 43,</u> 899-91

Pendergast, R.A., Jr. (1997). Back pain. In R.A. Hoekelman (Ed.), <u>Primary pediatric care</u>. St. Louis: Mosby.

Pissutillo, P.D. (1997). <u>Pediatric orthopaedics in primary practice.</u> McGraw-Hill: New York.

Reilly, B.M. (1991). Low back pain. In B.M. Reilly (Ed.), <u>Practical strategies in outpatient medicine</u>. Philadelphia: Saunders. Saunders.

Rothenberg, M.I., & Graf, B.K. (1993). Evaluation of acute knee injuries. <u>Postgraduate Medicine, 93</u> 75-86.

Saperstein, A.L., & Nicholas, S.J. (1996). Pediatric and adolescent sports medicine. <u>Pediatric Clinics of North America, 43,</u> 1013-1032.

Schaller, J.G. (1997). Juvenile rheumatoid arthritis. <u>Pediatrics in Review, 18,</u> 337-349.

Sills, E.M. (1999). Back pain. In R.A. Dershewitz (Ed.), <u>Ambulatory pediatric care</u> (3rd ed.). Philadelphia: Lippincott-Raven.

Sponseller, P.D. (1996). Evaluating the child with back pain. <u>American Family Physician, 54,</u> 1933-1942.

Stiell, I.G., Wells, G.A., Hoag, R.H., et al. (1993). Decision rules for the use of radiography in acute ankle injuries: Refinement and prospective validation. <u>Journal of American Medical Association, 269,</u> 1127-1132.

Tan, E.M., Cohen, A.S., Fries, J.F., et al. (1982). The 1982 revised criteria for the classification of systemic lupus erythematosus. <u>Arthritis Rheumatology, 25,</u> 1275-1277.

Tolo, V.T., & Wood, B. (1993). <u>Pediatric orthopaedics in primary care</u>. Baltimore: Williams & Wilkins.

Trovato, D., Mroczek, K.J., & Splain, S. (1998, March). The painful shoulder. <u>Emergency Medicine</u>, 78-100.

Waddell, G., Feder, G., & Lewis, M. (1997). Systematic reviews of bed rest and advice to stay active for acute low back pain. <u>British Journal of General Practice, 47,</u> 647-652.

Ward, W.T., Davis, H.W., & Hanley, Jr., E.N. (1992). Orthopedics. In B.J. Zitelli & H.W. Davis (Eds.), <u>Atlas of pediatric physical diagnosis</u>. Philadelphia: Lippincott.

Warren, R.W. (1998). Juvenile rheumatoid arthritis. In R.E. Rakel (Ed.). <u>1998 Conn's current therapy</u>. Philadelphia: Saunders.

Wexler, R.K. (1998). The injured ankle. <u>American Family Physician, 57,</u> 474-480.

Wheeler, A.H. (1995). Diagnosis and management of low back pain and sciatica. <u>American Family Physician, 52,</u> 1333-1341.

Wolfe, F., et al. (1990). The American College of Rheumatology 1990 criteria for the classification of fibromyalgia. <u>Arthritis and Rheumatism, 33</u>(2), 160-172.

610

Neurologic Problems

BELL'S PALSY (PERIPHERAL FACIAL PALSY)

I. Definition: Acute, unilateral paralysis of facial muscles due to inflammation and swelling of the 7th (the facial) cranial nerve

II. Pathogenesis

    A. An Idiopathic lower motor neuron disease that is acute in onset

    B. Condition is believed to be viral in origin and may be related to reactivation of herpes simplex virus (HSV)

    C. Damage to the intraneural capillaries is believed to be caused by viral infection of the nerve
        1. Fluid effusion is generated
        2. Subsequently, edema induces paralysis

III. Clinical Presentation

    A. Most often, the child awakens with a unilateral facial droop

    B. May have ear or facial pain on affected side for approximately 24 hours prior to onset of weakness

    C. The facial pain is usually transient and may have resolved by time of presentation

    D. Typical presentation is loss of facial expression, loss of voluntary movement of facial and scalp muscles on affected side, inability to close one eye, and numbness of the face

    E. Food may escape from the child's mouth, the affected eye will not close, and there may be excessive tearing

    F. The facial weakness may not be apparent when child's face is at rest, but asymmetry becomes apparent when the child cries, speaks, or attempts to close eyes
        1. During crying, the affected side is the one that is **not** moving even though it appears normal
        2. On the other hand, the unaffected side (during crying) shows downward movement of the lips and lid closure

    G. Most patients recover completely within weeks to a few months, but some have residual effects

    H. Recurrent facial nerve palsy is unusual and if patient has more than two episodes of the condition, the possibility of sarcoidosis, leukemia, or tumor should be suspected

IV. Diagnosis/Evaluation

    A. History
        1. Question about onset of symptoms as paralysis in Bell's palsy is **abrupt** and does not occur gradually over days or weeks
        2. Include careful questioning about neurological symptoms in other areas of face and body
        3. Ask about predisposing factors such as infection or trauma

    B. Physical Examination
        1. Measure vital signs, noting elevations in blood pressure and temperature
        2. Observe general appearance including gait, evidence of trauma or distress
        3. Inspect skin for herpetic lesions or characteristic lesions of Lyme disease
        4. Carefully examine the head, ears, eyes, nose, and throat

5. Special attention should be given to assessment of the cranial nerves and the neurological examination
    a. Eye movements should be normal and corneal sensation should be intact
    b. Jaw strength (motor division of 5th nerve) should be normal
    c. Hearing and balance (vestibular branch of 8th nerve) should be normal
6. To differentiate between Bell's palsy and a central lesion (an ominous cause of facial weakness) have patient raise eyebrows and wrinkle forehead
    a. With **peripheral** lesions, both the upper and lower face is affected (cannot wrinkle forehead)
    b. With **central** lesions, mainly the lower face is affected (can wrinkle forehead)
    c. Thus, patients with facial nerve involvement have weakness or paralysis of the entire side that is affected, including the forehead; patients with a central nervous system lesion usually have intact function of the upper face on both sides and can therefore wrinkle forehead
7. Use a grading system such as the one in the following table to classify paralysis of the face

GRADING SYSTEM TO CLASSIFY FACIAL PARALYSIS	
Grade 1	• Normal
Grade 2	• No synkinesis (movement in a paralyzed muscle accompanying motion in another part) • Good facial and scalp movement with preserved eyelid closure
Garde 3	• Dyskinesis, or difficulty in performing voluntary movements may or may not be present • Differences between sides of face are apparent
Grade 4	• Incomplete eye closure is present (eyes normal at rest)
Grade 5	• Incomplete eye closure is present (eyes are asymmetric at rest)
Grade 6	• Complete paralysis

C. Differential Diagnosis: Simultaneous bilateral facial palsies, unilateral facial weakness that slowly progresses over 3 weeks with or without facial hyperkinesis, and failure of facial function to return within 6 months after acute onset suggests a diagnosis other than Bell's palsy; possible alternative diagnoses are the following
   1. Tumor
   2. Infectious processes, viral, bacterial, or spirochete
   3. Trauma
   4. Guillain-Barré syndrome (typically has symmetric bilateral weakness)
   5. Neurofibromatosis (typically has café au lait spots and cutaneous neurofibromas)

D. Diagnostic Tests
   1. Diagnostic tests are not needed unless there is uncertainty about the diagnosis
   2. Obtain Lyme titer if there is a history of exposure to ticks or a rash suggestive of Lyme disease
   3. Consider computerized tomography (CT) scan or magnetic resonance imaging (MRI) to rule out tumor if history and physical exam are inconclusive
   4. Electromyographic (EMG) testing occasionally is done to predict prognosis and progression of disease but is usually not required

V. Plan/Management

A. Explain to the patient and parents that symptoms usually resolve in 3-4 weeks without any treatment and with no sequelae in up to 95% of patients

B. Maintain normal conjunctival moisture when there is loss of lid function with eye drops such as Tears Naturale II ophthalmic solution, 1-2 drops as needed

C. Affected eye may need to be taped, especially at night, to reduce eye damage

D. A physical therapy referral may be beneficial; usually involves heat therapy, electrical stimulation, or massage

E. Use of corticosteroids is controversial, but is commonly used nonetheless, particularly in patients who present within 48-72 hours after onset of facial weakness
   1. If there are no contraindications, initiate short-term treatment with prednisone (2 mg/kg per day for one week)
   2. Then taper and discontinue over the next week (for a total of 14 days of treatment)

F. Follow Up
   1. For patients with moderate or severe symptoms, reevaluate in at 3-4 days, and then in 2-4 weeks
   2. Patients taking steroids should be seen after completion of course of therapy
   3. Patients with mild symptoms should be told to return immediately if symptoms worsen or do not resolve completely in 3-4 weeks
   4. Patients who have delayed or incomplete recovery or who have recurrent Bell's palsy should be referred to a specialist for treatment

FEBRILE SEIZURE

I. Definition: Seizures accompanied by fever without central nervous system infection, occurring in infants and children between 6 months and 5 years of age

II. Pathogenesis

A. There is no clear etiology but age is one of the most important factors governing seizure threshold
   1. The cortex becomes increasingly prone to seizures during the early months of life
   2. At about three to six years of age, the neuronal excitability diminishes and children outgrow the tendency toward febrile seizures

B. The threshold of seizure activity may be exceeded in the presence of fever in infants and young children

C. Genetic factors may be linked as there is increased incidence of febrile seizures in first-degree relatives of affected children

III. Clinical Presentation

A. Occur in 2% to 4% of children between 6 months and 5 years of age, and are the most common convulsive event in children younger than 5 years of age, with boys being more susceptible than girls

B. Simple febrile seizures are benign events with an excellent prognosis

C. Simple (benign) febrile seizures are by far the most common type
   1. Seizures are generalized and last <10 minutes with most lasting only 1 or 2 minutes
   2. They do not recur within 24 hours
   3. Seizures usually occur in first few hours of child's illness
   4. EEG obtained 2 weeks after seizure is normal
   5. Otherwise healthy child with no central nervous system infection or abnormality

D. Complex febrile seizures are much less common
   1. Seizures are focal rather than generalized
   2. Seizures last >10 minutes (prolonged) and/or occur more than once in a 24-hour period (repetitive)

IV. Diagnosis/Evaluation

   A. History
      1. Inquire about onset, duration, degree of fever, and parent's management of child's fever (i.e., antipyretic use)
      2. Carefully determine characteristics (i.e., focal vs. generalized), and duration of seizure
      3. Review of systems should concentrate on uncovering concomitant infection
      4. Question about family history of febrile seizures and epilepsy
      5. Assess developmental milestones

   B. Physical Examination
      1. Assess alertness, color, and vital signs
      2. Perform a careful neurological examination
      3. Assess for meningeal signs and symptoms
      4. Complete physical examination is often needed to discover source of fever

   C. Differential Diagnosis
      1. Epilepsy
      2. Meningitis or Encephalitis
      3. Metabolic disorder

   D. Diagnostic Tests
      1. Order diagnostic tests such as CBC, urinalysis, blood cultures, chest x-ray if source of fever is unknown (**Note**: The purpose of these diagnostic tests is to diagnose and treat the cause of the fever, not to identify the cause of the seizure)
      2. After the first seizure with fever in infants younger than 12 months of age, performance of a lumbar puncture should be **strongly** considered because clinical signs and symptoms of meningitis in this age group may be minimal or absent; LP should also be considered in children between 12 and 18 months of age
      3. EEG is not indicated as part of the evaluation of a neurologically healthy child with a first simple febrile seizure

V. Plan/Management

   A. Children with simple febrile seizures lasting only a few minutes, with no focal neurologic deficits, and who have no (or a minimal) postictal period need no further therapy relating to the seizure
      1. Counsel family regarding benign nature of simple febrile seizures
      2. Family education should include use of antipyretics at onset of fever and first aid for seizures; warn the parents that use of antipyretics must be appropriate and that high doses of antipyretics do not reduce the seizure recurrence rate and do involve the risk of toxicity from overmedication
      3. The risk for at least one recurrence after a first febrile seizure is about 30%

   B. Children with prolonged febrile seizures (>10 minutes), focal deficits, a prolonged postictal time, or neurologic deficits must be referred to a pediatric neurologist for immediate/emergent care

   C. Children with new-onset seizure that is not associated with a fever should be referred to a pediatric neurologist for immediate/emergent care

   D. Prophylactic antiepileptic drugs are not recommended unless there are strong risk factors predicting a reoccurrence or the child has a medical problem such as cardiac disease which would be aggravated by a seizure

   E. Follow Up
      1. For children with simple febrile seizure, telephone follow up within first 24-48 hours to ascertain that child is alert, active, and has no additional symptoms
      2. For children with seizures that cannot be classified as a simple febrile seizure, follow up should be by the pediatric neurologist to whom the child was referred

HEADACHES

I. Definition: Diffuse pain in the head

II. Pathogenesis

    A. Primary headaches are caused by traction on pain sensitive structures, inflammation of vessels and meninges, vascular dilation, excessive muscle contraction, and dysregulation of the ascending brain stem serotonergic system

    B. Secondary headaches are due to an underlying organic cause; less than 2-10% of headaches are secondary

    C. International Headache Society Classification (1988)
        1. Migraine with aura and unaccompanied by aura
        2. Tension-type headache
        3. Cluster and chronic paroxysmal hemicrania
        4. Head trauma and post-traumatic headache
        5. Vascular disorders such as severe hypertension, temporal arteritis
        6. Nonvascular intracranial disorders such as brain tumor
        7. Substances or their withdrawal such as pain from caffeine withdrawal or use of nitrates
        8. Noncephalic infections such as otitis media, sinusitis, influenza
        9. Metabolic disorders such as pheochromocytoma
        10. Disorders of face, neck or cranial structures such as cervical radiculopathy, temporomandibular joint (TMJ) dysfunction, eyestrain, acute narrow angle glaucoma, dental problems
        11. Cranial neuralgias such as trigeminal neuralgia
        12. Other types such as psychogenic headaches

    D. Headaches are more common in children than previously recognized; children may experience all three types of primary headaches; organic causes are more likely in children <2 years of age

III. Clinical Presentation of Primary Headaches

    A. Migraines
        1. More common in females than males
        2. Episodes often begin in adolescence or early adulthood but are quite common in childhood beginning as early as age 5-6 years; often remit by age 50 or 60
        3. Frequently there is a positive family history
        4. Females often report a relationship between the migraine and their menses; headaches often remit after menopause
        5. Often unilateral, throbbing and accompanied with nausea, vomiting, phonophobia, photophobia, and perspiration; children often have bilateral headaches and have trouble localizing the pain
        6. Children may become quiet, pale and irritable before onset of headache
        7. Subdivided into two categories:
            a. Migraine accompanied with an aura such as visual prodromes (flashing lights, zigzags, illusions of distorted shapes, strange odors, or paresthesias); previously referred to as a classic migraine
            b. Migraine without an aura; previously referred to as common or nonclassic migraine
        8. Migraine variants are more prevalent in children and adolescents and include altered sensorium and confusion
        9. Complicated migraines are characterized by persistent neurologic symptoms
        10. Research indicates that migraines may increase stroke risk

B. Tension-type
   1. Most common headache type, with a lifetime prevalence of 69% in males and 88% in females; common in children beginning about 8-12 years
   2. Often slowly progressing, bilateral, non-throbbing, or patient complains of dull pressure or band-like sensation about head
   3. Pain is usually mild to moderate
   4. Patients usually do not get nausea, vomiting, photophobia, or phonophobia and headache is not aggravated by physical activity
   5. The International Headache Society distinguishes between patients with episodic tension-type headaches and chronic tension-type headaches (head pain must be present for 15 days a month for at least 6 month to be considered chronic)
   6. Depression, anxiety, and chronic headaches may coexist together
   7. May have combination migraine and tension-type headache

C. Cluster
   1. Severe, unilateral burning or stabbing pain behind eye
   2. Accompanied with at least one of the following on the headache side: ptosis, miosis, redness/edema of eyelid, conjunctival injection, lacrimation, nasal congestion, rhinorrhea, forehead and facial sweating
   3. Cluster headaches often begin in the 4th decade of life (30s), but may begin in children >10 years particularly older adolescent males
   4. Attacks occur in a series which may last months to weeks
   5. Attacks may be as short as 15 minutes or last more than 2-3 hours; attacks may occur once a day or as frequently as 8 times a day

D. Any type of recurrent headache can result in behavioral problems, depression and poor school or work performance

IV. Diagnosis/Evaluation

A. History
   1. Ask about onset of headache; ask about the patient's age at the time of their first headache
   2. Ask older children and adolescents to rate their headaches on a scale from 1 to 10
   3. Question about symptoms which are related to ominous causes (see section V.A.)
   4. Focus on temporal pattern of headaches, associated symptoms, and characteristics of pain such as location and whether headache is throbbing, dull, or burning
   5. Inquire about an aura and prodromal symptoms
   6. Determine whether there is a seasonal relationship to the headaches
   7. Ask about precipitating factors such as stress, diet, physical exertion, sleep problems, or menses
   8. Inquire about medication use, particularly birth control pills, which often cause headaches
   9. Ask about previous trauma to the head
   10. Determine how much caffeine is consumed each day
   11. Question about past medical history including mental health problems
   12. Carefully document family medical history, especially history of migraine headaches
   13. Explore present and previous treatments and responses to treatments including over-the-counter medications and home remedies
   14. Determine impact of headaches on patient's quality of life, daily functioning, and work and/or school performance
   15. Ask about symptoms of depression
   16. Patients with chronic headaches should keep a diary documenting their symptoms and the circumstances surrounding the symptoms

B. Physical Examination
   1. Observe general appearance, noting signs of acute distress, anxiety, or depression
   2. Measure temperature, blood pressure, pulse, pulse pressure
   3. In younger child, measure head circumference
   4. Inspect head for signs of trauma and deformities

5. Palpate temporal arteries for tenderness (patients with temporal arteritis have firm, tender, enlarged arteries)
6. Palpate sinuses and temporomandibular joint (TMJ)
7. Perform complete eye exam with funduscopy; check pupils for size, shape, accommodation, and response to light
8. Examine mouth and teeth
9. Check for nuchal rigidity, cervical bruits, cervical vertebrae radiculopathy
10. Auscultate and palpate peripheral pulses
11. Perform complete neurological exam including careful assessment of cranial nerves

C. Differential Diagnosis:
1. In children, many acute or subacute headaches are a result of non-CNS infections or febrile illnesses
2. Uncommon causes of headaches in children include hypertension, substance abuse or ocular diseases
3. Determine whether headache is a secondary headache due to an organic cause or a primary headache; consider the following questions:
   a. Does the patient have risk for secondary causes such as diabetes and hyperlipidemia which may be associated with headaches due to stroke?
   b. Do the associated symptoms suggest a secondary cause?
      (1) Meningitis/encephalitis (fever, nuchal rigidity)
      (2) Sinusitis (frontal tenderness, fever, nasal discharge)
      (3) Narrow angle glaucoma (cloudy vision)
      (4) TMJ syndrome (pain with chewing)
      (5) Cervical radiculopathy (pain with neck movement)
   c. Are the headaches related to precipitating factors such as cold or hot foods and drinks which may be associated with trigeminal neuralgia?
4. Brain tumors are always a consideration; patients with traction headaches due to intracranial lesions have the following signs and symptoms:
   a. Gradual onset of deep, aching pain which is often worse in morning and aggravated by coughing or straining for stool
   b. May have signs of increased intracranial pressure such as papilledema, and widening pulse pressure
5. Headaches that are sudden in onset and described as the "worst headache" may be due to a subarchnoid hemorrhage
6. If the secondary cause of headache is excluded, determine which type of primary headache is causing the pain

D. Diagnostic Tests; choice of test depends on history and physical findings; majority of patients with primary headaches do not require diagnostic tests
1. An electroencephalogram should be considered if the patient has lost consciousness or has altered consciousness
2. Order computerized tomography (CT) scan or magnetic resonance imaging (MRI):
   a. When there is suspicion of the following: intracranial tumor, cerebellar hemorrhage or infarction, stroke, intracerebral hemorrhage
   b. When there has been head trauma with findings of increased intracranial pressure, depressed or open skull fracture, and penetrating head injury
3. Other diagnostic tests should be ordered on the basis of the history and physical examination; the following are examples, but not an exhaustive list of possible tests:
   a. CBC with differential and immediate lumbar puncture if infection is suspected
   b. Erythrocyte sedimentation rate and antinuclear antibody to detect a collagen disease
   c. Magnetic resonance angiography if aneurysm is suspected
   d. X-rays of the temporomandibular joints if TMJ syndrome is suspected
4. CT, MRI, spectroscopy and PET are sometimes ordered for headaches without clinical findings when the diagnosis is uncertain

V. Plan/Management

    A.   Consider referral to a specialist if the patient has a complicated migraine or any of the following ominous signs (see table)

OMINOUS SIGNS OF HEADACHE
❖ Abnormal physical signs ❖ New-onset, unilateral headache, particularly in patients over age 35 ❖ Severe headache or headache different from previous ones ❖ Headaches becoming more continuous and intense ❖ Headaches accompanied by vomiting but not nausea

    B.   In children <18 years, the recommended acute treatment of a migraine headache is controversial

        1.   Recent study found ibuprofen (Children's Motrin) 10 mg/kg/dose every 6 hours or acetaminophen (Tylenol) 15 mg/kg/dose every 4 hours to be effective in relieving even severe migraines

        2.   Some experts recommend cyproheptadine (Periactin) 0.2-0.4 mg/kg per day in 2-3 divided doses in combination with Tylenol or ibuprofen for acute attacks

        3.   Other abortive agents are not recommended in children <18 years but are sometimes cautiously used such as sumatriptan, ergotamine, dihydroergotamine mesylate, butalbital; consult pediatric neurologist for dosing recommendations

        4.   For nausea prescribe prochlorperazine (Compazine) in one of the following routes:

            a.   PO doses in children: 20-29 lbs. use 2.5 mg QD/BID; 30-39 lbs. use 2.5 mg BID/TID; 40-85 lbs. use 2.5 mg TID or 5 mg BID (not recommended for children <2 years or <20 lbs.)

            b.   IM dose in children >2 years or 20 lb.: 0.06mg/lb IM

    C.   Acute therapy for migraines in patients ≥18 years

        1.   Limit all medications to those absolutely necessary to prevent transforming migraines to chronic, daily, intractable head pain or to avoid rebound headaches

        2.   Antiemetics administered orally, intramuscularly or by rectal suppository may offset nausea and enhance the effectiveness of analgesic drugs; prescribe one of the following:

            a.   Metoclopramide (Reglan) 10 mg PO every 6 hours increases gut motility which may counteract the gastric stasis that often accompanies migraine attacks; use sparingly because of possible dystonia effects

            b.   Alternatively, prescribe prochlorperazine (Compazine) 5-10 mg TID/QID PO, 5-10 mg IM every 3-4 hours, or 25 mg BID rectally

        3.   For mild attacks prescribe one of the following:

            a.   Aspirin 325-400 mg tablets, 2 tablets PO every 4 hours

            b.   Excedrin Migraine which contains 250 mg acetaminophen, 250 mg aspirin, 65 mg caffeine is the first over-the-counter analgesic to be cleared by the FDA for treatment of mild-to-moderate migraine pain; for adults and children >12 years give 2 tabs every 6 hours as needed with maximum of 8 tabs per day

            c.   Nonsteroidal anti-inflammatory drugs (NSAIDs) such as naproxen sodium (Anaprox), 275 mg tablets, 2 tabs initially followed by 1 tab every 6-8 hours

        4.   For moderate and severe attacks prescribe one of the following drugs:

            a.   Sumatriptan (Imitrex), a selective serotonin 5-HT 1D receptor agonist, is the agent of choice for adolescents

                (1)   Prescribe one of the following administration routes:

                      (a)   6 mg subcutaneous injection (available 6mg/0.5 mL); onset of action is rapid; may repeat injection in 1 hour, with a maximum of 2 doses in 24 hours

                      (b)   25-100 mg PO (available 25 & 50 mg tabs) -- 50 mg dose recently found to be most effective; may give second dose 2 hours after first with additional doses at two hour intervals if needed; maximum is 300 mg/day or 200 mg/day if injection was also used; take with fluids

                      (c)   5 mg, 10 mg, or 20 mg intranasally (available 5 mg & 20 mg per spray); may repeat dose once after 2 hours; maximum of 40 mg/day and treatment of 4 headaches within 30 days

619

(2) First dose of injectable sumatriptan should be given under medical supervision and possibly monitored with an electrocardiogram; cautiously prescribe to patients who are likely to have unrecognized coronary artery disease, such as patients with risk factors for coronary vascular disease

(3) Contraindicated in patients with history of myocardial infarction, symptomatic ischemic heart disease, Prinzmetal's angina or uncontrolled hypertension

(4) Do not use sumatriptan with vasoconstrictor drugs or within 2 weeks of therapy with monoamine oxidase inhibitors, and use of ergotamine derivatives within the previous 24 hours

(5) Advantages: medication is effective in relieving pain when given at any time during the attack and it is helpful in relieving nausea

(6) Disadvantages are that it is expensive, headaches tend to recur, and side effects such as flushing, throat discomfort, neck and chest tightness or pain, tingling can occur

b. Other selective serotonin 5-HT 1D receptor agonists are available for patients categorized as poor responders to other treatments including sumatriptan (see following table)

COMPARISON OF NEW TRIPTANS			
Drug	**Dosing**	**Administration**	**Comment**
Naratriptan tablets (Amerge)	1 or 2.5 mg with fluid. Repeat once after 4 h when necessary. Maximum dosage: 5 mg/24 h	Maximum dosage in patients with mild to moderate renal or hepatic impairment is 2.5 mg/24 h. Consider a lower starting dose. Contraindicated in patients with severe kidney or liver disease.	Long onset of action; long elimination half life; helpful for patients with long migrainous episodes; may have slightly lower rate of recurrence of migraine than other triptans; favorable side effect profile.
Rizatriptan (MAXALT, MAXALT-MLT)	5 or 10 mg by mouth. Repeat once after at least 2 h when necessary. Maximum dosage: 30 mg/24 h; for patients using propranolol, 15 mg/24 h.	Patients should be advised to consult the health care provider before administering a second dose if the first has had no effect. Make sure patients know that the conventional tablet must be swallowed with liquid. The fast-melting form, packaged in blisters, will dissolve with saliva.	More rapid onset of action than oral sumatriptan.
Zolmitriptan tablets (Zomig)	2.5 mg or less to start-- tablets can be broken in half, but response is better with 2.5- or 5-mg strengths. Dose can be repeated after 2 h. Maximum dosage: 10 mg/24 h.	Liver disease hinders clearance of zolmitriptan, a situation that can push up BP. Caution is warranted in patients with hepatic dysfunction-- individual doses should be <2.5 mg.	More rapid onset of action than oral sumatriptan; favorable side effect profile.

Adapted from Starr, C. (1998). Emerging migraine treatments. Patient Care Nurse Practitioner, 10-26.

c. Ergotamine tartrate, a serotonin agonist, is a second-line abortive agent

(1) Prescribed one of the following administration routes (rectal route may be best if patient is nauseous):

(a) Ergotamine tartrate with caffeine (Cafergot) 1 suppository per rectum; may insert 2nd suppository after 60 minutes up to 2 per day or 5 per week; best absorbed of all nonparenteral preparations

(b) Ergotamine tartrate 1 mg, caffeine 100 mg (Wigraine): take 2 tabs; may repeat 1 tab every 30 minutes up to 6 mg per attack or 10 mg per week

(c) Ergotamine tartrate (Ergostat): 2 mg under tongue; may repeat every 30 minutes up to 6 mg per day or 10 mg per week

(2) Must take these agents early in the attack to be effective

(3) With all routes of administration, there should be a 5-day hiatus between treatment days

        (4)   Not adhering to dosage guidelines should be avoided to prevent rebound headaches which are common with these agents

        (5)   Contraindications include coronary or peripheral vascular disease, uncontrolled hypertension, impaired hepatic or renal disorders

        (6)   Side effects include nausea, vomiting, diarrhea, cramping dizziness, transient paresthesias, vasoconstrictive complications, tachycardia, bradycardia, localized edema or itching

   d.   Dihydroergotamine mesylate (D.H.E. 45, Migranal) is a derivative of ergotamine and is used for rapid control of migraines

        (1)   Dosage is dependent on route of administration

            (a)   D.H.E. 45: Give 1 mL IM or IV at onset of attack then 1 mL after one hour as needed; maximum is 2 mL IV or 3 mL IM per attack

            (b)   Migranal: One spray in each nostril; repeat 15 minutes later with maximum of 6 sprays in 24 hours and 8 sprays per week

        (2)   Contraindications and side effects are similar to ergotamine

   e.   Isometheptene mucate 65 mg, dichloralphenazone 100 mg, acetaminophen 325 mg tablets (Midrin) is a cerebral vasoconstrictor and a third-line agent

        (1)   Usually recommended for patients who can't take sumatriptan or ergotamine

        (2)   Less beneficial in patients with severe headaches

        (3)   Prescribe 2 tabs initially followed by 1 every hour, maximum 5 per 12 hours

        (4)   Contraindications: Glaucoma, severe renal, cardiac, hypertensive, or hepatic disease, concurrent MAOIs

        (5)   Has fewer side effects than sumatriptan and ergotamine

   f.   Analgesics and sedatives are sometimes helpful but it is best to avoid regular use of them

        (1)   Butorphanol tartrate nasal spray (Stadol NS) 1 mg: Spray in one nostril; if relief is not provided within 60-90 minutes an additional 1 mg may be given; repeat every 3-4 hours as needed

        (2)   Fiorinal (combination of aspirin 325 mg, caffeine 40 mg, barbiturate 50 mg): Prescribe one to two tabs every four hours

        (3)   Parenteral narcotics can be used for pain relief and to enable patient to sleep through the attack; minimize use to prevent abuse

D.   Treatment of severe, intractable migraine attacks

   1.   Ketorolac (Toradol) 30-60 mg IM is often used in emergency departments

   2.   Three dopamine-antagonist drugs given intravenously may be beneficial: metoclopramide (Reglan), chlorpromazine (Thorazine), prochlorperazine (Compazine)

   3.   IV dihydroergotamine and/or corticosteroid therapy (IM or IV) along with metoclopramide or another antiemetic may break the headache cycle

E.   Migraine prevention in patients <18 years: prescribe one of the following when patient has >3 attacks per month

   1.   Propranolol hydrochloride (Inderal), start with 0.5-1 mg/kg BID and gradually increase until a therapeutic response is achieved

   2.   Cyproheptadine (Periactin) 0.5-1 mg/kg/day, divided every 6-8 hours or at bedtime

   3.   Tricyclic antidepressants such as amitriptyline (Elavil) 0.1 to 2.0 mg/kg at bedtime are effective, especially in older children and adolescents

   4.   The efficacy of calcium channel blockers has been variable in children

F.   Migraine preventive therapy in patients ≥18 years

   1.   Consider preventive therapy when the patient has >2 attacks per month, when attacks are severe or predictable, or when other therapies have failed or had serious side effects

   2.   General principles to follow when ordering preventive therapy:

      a.   Females of childbearing age should use barrier methods of contraception rather than oral birth control pills which often trigger headaches

      b.   Patients should discontinue all prior headache medications before prophylaxis therapy because previous medications may compete for monoamine-receptor sites with preventive drugs

       c.   Each preventive medication should be given for an adequate time to judge its effectiveness (i.e., 2-3 months)

       d.   Preventive medication is usually given for 6 months and then gradually withdrawn after the frequency of headaches diminishes

   3.   Common preventive medications are the following:

       a.   Aspirin 325-400 mg tabs, 1-2 tabs PO HS

       b.   Adrenergic blocking agents are especially beneficial for patients with concomitant hypertension, angina pectoris or thyrotoxicosis (avoid agents with intrinsic sympathomimetic activity)

          (1)   Contraindicated in patients with bronchospasm, congestive heart failure, cardiac arrhythmias, or a history of depression

          (2)   Propranolol (Inderal) is considered drug of choice: Start with 20 mg PO BID and increase gradually to maximum 160 mg/day

          (3)   Alternative drug is timolol (Blocadren): 10-20 mg/day

          (4)   Alternative drug (especially for asthmatics): Metoprolol (Lopressor) 100-200 mg/day in two divided doses

       c.   Divalproex sodium (Depakote), an anticonvulsant, is the first-line therapy for patients with concomitant seizures, mania, or anxiety; may also be given to patients without history of seizures

          (1)   Begin with 125-250 mg TID and increase gradually; average dose is 250-500 mg TID; prescribe twice daily for patients without seizures

          (2)   Order baseline CBC and liver function tests at frequent intervals, particularly in first 6 months

          (3)   Dose-related side effects are nausea, tremor, weight gain, hair loss

       d.   Tricyclic antidepressants such as amitriptyline (Elavil) 50-100 mg po HS are not first-line agents, but may be beneficial, particularly for patients with coexisting migraine and tension-type headaches

       e.   Calcium channel blockers are usually used after trials of the more effective beta blockers or amitriptyline; alternative to beta blockers in patients with asthma or chronic obstructive pulmonary disease; effective in patients with neurologic symptoms

          (1)   Verapamil (Calan) is the best studied agent in this class; prescribe 120-480 mg/day

          (2)   Use these agents with caution in patients with congestive heart failure

          (3)   Avoid abrupt withdrawal of these agents because of the potential to induce chest pain, rebound angina, or exacerbation of symptoms

       f.   For headaches unresponsive to above therapies, consider use of methysergide (Sansert), 2 mg PO TID/QID

          (1)   One of most effective agents but can cause retroperitoneal, pleural, and pulmonary valve fibrosis with extended use; monitor patient by assessing peripheral pulses and auscultating the chest monthly

          (2)   Contraindicated in patients with vascular disease because of its vasoconstrictor action

          (3)   Continue for 4 months then reduce slowly with gradual substitution of another prophylactic agent, so that one month elapses before resumption.

       g.   Other classes of drugs that may be used are nonsteroidal anti-inflammatory drugs (NSAIDs), clonidine (Catapres), and selective serotonin reuptake inhibitors (SSRIs) such as fluoxetine (Prozac)

G.   Patients with menstrual migraines

   1.   Acute therapy is similar to treatment of migraines not associated with menses (see V.B. and V.C.)

   2.   Prophylaxis with one of following drugs may be helpful when administered for one week during the luteal phase of the menses in patients ≥18 years

       a.   Percutaneous estrogen in gel form or transdermal patches containing 0.05 mg of ethinyl estradiol (Climara, Estroderm) because migraines may be triggered by falling estrogen levels (start 2-3 days before expected headaches)

       b.   NSAIDs such as mefenamic acid (Ponstel) 250 mg BID/TID

       c.   Propranolol (Inderal) 20-120mg PO BID

   d. Amitriptyline 50-100 mg po HS
   e. Antiestrogen tamoxifen citrate (Nolvadex) 5-15 mg/day
   f. Bromocryptine mesylate (Parlodel) 2.5-5 mg/day
   g. Androgen derivative danazol (Danocrine) 200-600 mg/day

H. Migraine: Patient Education
 1. Reduce precipitating factors such as stress, foods with nitrites (hot dogs), foods with monosodium glutamate (Chinese food), and tyramine containing foods (cheese, chocolate, red wine)
 2. Limit caffeine to 2 beverages/day
 3. Avoid alcoholic beverages, undersleeping, oversleeping, missing meals, smoking
 4. Avoid craning neck forward
 5. Avoid possible triggers such as glare or exposure to flickering lights, noise, or strong odors
 6. Avoid analgesic, ergotamine, and decongestant overuse
 7. Oral contraceptives should be discontinued
 8. Get regular aerobic exercise
 9. Biofeedback, relaxation therapy
 10. Rest in quiet dark room with topical ice to head or neck

I. Tension-type Headache Treatment
 1. Because of chronic nature of these headaches, try nonpharmacological approaches such as biofeedback, stress management, relaxation and exercise first
 2. Initiate drug therapy with least potent and least addictive medications such as acetaminophen, aspirin, and NSAIDS
 3. Use drugs for brief time period and limit to <15 pills per week; overuse of analgesics can lead to rebound headaches
 4. Chronic tension headache sufferers need evaluation for underlying anxiety and depression; antidepressant therapy with amitriptyline (Elavil) or specific serotonin reuptake inhibitors such as Prozac may be a beneficial

J. Cluster Headache Treatment
 1. Inhalation of 100% oxygen administered no longer than 15 minutes at 6-8 liters/minute flow rate
 2. For acute therapy in patients $\geq$18 years, sumatriptan and ergotamine are often used as well as the other medications recommended for treatment of migraine headaches (see V.B. and V.C.)
 3. For preventive therapy in patients <18 years, use medications recommended for prevention of migraines (V.E.)
 4. For preventive therapy in patients $\geq$18 years, the following are recommended:
   a. Verapamil (Calan) 80-120 mg TID
   b. Lithium initiated at 300-600 mg/day and increased to 600-1200 mg/day as needed in 2-4 divided dosed is effective
   c. Methysergide 2 mg QID is effective in shortening the course of headaches; doses should be tapered after 2-3 weeks of freedom from headaches
   d. Injectable or oral corticosteroids may be given for patients who do not respond to above preventive therapies; initiate prednisone at dose range of 40-60 mg per day in divided doses and taper over 1 month
   e. Other medications listed under preventive therapy for migraine headaches may also be effective for cluster headaches

K. Other therapies such as intranasal lidocaine and capsaicin nasal application have been effective in a few studies, but more research is needed before they can be recommended

L. Follow up for all types of headaches is to return if headache is unrelieved or if it increases in severity, duration or frequency from usual pattern

SEIZURES AND EPILEPSY

I.   Definitions

    A.   Seizures: Paroxysmal alteration in consciousness or other cerebral cortical function

    B.   Epilepsy: More than one unprovoked seizure in lifetime

II. Pathogenesis

    A.   Initiated by electrochemical abnormalities in brain such as alterations in concentration of excitatory or inhibitory neurotransmitter

    B.   Abnormal electrical discharge from one site is rapidly transmitted to other parts of the brain, producing disturbances in perception, motor control, attention, and consciousness

    C.   Major causes of seizure by age group are as follows
        1.   Newborns and infants
            a.   Birth trauma, congenital malformations
            b.   Febrile
            c.   Metabolic disorders
        2.   Children, adolescents, and young adults
            a.   Idiopathic
            b.   Alcohol or drug related
            c.   Traumatic
            d.   Infection

III. Clinical Presentation

    A.   Seizures affect about 1% of the population in the US

    B.   Children and adolescents are most likely to have idiopathic seizures or seizure secondary to infection, trauma, or drug use
        1.   Idiopathic seizures, known as epilepsy, often begin in childhood and adolescence
            a.   Cause is unknown, but there may be a hereditary predisposition
            b.   In many patients with idiopathic epilepsy, the physical, neurologic, and laboratory evaluations are normal
        2.   Traumatic causes, most often from accidental injuries
            a.   Birth and perinatal injuries can cause seizures but these are usually diagnosed early in life
            b.   Head trauma from MVAs, falls, and sports injuries are common causes, with the more severe the head injury, the greater the likelihood of developing posttraumatic seizures
        3.   Infectious causes, including infection of the brain, encephalitis; septic emboli and abscesses associated with endocarditis
            a.   Presence of an epidemic of encephalitis, recent history of febrile illness, and changes in mental status suggest an infectious cause
            b.   History of parenteral drug use, AIDS, recent dental work, and murmur or valvular heart disease also point to an infectious cause
        4.   Alcohol and drug related seizures occur via a number of mechanisms
            a.   Alcohol can cause seizures due to malnutrition, increased risk of head trauma, and during withdrawal
            b.   Cocaine and other stimulants are associated with increased risk of seizure; withdrawal from barbiturates can also cause seizures

INTERNATIONAL CLASSIFICATION OF EPILEPTIC SEIZURES BY MODE OF ONSET AND SPREAD	
Partial Seizures (seizures begin focally)	**Partial seizure with simple symptoms (no alteration/impairment of consciousness)** ✻ With motor symptoms (often begin in single muscle group and spread to entire side of body) ✻ With somatosensory symptoms (paresthesia, flashing lights visualized) ✻ With autonomic symptoms (tachycardia, loss of bowel/bladder control) ✻ With psychic symptoms (hallucinations) **Complex partial seizures always involve impairment of consciousness** ✻ Simple partial onset progressing to impairment of consciousness ✻ With impairment of consciousness at onset **Partial seizures evolving to secondarily generalized seizures** ✻ Simple partial seizures evolving to generalized seizures ✻ Complex partial seizures evolving to generalized seizures ✻ Simple partial seizures evolving to complex partial seizures to generalized seizures
Generalized seizures (convulsive or nonconvulsive)	✻ Absence seizures ✻ Myoclonic seizures ✻ Clonic seizures ✻ Tonic seizures ✻ Tonic-clonic seizures ✻ Atonic seizures
Unclassified epileptic seizures	✻ Includes all seizures whose classification is hampered by inadequate or incomplete data

Adapted from Commission on Classification and Terminology of the International League Against Epilepsy. (1981). Proposal for revised clinical and electroencephalographic classification of epileptic seizures. Epilepsia, 22, 489.

C. Partial seizures begin in one hemisphere of the brain and result in an asymmetric seizure (unless there is secondary generalization); this type seizure usually begins with an aura (commonly reflecting the focal nature of the epileptic discharge at its onset)

    1. Present as alterations in motor functions, sensory or somatosensory symptoms, or autonomic symptoms

    2. Are classified as simple, partial, complex partial depending on whether there is an impairment of consciousness, and partial seizures with secondary generalization

    3. Partial seizures are the most common type of seizure

D. Generalized seizures involve both hemispheres with motor involvement that is bilateral and there is an impairment in consciousness; types of generalized seizures are listed below

    1. Absence seizures are manifest by sudden onset, an interruption of activity in which the person is engaged, and a blank stare (also called behavior arrest)

    2. Tonic-clonic seizures are manifest by loss of consciousness; most often without warning, but with an aura in some patients; tonic refers to stiffening and clonic to contraction with tonic stiffening usually occurring first followed by clonic contractions; patient may fall, lose sphincter control, bite tongue, or develop cyanosis; a patient frequently falls into deep sleep after the seizure

    3. Tonic and clonic seizures may occur separately and thus are classified as separate types

    4. Myoclonic seizures are brief shock-like muscular contractions of the face, trunk, and extremities; may be isolated events or occur repetitively

    5. Atonic seizures are characterized by sudden loss of muscle tone; may be a head drop, a limb drop, or total body drop to the floor or ground

E. Unclassified seizures include all seizures that cannot be classified because of inadequate or incomplete data

IV. Diagnosis/Evaluation

A. History

    1. History should include information to help determine if a seizure has occurred and the probable type of seizure

        a. Important to question parents and witnesses as well as patient (for much of the history, witnesses are better sources than patients, but patients are the best source for presence and type of aura)

        b. Explore precipitating factors

        c. Describe the focal onset, duration, and seizure characteristics

        d. Inquire about the setting in which episode occurred

  e. Determine whether the patient completely lost consciousness and/or was incontinent

  f. Determine if there was an aura, antigrade amnesia, or postical period

 2. Ask if there was a history of trauma; ask about alcohol or drug use and withdrawal from alcohol or drugs; enquire about exposures to toxins, including occupational, recreation, or accidental exposures

 3. Obtain complete medical history, including history of any pulmonary, hepatic, cardiac, renal, or endocrine disease; ask about history of cancer

 4. Obtain complete medication history and ask about allergies

 5. Question about family history of seizures

 6. Obtain birth history and attainment of developmental milestones

 7. For patients with known epilepsy who present with seizures, determine the following:

  a. Precipitating factors

  b. Similarity and differences between these seizures and ones in the past

  c. Medications currently taking and adherence with regime

  d. If the seizures are occurring more frequently

B. Physical Examination

 1. Assess vital signs and evaluate for orthostatic hypotension

 2. Perform a complete physical examination with a focus on cardiovascular and neurological systems

  a. Examine the heart for signs of valvular disease and arrhythmia

  b. Perform a neurologic exam including assessment of the head, eye grounds, cranial nerves, neck, speech, gait, mental status, motor (including cerebellar), sensory, and deep tendon reflexes (**Note**: A normal neurologic exam is often found in persons with idiopathic seizures)

C. Differential Diagnosis

 1. Most common causes of seizures are listed under II.C. above and must be considered

 2. Syncope does not cause seizures but is often confused with this disorder

  a. Whereas patients with syncope may exhibit repetitive clonic, myoclonic, or dystonic movements, these movements rarely last beyond 5-10 seconds and do not exhibit the organized progression from tonic to clonic phase seen in convulsive seizures

  b. Incontinence does not occur with syncope but may occur with seizures

  c. Tongue biting does not occur with syncope but may occur with seizures

  d. A few minutes of confusion immediately following the event is not likely with syncope but is likely with seizures

D. Diagnostic Tests

 1. Basic laboratory evaluation should focus on detecting systemic disorders sometimes associated with seizures

  a. CBC

  b. Chemistry profile

  c. Liver function tests

  d. Toxicology screen

  e. Electroencephalography (EEG) [Multiple EEGs increase their diagnostic utility]

 2. Most authorities recommend that all patients who experience an unprovoked seizure undergo a brain imaging study to detect any cerebral lesions (tumor, abscess, vascular malformation, stroke, traumatic injury)

  a. In nonurgent presentations, the imaging study of choice is magnetic resonance imaging (MRI) because it is more sensitive than computed tomography (CT)

  b. In emergent cases, in which the history or physical examination suggest new focal deficits, altered mental status, fever, persistent headache, recent trauma, history of cancer, immunosuppression, emergency imaging is required, most often with a CT scan (better at detection of acute hemorrhage than MRI)

  c. If an infection in the nervous system is suspected, lumbar puncture should be performed

V.   Plan/Management

A.   Some seizures are from correctable etiologies and the underlying problem must be identified and corrected in those cases

B.   Goal of treatment of patients with epilepsy is to provide optimal control of seizures without producing unacceptable side effects

C.   Decision to treat **initial or first-time** seizures with medications is controversial and patients with first seizure should be referred to a neurologist in the following instances
1.   There is uncertainty regarding whether event was actually a seizure
2.   For evaluation of focal seizures
3.   If the neurologic examinations is abnormal
4.   When the EEG shows focality
5.   When special diagnostic procedures are indicated (MRI, CT scan, sleep-deprived EEG)
6.   Children are **rarely** treated for a first-time seizure

D.   Selection of an antiepileptic drug (AED) that is appropriate for the patient's type of epilepsy is the cornerstone of treatment
1.   From the appropriate drugs, select one that best fits the patient based on both patient and medication characteristics including side-effect profile
2.   Initiate and titrate the medication at the correct dosage, and make incremental changes that will enhance effectiveness and tolerability
3.   A general rule of thumb is to initiate therapy with one-fourth to one-third of the anticipated maintenance dose and increase the dose to maintenance over a 3-4 week period
4.   Increase the medication dosing until complete seizure control occurs or until side effects that are persistent and nontolerable occur
5.   If adequate seizure control--defined as complete seizure control for most persons--is not attained at the maximum tolerated dosage of the first medication that is prescribed two approaches can be considered
a.   First, consideration should be given to referring the patient for neurologic consultation if such consultation has not already been sought
b.   A second option is to start a second drug and taper the first. As the dosage of the new medication is titrated up, the original medication is gradually tapered until monotherapy with the new agent is achieved. If control is not obtained with monotherapy with a second drug, then refer to a neurologist (**Note:** Dual therapy should never be used until adequate trials of at least two or three drugs as monotherapy have been attempted)
c.   Never abruptly withdraw any drug; gradually taper

E.   Treatment should begin with one AED, preferably the drug of choice
1.   Common epilepsy types with the first- and second-choice AED treatments are listed in the following table
2.   The advantage of using one drug is that patient adherence is increased, the management of toxicity is easier, side effects are easier to monitor and control, drug interactions are avoided, and it is less expensive

DRUGS OF CHOICE ACCORDING TO SEIZURE TYPE		
Seizure Type	**Drugs of Choice**	**Alternative Drugs**
Generalized Seizures		
Primary generalized, tonic-clonic	Valproic acid (Depakene)	Carbamazepine (Tegretol), Phenytoin (Dilantin), Primidone (Mysoline), Phenobarbital
Primary generalized, absence	Ethosuximide (Zarontin), valproic acid	Clonazepam (Klonopin)
Primary myoclonic	Valproic acid, clonazepam	Phenytoin, phenobarbital
Partial Seizures		
Partial simple and complex, and secondarily generalized epilepsy	Carbamazepine, phenytoin	Valproic acid, phenobarbital, primidone
Mixed Forms	Valproic acid, clonazepam	Carbamazepine, phenytoin, phenobarbital

F. Patient's age, seizure type, daily activities, and economic considerations should influence selection of AED
    1. Primidone and phenobarbital cause excess sedation, behavioral problems such as irritability, and cognitive impairment, particularly in schoolchildren
    2. Phenytoin is a poor first choice for children and adolescents because of the consequences of long-term use which may include coarsening of the facial features, gingival hyperplasia, hirsutism, and enlargement of the lips
    3. Carbamazepine, particularly the new extended-release preparation, is a good choice for many children with focal seizures

G. The newer AEDs include tiagabine, gabapentin, lamotigine, felbamate, and topiramate; these drugs are used primarily as adjunctive therapy in refractory patients
    1. Tiagabine (Gabitril) is used as adjunctive therapy in patients ≥12 years of age with localization-related epilepsy; drug selectively inhibits uptake of gamma aminobutyric acid (GABA) and prolongs the duration of inhibitory activity at postsynaptic receptors
    2. Gabapentin (Neurontin) is used as adjunctive therapy in patients ≥12 years of age with localization-related epilepsy; works well in patients in whom drug-drug interactions must be avoided such as persons with comorbidities and the elderly on multiple medications
    3. Lamotrigine (Lamictal) is used as adjunctive therapy in adults with localization-related epilepsy and also as an alternative in patients with localization-related or generalized epilepsies; has been associated with severe, potentially life-threatening rashes, including Stevens-Johnson syndrome and toxic epidermal necrolysis; not licensed for use in children
    4. Felbamate (Felbatol) is used as adjunctive therapy or monotherapy in adults with localization-related epilepsy and as adjunctive therapy in children with Lennox-Gastaut syndrome (symptomatic generalized epilepsy consisting of multiple types of generalized seizures); felbamate has been associated with aplastic anemia and fulminant hepatic failure and this drug should only be used by an epileptologist in patients in whom the benefits outweigh the risks
    5. Topiramine (Topamax) is used as adjunctive therapy in adults with localization-related epilepsy and may also be useful in some patients with certain types of generalized epilepsies; cognitive effects constitute the main dose-limiting toxicity that is known at this time

H. Dosages for the most commonly used AEDs
    1. Carbamazepine : Tegretol, 100, 200 mg tabs, and 100 mg chewable tabs; Tegretol suspension, 100 mg/5 mL
        a. Children: > 6 years of age: Begin with 100 mg BID and increase weekly by 100 mg/day in 3-4 divided doses (Maximum daily dose is 1 g)
        b. Children <6 years of age: Begin with 10 mg/kg/day, in 3 divided doses; increase weekly if needed to 20 mg/kg/day, in 3 divided doses
        c. Tegretol-XR, 100, 200, 400 mg tabs: Same beginning dose and weekly rate of increase as described above for children >6 years of age **except** dosing should be BID
    2. Phenytoin: Dilantin, 30, 100 mg caps, and 50 mg chewable tabs; Dilantin suspension, 125 mg/5 mL

      a.   Children: 5mg/kg/day in 2-3 divided doses and increase weekly if needed

      b.   Maintenance dose is usually 4-8 mg/kg/day with a maximum of 300 mg daily

3.   Ethosuximide: Zarontin, 250 mg caps; Zarontin suspension, 250 mg/5mL

      a.   Children: 3-6 years, initially 250 mg/day

      b.   >6 years, initially 500 mg/day

      c.   In both age groups, increase every 4-7 days by 250 mg/daily according to response

      d.   Usual maintenance dose is 20 mg/kg/day in divided doses (Maximum dose is 1.5 mg/day in divided doses)

      e.   Used only for absence seizures

4.   Valproic acid: Depakene 250 mg caps; Depakene syrup, 250 mg/5 mL

      a.   Initially, 15 mg/kg/day in 3 divided doses; increase weekly if needed by 5-10 mg/kg/day

      b.   Maximum daily dose is 60 mg/kg/day in divided doses

5.   Clonazepam: Klonopin, 0.5, 1, 2 mg tabs

      a.   Children: <10 years (or 30 kg); initially, 0.01-0.03 mg/kg/day in 2-3 divided doses

      b.   Increase if needed every 3 days by 0.25-0.5 mg daily

      c.   Maintenance dose is usually 0.1 -0.2 mg/kg/day in 3 equally divided doses

6.   Phenobarbital

      a.   Begin with 15 mg BID

      b.   Maintenance dose is usually 3-5 mg/kg/day given in a single dose

7.   Titrate dosages to achieve adequate blood concentrations

      a.   Because all drugs have central nervous system effects, begin therapy with low doses

      b.   Use therapeutic range in combination with clinical response to determine appropriate dosage

8.   Patients at high risk for recurrent seizures should be treated for two year period

9.   Prior to initiation of any antiepileptic medication, the following laboratory studies should be done: CBC with differential and platelet count, electrolytes, and liver enzymes

10.   Repeat studies during the early weeks of treatment (for example, at one and three months) are also recommended

I.   Patient and parent education is summarized below

1.   Understanding the disorder and the prescribed medications by both the patient and family is of the utmost importance; non-adherence to the medication regime has been identified as the single most common reason for treatment failure

      a.   Teach parent and patient regarding dosing, actions, side effects, and drug interactions of the particular AED that is being prescribed

      b.   For females of childbearing age or who are taking oral contraceptives, emphasize that AEDs are teratogenic and that they also reduce the effectiveness of oral contraceptives

      c.   Patient education must be continuous and must be addressed on every visit

2.   Instruct families regarding the fundamentals of emergency management of seizures

3.   Review the law in your state concerning operating a motor vehicle by persons with seizure disorders

4.   If patient has good control of seizures, minimum restrictions are needed such as swimming with a buddy or wearing a helmet with some sports

5.   Review factors that are sometimes associated with seizures such as stimulants, alcohol, caffeine, inadequate sleep or fever

6.   Discuss the emotional stress that often occurs in family related to social stigma and unpredictability of seizure activity in some patients

7.   Children who are not well-controlled should not be given the pertussis vaccine (As soon as the child is well controlled, he/she should be vaccinated with the acellular pertussis vaccine)

8.   Parents may ask about the ketogenic diet, a diet that mimics the mebatolic effects of fasting that is sometimes used in the treatment of children (and more recently adults) to treat refractory epilepsy; this diet must be supervised by experts and used only in patients with refractory epilepsy

9.   Refer the patient and family to the Epilepsy Foundation of American (EFA), an organization dedicated to countering societal misconceptions and prejudices about epilepsy as well as improving the quality of life for persons affected by seizures

          a.   The national office can be contacted by writing EFA, 4351 Garden City Drive, Landover, MD 20785-2267 or by calling 301/459-3700 or 1-800-EFA-1000

          b.   The Internet Web sites is htt://www.efa.org

          c.   Most states have local affiliates which provide community outreach programs, support groups, information and referral, employment services, respite care for families, and help with living arrangements

J.   Follow Up

    1.   Follow-up visits should be weekly during period of adjusting medication dose, then every 3 months for the next 6 months, and then every six months thereafter

    2.   AEDs may not need to be given for a lifetime

          a.   Factors promoting complete withdrawal from medication include a seizure-free period of 2-4 years, complete seizure control within 1 year of onset, an onset of seizures after age 2 but before age 35, and a normal EEG

          b.   The withdrawal of therapy should be gradual and at a mutually agreed upon time with the patient

          c.   Review state laws regarding operation of a motor vehicle as related to tapering of seizure medication

    3.   In children, the current practice is to discontinue therapy one to two years after the last seizure

    4.   Patients on carbamazepine

          a.   May need to monitor more frequently than recommended under V.H. (above); consult PDR for recommendations

          b.   Leukopenia is the most common hematologic side effect of carbamazepine

    5.   Patients on phenytoin

          a.   Monitor serum drug concentrations 2-4 weeks after any dose increase

          b.   Obtain periodic serum drug concentrations

          c.   Annual CBC, LFTs and platelet

    6.   Patients on long-term phenobarbital: Annual CBC and LFTs

    7.   Patients on long-term ethosuximide: Periodic CBC

    8.   Patients on long-term Valproic acid: Baseline LFTs; repeat every 2-3 months x 2

SLEEP PROBLEMS IN INFANTS AND YOUNG CHILDREN

I.   Definition: Sleep problems are difficulty falling asleep or staying asleep as perceived by the parent; excessive daytime sleepiness (hypersomnolence) and abnormal behaviors associated with sleep (parasomnias) such as night terrors, sleepwalking, bruxism, and enuresis are not considered here

II.   Pathogenesis

    A.   Sleep patterns are carefully controlled by underlying circadian pacemakers

        1.   The task of the newborn is twofold: To organize behavior into specific states--waking, non-rapid eye movement (NREM) sleep and rapid eye movement (REM) sleep--and to organize these states into a 24-hour rhythmic pattern

        2.   Over a period of 24 hours, newborns sleep 16-17 hours; by 16 weeks of age, total sleep time has slowly decreased to 14-15 hours, and by 6-8 months of age, has decreased even further to about 13-14 hours per day

        3.   By 3 weeks of age, sleep is spread out over the 24-hour day in approximately equal segments between feedings

        4.   By about 6 weeks of age, a clear diurnal/nocturnal distribution of wake and sleep emerges in most infants

        5.   By 3 months of age, day/night differentiation is defined in most infants; sleep is largely distributed in the night hours and daytime sleep becomes consolidated into better defined daytime naps; thus waking periods also become longer

6. By 4 months of age, the infant lengthens his/her longest sleeping period; between birth and 4 months, the sleeping stretch usually doubles to about 8 hours
7. By 6 to 9 months of age, most infants have developed pattern of well-consolidated nighttime sleep, a significant milestone in the infant's development of a mature sleeping pattern
8. Between 2 and 5 years of age, REM sleep decreases from between 30-35% of total sleep time to the adult level of 20-25%; the total sleep time decreases for most children during the preschool years from about 14 hours to 12 hours per day
9. From entry to first grade (at age 6 years) to the beginning of adolescence, the total amount of sleep steadily decreases from about 10 hours to 8-9 hours
10. Daytime sleep or napping changes substantially during infancy and early childhood
    a. Infants at 4 months of age take two to three naps each day and about half of 15 month old toddlers take one nap per day, most often in the morning
    b. Most preschoolers continue to nap, with 90% of 3 years olds, over half of 4 year olds, and about one-fourth of 5 year olds taking one nap on most days of the week
    c. Little is know about napping patterns in school-aged children, but napping behavior is believed to be uncommon among this age group

B. Night wakings are an important aspect of infant and toddler development and follow a predictable pattern
   1. Brief awakening from sleep are more frequent during the early months than at older ages in infancy
   2. Most infants awaken for brief periods throughout the night and return to sleep without their parents being aware that wakings have occurred
   3. Infants who put themselves back to sleep without their parents' knowledge are called *self-soothers*; infants who cry to awaken their parents are called *signalers*
   4. *Settling* is defined as sleeping throughout most of the night, with self-soothing behaviors used to return to sleep on one's own
   5. In general, as infants mature, they become increasingly more able to settle into sleep without signaling the parent
   6. Development of the ability to settle by infants is believed to be affected by parenting practices, feeding and soothing styles, as well as by individual characteristics of the infant
   7. Good sleepers are able to soothe themsleves to sleep after waking up, whereas night wakers require the parent's presence to return to sleep

C. Problems with sleep have many causes, but there are five major areas that must be considered
   1. Parental misperceptions regarding age-appropriate sleep patterns in infants and children
   2. Parental behaviors that are well-intended but that promote disrupted sleep in the infant or child
   3. Transient physical discomfort associated with colic, teething, or other minor illness
   4. Serious medical problems causing disturbed sleep via the mechanism of partial or complete airway obstruction during sleep
   5. Family problems such as marital discord or maternal guilt that create or maintain a sleep disturbance for the child

III. Clinical Presentation

A. Sleep occupies a major portion of young children's lives with newborn infants spending almost 70% of the first few weeks in the sleep state

B. Sleep comprises such a significant part of the infant and young child's life that it is assumed to play a critical role in the child's development

C. The complaint of sleep disturbance almost always comes from the parent and not from the child, even when the child is an adolescent

D. Night wakings, prolonged bedtime routines, and other sleep/wake behaviors often concern parents, either because the behaviors themselves are inconvenient and disturb the parents' sleep, or because they may be considered symptomatic of more serious difficulties

E.	On occasion, infants' and young children's sleep is disrupted because of physical problems such as colic, discomfort from teething, or respiratory tract infections; more often, however, there is no physical cause for disrupted sleep

F.	The most common cause of disturbed sleep in infants, toddlers, and preschoolers is parental mismanagement

IV.	Diagnosis/Evaluation

A.	History
1.	Ask parent to give an overview of the problem as a beginning point (the focus should be on exactly what happens most nights and days and under what circumstances)
a.	Parents tend to say the child "never sleeps," so they must be assisted in focusing their account on specifics rather than on generalizations
b.	Keep in mind that parents often like to describe worst-case scenarios, and may have difficulty relating what patterns the infant or child typically follows, saying "There is **not** one"
c.	Focus on the current pattern of sleep; past patterns are important, but the current problem is most relevant
2.	If the child is at least 4 years of age, include him/her as appropriate in the history taking process (for example, determine how he/she views the problem [if it is viewed as a problem])
3.	Ask about evening routines in the family such as what time the evening meal is consumed (in infants, what time the last feeding is provided), what time the child is placed in (or goes to) bed, what sorts of bedtime rituals there are prior to, and after child is placed in (or goes to) bed, how long the child takes to fall asleep, what problems occur with sleep onset and how these are handled by the parent
4.	Ask about the sleep environment, specifically determine **where** the child sleeps and who else sleeps in the room or in the bed with the child; ask about the lighting in the room at night; ask about nighttime noises (are there lullaby tapes, radios, televisions on in the room?)[Note: Unsupervised watching of TV in bed is a common cause for sleep disturbances in school-aged children]
5.	In infants and toddlers, ask about the use of pacifiers, the use and significance of transitional objects such as blankets and stuffed toys; ask if infant/toddler is placed in bed with a bottle and what liquid is in the bottle (water, milk, juice)
6.	Ask about the number of night wakings, the interventions used, and the effectiveness of these interventions
a.	Ascertain the timing and length of wakings
b.	Ask if interventions result in rapid return to sleep or if wakings are extended regardless of the intervention
7.	Ask about morning awakening
a.	What time does it occur?
b.	Is it spontaneous or does the child have to be awakened?
8.	Obtain daytime schedule for weekdays and weekends (which are different for children in daycare or school), with a focus on amount of daytime sleep (how many naps, what time the naps occur, and how long the naps last)
9.	Ask about bedwetting (in children over 3 in whom nighttime dryness has usually been established), walking or talking while asleep, nightmares, teeth grinding, snoring, complaints of nighttime leg discomfort, head banging while in bed
10.	Obtain developmental history and psychosocial history
a.	Ascertain that the child's development is age appropriate; perform a screening test such as the Denver II
b.	Interaction between social problems and sleep problems are well documented
c.	A parent with problems with alcohol, drugs, depression or anxiety creates tension within the family that may be expressed as disordered sleep in the child
d.	Sleep problems in the child may be an early symptom of an emerging psychiatric disturbance, but this is very uncommon
11.	Obtain past medical history, and ask what medications, if any, are presently being taken by the child

B. Physical Examination
   1. The focus of the exam should be to establish normality and to rule out any underlying medical problems (**Note**: Physical findings to explain sleeplessness in an infant and child are rare)
   2. Obtain weight, length (or height for children ≥2 years), head circumference (for children ≤24 months of age), weight for length; plot on the child's growth chart, and compare it with previous recordings to determine if child is following his/her growth curve
   3. Observe the child for any facial abnormalities
   4. Assess the nose and throat to evaluate nasal airflow, tonsillar size
   5. Perform a cardiopulmonary assessment including blood pressure measurement
   6. Perform a neurologic assessment

C. Differential Diagnosis
   1. Underlying behavioral or emotional problem in which disturbed sleep is an associated feature
   2. Medical problem including allergies, large adenoids or tonsils, or birth defects–all of these conditions can cause partial or complete airway obstruction during sleep
   3. Problems between the parents or within the family

D. Diagnostic Testing
   1. None indicated unless underlying medical problem is suspected
   2. If there are suspected respiratory deficits, referral to a pediatric sleep specialist for sleep studies to evaluate the quality of breathing during sleep or referral to an otolaryngologist (if allergies or enlarged adenoids or tonsils are believed to be the problem) is indicated

V. Plan/Management

A. The exact management strategy should be geared to the developmental level of the child and to the particular circumstances of the individual child and family

B. The following tables contain age-specific sleep patterns and parental behaviors that can promote good sleep habits in infants and children

BIRTH TO 4 MONTHS
↦ Parents should understand the usual cycles of sleep/waking in the newborn and early infant period; babies should always be fed when they are hungry and consoled when they cry; parents should anticipate when the baby will become drowsy and prepare for these periods of sleep
↦ When the infant is ready for sleep, some parents prefer to soothe the baby for several minutes, and then put the baby in the crib whether or not he or she is asleep; other parents prefer to always hold the baby until he or she is in a deep sleep, and then put the baby in the crib asleep
↦ Either of the methods described above is acceptable but it is probably best for parents to allow infant to learn to get to sleep in bed rather than in parent's arms so that the infant learns to fall asleep without parent present
↦ Establishment of bedtime routines should be started during this time period–bedtime song or music box, use of a pacifier or blanket for comfort
↦ The goal in this age group is not to impose a rigid sleep schedule but instead to synchronize care giving with the infant's circadian sleep-wake rhythms and to develop an orderly routine that is predictable and helps the infant achieve the developmental task of trust
↦ Parents should expect newborns and infants to awaken every 3-4 hours during the night for feedings (breast fed infants may awaken every 2-3 hours during the neonatal period)
↦ Parents of colicky infants should expect to spend more time holding and soothing the infant than parents of noncolicky infants

INFANTS 4 TO 9 MONTHS OF AGE

- Circadian rhythms continue to mature during this age period, and parents can begin to look more to clock time as an aid to predict nap time, bed time, and morning awakening time
- By 9 months of age, most infants take lengthy naps at 9 AM and 1 PM and then fall asleep at around 7 or 8 PM; babies often wake up for a feeding once or twice each night until 9 months of age
- If there is a night-waking problem during this age period, parents should be advised to stop attending to all but one or two night wakings
  - If infant is overtired, parent can try an earlier bedtime and put their infant in bed either awake or asleep after the established soothing period and bedtime rituals (story, song, pacifier, blanket)
  - If this schedule is maintained, protest crying at bedtime or a night-waking should rapidly (over 3-4 nights) disappear
  - Remind the parent that consistency is the key; intermittent reinforcement by the parent has the effect of increasing crying in the infant

INFANTS 9 TO 15 MONTHS OF AGE

- Children in this age group should have consolidated night sleep with no night waking and one or two naps during the day, at 9 AM and 1 PM; 90% of 9 month olds, 80% of 12 month olds, and 45% of 15 month olds take two naps a day (total duration of naps during the day is 2-3 hours)
- Bed time does not have to be on a rigid schedule; it can be variable, but always early, and based on the child's apparent degree of tiredness, whether naps occurred, and nap duration
- Soothing to sleep rituals should always be regular and predictable in terms of what the parent does to soothe the child to sleep; by this time, bedtime rituals should be firmly in place, with changes in the rituals based on developmental level (for example, reading a story is not as appropriate for a 3 month old as it is for a 15 month old)
- Children in this age group have more persistence, autonomy, and willfulness; sleep problems are likely to be more common and more easily mismanaged by the parent
- Desire for the parent's company may prompt child to cry or call out for the parent; it is important that parents not respond once they have assured themselves that the child is not ill

TODDLERS 15 TO 24 MONTHS OF AGE

- Toddlers in this age group should be taking one nap per day in the early afternoon
- Toddlers who have difficulty transitioning from two to one nap per day should have an earlier bedtime; parents should be told that an earlier bedtime does not mean an earlier wake-up time
- Consistency in bedtime rituals at sleep times and reasonable regularity when the child is tired help to establish structured sleep habits
- Toddlers who get out of crib or bed should be firmly and silently placed back in the bed to teach the child that this behavior is not acceptable
- Silence and an unemotional attitude reduce the social rewards that reinforce night waking
- Parents should understand that they cannot force the child to sleep but that they can insist that the child remain in his/her crib or bed

CHILDREN 2 TO 3 YEARS OF AGE

- ↦ Between ages two and three years of age, children sleep an average of 14 hours a day
- ↦ Virtually all children are napping at 2 (most often around lunch time for 2-3 hours) but about 10% have discontinued napping by age 3
- ↦ Children in this age group resist going to sleep even when going-to-sleep rituals have been firmly established
- ↦ To provide the toddler with feelings of control (and thereby promote his feelings of autonomy), encourage parents to let him make as many choices as possible at bedtime–let him select which book to read, which stuffed toy to take to bed, etc.; make certain the night light is on as this promotes feelings of security
  - ◆ If the child cries when the parent leaves the room, the parent should wait 10 minutes, then return to settle him down again
  - ◆ Parent should be advised not to reinforce this behavior by giving child food or their company. If the child cries again, wait 10 minutes to give him the opportunity to settle down, then repeat the process
  - ◆ The child should not be scolded or punished, but firmly settled down and left alone to get to sleep
- ↦ By age 3, sleep rules can be instituted to help motivate the child in good sleep hygiene; a poster can be made with the sleep rules and placed in the child's room
  - ◆ The sleep rules are simple ones that a 3 year old can understand and can consist of the following: "At sleep time, we stay in bed, we close our eyes, and we rest"
  - ◆ Parents can recite these rules with child at nap time and at bed time
  - ◆ The child is rewarded for following the rules (the reward needs to be highly motivational and should not involve food)
  - ◆ Children younger than 3 who do not understand sleep rules should be silently and unemotionally returned to bed
- ↦ Children in this age group are often very demanding and parents find themselves spending more and more time in bedtime routines and soothing behaviors; to limit this, parents can place a timer (with a very soft bell or pleasing musical sound) on the night stand set to go off after a reasonable period
- ↦ **A word about nightmares**: When nightmares awaken the toddler, it is important that the parent comfort the child by holding him, asking him to tell you about the dream (a 3 year old may be able to do this), and stay with him until he is calm enough to fall asleep

CHILDREN 4 TO 5 YEARS OF AGE

- ↦ During this age period, the total sleep time decreases for most children from about 14 hours a day to 11 to 12 hours per day
- ↦ By the end of this period, most children have a single consolidated nighttime sleep period with no napping during the day
- ↦ Preschoolers often resist going to bed, especially when there are older sibling in the family who stay up later
- ↦ Reading the preschooler a story is the best way to prepare her for sleep; avoid letting her roughhouse right before bedtime as the calmer the activity before bedtime, the more prepared she will be for sleep
- ↦ Once story time is over, the parent should say goodnight and should not remain in the room until the child falls asleep
- ↦ For the 5 year old (or the mature 4 year old) books about sleep and dreams may be helpful; classic children's books on these topics are listed in the table that follows
- ↦ For children in this age group who awaken during the night and the parent is certain that the child is not having a nightmare, advise the parent to give the child 10 minutes to settle back to sleep on her own; after that time, go to the child, reassure her, and leave. Parents should avoid rewarding this behavior with food or with taking the child to the parents' bed for the rest of the night

CHILDREN'S BOOKS ABOUT DREAMS AND SLEEP

In the Night Kitchen by Maurice Sendak
Bedtime for Frances by Russell Hoban
There's a Nightmare in My Closet by Mercer Mayer
Ben's Dreams by Chris van Allsberg

C. Consider referral to a pediatric sleep specialist if the problem is chronic and severe, or if the problem has seriously disrupted the family and there is lack of agreement between the parents regarding how to deal with the problem

D. Follow Up: Telephone follow up once a week or so for a month can be very helpful to parents who are dealing with sleep problems in their child; visits should be scheduled on an as-needed basis

VERTIGO

I. Definition: Sensation of abnormal movements of the body or surroundings

II. Pathogenesis

A. Usually a disturbance of the peripheral or central vestibular system which assists in the maintenance of spatial orientation and posture

B. **Peripheral origin**: Dysfunction of structures peripheral to the brain stem
    1. Vestibular neuritis: May be of viral origin; affects the vestibular nerve
    2. Labyrinthitis: Presumed to be of viral origin with bacterial labyrinthitis extremely rare; may also occur secondary to trauma
    3. Meniere's disease: Unknown cause, but dilation of the endolymphatic systems of middle ear occurs
    4. Benign paroxysmal positional vertigo: Believed to result from calcium carbonate crystal deposition in inner ear
    5. Drug induced vertigo: Related to vestibulotoxic drugs such as furosemide, NSAIDs (especially indomethacin), cytotoxic agents, anticonvulsant (phenytoin, carbamazepine, and ethosuximide), and aminoglycosides

C. **Central origin**: Involves disease processes affecting brain stem or cerebellum
    1. Acoustic schwannomas or meningiomas: Tumor affecting cranial nerve VIII
    2. Cerebellar pontine angle tumors: Tumors affecting cranial nerves V, VII, IX, and XII
    3. Cerebellar infarction
    4. Cerebellar hemorrhage
    5. Vertebrobasilar insufficiency

III. Clinical Presentation of disorders based on origin--peripheral or central

A. Vertigo occurs much less often in the adolescent than does nonspecific dizziness, lightheadedness, or syncope

B. Clinical presentation of vertigo disorders is summarized in the table that follows

CLINICAL PRESENTATION OF VERTIGO DISORDERS	
Type of Vertigo	**Typical Presentation**
Peripheral Vertigo	
Vestibular neuritis	Acute onset of intense vertigo with associated nausea and vomiting Head positioning worsens the symptoms; may be preceded by URI Usually results from viral, bacterial infection or from trauma No hearing loss Vertigo may last for days or weeks
Labyrinthitis	Vertigo with associated hearing loss May occur (rarely) secondary to bacterial infection such as otitis media, mastoiditis May also occur secondary to trauma
Benign paroxysmal positional vertigo	Characterized by spinning sensation Occurs when patient moves head or body quickly No associated hearing loss, tinnitus, or nausea/vomiting Cause is unknown in most patients
Drug induced vertigo	Acute onset related to medication use Nausea and vomiting are common Transient or permanent hearing loss can occur

(continued)

636

CLINICAL PRESENTATION OF VERTIGO DISORDERS (CONTINUED)	
Type of Vertigo	**Typical Presentation**
Motion sickness	Occurs when riding in car, on boat or train
Central Vertigo Acoustic schwannomas	Tumors have highest incidence in 5th decade of life Gradual onset of vertigo preceded by hearing loss
Cerebellar pontine angle tumors	Vertigo, hearing loss, and nystagmus Onset of symptoms is gradual
Cerebellar infarction	Sudden onset of vertigo Cranial nerve deficits are present as well as cerebellar signs
Cerebellar hemorrhage	Vertigo and an occipital headache Gaze is affected; patient cannot look toward side of lesion Other cranial nerves (in addition to the sixth) are often affected
Vertebrobasilar insufficiency	Disruption of both cranial nerve and cerebellar function Vertigo may occur

IV. Diagnosis/Evaluation

    A. History
1. Ask patient to describe in a few words the sensation he/she experiences
   a. Vertigo always has a sensation of motion that things are spinning around the patient or that the patient is spinning around the environment
   b. Lightheadedness or feeling that one is about to faint is referred to as syncope or near syncope (see section on SYNCOPE/NEAR SYNCOPE)
   c. Disequilibrium or a sensation of feeling drunk, unsteady on one's feet, or imbalance suggests a syndrome of multiple sensory deficits, vertebrobasilar insufficiency, anxiety, or motor gait disorders
2. Ask about symptom patterns
3. If possible obtain a description of the episode and events preceding the vertigo from a witness
4. Inquire about past medical history including past episodes of vertigo, recent respiratory, gastrointestinal, or ear infections, trauma, risk factors for cardiovascular disease such as smoking, diabetes, hyperlipidemia
5. Obtain a complete medication history with a focus on medications known to produce vertigo

    B. Physical Examination
1. Measure blood pressure in both arms (to assess for subclavian steal syndrome); assess for orthostatic hypotension (see section on SYNCOPE for measurement procedure)
2. Complete ear examination
   a. Observe TM for loss of landmarks, erythema, or cholesteatoma
   b. Perform hearing, Rinne and Weber tests
3. Nystagmus is objective marker for new onset vertigo
   a. Look for spontaneous nystagmus in 5 positions of gaze
   b. Reproduce nystagmus with Bárány maneuver. (Sitting, turn head to right and quickly lower to supine position with head over edge 30° below horizontal level and observe for nystagmus. Repeat on other side) [see Figure 18.1]

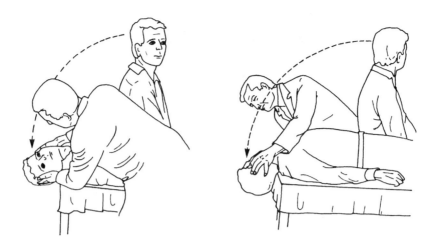

Figure 18.1. Nylen-Bárány Maneuver.

Source: Reilly, B.M. (1991). <u>Practical strategies in outpatient medicine</u>. Philadelphia: Saunders, p. 204. Reprinted by permission.

    4.   Auscultate neck for carotid bruits
    5.   Perform a complete cardiovascular exam
    6.   Do a careful neurological examination to determine if the condition is central or peripheral in origin
        a.   Test cranial nerves for deficits **(Note**: Any cranial nerve abnormality suggests a central process)
        b.   Test cerebellar function and the Romberg test
        c.   Perform funduscopic exam
        d.   Check tendon reflexes for loss, asymmetry, hyperreflexia
        e.   Evaluate for sensory abnormalities
    7.   Symptom reproduction with hyperventilation may also be helpful

  C.   Differential Diagnosis
    1.   Includes all conditions listed under pathogenesis as well as syncope, multiple sensory defects, and various neurologic disorders
    2.   The major challenge is differentiating peripheral and central vertigo; clinical features of both types are compared in the following table

DIFFERENTIATING PERIPHERAL AND CENTRAL VERTIGO		
Characteristics	**Peripheral Vertigo**	**Central Vertigo**
Onset	Abrupt	Insidious
Intensity	Moderate to severe	Mild to moderate (seldom severe)
Nausea & Vomiting	Common	Not common
Positionally related	Usually	Not usually
Hearing loss	Common	Not common
Focal neurologic deficits	No	Yes
Nystagmus	Fatigable and inhibited by ocular fixation	Nonfatigable Not inhibited by ocular fixation

D.   Diagnostic Tests
1.   Cerebral imaging is required for patients with central vertigo to rule out tumor, hemorrhage, or infarction; MRI is usually the test of choice
2.   For patients in whom a peripheral etiology is suspected, the following testing may be considered
a.   Audiometry may be ordered and is abnormal with Meniere's disease and acoustic neuroma
b.   Special vestibular function tests may be ordered
(1)   Caloric stimulation
(2)   Electronystagmography

V.   Plan/Management

A.   Patients with central vertigo require immediate referral to a neurologist/neurosurgeon for management

B.   Patients with peripheral vertigo usually benefit from hydration, symptomatic therapy with antivertiginous and antiemetic drugs, and vestibular exercises
1.   Patients need counseling and reassurance that their symptoms are benign but may be protracted
2.   Counsel patients on proper hydration by providing very explicit instructions regarding fluid intake
3.   Use of medications should be limited to the acute phase
4.   Vestibular exercises offer the best approach to recovery and should be instituted as soon as possible

C.   Antivertiginous drugs, through a number of mechanisms, decrease the imbalance resulting from a vestibular disorder; prescribe one of the following:
1.   Meclizine (Antivert) 12.5-25 PO QD or QID with dosage tapered as symptoms improve (adolescents only)
2.   Dimenhydrinate (Dramamine)
a.   Children <12: 12.5-25 mg PO Q 8 hours
b.   Children >12: 50 mg PO Q 4-6 hours
3.   Scopolamine transdermal disc (Transderm-Scop) 1 disc applied behind ear, leave in place for 3 days (adolescents only)

D.   Antiemetic drugs suppress the brain emetic centers or input to these centers, including signals from the vestibular nuclei; prescribe one of the following if nausea and vomiting are a problem; can be combined with an antivertiginous medication
1.   Prochlorperazine (Compazine)
a.   Children <12: Dose by weight (see PDR)
b.   Children >12: 5-10 mg PO Q 6 hours as needed
2.   Promethazine (Phenergan)
a.   Children <12: 12.5 mg PO Q12 hours
b.   Children >12: 25 mg PO Q 6 hours; also available in suppository form: 50 mg Q 12 hours as needed

E.   Vestibular exercises are designed to speed the compensation for interruptions in vestibular input
1.   Should be begun as soon as possible after the acute stage of nausea and vomiting has resolved
2.   Many of the exercises result in dizziness, a sensation that is a necessary stimulus for developing compensatory mechanisms
3.   The exercises should be done under the supervision of a trained therapist
4.   Compensation development often requires 2 to 6 months

F.   Follow Up: Symptoms that fail to improve with pharmacologic therapy and vestibular exercises should be reevaluated in 2-4 weeks; patients who develop worsening symptoms should return immediately for further evaluation

REFERENCES

American Academy of Pediatrics. Caring from your baby and young child: Birth to age 5. New York: Bantam Books.

American Academy of Pediatrics, Provisional Committee on Quality Improvement, Subcommittee on Febrile Seizures. (1996). Practice parameter: The neurodiagnostic evaluation of the child with a first simple febrile seizure. Pediatrics, 97(5), 769-771.

American Psychiatric Association. (1994). Diagnostic and statistical manual of mental disorders, (4th ed.). Washington, DC: Author.

Commission on Classification and Terminology of the International League Against Epilepsy. (1981). Proposal for revised clinical and electroencephalographic classification of epileptic seizures. Epilepsia, 22, 480-490.

Curry, W.J., & Kulling, D.I. (1998). Newer antiepileptic drugs: Gabapentin, lamotrigine, felbamate, topiramte and fosphenytoin. American Family Physician, 57, 513-520.

Davis, W.M. (1997, November). Advances in the pathophysiology and pharmacotherapy of epilepsy. Drug Topics, 110-117.

Diamond, S., & Diamond, M.L. (1997). Emergency treatment of migraine: Insights into current options. Postgraduate Medicine, 101, 169-179.

Ferber, R. (1966). Clinical assessment of child and adolescent sleep disorders. Child and Adolescent Psychiatric Clinics of North America, 5(3), 569-578.

Fettes, I. (1997). Menstrual migraine: Methods of prevention and control. Postgraduate Medicine, 101, 67-75.

France, K.G., Henderson, J.M.T., & Hudson, S.M. (1996). Fact, act, and tact: A three-stage approach to treating the sleep problems of infants and young children. Child and Adolescent Psychiatric Clinics of North America, 5(3), 581-599.

Freeman, J.M., & Vinning, E.P. (1995). Febrile seizures: A decision-making analysis. American Family Physician, 52, 1401-1406.

Hamalainen, M.L., et al. (1997). Ibuprofen or acetaminophen for the acute treatment of migraine in children. Neurology, 46, 103-107.

Headache Classification Committee of the International Headache Society. (1988). Classification and diagnostic criteria for headache disorders, cranial neuralgias and facial pain. Cephalalgia, 8 (Suppl. 7), 1-96.

Leston, J.A. (1996). Migraine and tension-type headache are not separate disorders. Cephalagia, 16 (4), 220-222.

Marks, W.J., & Garcia. (1998). Management of seizures and epilepsy. American Family Physician, 57, 1589-1600.

Merikangas, K., et al. (1997). Association between migraine and stroke in a large-scale epidemiological study of the United States. Archives of Neurology, 54, 362-368.

Mindell, J.A. (1996). Treatment of child and adolescent sleep disorders. Child and Adolescent Psychiatric Clinics of North America, 5(3), 571-751.

Moore, K.L. (1997). Drug treatment of migraine: Part I. Acute therapy and drug-rebound headache. American Family Physician, 56, 2039-2048.

Noble, S.L. & Moore, K.L. (1997) Drug treatment of migraine: Part II. Preventive therapy. American Family Physician, 56, 2279-2287.

O'Hara, J. & Koch, T.K. (1998). Heading off headaches. Contemporary Pediatrics, 15, 97-116.

Plantz, S.H., & Adler, J.N. (1998). Emergency medicine. Baltimore: Williams & Wilkins.***Chapter Name?

Reilly, B.M. (1991). Practical strategies in outpatient medicine. Philadelphia: Saunders.***Chapter Name?

Roddy, S.M., & McBride, M.C. (1997). Seizure disorders. In R.A. Hoekelman (Ed.). Primary pediatric care. St. Louis: Mosby.

Rothner, A.D. (1999). Headaches. In R.A. Dershewitz (Ed.). Ambulatory pediatric care (3rd ed.). Philadelphia: Lippincott-Raven.

Weissbluth, M. (1999). Sleep disturbances in young children. In R.A. Dershewitz (Ed.). Ambulatory pediatric care. Philadelphia: Lippincott.

Wells, B.G. (Ed.). (1998). Headache: Migraine and cluster. In B.G. Wells, J.T. DiPiro, T.L. Schwinghammer, & C.W. Hamilton (Eds.). Pharmacotherapy Handbook. Stamford, Connecticut: Appleton & Lange.

Wells, B.G. (1998). Epilepsy. In B.G. Wells, J.T. DiPiro, T.L. Schwinghammer, & C.W. Hamiliton (Eds.). Pharmacotherapy handbook. Stamford, CT: Appleton & Lange.

Winner, P.K. (1997). Headaches in children: When is a complete diagnostic workup indicated? Postgraduate Medicine, 101 (5), 81-90.

Wolfson, A.R. (1996). Sleeping patterns of children and adolescents: Developmental trends, disruptions, and adaptations. Child and Adolescent Psychiatric Clinics of North America, 5(3), 549-566.

CHAPTER 19

Hematologic Problems

Iron Deficiency Anemia

Table: *Maximum Hemoglobin Concentration and Hematocrit Values for Anemia*

IRON DEFICIENCY ANEMIA

I. Definition: Anemia characterized by small (microcytic), pale (hypochromic), red blood cells (RBCs), and depletion of iron (Fe) stores

II. Pathogenesis

    A. Iron loss exceeds intake so that storage iron (as measured by serum ferritin concentration) is progressively depleted

    B. As storage iron is depleted, a compensatory increase in absorption of dietary Fe and in the concentration of transport iron (as measured by transferrin saturation) occurs

    C. Iron stores are no longer able to meet the needs of the erythroid marrow; the plasma-transferrin level increases, the serum Fe concentration declines, resulting in a decrease in Fe available for RBC formation

    D. The shortage of iron leads to underproduction of iron-containing functional compounds, including hemoglobin

    E. The RBCs of persons who have iron-deficiency anemia (IDA) are microcytic and hypochromic

    F. In early childhood and adolescence, poor dietary intake and increased demand are the most common causes

III. Clinical Presentation

    A. Iron deficiency anemia is the most common hematologic disease of infancy and childhood and usually results from inadequate intake of dietary iron; increased demands related to periods of rapid growth (as occurs in infancy and adolescence) can also cause anemia
        1. A rapid rate of growth together with dietary intake that is frequently inadequate in dietary iron places children less than 24 months (especially those between 9-18 months of age) at the highest risk of any age group for iron deficiency
        2. After 24 months of age, with the slowing of growth and increased diversification of diet, the risk for iron deficiency declines
        3. In children ≥36 months of age, dietary iron and iron status are usually adequate; risk for iron deficiency among children in this age group includes low family income, a low iron or other specialized diet, and medical conditions that affect iron status (inflammatory or bleeding disorders)
        4. During adolescence (defined here as ages 12 to <18 years of age), iron requirements and thus the risk for iron deficiency increase because of rapid growth
            a. Among males, the risk essentially ends after the peak pubertal growth period
            b. Among females, menstruation increases the risk for iron deficiency thoughout the childbearing years
                (1) Use of an intrauterine device is also a risk factor
                (2) Use of oral contraceptives is associated with a ***decreased*** risk for iron deficiency

    B. Iron stores of full-term infants can meet infants' iron requirements until ages 4-6 months, and iron deficiency anemia usually does not develop until about 9 months of age

    C. Preterm and low-birth weight infants are at greater risk for IDA than are full-term and appropriate weight infants

    D. Iron bioavailability depends on dietary composition
        1. Heme iron, found only in meat, poultry, and fish is 2-3 times more absorbable than non-heme iron which is found in plants and iron-fortified foods

2. The bioavailability of non-heme iron is affected by the kind of other foods ingested at the same meal
3. Enhancers of iron absorption are vitamin C and heme iron
4. Inhibitors of iron absorption include polyphenols (found in some vegetables), tannins (in tea), phytates (in bran), and calcium (in dairy products)

E. An infant's diet is a predictor of iron status in late infancy and early childhood
   1. Approximately 30% of infants fed only non-iron fortified formula or whole cow's milk and about 20% of breast-fed infants are at risk for iron deficiency by ages 9-12 months
   2. Infants fed mainly iron-fortified formula are not likely to have iron deficiency at age 9 months
   3. Among exclusively breast-fed infants, intake of iron-fortified cereal (beginning at 6 months of age) protects against iron deficiency
   4. Early introduction (prior to one year of age) of whole cow's milk and consumption of greater than 24 ounces/day of whole cow's milk after age one year are risk factors of iron deficiency for two reasons:
      a. First, whole cow's milk has little iron and may replace foods with higher iron content
      b. Second, whole cow's milk may cause occult gastrointestinal bleeding

F. Iron deficiency represents a spectrum ranging from iron depletion which causes alterations in physiologic function, to iron-deficiency anemia which affects the functioning of several body systems

G. Prevalence of IDA is higher among children living at or below the poverty level and among Black and Mexican-American children

H. Long-term residency at high altitude ($\geq$3,000 feet), and cigarette smoking cause a generalized upward shift in Hb concentration and Hct

I. Iron deficiency anemia also contributes to lead poisoning in children by increasing the gastrointestinal tract's ability to absorb heavy metals such as lead

J. Iron deficiency anemia is usually slow in onset, allowing for compensatory mechanisms to develop so that symptoms may be minimal until significant anemia develops

K. Clinical presentation depends on severity, age, and ability of the cardiovascular and pulmonary systems to compensate for decreasing oxygen carrying capacity of the blood

L. There are few symptoms when hematocrit (Hct) is 30 or above in otherwise healthy individuals and anemia is frequently discovered during routine health maintenance visits; as Hct falls, dyspnea and mild fatigue with exercise may occur

M. Nonspecific complaints of headache, poor concentration, palpitations, anorexia can also occur

N. In infants and young children, irritability and anorexia may be observed or the child may be entirely asymptomatic

O. Signs of anemia include pallor, best seen in the conjunctiva

P. In very severe anemia, atrophic glossitis, cheilitis, and koilonychia may appear

Q. Cut off values for the diagnosis of iron deficiency anemia for each age group are contained under section V.B.

R. Laboratory indices that reflect an iron-deficient state are listed here
   1. A low mean red cell volume
   2. A reduced serum ferritin level
   3. A reduced serum iron level
   4. An increased serum iron-binding capacity
   5. An increase in hemoglobin concentration after the institution of iron therapy

S. The earliest laboratory change associated with iron-deficiency anemia is decreased serum ferritin; the absence of storage iron, as defined as a serum ferritin level below 20 μg per liter in an anemic patient is **conclusive evidence** of iron deficiency anemia

T. In mild forms of iron-deficiency anemia, the laboratory values of iron-deficiency and iron-sufficiency may overlap considerably, thus presenting a diagnostic challenge

IV. Diagnosis/Evaluation

A. History
1. Inquire about onset and duration of symptoms
2. In infants, determine if premature, and obtain data related to feeding, including type, (if formula fed, specifically ask if iron-fortified formula is being fed to infant), amount, and frequency; ask if whole cow's milk is being given to infant [can cause gastrointestinal blood loss]
3. In infants and children, obtain dietary history with focus on types and amounts of iron enriched food consumed
4. In adolescents, ask if there has recently been an unintended weight loss
5. In both children and adolescents, obtain a careful history of gastrointestinal complaints that might suggest gastritis, peptic ulcer disease, or other conditions that might produce gastrointestinal bleeding
6. Ask if there has been change in stool patterns or color and if there are hemorrhoids present (**Note**: Black tarry stools usually indicate an upper GI source of bleeding, while stool streaked with red blood is more often associated with colorectal bleeding [or bleeding from hemorrhoids])
7. In menstruating females, ask about blood loss during menses
8. Ask about dietary intake of iron rich foods and pica
9. Obtain medication history, particularly use of aspirin and other NSAIDs; ask about past history of GI bleeding

B. Physical Examination
1. In infants and children, obtain height and weight, plot on growth chart, and compare with previous parameters
2. In adolescents, obtain weight and compare with previous weight
3. Observe for pallor, particularly the conjunctiva
4. Examine tongue, corners of mouth, and nails for characteristic changes
5. Perform abdominal exam for tenderness on palpation and enlargement of the spleen
6. Auscultate heart for systolic flow murmurs
7. Obtain stool for occult blood if history suggests that blood loss from the GI tract is a possibility

C. Differential Diagnosis
1. Inadequate intake of iron
2. Any condition that causes acute or chronic blood loss
3. Hemolytic diseases such as sickle cell

D. Diagnostic tests to detect anemia and assess iron status
1. The test used to detect iron deficiency anemia in infants and children is the measurement of either hemoglobin or hematocrit
   a. **Hemoglobin**: Concentration of the iron-containing protein Hb in circulating red blood cells and a more direct and sensitive measure than Hct
   b. **Hematocrit**: Proportion of whole blood occupied by the red blood cells; it falls only after the Hb concentration
2. If the H & H meet the criteria for the diagnosis of anemia as outlined in the table MAXIMUM HEMOGLOBIN CONCENTRATION AND HEMATOCRIT VALUES FOR ANEMIA under V. below, the next step recommended by the Centers for Disease Control and Prevention (CDC) in their *Recommendations to Prevent and Control Iron Deficiency in the United States* [1998] is to repeat the hemoglobin concentration or hematocrit test; if the tests agree and the child is not ill, a presumptive diagnosis or IDA can be made and treatment begun

3. If a more definitive diagnosis is desired prior to the initiation of treatment, perform a complete blood count (CBC), which includes red blood cell indices, and a reticulocyte count

 a. **Mean cell volume (MCV)**: Average volume of red blood cells, measured in femtoliters using an electronic counter. MCV is highest at birth, decreases during the first 6 months of life, then gradually increases during childhood to adult levels; a low MCV indicates microcytic anemia (Lead poisoning, anemias of infection, chronic disease, and thalassemia minor can also cause a reduction in MCV)

 b. **Red blood cell distribution width (RDW)**: Indication of variation in cell size. IDA usually causes greater variation in red blood cell size than do conditions such as thalassemia minor

4. Finally, further evaluation of anemia is indicted **if the child does not respond to iron treatment despite compliance with the iron supplementation regimen**

 a. **Serum ferritin concentration**: Nearly all ferritin in the body is intracellular, but a small amount circulates in the plasma. A direct relationship exists between serum ferritin concentration and the amount of iron stored in the body (1 μL of serum ferritin concentration is equivalent to approximately 10 mg of stored iron). Serum ferritin concentration is an early indicator of the status of iron stores and is the **most specific indicator** available of depleted iron stores

 b. **Erythrocyte protoporphyrin concentration**: The concentration of erythrocyte protoporphyrin in blood increases when insufficient iron is available for hemoglobin production; infection, inflammation, and lead poisoning can also elevate erythrocyte protoporphyrin concentration

 c. **Transferrin saturation**: An indicator of the extent to which transferrin has vacant iron-binding sites (**low** transferrin saturation indicates a **high** proportion of vacant iron-binding sites)

  (1) Saturation is highest in neonates, declines by age 4 months, and then increases throughout childhood until adulthood

  (2) Transferrin saturation is based on two laboratory measures–serum iron concentration and total iron-binding capacity (TIBC)

  (3) Transferrin saturation is calculated dy dividing serum iron concentration by TIBC and multiplying by 100 to express the result as a percentage

  (4) Transferrin saturation (%) = [serum iron concentration (μg/dL)/TIBC (μg/dL)] x 100

 d. **Serum iron concentration**: Measures the total amount of iron in the serum (concentration increases after each meal, rises in the AM and falls at night, and decreases with infections and inflammations); more variation of this measure than with Hb and Hct

 e. **Total iron binding capacity (TIBC)**: Measures the iron-binding capacity within the serum and reflects the availability of iron-binding sites on transferrin; TIBC increases when serum iron concentration and stored iron is low and decreases when serum iron concentration and stored iron is high. **Note:** factors other than iron status that can affect this measure are inflammation and chronic infection (result in lower TIBC); oral contraceptives and pregancy can elevate this measure; however, a more stable measure than serum iron concentration. Changes in TIBC occur after iron stores are depleted

V. Plan/Treatment

 A. Check a positive anemia screening result by performing a repeat Hb or Hct test; if the tests agree and child is not ill, a presumptive diagnosis of IDA can be made and treatment can be begun

B. See the following table for diagnosing anemia based on hemoglobin and hematocrit levels for children in various age groups

MAXIMUM HEMOGLOBIN CONCENTRATION AND HEMATOCRIT VALUES FOR ANEMIA			
Gender	Age, y	Hemoglobin, g/dL	Hematocrit, %
Both Genders	1-<2	11.0	32.9
	2-<5	11.1	33.0
	5-<8	11.5	34.5
	8-<12	11.9	35.4
Females	12-<15	11.8	35.7
	15-<18	12.0	35.9
	≥18	12.0	35.7
Males	12-<15	12.5	37.3
	15-<18	13.3	39.7
	≥18	13.5	39.9

NOTE: The values listed for children ages 1-<2 years can be used for infants aged 6-12 months.

Source: Centers for Disease Control and Prevention. (1998). Recommendations to prevent and control iron deficiency in the United States. MMWR, 47, (RR-3), p. 12

C. A therapeutic trial of oral iron therapy is justified for infants and children who are determined to be anemic based on the values listed above

D. Treat presumptive iron deficiency anemia with 3 mg/kg/day of elemental iron
   1. Products available include Nu-Iron Elixir which contains 100 mg of elemental iron per 5 mL (and may be dosed once daily) and Feosol Elixir which contains 44 mg of elemental iron per 5 mL and is divided into 3 doses/day
   2. Advise parent regarding the following
      a. Give iron between meals for better absorption and place medication in back of mouth to reduce staining of teeth (in infants and small children)
      b. Toddlers and older children can be given iron with vitamin C containing juice which boosts absorption

E. Treatment requires change in diet to provide adequate iron as well as administration of iron replacement
   1. All infants must be on iron-fortified formula or breast-milk; whole cow's milk is not appropriate for children <12 months of age
   2. Counsel parent regarding iron rich foods that are age-appropriate (e.g., fortified infant cereals for infants; iron-fortified bran for toddlers/children, dried fruit for older children, red meat, beans, and so on)
   3. Beverages consumed with meals have a dramatic effect on iron absorption from food
      a. Orange juice with meals doubles the absorption of iron from the meal
      b. Tea or milk with meals can reduce absorption to less than one-half
      c. Milk and tea should be consumed in moderation between meals
   4. Refer to nutritionist or Special Supplemental Food Program for Women, Infants, and Children (WIC) for counseling, if available

F. In adolescents, iron deficiency anemia is treated with 200 mg of elemental iron per day
   1. Products available include Nu-Iron 150 capsules which contain 150 mg of elemental iron and may be dosed once daily OR
   2. Feosol tablets which contain 65 mg of elemental iron and is given TID

G. Follow Up
    1. In 4 weeks for repeat examination and hemoglobin or hematocrit testing
        a. A hemoglobin response of ≥1 g/dL or Hct ≥3% over a 4-week period confirms the diagnosis of IDA
        b. Restoration of iron stores is the goal of iron replacement therapy; the time required to accomplish this goal varies from patient to patient; in general, approximately 3 months of therapy is necessary
        c. Recheck Hb or Hct after 2 more months; then reassess again about 6 months after treatment is completed
    2. A reticulocytosis occurs within 7-10 days after initiation of iron therapy, but a reticulocyte count is not usually ordered unless there are concerns about the diagnosis; if the patient does not develop reticulocytosis, the diagnosis should be reevaluated
    3. Common causes of treatment failure include noncompliance with therapy, misdiagnosis, and malabsorption
    4. The therapeutic trial should not be continued beyond 1 month if the hemoglobin concentration has not increased appropriately and the patient has been compliant with the treatment regimen; further evaluation is indicated (see IV.D.)

H. Primary prevention of iron deficiency among infants and children is contained in the table that follows

---

PRIMARY PREVENTION OF IRON DEFICIENCY AMONG INFANTS AND CHILDREN

❖ Encourage breastfeeding of all infants for the first 12 months of life

❖ Encourage exclusive breastfeeding (without supplementary liquid, formula, or food) for the first 6 months of life

❖ When exclusive breastfeeding is discontinued, encourage use of an additional source of iron (approximately 1 mg/kg/day or iron) from supplementary foods such as iron fortified infant cereal (Two or more servings per day of iron-fortified infant cereal can meet an infants' requirements for iron)

❖ For breastfed infants who were preterm or had a low birthweight, recommend 2/4 mg/kg/day of iron drops (to a maximum of 15 mg/day) starting at 1 month after birth and continuing until 12 months after birth

❖ Suggest that children aged 1-5 years consume no more than 24 ounces of cow's milk, goat's milk, or soy milk each day

❖ At age 6 months of age, when the extrusion reflex diasppears, recommend that infants be introduced to plain, iron-fortified infant cereal

❖ By approximately age 6 months, encourage one feeding per day of foods rich in vitamin C to improve iron absorption, preferably with meals

❖ Suggest introducing plain, pureed meats after 6 months of age (when the infant is developmentally ready to consume such foods)

REFERENCES

Barkin, J.S., Green, R., Johnson, B., & Krantz, S. (1998, March). A practical workup for the patient with anemia. Patient Care, 70-90.

Borman, R.J., & McGuire, S.M. (1997). In R.B. Taylor (Ed.), Manual of family practice. Boston: Little, Brown.

Centers of Disease Control and Prevention. (1998). Recommendations to prevent and control iron deficiency in the United States. MMWR, 47, RR-3, 1-36.

Hamilton, C.W. (1998). Hematologic disorders. In B.G. Wells, J.T. DiPiro, T.L. Schwinghammer, & C.W. Hamilton (Eds.), Pharmacotherapy handbook. Stamford, CT: Appleton & Lange.

Oski, F.A. (1993). Iron deficiency in infancy and childhood. The New England Journal of Medicine, 329(3), 190-193.

Platt, O.S. (1999). Anemia. In R.A. Dershewitz (Ed.), <u>Ambulatory pediatric care</u>. Philadelphia: Lippincott.

Shine, J.W. (1997). Microcytic anemia. <u>American Family Physician, 55</u>, 2455-2462.

Spruill, W.J., & Wade, W.E. (1997). Anemia. In J.T. DiPiro, R.L. Talbert, G.C. Yee, G.R. Matzke, B.G. Wells, & L. M. Posey (Eds.), <u>Pharmacotherapy: A pathophysiologic approach</u>. Stamford, CT: Appleton & Lange.

US Department of Health and Human Services. (1994). <u>Clinician's handbook of preventive services: Put prevention into practice</u>. Washington, DC: Author.

US Preventive Services Task Force. (1996). <u>Guide to clinical preventive services</u>. Baltimore: Williams & Wilkins.

Emergencies

AVULSED TOOTH

I. Definition: A total displacement of a tooth out of its socket

II. Pathogenesis

   A. Trauma to mouth resulting in displacement of tooth

   B. Teeth not fully erupted have loosely structured periodontal ligaments; thus these are the teeth most likely to be displaced when trauma to mouth occurs

III. Clinical Presentation

   A. An upper central incisor is the most frequently avulsed tooth

   B. Children are more likely to have avulsed teeth, but avulsion can also occur in adults

IV. Diagnosis/Evaluation

   A. Determine if the avulsed tooth is a primary or a secondary tooth; primary teeth should not be reimplanted because they often ankylose or fuse to the bone

   B. Defer history and physical since immediate reimplantation of the tooth is necessary to maintain vitality of the tooth (each minute the tooth remains out if its socket greatly reduces the likelihood that implantation will be successful)

   C. Go immediately to treatment

V. Plan/Treatment

   A. The avulsed tooth should be replanted immediately if possible
      1. If the tooth was displaced from the mouth and has collected debris from the ground or floor, rinse gently with sterile water holding the tooth by the crown. (DO NOT TOUCH ROOT SURFACE)
      2. Holding the tooth by the crown, gently tease it back onto the socket and cover with gauze; instruct patient to gently bite down on gauze during transport to dentist office
      3. If the avulsed tooth cannot be placed into socket for transport, store tooth in physiologic medium to preserve vitality of tooth
      4. Milk is an ideal storage medium; physiologic saline is also a satisfactory storage medium
      5. Saliva is a less desirable storage medium, but if milk and saline are not available, and placement back into socket cannot be done, placement of the tooth under the patient's tongue is better than allowing to air dry which is destructive to the tooth (irreversible damage to the periodontal cells occurs in 30 minutes of air drying)
      6. Transport to the dentist must be immediate

   B. Follow Up: By dentist to whom the patient was referred for reimplantation

BITE WOUNDS

I.   Definition: Mechanical trauma to skin and/or underlying tissue from bite of an animal or human

II. Pathogenesis

A. Transmission of bacteria from animal's or human's mouth into wound may produce infection
   1. *Pasteurella multocida* is the causative agent in 20-50% of infections from dog bites and 80% of infections from cat bites
   2. Dog and cat bites also become infected with *Staphylococcus aureus*, *Streptococcus epidermidis*, and *Enterobacter* species
   3. Enteric Gram-negative bacteria and anaerobes are likely to cause infection from reptile bites
   4. Rats and mice bites may become infected from *Streptobacillus moniliformis*
   5. Streptococci, *Staphylococcus aureus*, *Eikenella corrodens*, or anaerobes are likely to cause infection from human bites
      a. Hepatitis B can be transmitted by human bites; especially consider this if the biter is within a high-risk group
      b. Transmission of human immunodeficiency virus (HIV) is low but is a risk if the biter is HIV infected; especially consider this if biter is from a high-risk group

B. Rabies, an acute viral illness, may be transmitted to human beings by infected saliva or other secretions after an animal bite or by licking mucosa of an open wound; airborne transmission has been reported in bat-infested caves

III. Clinical Presentation

A. Dog bites account for over 90% of mammal bites

B. Most bites are minor and may include scratches, abrasions, lacerations, and puncture wounds

C. Human bites may occur, particularly in children
   1. A common injury in children is a tooth penetrating from the lower lip during a fall
   2. "Clenched-fist" injuries that occur during fistfights can cause potential tendon or joint capsule injuries and often require hospitalization

D. Potential complications of bites include to the following:
   1. Infection is the most common problem
      a. Cat bites become infected more frequently than dog bites because they are often deep puncture wounds
      b. Bites on the hand have the highest infection rate; bites on the face have the lowest infection rate
      c. Cellulitis and abscesses are common; infections of tendons, periosteum, and joint spaces can be devastating infections
   2. Rabies may occur after a bite
      a. Rabies in small rodents is rare
      b. Rabies in domestic animals has been decreasing, but rabies in wild animals is on the increase
      c. Skunks, bats, raccoons, bobcats, coyotes, and foxes may harbor the virus and may also bite and infect domestic dogs, cats, horses, and cows
      d. Infection with rabies produces an acute febrile illness with central nervous system problems and death if untreated
   3. Bites of large dogs and other animals may produce crush injuries, avulsions, and fractures

IV. Diagnosis/Evaluation

    A. History
       1. Inquire about type of mammal which bit patient
       2. Ask if attack was provoked or unprovoked
       3. If animal is known to the patient, obtain name and telephone number(s) of owner
       4. Ask about condition of animal such as was animal acting strangely or did animal appear ill
       5. Determine the amount of time which has elapsed since the bite
       6. If patient receives a human bite, determine whether the biter is HIV infected or has hepatitis B or if biter is from a high risk group
       7. Inquire about all self-treatments of injury
       8. Determine immune status of the animal or human biter
       9. Inquire about tetanus immunization status and prior rabies immunizations
      10. Inquire about patient's past medical history, especially diseases such as diabetes mellitus and immunodeficiencies which would place patient at risk for infection

    B. Physical Examination
       1. Check distal to the injured site for neurovascular status and motor function
       2. Determine extent and depth of wound; check for foreign body
       3. In patients with old wounds, check for signs of infection

    C. Differential Diagnosis: See Pathogenesis

    D. Diagnostic Tests
       1. Order x-rays if bony injury or presence of a foreign body such as tooth is suspected
       2. Obtain wound cultures in following cases:
          a. If wound is ≥8 hours and <24 hours from time of injury
          b. All cases in which there are signs of infections regardless of time from injury
       3. To determine if an animal is rabid, brain tissue can be examined by fluorescent microscopy

V. Plan/Management

    A. Wound care
       1. Sponge away visible dirt
       2. Irrigate wound with copious amounts of saline; do not irrigate puncture wounds
          a. Irrigate under pressure with either a 18 gauge needle and a 35 mL syringe or a Water-Pik
          b. Use at least 500-1000 mL of solution for irrigation and direct stream at all surfaces of wound
       3. Scrub the surrounding area
       4. Debride all wounds to reduce risk of infection unless they are small and superficial
       5. Trim jagged edge of wound

    B. Open-wound management versus sutures
       1. Do not suture wounds that are likely to become infected such as the following:
          a. Hand bites
          b. Bites that are older than 8 hours
          c. Deep or puncture bites
          d. Bites with extensive injury
       2. See section on WOUNDS for suturing procedure

    C. Antibiotic prophylaxis of bite wounds to prevent infection
       1. Following type of wounds need prophylaxis
          a. All wounds with signs of infections
          b. Moderate or severe wounds, especially if edema or crush injury is present
          c. Puncture wounds, especially if bone, tendon sheath, or joint penetration may have occurred
          d. Facial bites
          e. Hand and foot bites
          f. Genital area bites
          g. Wounds in immunocompromised and asplenic persons

2. Selection of antimicrobial agent is based on organism likely to cause infection and should be modified after culture results (see following table for antibiotics)

ANTIBIOTICS FOR ANIMAL OR HUMAN BITE WOUNDS

	Dog/Cat	Reptile	Human
Oral Route	Amoxicillin-clavulanate**	Amoxicillin-clavulanate**	Amoxicillin-clavulanate**
Oral Alternatives for Penicillin-Allergic Patients*	Extended spectrum cephalosporin or trimethoprim-sulfamethoxazole **PLUS** clindamycin	Extended spectrum cephalosporin or trimethoprim-sulfamethoxazole **PLUS** clindamycin	Trimethoprim-sulfamethoxazole **PLUS** clindamycin
Intravenous Route	Ampicillin-sulbactam	Ampicillin-sulbactam **PLUS** gentamicin **OR** ticarcillin-clavulanate	Ampicillin-sulbactam
Intravenous Alternative for Penicillin-Allergic Patients*	Extended spectrum cephalosporin or trimethoprim-sulfamethoxazole **PLUS** clindamycin	Clindamycin **PLUS** gentamicin	Extended spectrum cephalosporin or trimethoprim-sulfamethoxazole **PLUS** clindamycin

*In patients with history of allergy to penicillin, a cephalosporin or other β-lactam class drug may be acceptable. However, these drugs should not be used in patients with an immediate hypersensitivity (anaphylaxis) to penicillin because approximately 5% to 15% of penicillin-allergic patients also will be allergic to the cephalosporins.
**Prescribe amoxicillin/clavulanate (Augmentin) 250-500 mg every 8 hours; in children prescribe 20-40 mg/kg/dose in 3 divided doses for 3-7 days. Available 125 mg/5 mL and 250 mg/5 mL liquids

Adapted from American Academy of Pediatrics. (1997). Bite wounds. In G. Peter (Ed.). Red book: Report of the committee on infectious diseases (24th ed., pp. 125). Elk Grove Village, IL: American Academy of Pediatrics.

D. Prescribe appropriate tetanus prophylaxis; see WOUND section for guidelines

E. If there is a high risk or known exposure to hepatitis B after a human bite, provide passive prophylaxis with hepatitis B immune globulin (HBIG) 0.06 mL/kg intramuscularly and begin hepatitis B vaccination three-shot series

F. Consult infectious disease specialist if there is a high risk or known exposure to HIV after a human bite

G. Control measures related to rabies
   1. Contact personnel in local health department who can provide information on the risk of rabies in a particular area for each species of animals (unprovoked attack is more suggestive of rabid animal than provoked attack; properly immunized domestic animals have only a minimal chance of developing rabies)
   2. A suspected domestic animal should be caught, confined, and observed by a veterinarian for 10 days; if animal develops signs of rabies it should be killed and its head removed and shipped to laboratory for examination. No treatment is necessary if examination of brain is negative
   3. A suspected wild animal should be killed and its brain examined for evidence of rabies. No treatment is necessary if examination of brain is negative
   4. Patients with bites from bats and wild carnivores need rabies prophylaxis if the offending animal cannot be caught

H. Care of patients exposed to rabies; after local wound care, use both passive and active immunoprophylaxis as soon as possible after exposure, ideally within 24 hours, but even patients who have been exposed >24 hours should still be given therapy
   1. Active immunization: Human diploid cell vaccine (HDCV) or rhesus diploid cell vaccine, rabies vaccine absorbed (RVA) 1.0 mL is given intramuscularly in the deltoid on first day of treatment, and repeat doses are administered on days 3, 7, 14, and 28
   2. Passive immunization: Rabies immune globulin (Human) (RIG) should be used simultaneously with first dose of HDCV or RVA; recommended dose 20 IU of RIG per kilogram of weight; approximately one half of RIG is infiltrated into wound and the remainder is given intramuscularly

I.   Patient Education
      1.   Teach patient to watch for signs of infection
      2.   Educate about bite prevention
            a.   Caution against approaching unknown dogs, cats, and wild animals and avoid contact when animals are eating
            b.   Young children should not be left alone with a pet
            c.   Secure garbage containers so that raccoons and other animals will not be attracted to home and areas where children may play
            d.   Chimneys and other potential portals of entry for wild animals should be identified and covered

J.   Referral/consultation is needed in the following cases:
      1.   Bites of ears, face, genitalia, hands and feet
      2.   Large, contaminated wounds

K.   Follow Up: Inspect wound for signs of infection within 48 hours

BURNS, MINOR

I.   Definition: Lesions caused by heat or other cauterizing agents; the following are considered minor burns:

      A.   First- or second-degree burns covering <10% percent of the total body surface area (TBSA) in children and <15% in adults

      B.   In addition, third-degree burns of less <2% TBSA when they do not involve the eyes, ears, face or genitalia

II.   Pathogenesis

      A.   As a result of excessive heat energy which is transferred into the skin, cellular protein coagulation and destruction of enzyme systems occur

      B.   Common agents causing burns include the following:
            1.   Scalds or burns from wet heat
            2.   Direct burns from flames; matches and cigarettes are common sources; irons and ovens are other sources
            3.   Chemicals
            4.   Electricity
            5.   Radiation; burns caused by exposure to sunlight

III. Clinical Presentation

      A.   Depth of burn will depend on the intensity of the burning agent and the amount of time the burning agent is in contact with skin
            1.   First degree burns cause no skin loss and have erythema only; heal without scarring
            2.   Second degree burns (partial thickness) involve the upper layers of the epidermis and present with tender, erythematous, weeping skin and blisters
            3.   Third degree burns (full thickness) involve the entire thickness of the skin down to the subcutaneous tissues; sensation is absent and skin is charred or whitish in appearance

B. Scalds are the most common type of burn injury and generally result in superficial skin loss

C. Burns from flames are the second most common cause of burns; burns in which clothing is caught on fire is almost always third degree and serious

D. The severity of chemical burns depends on the type of chemical, its concentration and the contact time; cement and phenol are common sources

E. Electricity burns often cause small, punctate, deep burns at the entry point; electrical burns across the chest can cause cardiac problems

F. Radiation burns due to sun exposure are always superficial but can be extensive, painful, and result in hospitalization

G. Minor burns do not result in systemic problems (shock, acute renal failure, hypothermia, and severe depression of the immune systems) which may occur with severe burns

H. Other injuries may accompany minor burns and include trauma and smoke inhalation; carbon monoxide and cyanide poisoning may occur with more extensive burns

I. Bacterial infection is a complication of minor burns

IV. Diagnosis/Evaluation

A. History
   1. Ask what caused the burn or how the burn was acquired
   2. Query about length of the time the skin was in contact with the burning agent
   3. Determine how much time has elapsed from burn occurrence to seeking of treatment
   4. Question about occurrence of smoke inhalation
   5. Ask about associated injuries
   6. When chemicals are involved ask the name and concentration of the chemical
   7. Ask patients with electrical injury about the amount of voltage involved and whether there was loss of consciousness at time of injury
   8. Ask about tetanus status
   9. Ask about past medical history, particularly cardiac valvular disease
   10. Inquire about history of alcohol and narcotic abuse; this information is important in managing the patient's pain
   11. Ask about recent streptococcal infection
   12. Because of possibilities of abuse and neglect, ask about prior injuries and burns; documentation of quotes should be recorded

B. Physical Examination; important to remove all clothing, dressings, jewelry, dentures and prostheses to thoroughly assess burns and any associated injuries
   1. Observe general appearance for distress
   2. Observe for any signs that suggest abuse such as scald burns consistent with "dipping" injuries of the buttocks or arms and legs, cigarette burns, and iron burns
   3. Measure vital signs
   4. Estimate the area of burn from Lund-Browder burn charts
   5. Determine depth of burn
   6. Assess sensation in the burn area by using a blunt sterile needle or pin
   7. Check distal to the burn site for neurovascular status and motor function
   8. Perform a complete exam of the lung and heart
   9. Other body systems should be examined depending on location and extent of burn and to determine any associated injuries such as fractures and dislocations from jumping from windows in house fires
   10. In old burns, assess for signs of infection

C. Differential Diagnosis: Always consider possibility of abuse or neglect, particularly if location of burn is inconsistent with the history

D. Diagnostic Tests: None usually needed

V.   Plan/Management

A.   Refer following patients to a burn center
1.   Patients 11-49 years with partial-thickness burns ≥20% TBSA
2.   Patients <10 years and/or >50 years with partial-thickness burns ≥10% TBSA
3.   Patients of any age with full-thickness burns ≥5% TBSA
4.   Patients with partial- or full-thickness burns to hands, feet, face, eyes, ears, perineum and/or major joints
5.   Patients with electrical injuries, including lightning injuries
6.   Patients with significant burns from caustic chemicals
7.   Patients with burns complicated by multiple trauma in which the burn poses the greatest risk of morbidity
8.   Patients with significant inhalation injury
9.   Patients with co-morbid conditions that could complicate the management
10.   Patients who need social or emotional support and/or long-term rehabilitative support including suspected family violence

B.   Emergency treatment of severe burns while waiting transport of the patient to a burn center or an emergency department includes prompt IV fluid resuscitation with lactated Ringer's solution, elevating the burned areas, and administering 100% oxygen if inhalation injury is present

C.   First aid consists of removing the burning agent and lavaging burned area with cool water or normal saline; chemical burns require extensive lavaging (at least 15 minutes)

D.   Treatment of first degree burns from all causes except radiation
1.   Cleanse with mild detergent such as phisohex and water or saline
2.   May use topical anesthetic such as dibucaine (Nupercainal) cream or benzocaine (Americaine) spray 3-4 times a day as needed for pain
3.   No dressings needed

E.   Treatment of second degree burns from all causes except radiation
1.   Cleanse burned areas with mild detergent such as phisoHex and sterile saline (may need to sedate patient with codeine or chloral hydrate 30 minutes before cleansing and debridement)
2.   Leave blisters intact unless they are large and thin-walled (may aspirate blister with 19-gauge hypodermic needle)
3.   Remove blistered skin that is almost detached and other devitalized skin
4.   For small burns on face cover with bacitracin ointment and leave open; for other small burns cover with bacitracin and apply nonadherent dressing and a bulky dressing to absorb drainage from burn
5.   For larger burns:
      a.   Cover burned area with a thin layer of silver sulfadiazine 1% cream (Silvadene)
      b.   For sulfa-allergic patients, use nitrofurazone (Furacin) cream
      c.   Apply nonadherent gauze and bulky dressing to absorb drainage from burn
      d.   Other appropriate dressings include transparent adhesive dressings (OpSite, Tegaderm) or a biosynthetic compound (Biobrane) that is applied directly to burn and wrapped in gauze

F.   For mild sunburns use cool compresses and topical, dexamethasone aerosol spray every 3 hours; most effective if treatment is started within 12 hours of injury

G.   Pain management of all types of burns is important; recommend regular use of aspirin, acetaminophen or a nonsteroidal anti-inflammatory drug

H.   Tetanus prophylaxis is needed if the patient has not received either a course of immunizations or a booster within 10 years; see guidelines for tetanus prophylaxis in the WOUND section

I.   Systemic antibiotics are given only if patient has a valvular disease or a concomitant streptococcal infection

J. Patient Education
1. Teach patient or parent to clean burned area completely twice a day with gentle soap and water, dry burn well, and reapply ointment or cream and dressing
2. Keep dressing and/or burn clean and dry
3. Increase fluid intake
4. Elevate affected parts
5. Maintain active range of motion of all joints with overlying burns
6. Teach signs and symptoms of infection and need to return to provider if they occur

K. Follow Up
1. Patients should be reevaluated in 24-48 hours for evidence of infection and change of dressing
2. At least once a week, burn should be assessed for signs of complications at the health care site

CORNEAL ABRASION

I. Definition: Partial or complete removal of a focal area of epithelium on the cornea

II. Pathogenesis

A. The cornea is composed of three principal layers: epithelium (the outer layer), stroma, and endothelium

B. Disruption of the epithelium on the cornea by mechanical or chemical factors results in corneal abrasion

C. Because the epithelium is richly innervated with sensory nerve endings, even the tiniest injuries are painful

III. Clinical Presentation

A. Corneal injuries are very painful, with the degree of pain generally related to the amount of epithelial disruption

B. Patients usually complain of a scratchy, gritty sensation (foreign body sensation) that develops suddenly and worsens with blinking

C. Redness of the eye follows corneal insult due to the reactive conjunctival vasodilation (injection)

D. Photophobia is often present and occurs because the disruption in the optical surface causes light to be scattered within the eye rather than focused so that bright light sources have a glaring appearance

IV. Diagnosis/Evaluation

A. History
1. Ask which eye is injured
2. Determine how, when, and where the eye was injured
3. Ascertain if eye pain or vision loss is present
4. Ask if any eye protection was being used at time of injury and if anyone witnessed the injury
5. Ask if contact lenses are being worn (or were being worn at time of injury)
6. Ask about tetanus immunization status

B. Physical Examination
    1. Measure visual acuity (**Note**: Even in the case of trauma, it is critically important to know visual ability is present; if patient is unable to read chart, acuity may be grossly evaluated by finger counting)
    2. Evert the eyelids and examine the conjunctival fornices for foreign body (The presence of a foreign body under the upper lid should <u>always</u> be looked for in the presence of a suspected corneal abrasion)
    3. Examine cornea for abrasions using the technique described in the following table:

FLUORESCEIN STAINING TO ASSESS CORNEAL EPITHELIAL INTEGRITY

<u>Technique</u>

▲ Instill 1 or 2 drops of a rapid onset and short duration topical anesthetic (e.g., proparacaine HCl 0.5% [Ophthetic])

▲ Moisten the fluorescein strip with sterile normal saline (can also touch strip to the tear film in the lower cul de sac of affected eye)

▲ Touch moistened fluorescein strip to lower conjunctiva of the eye being inspected (If used tear film to moisten, this step is unnecessary as dye has already been placed in eye)

▲ Ask patient to blink eye

▲ Illuminate the eye with cobalt blue light and inspect for patterns of fluorescence

▲ Remove excess dye with sterile saline and remind patient not to rub eye

<u>Interpretation</u>

▲ If the corneal epithelium has been disturbed, fluorescein will pool within these areas and stain the hydrophilic stroma; the resultant brighter fluorescence of these pools will delineate the corneal abrasion from surrounding intact epithelium

▲ The size and pattern of the defect depends on nature and extent of injury

▲ A characteristic pattern that suggests the presence of a foreign body trapped underneath the upper lid is a faint vertically- oriented pattern on the cornea

---

C. Differential Diagnosis
    1. Corneal foreign body
    2. Viral keratitis
    3. Corneal laceration

D. Diagnostic Tests: None indicated beyond fluorescein staining described above

V. Plan/Management

    A. Instil an antibiotic ointment such as erythromycin ophthalmic ointment (Ilotycin) OR gentamicin ophthalmic ointment (Garamycin) into the affected eye

    B. Instruct patient to close injured eye and then apply a two-pad pressure dressing over the closed lids of the affected eye
        1. The patch must be firm and tight such that the eye cannot be opened beneath it
        2. Leave pad in place for 24 hours
        3. Instruct patient to return to clinic after 24 hours for removal of dressing
        4. Prescribe topical antibiotic ointment such as either of the ointments listed above, or drops such as sulfacetamide sodium solution (Sulamyd). Small amount of ointment or 2-3 drops should be used 4x/day x 5 days
        5. Administer tetanus immunization if indicated

    C. If the type of injury sustained is chemical, thermal, or a mechanical injury that has qualities of both blunt and sharp trauma, immediate transport to an ophthalmologist is required because of threat to vision

    D. Follow Up: In 24 hours to remove patch and evaluate healing

HEAD TRAUMA, MINIMAL AND MILD

I. Definition: Trauma to the head; simple linear skull fractures and concussions are the most common examples of minor head injuries

   A. Simple linear skull fractures: small break in skull that is not associated with depressed bone fragments and underlying brain injury

   B. Concussion: Trauma-induced alteration in mental status that may or may not involve loss of consciousness (previously, to be diagnosed with a concussion, the patient had to have a loss of consciousness)

   C. Classification of head injuries (see following table)

CLASSIFICATION OF HEAD INJURIES		
Minimal	**Mild**	**Moderately or Potentially Severe**
All of the following:	Any of the following:	Any of the following:
* No loss of consciousness or amnesia * Glasgow Coma Scale score of 15 * Normal alertness and memory * No focal neurologic deficit * No palpable depressed skull fracture	* Brief (<5 min.) loss of consciousness * Amnesia for the event * Glasgow Coma Scale score of 14 * Impaired alertness and memory	* Prolonged (>5 min.) loss of consciousness * Glasgow Coma Scale score of <14 * Focal neurologic deficit * Posttraumatic seizure * Intracranial lesion detected on CT scan

Adapted from Smith, E.E. (1993). Minor head injury: A proposed strategy for emergency management. <u>Annals of Emergency Medicine, 22,</u> 1193-1196.

II. Pathogenesis:

   A. The most common cause of traumatic head injuries in all ages is falls
      1. In infants, head injuries are often associated with falls and abuse; "shaken baby syndrome" should always be considered
      2. In preschool and school-age children, auto accidents are frequent
      3. In adolescents, sports injuries and assault become more important etiologic factors
      4. In adults, auto accidents, falls, and assaults are causative factors
      5. In the elderly, falls are the most common cause

   B. Outcomes following head trauma:
      1. Seriousness of the head injury is related to the nature and extent of the cerebral injury rather than the damage to the overlying scalp or skull structures
      2. Clinical course is dependent on the degree of acute injury to brain at the time of the accident (primary brain injury) and to delayed neurochemical and metabolic changes that result during the initial hours and days after the injury (secondary brain injury)
      3. Even minimal head injuries can result in a secondary brain injury which involves tissue injury, swelling, and ischemia
         a. Delayed cerebral edema may occur within 8-12 hours
         b. Maximal cerebral edema occurs within 48-72 hours after the injury
      4. "Second impact syndrome" occurs when a person (particularly an athlete) has a second concussion without recovering from the first; may lead to massive acute-brain swelling and ultimately, death; multiple head injuries can result in chronic impairment of brain function

III.   Clinical Presentation

   A.   Epidemiology
         1.   Head injury is the most common cause of traumatic mortality in the U.S.
         2.   Most patients with head injuries are between 15-24 years of age
         3.   Males are 2-3 times more likely to have a head injury than females
         4.   In 50-60% of adult cases with head injuries, a positive blood alcohol is detected

   B.   Head injuries in infants and children are different than those in adults
         1.   "Shaken baby syndrome" is often fatal
               a.   Typically, the baby is held by shoulders and shaken vigorously
               b.   Diffuse cerebral swelling is often present
               c.   Infants with minimal external signs of trauma with neurologic deficits should be suspected of this injury
         2.   Children typically have a better prognosis than adults, especially elderly persons, with similar head injuries for the following reasons:
               a.   The skull in younger children is thin and, in infants, the sutures are not fused which allows the skull to expand and decreases likelihood of increased intracranial pressure
               b.   The base of children's skulls are smoother than in adults which reduces the incidence of basilar contusions and contré coup injuries

   C.   Simple or linear skull fractures
         1.   Approximately 75% of skull fractures in children are linear
         2.   Patients with linear fractures are usually asymptomatic, but any fracture requires close observation because the force required to fracture a skull, particularly a child's skull, is significant
         3.   Skull fractures with underlying lacerations may predispose the patient to meningitis
         4.   Infants can lose a significant amount of blood from skull fractures
         5.   In children, a rare complication is a leptomeningeal cyst or "growing fracture" which presents as an enlarging bony defect due to a portion of leptomeninges squeezing between the edges of the fracture

   D.   Concussion
         1.   Hallmarks are confusion and amnesia which occur immediately after injury or several minutes later
         2.   Early symptoms (first few minutes or hours) include headache, dizziness or vertigo, lack of awareness of surroundings, and nausea and vomiting
         3.   Postconcussive syndrome may occur and includes low-grade headaches, light-headedness, poor attention and concentration, memory dysfunction, reduced energy levels, intolerance of bright lights and noise, sleep disturbances, and irritability and depression; symptoms may last as long as 3 months post injury
         4.   A grading scale based on severity of the injury is in the following table:

SCALE FOR GRADING THE SEVERITY OF CONCUSSION		
Grade 1	Grade 2	Grade 3
1. Transient confusion 2. No loss of consciousness 3. Concussion symptoms or mental status abnormalities on examination **resolve in *less* than 15 minutes**. Grade 1 concussion is the most common yet the most difficult form to recognize.	1. Transient confusion 2. No loss of consciousness 3. Concussion symptoms or mental status abnormalities on examination **last *more* than 15 minutes**. Grade 2 symptoms (greater than 1 hour) warrant medical observation.	1. Any loss of consciousness either brief (seconds) or prolonged (minutes). Grade 3 concussion is usually easy to recognize--the patient is unconscious for any period of time.

Adapted from American Academy of Neurology, Quality Standards Subcommittee: Practice parameter. (1997). The management of concussion in sports (summary statement). Neurology, 48, 581-585.

IV. Diagnosis/Evaluation

A. History: Important to obtain information from the patient as well as a person at the scene of the injury as the patient may be amnestic or confused
1. Determine how the injury occurred and the incidents surrounding the injury
2. Ask whether the patient had a loss of consciousness and amnesia
3. Inquire about symptoms after the injury such as vomiting, headaches, confusion, drowsiness, or abnormal behaviors
4. Determine if there is any neck pain or pain in other areas of the body
5. Inquire about other injuries
6. Ask about self treatments
7. Always ask about previous head injuries, particularly in athletes, to determine "second impact syndrome"

B. Physical Examination
1. To quickly rule out a serious injury which needs immediate intervention, perform the following
a. Assess airway patency, breathing, and circulation
b. Assess level of consciousness
c. Measure vital signs
d. Stabilize neck and check for signs of neck injury which often accompany head trauma
e. Assess the thorax for hemothorax and pneumothorax
f. Examine abdomen for signs of bleeding such as fullness and rigidity
g. Signs of increased intracranial pressure are listed in the following table

SIGNS OF INCREASED INTRACRANIAL PRESSURE[†]	
* Papilledema	* Decreased pulse
* Elevated systolic pressure	* Slow respirations
* Wide pulse pressure	

[†] In young children a full fontanelle (even when upright) and separation of cranial sutures are signs

2. A rapid system for evaluating athletes who suffer injuries during an event is presented in the following table

QUICK EVALUATION OF ATHLETES WITH HEAD INJURIES DURING THE SPORTS EVENT	
Mental Status Testing	
Orientation	Time, place, person, and situation (circumstances of injury)
Concentration	Digits backward (e.g., 3-1-7, 4-6-8-2, 5-3-0-7-4) Months of the year in reverse order
Memory	Names of teams in prior contest; recall of 3 words and 3 objects at 0 and 5 minutes Recent newsworthy events; details of the contest (plays, moves, strategies, etc)
External Provocative Testing	40-yard sprint; 5 push ups; 5 sit ups; 5 knee bends (any appearance of associated symptoms is abnormal, e.g., headaches, dizziness, nausea, unsteadiness, photophobia, blurred or double vision, emotional lability, or mental status changes)
Neurologic Tests	
Pupils	Symmetry and reaction
Coordination	Finger-nose-finger, tandem gait
Sensation	Finger-nose (eyes closed) and Romberg

Source: McCrea, M., Kelly, J.P., Kluge, J., Ackley, B., & Randolph, C. (1997). Standardized assessment of concussion in football players. Neurology, 48, 586-588.

3. After determining that the patient is not in acute distress, perform the following at frequent intervals:
   a. Use the Glasgow coma scale to quantitate mental status which can be used later to evaluate the patient's progress (see following table)

GLASGOW COMA SCALE FOR EVALUATING CHILDREN AND ADULTS*		
Eye-Opening Response		
Score	**Children <1 Year**	**Children >1 Year and Adults**
4	Spontaneous	Spontaneous
3	To shout	To verbal command
2	To pain	To pain
1	None	None
Motor Response		
Score	**Children <1 Year**	**Children >1 Year and Adults**
6	Spontaneous response	Obeys commands
5	Localizes pain	Localizes pain
4	Withdraws from pain	Withdraws from pain
3	Displays abnormal flexion to pain (decorticate rigidity)	Displays abnormal flexion to pain (decorticate rigidity)
2	Displays abnormal extension to pain (decerebrate rigidity)	Displays abnormal extension to pain (decerebrate rigidity)
1	None	None

Verbal Response		
Score **Children <2 Years**	**Children 2-5 Years**	**Children >5 Years and Adults**
5 Babbles, coos appropriately	Uses appropriate words and phrases	Is oriented and converses
4 Cries, but is consolable	Use inappropriate words	Conversation is confused
3 Cries or screams persistently to pain	Cries or screams persistently to pain	Words are inappropriate
2 Grunts or moans to pain	Grunts or moans to pain	Sounds are incomprehensible
1 None	None	None

Score of less than 8 denotes severe head injury

Adapted from Simon, J. (1992). Accidental injury and emergency medical services for children. In R.E. Behrman (Ed.). Nelson textbook of pediatrics. Philadelphia: WB Saunders.

   b. Observe gait
   c. Examine the eyes
      (1) Evaluate pupillary size, equality, and reaction to light
      (2) Perform funduscopy to detect retinal hemorrhage and papilledema
   d. Carefully inspect and palpate head, noting wounds, indentations
   e. Examine nasopharynx and ears for evidence of fresh blood
4. Palpate abdomen for signs of bleeding
5. Perform a complete neurologic examination including assessment of cranial nerves, reflexes, motor functioning, sensory functioning, and coordination
6. Assess mental status
7. Assess memory

C. Differential Diagnosis: Crucial to identify persons who are at risk for development of complications such as intracranial mass lesions, intracranial edema, and delayed neurological deterioration
   1. Age, co-morbidity, and mechanism of the injury are potential risk factors for severe head injuries (see following table)

RISK FACTORS FOR SEVERE HEAD INJURIES		
Mechanism	**Age**	**Medical Condition**
* High speed motor vehicle accident * Fall of more than 8 feet * Injury with extensive damage to other areas of body	* Greater than 65 years	* Long-term anticoagulant therapy * Presence of cerebrovascular malformation

Adapted from Marion, D.W. (1998). Acute head injuries in adults. In R.E. Rakel (Ed.), 1998 Conn's current therapy. Philadelphia: WB Saunders.

2. Common causes of serious head trauma include the following:
  a. Basilar skull fractures
    (1) Bruising around the eye (raccoon sign), blood in external auditory canal (Battle's sign), cerebrospinal fluid leakage in the ear or nose, and cranial nerve palsies often occur
    (2) Fractures may not be present on plain x-rays, but are apparent on computed tomography (CT)
  b. Cerebral contusion or laceration results from edema, hemorrhage and possibly necrosis
    (1) Associated with trauma directly beneath the site of blunt or penetrating injury (coup) or may result from indirect trauma contralateral to the injury (contré coup)
    (2) Typically, the patient has loss of consciousness for >2 minutes
    (3) May result in death or severe residual neurologic deficits such as post-traumatic epilepsy
  c. Acute epidural hemorrhage results from a tear in the meningeal artery, vein, or dural sinus and is usually associated with a skull fracture
    (1) Several hours after injury the patient may have a headache, confusion, somnolence, seizures, or focal deficits
    (2) Without treatment, coma, respiratory arrest, and death follow
  d. Acute subdural hematoma is due to a tear in veins from cortex to superior sagittal sinus or from cerebral laceration
    (1) More common injury than acute epidural hemorrhage
    (2) The symptoms and complications are similar to an epidural hemorrhage but the interval before onset of symptoms is longer
  e. Cerebral hemorrhage develops immediately after the injury with symptoms of intracranial pressures and distress; a hematoma is usually visible on CT scan
3. Typical characteristics of severe head injuries include the following:
  a. Loss of consciousness associated with one or more neurologic deficits
  b. Glasgow Coma Scale score of less than 8
  c. Alterations in mental status
  d. Prolonged memory deficit
  e. Persistent vomiting and severe headache
  f. Seizures
  g. Signs of primary brainstem injury include coma, irregular breathing, fixation of pupils to light, and diffuse motor flaccidity
4. Child abuse or family violence should always be included in differential diagnosis

D. Diagnostic Tests:
  1. No tests are needed in patients with minimal head trauma (see classification system in I.C.) who have no abnormal neurological signs but monitoring for neurological abnormalities should extend for at least 48 hours after the injury
  2. CT scan is the most efficacious test for detecting intracranial injury but a skull x-ray is helpful in the following cases: penetrating injuries, possible depressed fractures, or suspected nonaccidental injuries; consider ordering skull x-rays in patients who have point tenderness or scalp hematomas
  3. Order CT scans in patients who are classified as having mild, moderate, or severe head injuries (see I.C.) and patients with minimal head trauma if they have evidence of a skull fracture on x-ray or if they later develop abnormal neurological symptoms and signs

4. Always consider ordering cervical spine films or other radiographs for any patient depending on the mechanism and circumstances surrounding the injury
5. Consider ordering a blood alcohol
6. Obtain serial CBCs in young children with skull fractures

V. Plan/Management

A. Hospitalization
1. For patients with simple fractures and concussions without abnormal neurologic signs and symptoms, hospitalization is not required unless the patient is an infant who is predisposed to losing a significant amount of blood
2. Hospitalization is recommended in the following situations:
a. Suspicion of child abuse or family violence
b. All head injuries categorized as mild, moderate, or severe
c. Injuries accompanied with a neurologic deficit
d. Any mechanism severe enough to cause concern of secondary brain injury

B. For patients who are not hospitalized, careful monitoring for delayed abnormal signs and symptoms is essential; patient education includes the following:
1. Teach family members that there is a need for thorough, frequent observation and precautions for at least 48 hours after the injury; recommend the following:
a. Check whether pupils are equal and react to light
b. Determine arousability and coherence by waking patient every 4 hours
c. Time respiratory rate and check whether respiratory pattern is regular
2. Call health care provider for any of the following:
a. Headaches which worsen
b. Vomiting becomes more frequent
c. Pupils are unequal or do not react to light
d. Symptoms such as seizures, neck pain, drowsiness, confusion, difficulty walking, talking, or visualizing occur
3. Instruct family members that patient should be observed for the development of complications for at least 2 weeks after the injury; signs of complications include drowsiness, vomiting, gait disturbance, or severe headache
4. Emphasize to family members of athletes, that repeat head injuries can lead to permanent brain damage

C. Guidelines for the management of sports-related concussions were developed by the American Academy of Neurology
1. Initial management following the head injury depends on the grade of the concussion (see III.D.4)
a. Athletes with Grade 1 injuries may return to play the same day if the following are met: Normal on-site evaluation (see IV.B.2) while at rest and with exertion, including a normal, detailed mental status examination
b. Athletes with Grade 2 and Grade 3 injuries must have a complete neurologic examination and may not return to play the same day
2. Decisions on when to return to play after removal from the athletic event are based on grade of the concussion and whether previous head injuries have occurred (see table that follows)

Grade of Concussion	Time Until Return to Play*
Multiple Grade 1 concussion	1 week
Grade 2 concussion	1 week
Multiple Grade 2 concussions	2 weeks
Grade 3--brief loss of consciousness (seconds)	1 week
Grade 3--brief loss of consciousness (minutes)	2 weeks
Multiple Grade 3 concussions	1 month or longer, based on clinical decision of evaluating health care provider

*Only after being asymptomatic with normal neurologic assessment at rest and with exercise.

Adapted from American Academy of Neurology, Quality Standards Subcommittee: Practice parameter. (1997). The management of concussion in sports (summary statement). Neurology, 48, 581-585.

D. Prevention of head injuries
    1. Remind patients to wear safety belts in motor vehicles and helmets when riding a bike or motorcycle
    2. Proper safety equipment is needed for even recreational sports
    3. Measures to prevent falls in the household such as removing loose carpets and maintaining uncluttered, well-lit walkways is important

E. Follow Up
    1. Frequent monitoring of all head injuries is important
    2. Communicate with family members within first 4-12 hours after the injury and then periodically depending on the clinical condition of the patient

INSECT STING AND BROWN RECLUSE SPIDER BITE

I. Definition: A sting or bite in which there is secretion of venom into skin by insect or spider

II. Pathogenesis

A. Insect Sting
    1. Honeybees, bumblebees, wasps, hornets, and yellow-jackets (hymenoptera) embed a firm, sharp stinger in the skin; venom is secreted
    2. Honeybees leave their stingers in the skin (with venom sac attached; other hymenoptera have a retractable stinger and thus may sting many times)
    3. The injected venoms are proteins with enzyme activity that can cause local or general reactions, or both; reactions are classified as toxic or allergic

B. Brown Recluse Spider Bite
    1. Of the 50 or so species known to bite humans, the brown recluse spider (Loxosceles reclusa) is one of two species in the US (black widow is the other) capable of producing severe reactions
    2. Brown recluse spider is small (1.5 cm or less) light brown, and lives in dark areas such as closets, under porches, or in basements; usually found in river country of mid-America, most commonly in the south-central US
    3. Spider venom is composed of enzyme-spreading factor hyaluronidase, and a toxin distributed by the enzyme
    4. The venom of the spider is antigenic and once a person has been bitten, subsequent bites are not severe
    5. Spider bite can cause local or general reactions, but does not cause allergic reactions

III.   Clinical Presentation

    A.   Insect Sting
        1.   A sharp, pinprick sensation is felt at the instant of stinging followed by burning pain at site
        2.   A red papule or weal appears, enlarges, then subsides within hours
        3.   Multiple stings can cause a toxic reaction producing symptoms such as syncope, dizziness, vomiting, diarrhea, and headache because of the large toxin load
        4.   Allergic reactions begin as localized toxic reactions but quickly (within minutes or hours) produce an exaggerated urticarial response
        5.   Generalized reactions begin 2-60 minutes after sting and range from a few hives to anaphylaxis; forty percent of persons with generalized allergic reactions have a previous history of similar reaction
        6.   Anaphylaxis symptoms include generalized itching, hypotension, shortness of breath, and wheezing which may subside spontaneously or progress to edema of upper airway causing obstruction and death

    B.   Brown Recluse Spider Bite
        1.   Bite may feel sharp, or it might cause little or no pain; subsequent minor swelling and erythema at site often occur
        2.   Severity of local reaction appears to depend on site of bite with fatty areas of body developing more severe reactions
        3.   Tissue necrosis in bite area may develop as early as four hours after bite
        4.   Cutaneous changes at the site include a blue-gray, macular halo around puncture site; emergence of pustule, or vesicle/bulla at site; widening of macule and sinking of center of lesions producing a "sinking infarct;" sloughing of tissue leaving a deep ulcer which takes weeks or months to heal
        5.   In a few cases, within 12 hours after bite, systemic symptoms of fever, chills, nausea, vomiting, and generalized weakness may appear; rarely severe systemic reactions of generalized hemolysis, disseminated intravascular coagulation, and renal failure occur (usually only in children)

IV.   Diagnosis/Evaluation

    A.   History
        1.   Quickly question regarding type of bite or sting, time of occurrence, and location of bite/sting
        2.   If sting, quickly determine if allergic reaction is present (generalized itching, shortness of breath, and wheezing)
        3.   If sting, question about history of previous allergic reactions

---

*****   **ALERT**   *****
If allergic reaction is present or anticipated based on history, go immediately to treatment.

---

        4.   If bite, determine type of spider if patient can describe
        5.   If bite, ask about presence of systemic symptoms such as fever, chills, nausea, vomiting, and weakness

    B.   Physical Examination
        1.   If history suggests a severe anaphylactic reaction is imminent, do not complete exam or wait for symptoms to develop, institute treatment immediately (See V.B., below)
        2.   If sting with no allergic reaction evident or anticipated based on history, take pulse, respirations, and blood pressure
        3.   Examine site of bite or sting for characteristic erythema and edema. If spider bite which occurred within hours, examine for characteristic progression of site described under Brown Recluse Spider bite, above

    C.   Differential Diagnosis
        1.   Vasovagal attacks: May follow pain or upset and be accompanied by nausea, diaphoresis and hypotension; lasts only a few minutes and relieved by lying down

2. Hyperventilation episodes: Accompanied by tachypnea, perioral tingling, but BP is maintained and other signs of anaphylaxis are absent

D. Diagnostic Tests: None indicated for bites or stings with no systemic symptoms

V. Plan/Treatment

A. Treatment of anaphylactic reactions is based on type of reaction which can range from mild to life-threatening; in all cases, epinephrine is the drug of choice

B. Treatment of mild anaphylaxis is outlined in the table that follows

---

TREATMENT OF MILD ANAPHYLAXIS

For mild symptoms of pruritus, erythema, urticaria, and wheezing, treat with epinephrine injected subcutaneously, followed by diphenhydramine, hydroxyzine, or other antihistamine given orally or parenterally

Epinephrine, 1:1000 (aqueous) 0.01 mL/kg per dose, administered subcutaneously. Usual dose:

Infants: 0.05-0.1 mL   **Children:** 0.1-0.3 mL

Repeat in 10-20 minutes; monitor patient's condition constantly, and monitor BP every 10 minutes

Antihistamine: Give **one** of the following:
　Hydroxyzine, Oral or IM: Give 0.5-1 mg/kg/dose (100 mg maximum single dose)
　Diphenhydramine, Oral, or IM: Give 1-2 mg/kg/dose (100 mg maximum single dose)

If symptoms improve with this management, give a long-acting epinephrine injection (Sus-Phrine) as a single dose, 0.005 mL/gm. Usual dose:

Infants: 0.025-0.05 mL   **Children:** 0.05-0.15 mL

Also, give oral antihistamines for next 24 hours; see dosing above

Observe patient in clinic for several hours before discharging to home. Instruct patient to apply ice to site and elevate the affected extremity to control local reaction

Follow Up: By telephone in 12-24 hours.

C. For severe and potentially life-threatening systemic anaphylaxis (bronchospasm, laryngeal edema, hypotension, shock, and cardiovascular collapse) institute the following and call 911 for immediate transport

---

TREATMENT OF SEVERE ANAPHYLAXIS

Promptly institute airway maintenance and oxygen therapy
Give Intravenous (IV) epinephrine
A slow continuous infusion is preferable to repeated bolus administration. For a continuous infusion, add one milligram (1 mL) of 1:1000 dilution of epinephrine to 250 mL of 5% dextrose in water, resulting in a concentration of 4 μg/mL; initially infuse at a rate of 0.1 μg/kg/minute and increase gradually to 1.5 μg/kg/minute to maintain blood pressure

If bronchospasm is prominent, inhaled β_2 agonist: Albuterol (Ventolin) should be administered via nebulizer

Usual dose:　Children: 0.1-0.15 mg/kg in 2 cc of saline　Adolescents: 2.5 mg (0.5 cc of 0.5% solution) in 2 cc saline

Transport to emergency department

D. Prevention of recurrence in patients with mild to severe anaphylactic reactions
1. Refer patient for allergy testing with insect venom to identify the venom responsible for sensitization
2. Five venoms are commercially available for this purpose: honeybee, yellow jacket, yellow hornet, white-faced hornet, and Polistes wasps

3. If skin tests produce ambiguous results, a RAST can be performed to detect IgE antibody to venoms

4. Immunization with insect venom can prevent future systemic reactions in patients with a previously documented reaction

E. Emergency treatment kits (available by prescription) for self-treatment before reaching medical help should be obtained by all persons at risk for anaphylaxis from insect stings

    1. Patients should be prescribed 3 kits: one for home, one for car, and one to carry

    2. Ana-Kit (Hollister-Stier, Spokane, WA) contains a preloaded syringe; refill syringes (Ana-Guard) are available

    3. Epi-Pen or Epi-Pen Junior are spring-loaded automatic injectors for individuals reluctant to perform self-injection

F. Patients should also wear a medical alert tag

G. For insect stings which are localized with mild urticaria

    1. Remove stinger if present using forceps, or by scraping out (do not attempt to squeeze out)

    2. Wash the wound thoroughly and apply ice packs

    3. Prescribe oral antihistamines (see above for dosing of hydroxyzine and diphenhydramine) to relieve local reaction and discomfort

    4. Recommend continued use of ice packs and elevation for the next 8-12 hours

H. For moderate swelling, the interventions outlined above should be used. In addition, a short course (5 days) of oral steroids is also recommended

I. Treatment of the brown recluse bite is somewhat controversial; there are no accepted, conclusively established guidelines

    1. All experts recommend the following conservative treatment

        a. Gentle cleansing with soap and water

        b. Apply ice and elevate

        c. Avoid strenuous exercise

        d. AVOID APPLICATION OF HEAT

        e. Give tetanus toxoid if indicated

    2. Controversy surrounds which drugs, if any, are indicated

        a. No drug treatments are indicated, according to most experts (excellent outcomes usually occur without any pharmacologic interventions)

        b. Some experts recommend systemic steroids for adolescents who are seen within 24 hours of the bite; methylprednisolone, 100 mg IV, followed by oral prednisone for 5 days

        c. Some experts recommend Dapsone, 50-200 mg per day (adolescents >18 only), even though it has many side effects and must be used with extreme caution

        d. Antibiotic treatment may be helpful, but use is recommended only in treating secondary infection (prophylactic use has not been proven to be of any benefit); if secondary infection present, erythromycin is a good choice

            (1) Children: Erythromycin (as ethylsuccinate) suspension (Eryped 200 mg/5 mL, 400 mg/5 mL); give 30 mg/kg/day, divided into 4 doses x 10 days. Also available in 200 mg chewable tabs

            (2) Adolescents: Erythromycin (as base) [E-Mycin] 250 mg QID x 10 days

        e. Use of oral and intralesional steroids have not been shown to decrease progressive reaction in patients with clinically significant bites (necrosis >1 cm)

    3. In previous years, early debridement was the most commonly advocated brown recluse spider bite therapy; this is no longer done as no evidence supports the belief that this procedure promotes healing and reduces complications

J.   Follow Up
     1.   Stings: In 24-24 hours (may be by telephone) for patients with mild anaphylactic symptoms; none indicated for those with localized reactions only
     2.   Brown recluse spider bite: No follow up is needed, but patients must be instructed to report any systemic problems such as headache, myalgia, fever, chills, gastrointestinal complaints, rash and darkening of urine (the presentation of hemolysis is within the first weeks); complications of wound healing may occur at any time until resolution and patients must be instructed in signs and symptoms of wound infection

OCULAR FOREIGN BODY

I.   Definition: Presence of a foreign body in the cul-de-sacs and under the upper lid or on the cornea

II. Pathogenesis

     A.   A foreign body of the conjunctiva occurs when particles become entrapped under the upper lid or in the cul-de-sacs

     B.   Most often occurs with blowing dirt or sand; there is usually no trauma involved

     C.   A foreign body of the cornea occurs when substances become embedded in the corneal epithelium most often due to some traumatic event

     D.   A sudden event such as an explosion, or an accident involving metal grinding may scatter small fragments onto the cornea

III. Clinical Presentation

     A.   The most common conjunctival foreign bodies are dust, sand, and contact lenses

     B.   The most common foreign bodies found on the cornea are metallic, often rusty particles

     C.   Foreign bodies may be single or multiple, easily seen without magnification or barely detectable with slit-lamp examination

     D.   Symptoms are photophobia, lacrimation, and foreign body sensation

IV. Diagnosis/Evaluation

     A.   History
          1.   Ask which eye is injured
          2.   Determine how, when, and where the eye was injured
          3.   Ascertain if eye pain or vision loss is present
          4.   Ask if any eye protection was being used at time of injury and if anyone witnessed the injury (important for medicolegal reasons)
          5.   Ask if contact lenses are in place (or were in place at time of injury)
          6.   Ask about tetanus immunization status
          7.   Note: Based on history, if foreign body is result of explosion, blunt or sharp trauma, (i.e., if corneal foreign body is suspected) eye should be protected from further damage by placing eye shield over eye (or if shield not available, a paper cup to prevent rubbing eye) at this point and person transported for emergency care

     B.   Physical Examination
          1.   Measure visual acuity (Note: Even in the case of trauma, it is critically important to know visual ability is present; if patient is unable to read chart, acuity may be grossly evaluated by finger counting)

2. Evert the eyelids and examine for foreign body
3. Technique for everting the eyelid is as follows:

EVERSION OF THE UPPER LID

▲ Instill 1 or 2 drops of a rapid onset, short duration topical ophthalmologic anesthetic such as proparacaine HCl (Ophthetic, 0.5%) into the affected eye

▲ Ask patient to look down

▲ Grasp the lashes with one hand and apply gentle pressure on the lid above the tarsal plate with a cotton-tip applicator with the other hand

▲ Foreign bodies such as soft contact lenses and grit are often found in superior temporal cul-de-sac of the orbit

---

4. Examine the inferior cul-de-sac by having the person look up while the lower lid is pulled down

V. Plan/Management

A. When foreign body is visualized, sweep sterile cotton-tipped swab moistened with topical anesthetic across conjunctival area to remove the object
   1. If there is difficulty with removal or if patient complains of severe pain, attempts should be discontinued
   2. Refer to ophthalmologist

B. After removal of conjunctival foreign body (or if conjunctival foreign body cannot be located), determine if corneal abrasion present (See CORNEAL ABRASION)
   1. If no corneal abrasion present, prescribe topical antibiotic ointment or drops such as sulfacetamide sodium (Sulamyd); apply small amount of ointment or 2-3 drops to affected eye 4x/day x 5 days
   2. If corneal abrasion present, see CORNEAL ABRASION for treatment recommendations
   3. Provide tetanus immunization if indicated

C. Follow Up: In 24 hours

SUBCONJUNCTIVAL HEMORRHAGE

I. Definition: A flat, bright-red hemorrhage under the conjunctiva

II. Pathogenesis

A. May occur spontaneously, with raised venous pressure from a forced Valsalva maneuver (as in coughing, sneezing)

B. May occur with minor or major trauma

III. Clinical Presentation

A. Presents as a striking flat, deep-red hemorrhage under the conjunctiva and may become sufficiently severe to cause a "bag of blood" to protrude over lid margin

B. Subconjunctival hemorrhage is usually asymptomatic

IV. Diagnosis/Evaluation

    A. History
        1. Determine which eye affected how, when, and where the injury occurred
        2. Ascertain if eye pain, discharge of secretions, or vision loss is present
        3. Ask if patient has had previous symptoms or complaints similar to the current complaint

    B. Physical Examination
        1. Measure visual acuity
        2. Examine lids and the adnexa for symmetry, swelling, abnormal discharge, and erythema
        3. Palpate the soft tissue of the orbit, lids, and zygoma
        4. Inspect the conjunctiva and sclera for localized swelling, signs of hemorrhage
        5. Examine pupils for size, shape, reaction to light, and perform funduscopic exam

    C. Differential Diagnosis
        1. Conjunctivitis
        2. Conjunctival laceration

    D. Diagnostic Tests: None indicated

V. Plan/Management

    A. With no other signs and symptoms, no treatment is required; the patient should be reassured that the blood will clear over a 2-3 week period

    B. If trauma with a sharp object is suspected, or if there is impaired vision, eye pain, foreign body sensation, discharge of secretions from the eye, change in the appearance of the globe, patient should be referred to an ophthalmologist for evaluation

    C. Follow Up: None required; for patients with signs and symptoms described under V.B. above, follow-up should be by the ophthalmologist to whom the patient was referred

WOUNDS

I. Definition: Breach in the external surface of the body

II. Pathogenesis

    A. Wounds such as lacerations and abrasions typically heal through a 3 stage process: clotting, inflammatory and proliferative stages

    B. Devitalized tissue, oral secretions, toxic solutions, soil and dirt, and injurious forces can impede the healing process and possibly cause infection

    C. *Staphylococcus aureus* and β-hemolytic *streptococcus* are the most common pathogens causing wound infection

    D. Tetanus can also occur due to multiplication of *Clostridium tetani*, producing a toxin which can block motor neurons

III. Clinical Presentation

    A. Mechanism of injury is important in determining likelihood of infection and tissue damage
        1. Sharp objects often make smooth cuts which can penetrate deep structures
        2. Crushing injuries often damage underlying tissues and can result in fractures
        3. Human bites have the greatest risk of bacterial infection and can also transmit hepatitis B and possibly human immunodeficiency virus (HIV)

B. Location or environment in which the wound occurred suggests potential problems; wounds which occur in dirty soil such as farmyards are at risk for contamination with spores of *Clostridium tetani*

C. The time interval between when the wound first occurred to when the patient received appropriate care affects the chances of infection; if 6 hours have elapsed, bacterial multiplication is likely

D. Site of the wound influences rate of healing and potential for complications:
1. Due to rich vascular supply, wounds on face heal rapidly, but may create future cosmetic problems
2. Hands are used extensively; wounds on hands have increased risk for reinjury and infection

E. Certain types of wounds may be problematic
1. Dirty wounds are more at risk for infection
2. Deep wounds can cause underlying tissue destruction and also have increased risk of contamination
3. Wounds with untidy edges often heal slowly and may heal with disfigurement
4. Wounds with tissue necrosis have potential for infection and delayed healing

F. Characteristics of the patient are also factors in wound healing; elderly patients, undernourished patients, patients on corticosteroids and chemotherapeutic agents, and patients with underlying illnesses have the greatest risk for adverse sequela from wounds

G. Tetanus is a rare but dangerous complication of a wound and is characterized by trismus and severe muscular spasms

IV. Diagnosis/Evaluation

A. History
1. Ask patient to explicitly describe how the wound occurred
2. Determine where the injury was sustained
3. Question how much time has elapsed since the wound occurred
4. Ascertain tetanus immunization status
5. Ask about allergies to drugs, dressings, and local anesthetics
6. Ask about current medication use, especially steroid and anticoagulant therapy
7. Inquire about past medical history to determine if patient has underlying illness such as immunodeficiency which could affect healing process
8. Ask whether the patient has a tendency to form keloids, because this could result in a poor scar

B. Physical Examination: Always use sterile technique when examining wounds; it may be necessary to apply local or regional anesthesia prior to the examination
1. Measure wound
2. Assess depth of wound
3. Explore wound for foreign bodies
4. Fully examine underlying structures
5. Assess circulation, sensation and movement distal to wound
6. Palpate underlying bone
7. Assess range of motion and strength against resistance of all body parts surrounding wound site
8. Examination of the patient with an old wound includes the following:
   a. Carefully inspect wound and surrounding area
   b. Palpate for local lymphadenopathy
   c. Measure patient's temperature

C. Differential Diagnosis: Always consider the possibility of non-accidental injury (see following table)

INDICATORS OF POSSIBLE NON-ACCIDENTAL INJURY
• Delay between injury and seeking treatment
• The history of the accident does not match the observed injury
• The history changes
• Other injuries, especially if at different stages of healing
• Signs of general neglect or failure to thrive
• Signs of family tension or indications of alcohol or drug abuse

Adapted from Wardrope, J., & Smith, J.R.R. (1992). The Management of wounds and burns. New York: Oxford.

D. Diagnostic Tests
1. Order x-rays for crushing, and deep penetrating wounds
2. Obtain wound swabs for culture on any wound which is slow to heal; fresh wounds do not require a culture

V. Plan/Management

A. The following wounds should be managed by an health care provider with extensive experience in wound management
1. Wounds involving nerve, tendon, or bone damage
2. Wounds with full thickness skin loss
3. Facial and hand wounds (small, superficial wounds, however, may be treated in outpatient setting)

B. Wound-cleansing is the first step of wound care
1. Irrigate wound with one of the following:
   a. Normal saline is an economical and effective irritant
   b. Povidone-iodine, hydrogen peroxide, and other detergents can cause tissue toxicity and should not be used
   c. Use high-pressure irrigation which can be achieved with a 35- or 65-ml syringe and a 16- or 19- gauge needle; higher pressure may result in tissue trauma and should be reserved for highly contaminated wounds
2. Apply mechanical force to clean wound: may use a fine-pore sponge such as an Optipore with a surfactant such as poloxamer 188 (Shur Clens)

C. Preparation of the wound site is next
1. Debridement of devitalized tissue is important
2. Clip, do not shave, surrounding hair as close to skin surface as possible

D. After appropriately preparing the wound, the next step is to decide whether to apply sutures; the following wounds require open-wound management:
1. Abrasions and superficial lacerations
2. Wounds with a great deal of tissue damage
3. Wound which have a low risk for infection of >12-24 hours of age
4. Wounds which have a high risk for infection of >6 hours of age
5. Wounds contaminated by feces, human or animal saliva, or large amounts of soil or dirt
6. Abrasions or wounds involving large superficial denudement of skin

E. Wound dressings: Best environment for wounds which are not sutured is a moist one; the following occlusive or semiocclusive dressings can promote a moist environment and all are effective
1. Occlusive dressings such as duoderm, telfa, and Opsite can be used
2. Hydrocolloid dressing is another possible choice (good for leg ulcers and pressure sores)
3. Hydrogel dressing such a Vigilon may be selected
4. Foam dressings are another choice

F.   Closure of the wound with tape (Steri-strip) is appropriate if the wound is superficial, has little tension, the edges are well approximated, and the injured area has full range of motion

G.   Other wounds require sutures
1.   Anesthesia
a.   Inject 1% buffered lidocaine hydrochloride (Xylocaine) or 0.25% or 0.50% bupivacaine (may cause less discomfort than lidocaine)
b.   Topical anesthetics such a mixture of tetracaine, adrenaline, and cocaine (TAC) are generally not recommended because they are expensive, not reliable when used below the head, may be toxic to the tissue, and cause other complications
c.   Do not use any anesthetic containing epinephrine in an area in which circulation is easily compromised such as fingers, toes, nose, penis or ears
2.   Wound edge approximation should be achieved with little or no tension to the surrounding area. Tension would be indicated by puckering of the skin
a.   In patients with a history of keloid formation, close skin with minimal tension and consider applying a pressure dressing for 3-6 months
b.   Many different suture techniques are available; suturing technique will depend on site and extent of injury
c.   Different suture materials are available
(1)   Skin is usually closed with nonabsorbable suture material such as nylon, prolene, or silk
(2)   Subcutaneous tissue and mucosal surfaces are usually closed with absorbable material, such as Dexon, Vicryl, or plain or chromic gut
(3)   Rapidly dissolving suture forms may be used to close the skin in children to avoid the discomfort associated with follow up suture removal
3.   Delayed primary closures with sutures
a.   This technique is used for wounds that cannot be closed initially because of gross contamination, potential injury to joints or other deep structures, retained foreign bodies, host immune status or an inability to adequately cleanse the wound
b.   Consider closing wound in 3-5 days when the risk of infection decreases
4.   Care of wound after suturing
a.   For simple lacerations, place gauze over suture line and cover with occlusive dressing for 24-48 hours. For more complex lacerations, immobilize injured body part for 5-7 days and apply bulky dressing; some advocate wound closure tape directly over the sutures
b.   Splint sutured wounds which are over or around a joint
c.   Instruct patient to keep wound clean and dry for at least 48 hours

H.   Tissue adhesives or glue such as cyanoacrylates have been used in Europe and Canada and are under review by the Food and Drug Administration (FDA)
1.   Apply adhesive by approximating wound margins with one hand and applying adhesive with the other; apply just enough adhesive to close the wound
2.   Application is rapid and painless
3.   Suture removal is not necessary as adhesives slough off in 7-10 days
4.   Adhesives act as their own dressings and have antimicrobial effects against gram-positive organisms
5.   Disadvantages are that adhesives have lower tensile strength than sutures and may break over high-tension areas such as joints

I.   Certain types of wounds require different therapy
1.   Puncture wounds should have very high-powered irrigation with saline; do not close puncture wounds with sutures
2.   Flap wounds which have edges which are not approximated should be cleaned, non-viable fat should be removed, and steristrips should be applied to appose but not close the wound

J.   Topical antibiotic ointments can be applied to open or sutured wounds
1.   Polysporin, bacitracin, and mupirocin are appropriate choices
2.   Avoid neosporin because it may cause allergies

K. Oral antibiotics are sometimes used for prophylactic purposes to prevent infection
1. Prophylactic antibiotics should be given in the following cases:
   a. Most mammal bites (see section on BITE WOUNDS)
   b. Puncture wounds in which cleansing was difficult
   c. Patients with valvular disease or implants who are at risk for bacteremia
2. Also, consider prophylactic antibiotics in the following cases:
   a. Heavily contaminated wounds
   b. Wounds with delayed treatment
   c. Wounds with tissue necrosis
3. Choose one of the following antibiotics for prophylaxis
   a. Amoxicillin-clavulanate (Augmentin) can be used as prophylactic antibiotic; Prescribe 250-500 mg every 8 hours. For children prescribe 20-40 mg/kg/day of the amoxicillin component in 3 divided doses for 7-10 days. Available in 125 mg/5 mL or 250 mg/5 mL liquid.
   b. For patients with penicillin allergies, prescribe erythromycin (E-Mycin) 250 mg QID for 7-10 days; children (Eryped) 30-60 mg/kg/day QID for 7-10 days. Available in 200 mg/5 mL or 400 mg/5 mL liquid

L. Prevention of tetanus is important (following table provides guidelines on tetanus prophylaxis)

GUIDE TO TETANUS PROPHYLAXIS IN WOUND MANAGEMENT				
History of Tetanus Immunization (doses)	Clean, Minor Wounds		All Other Wounds**	
	Td*	TIG*	Td*	TIG*
Uncertain or <3	Yes	No	Yes	Yes
3 or More†	No‡	No	No§	No

*Td = adult-type tetanus and diphtheria toxoids. If the patient is younger than 7 years, DTP or DtaP is given. TIG = tetanus immune globulin.
**Such as, but not limited to, wounds contaminated with dirt, feces, soil, and saliva; puncture wounds; avulsions; and wounds resulting from missiles, crushing, burns, and frostbite
†If only 3 doses of fluid toxoid have been received, a fourth dose of toxoid, preferably an adsorbed toxoid, should be given.
‡Yes, if >10 years since the last dose.
§Yes, if >5 years since the last dose.

Adapted from American Academy of Pediatrics. (1997). Tetanus. In G. Peter (Ed.), 1997 red book: Report of the Committee on Infectious Disease. 24th ed. Elk Grove Village, IL: American Academy of Pediatrics.

M. Patient Education
1. Teach patient to return if wound is increasingly painful, if there is significant discharge or if there is spreading of redness around wound or a red streak developing from the wound in the direction of the heart
2. Inform patient that appearance of the wound and subsequent scar will change substantially during the year after the injury; thus, decisions for scar revision should be made after one year
3. Advise patients to avoid sun exposure of their wounds to reduce the risk of developing hyperpigmentation

N. Follow Up
1. On return visits evaluate and consider hospitalization or aggressive antimicrobial therapy if signs and symptoms of pyogenic abscess, cellulitis, and ascending lymphangitis (red line spreading proximally on a limb) are present
2. Return for reevaluation, dressing change and/or suture removal in 2 days
3. Time to remove sutures depends on wound location; apply surgical adhesives or tape after sutures are removed
   a. Facial wounds: 3-5 days
   b. Scalp wounds: 7-10 days
   c. Hand wounds: 10-14 days
   d. Lower legs: 14 days
   e. Other: 7-21 days

Allwood, J.S. (1995). The primary care management of burns. Nurse Practitioner, 20 (8), 74-87.

American Academy of Pediatrics. (1997). Bite wounds. In G. Peter (Ed.), Red book: Report of the Committee on Infectious Diseases (24th ed.). Elk Grove Village, IL: Author.

American Academy of Pediatrics. (1997). Rabies. In G. Peter (Ed.), Red book: Report of the Committee on Infectious Diseases (24th ed.). Elk Grove Village, IL: Author.

American Academy of Pediatrics. (1997). Tetanus. In G. Peter (Ed.), Red book: Report of the Committee on Infectious Diseases (24th ed.). Elk Grove Village, IL: Author.

American Academy of Pediatrics. (1997). Treatment of anaphylactic reations. In G. Peter (Ed.), Red book: Report of the committee on infectious diseases (24th ed.). Elk Grove Village, IL: Author.

American Burn Association. (1996). Guidelines for transfer of patients in burn centers. New York: American Burn Association.

American Academy of Neurology, Quality Standards Subcommittee: Practice parameter. (1997). The management of concussion in sports (summary statement). Neurology, 48, 581-585.

Anderson, P.C. (1997). Spider bites in the United States. Dermatologic Clinics, 15(2), 307-311.

Arminoff, M.J. (1998). Nervous system. In L.M. Tierney, S.J. McPhee, & M.A. Papadakis (Eds.), Current medical diagnosis and treatment 1998 (37th ed.). Stamford, CT: Appleton & Lange.

Cornell, S. (1997, August). When animals attack. Advance for Physician Assistants, 47-50.

Crown, L.A., Lofton, B., & Magill, E. (1998). A 20-year old woman with an insect bite. Family Practice Recertification, 20(4), 22-29.

Dershewitz, R.A., & Lewin, S. (1999). Animal and human bites. In R.A. Dershewitz (Ed.), Ambulatory pediatric care. Philadelphia: Lippincott.

Doody, D.P. (1999). Lacerations and abrasions. In R.A. Dershewitz (Ed.), Ambulatory pediatric care. Philadelphia: Lippincott.

Drowling, E.C. (1999). Head trauma. In R.A. Dershewitz (Ed.), Ambulatory pediatric care. Philadelphia: Lippincott.

Gruen, P., & Liu, C. (1998). Current trends in the management of head injury. Contemporary Issues in Trauma, 16, 63-83.

Hall, D.E. (1997). Head injuries. In R.A. Hoekelman (Ed.), Primary pediatric care (3rd ed.). St. Louis: Mosby.

Herbert, A.E. (1998). Acute head injuries in children. In R.E. Rakel (Ed.), 1998 Conn's current therapy. Philadelphia: WB Saunders.

Howell, J.M., & Chisholm, C.D. (1997). Wound care. Emergency Medical Clinics of North America, 15, 417-425.

Kelly, J.P., & Rosenberg, J.H. (1997). Diagnosis and management of concussion in sports. Neurology, 48, 575-580.

Lloyd, D.A., Carty, H., Patterson, M., Butcher, C.K., & Roe, D. (1997). Predictive value of skull radiography for intracranial injury in children with blunt head injury. Lancet, 349, 821-824.

Marion, D.W. (1998). Acute head injuries in adults. In R.E. Rakel (Ed.), 1998 Conn's current therapy. Philadelphia: WB Saunders.

McCrea, M., Kelly, J.P., Kluge, J., Ackley, B., & Randolph, C. (1997). Standardized assessment of concussion in football players. Neurology, 48, 586-588.

Monafo, W.W. (1996). Initial management of burns. New England Journal of Medicine, 335, 1581-1586.

National Association of State Public Health Veterinarians, Inc. (1997). Compendium of animal rabies control 1997. MMWR, 46 (RR-4), 1-15.

Presutti, R.J. (1997). Bite wounds: Early treatment and prophylaxis against infectious complications. Postgraduate Medicine, 101, 243-253.

Roddy, S.P., et al. (1998). Minimal head trauma in children revisited: Is routine hospitalization required? <u>Pediatrics, 101,</u> 575-577.

Singer, A.J., Hollander, J.E., & Quinn, J.V. (1997). Evaluation and management of traumatic lacerations. <u>New England Journal of Medicine, 337,</u> 1142-1148.

Smith, E.E. (1993). Minor head injury: A proposed strategy for emergency management. <u>Annals of Emergency Medicine, 22,</u> 1193-1196.

Trued, S.J. (1997). Minor soft tissue injuries and infections. In L. Dornbrand, A.J. Hoole, & R.H. Fletcher. (Eds.), <u>Manual of clinical problems in adult ambulatory care</u> (3rd ed.). Philadelphia: Lippincott-Raven.

Wardrope, J., & Smith, J.A.R. (1992). <u>The management of wounds and burns</u>. New York: Oxford University Press.

Widell, T. (1998). Eye, ear, nose, throat, and dental emergencies. In S. H. Plantz, & J.N. Adler (Eds.), <u>Emergency medicine</u>. Baltimore: Williams & Wilkins.

Wipfler, E.J. (1998). Insect and arachnid bites and stings. In S. H. Plantz, & J.N. Adler (Eds.), <u>Emergency medicine</u>. Baltimore: Williams & Wilkins.

Zaveruha, A., Bishop, D., St. Clair, A., & Moreau, K. (1997). Rabies update for primary-care practitioners. <u>Clinical Excellence for Nurse Practitioners, 1,</u> 367-375.

Index

BARMARRAE BOOKS, INC.

ORDERING INFORMATION

1-888-276-7780

Credit card orders (VISA or MasterCard) or institutional purchase orders may be placed toll free 8 A.M. - 5 P.M. EST weekdays at the above telephone number.

Credit card orders (VISA or MasterCard) or institutional purchase orders may be faxed 24 hours to **1-352-378-1441**

OR

Please photocopy or clip the order form below and mail with your check, money order, or purchase order to:

BARMARRAE BOOKS, INC.
3017 NW 62ND TERRACE
GAINESVILLE, FL 32606

Note to Book Sellers:
All book returns require written permission and label from the publisher. Write to the address above or fax to the number above for permission.

Please photocopy this form or cut and mail to
Barmarrae Books, Inc., 3017 NW 62nd Terrace, Gainesville, FL 32606

ORDER FORM
BARMARRAE BOOKS, INC.
3017 NW 62ND TERRACE
GAINESVILLE, FL 32606

Order by mail, phone, or fax

Title	Unit Price	Qty	Total
Clinical Guidelines in Family Practice ISBN 0-9646151-3-4	60.00		
Clinical Guidelines in Adult Health ISBN 0-9646151-5-0	55.00		
Clinical Guidelines in Child Health ISBN 0-9646151-4-2	55.00		
Subtotal			
Shipping and Handling (within the US)	5.00		
Shipping Outside US, add $15			
Florida residents, add 6% sales tax			
TOTAL DUE (US funds **ONLY**)			

Name: _____

Address: _____

City: _____ State/Zip _____

Area Code/Phone No.: _____

Form of Payment: ❑ Check ❑ Money Order
❑ Purchase Order (Institutions Only) ❑ MasterCard ❑VISA

Credit Card # _____

Expiration Date _____

Signature _____

Mail Order to: **BARMARRAE BOOKS, INC.**
3017 NW 62nd Terrace
Gainesville, FL 32606

Phone Order to: 1-888-276-7780 or
1- 352-378-5554

Fax Order to: 1-352-378-1441

BARMARRAE BOOKS, INC.

ORDERING INFORMATION

1-888-276-7780

Credit card orders (VISA or MasterCard) or institutional purchase orders may be placed toll free 8 A.M. - 5 P.M. EST weekdays at the above telephone number.

Credit card orders (VISA or MasterCard) or institutional purchase orders may be faxed 24 hours to **1-352-378-1441**

OR

Please photocopy or clip the order form below and mail with your check, money order, or purchase order to:

BARMARRAE BOOKS, INC.
3017 NW 62ND TERRACE
GAINESVILLE, FL 32606

Note to Book Sellers:
All book returns require written permission and label from the publisher. Write to the address above or fax to the number above for permission.

Please photocopy this form or cut and mail to
Barmarrae Books, Inc., 3017 NW 62nd Terrace, Gainesville, FL 32606

ORDER FORM
BARMARRAE BOOKS, INC.
3017 NW 62ND TERRACE
GAINESVILLE, FL 32606

Order by mail, phone, or fax

Title	Unit Price	Qty	Total
Clinical Guidelines in Family Practice ISBN 0-9646151-3-4	60.00		
Clinical Guidelines in Adult Health ISBN 0-9646151-5-0	55.00		
Clinical Guidelines in Child Health ISBN 0-9646151-4-2	55.00		

Name: _____

Address: _____

City: _____ State/Zip _____

Area Code/Phone No.: _____

Subtotal	
Shipping and Handling (within the US) 5.00	
Shipping Outside US, add $15	
Florida residents, add 6% sales tax	
TOTAL DUE (US funds **ONLY**)	

Form of Payment: ❑ Check   ❑ Money Order

❑ Purchase Order (Institutions Only) ❑ MasterCard ❑VISA

Credit Card # _____

Expiration Date _____

Signature _____

Mail Order to: BARMARRAE BOOKS, INC. 3017 NW 62nd Terrace Gainesville, FL 32606	**Phone Order to:** 1-888-276-7780 or 1- 352-378-5554 **Fax Order to:** 1-352-378-1441

BARMARRAE BOOKS, INC.

ORDERING INFORMATION

1-888-276-7780

Credit card orders (VISA or MasterCard) or institutional purchase orders may be placed toll free 8 A.M. - 5 P.M. EST weekdays at the above telephone number.

Credit card orders (VISA or MasterCard) or institutional purchase orders may be faxed 24 hours to 1-352-378-1441

OR

Please photocopy or clip the order form below and mail with your check, money order, or purchase order to:

BARMARRAE BOOKS, INC.
3017 NW 62ND TERRACE
GAINESVILLE, FL 32606

Note to Book Sellers:
All book returns require written permission and label from the publisher. Write to the address above or fax to the number above for permission.

Please photocopy this form or cut and mail to
Barmarrae Books, Inc., 3017 NW 62nd Terrace, Gainesville, FL 32606

ORDER FORM
BARMARRAE BOOKS, INC.
3017 NW 62ND TERRACE
GAINESVILLE, FL 32606

Order by mail, phone, or fax

Title	Unit Price	Qty	Total
Clinical Guidelines in Family Practice ISBN 0-9646151-3-4	60.00		
Clinical Guidelines in Adult Health ISBN 0-9646151-5-0	55.00		
Clinical Guidelines in Child Health ISBN 0-9646151-4-2	55.00		
Subtotal			
Shipping and Handling (within the US)	5.00		
Shipping Outside US, add $15			
Florida residents, add 6% sales tax			
TOTAL DUE (US funds ONLY)			

Name: _____

Address: _____

City: _____ State/Zip _____

Area Code/Phone No.: _____

Form of Payment: ❏ Check   ❏ Money Order

❏ Purchase Order (Institutions Only) ❏ MasterCard ❏ VISA

Credit Card # _____

Expiration Date _____

Signature _____

Mail Order to: BARMARRAE BOOKS, INC.
3017 NW 62nd Terrace
Gainesville, FL 32606

Phone Order to: 1-888-276-7780 or
1- 352-378-5554
Fax Order to: 1-352-378-1441

BARMARRAE BOOKS, INC.

ORDERING INFORMATION

1-888-276-7780

Credit card orders (VISA or MasterCard) or institutional purchase orders may be placed toll free 8 A.M. - 5 P.M. EST weekdays at the above telephone number.

Credit card orders (VISA or MasterCard) or institutional purchase orders may be faxed 24 hours to **1-352-378-1441**

OR

Please photocopy or clip the order form below and mail with your check, money order, or purchase order to:

**BARMARRAE BOOKS, INC.
3017 NW 62ND TERRACE
GAINESVILLE, FL 32606**

Note to Book Sellers:
All book returns require written permission and label from the publisher. Write to the address above or fax to the number above for permission.

**Please photocopy this form or cut and mail to
Barmarrae Books, Inc., 3017 NW 62nd Terrace, Gainesville, FL 32606**

ORDER FORM
BARMARRAE BOOKS, INC.
3017 NW 62ND TERRACE
GAINESVILLE, FL 32606

Order by mail, phone, or fax

Title	Unit Price	Qty	Total
Clinical Guidelines in Family Practice ISBN 0-9646151-3-4	60.00		
Clinical Guidelines in Adult Health ISBN 0-9646151-5-0	55.00		
Clinical Guidelines in Child Health ISBN 0-9646151-4-2	55.00		
Subtotal			
Shipping and Handling (within the US)	5.00		
Shipping Outside US, add $15			
Florida residents, add 6% sales tax			
TOTAL DUE (US funds **ONLY**)			

Name: _____

Address: _____

City: _____ State/Zip _____

Area Code/Phone No.: _____

Form of Payment: ❏ Check   ❏ Money Order

❏ Purchase Order (Institutions Only) ❏ MasterCard ❏VISA

Credit Card # _____

Expiration Date _____

Signature _____

Mail Order to: BARMARRAE BOOKS, INC.
3017 NW 62nd Terrace
Gainesville, FL 32606

Phone Order to: 1-888-276-7780 or 1- 352-378-5554

Fax Order to: 1-352-378-1441

BARMARRAE BOOKS, INC.

ORDERING INFORMATION

1-888-276-7780

Credit card orders (VISA or MasterCard) or institutional purchase orders may be placed toll free 8 A.M. - 5 P.M. EST weekdays at the above telephone number.

Credit card orders (VISA or MasterCard) or institutional purchase orders may be faxed 24 hours to **1-352-378-1441**

OR

Please photocopy or clip the order form below and mail with your check, money order, or purchase order to:

BARMARRAE BOOKS, INC.
3017 NW 62ND TERRACE
GAINESVILLE, FL 32606

Note to Book Sellers:
All book returns require written permission and label from the publisher. Write to the address above or fax to the number above for permission.

Please photocopy this form or cut and mail to
Barmarrae Books, Inc., 3017 NW 62nd Terrace, Gainesville, FL 32606

ORDER FORM
BARMARRAE BOOKS, INC.
3017 NW 62ND TERRACE
GAINESVILLE, FL 32606

Order by mail, phone, or fax

Title	Unit Price	Qty	Total	
Clinical Guidelines in Family Practice ISBN 0-9646151-3-4	60.00			**Name:** _____
Clinical Guidelines in Adult Health ISBN 0-9646151-5-0	55.00			**Address:** _____
Clinical Guidelines in Child Health ISBN 0-9646151-4-2	55.00			**City:** _____ **State/Zip** _____
				Area Code/Phone No.: _____
Subtotal				Form of Payment: ❏ Check ❏ Money Order
Shipping and Handling (within the US)	5.00			❏ Purchase Order (Institutions Only) ❏ MasterCard ❏VISA
Shipping Outside US, add $15				Credit Card # _____
Florida residents, add 6% sales tax				Expiration Date _____
TOTAL DUE (US funds **ONLY**)				Signature _____

Mail Order to: BARMARRAE BOOKS, INC. 3017 NW 62nd Terrace Gainesville, FL 32606	**Phone Order to:** 1-888-276-7780 or 1- 352-378-5554 **Fax Order to:** 1-352-378-1441

BARMARRAE BOOKS, INC.

ORDERING INFORMATION

1-888-276-7780

Credit card orders (VISA or MasterCard) or institutional purchase orders may be placed toll free 8 A.M. - 5 P.M. EST weekdays at the above telephone number.

Credit card orders (VISA or MasterCard) or institutional purchase orders may be faxed 24 hours to 1-352-378-1441

OR

Please photocopy or clip the order form below and mail with your check, money order, or purchase order to:

BARMARRAE BOOKS, INC.
3017 NW 62ND TERRACE
GAINESVILLE, FL 32606

Note to Book Sellers:
All book returns require written permission and label from the publisher. Write to the address above or fax to the number above for permission.

Please photocopy this form or cut and mail to
Barmarrae Books, Inc., 3017 NW 62nd Terrace, Gainesville, FL 32606

ORDER FORM
BARMARRAE BOOKS, INC.
3017 NW 62ND TERRACE
GAINESVILLE, FL 32606

Order by mail, phone, or fax

Title	Unit Price	Qty	Total
Clinical Guidelines in Family Practice ISBN 0-9646151-3-4	60.00		
Clinical Guidelines in Adult Health ISBN 0-9646151-5-0	55.00		
Clinical Guidelines in Child Health ISBN 0-9646151-4-2	55.00		

Name: _____

Address: _____

City: _____ State/Zip _____

Area Code/Phone No.: _____

Subtotal	
Shipping and Handling (within the US) 5.00	
Shipping Outside US, add $15	
Florida residents, add 6% sales tax	
TOTAL DUE (US funds **ONLY**)	

Form of Payment: ❏ Check   ❏ Money Order

❏ Purchase Order (Institutions Only) ❏ MasterCard   ❏VISA

Credit Card # _____

Expiration Date _____

Signature _____

Mail Order to: BARMARRAE BOOKS, INC.
3017 NW 62nd Terrace
Gainesville, FL 32606

Phone Order to: 1-888-276-7780 or
1- 352-378-5554

Fax Order to: 1-352-378-1441

BARMARRAE BOOKS, INC.

ORDERING INFORMATION

1-888-276-7780

Credit card orders (VISA or MasterCard) or institutional purchase orders may be placed toll free 8 A.M. - 5 P.M. EST weekdays at the above telephone number.

Credit card orders (VISA or MasterCard) or institutional purchase orders may be faxed 24 hours to **1-352-378-1441**

OR

Please photocopy or clip the order form below and mail with your check, money order, or purchase order to:

BARMARRAE BOOKS, INC.
3017 NW 62ND TERRACE
GAINESVILLE, FL 32606

Note to Book Sellers:
All book returns require written permission and label from the publisher. Write to the address above or fax to the number above for permission.

Please photocopy this form or cut and mail to
Barmarrae Books, Inc., 3017 NW 62nd Terrace, Gainesville, FL 32606

ORDER FORM
BARMARRAE BOOKS, INC.
3017 NW 62ND TERRACE
GAINESVILLE, FL 32606

Order by mail, phone, or fax

Title	Unit Price	Qty	Total	
Clinical Guidelines in Family Practice ISBN 0-9646151-3-4	60.00			Name: _____
Clinical Guidelines in Adult Health ISBN 0-9646151-5-0	55.00			Address: _____
Clinical Guidelines in Child Health ISBN 0-9646151-4-2	55.00			City: _____ State/Zip _____
				Area Code/Phone No.: _____

Subtotal		Form of Payment: ❏ Check ❏ Money Order
Shipping and Handling (within the US)	5.00	❏ Purchase Order (Institutions Only) ❏ MasterCard ❏VISA
Shipping Outside US, add $15		Credit Card # _____
Florida residents, add 6% sales tax		Expiration Date _____
TOTAL DUE (US funds **ONLY**)		Signature _____

Mail Order to: BARMARRAE BOOKS, INC. 3017 NW 62nd Terrace Gainesville, FL 32606	**Phone Order to:** 1-888-276-7780 or 1- 352-378-5554 **Fax Order to:** 1-352-378-1441

BARMARRAE BOOKS, INC.

ORDERING INFORMATION

1-888-276-7780

Credit card orders (VISA or MasterCard) or institutional purchase orders may be placed toll free 8 A.M. - 5 P.M. EST weekdays at the above telephone number.

Credit card orders (VISA or MasterCard) or institutional purchase orders may be faxed 24 hours to
1-352-378-1441

OR

Please photocopy or clip the order form below and mail with your check, money order, or purchase order to:

BARMARRAE BOOKS, INC.
3017 NW 62ND TERRACE
GAINESVILLE, FL 32606

Note to Book Sellers:
All book returns require written permission and label from the publisher. Write to the address above or fax to the number above for permission.

Please photocopy this form or cut and mail to
Barmarrae Books, Inc., 3017 NW 62nd Terrace, Gainesville, FL 32606

ORDER FORM
BARMARRAE BOOKS, INC.
3017 NW 62ND TERRACE
GAINESVILLE, FL 32606

Order by mail, phone, or fax

Title	Unit Price	Qty	Total
Clinical Guidelines in Family Practice ISBN 0-9646151-3-4	60.00		
Clinical Guidelines in Adult Health ISBN 0-9646151-5-0	55.00		
Clinical Guidelines in Child Health ISBN 0-9646151-4-2	55.00		

Subtotal	
Shipping and Handling (within the US)	5.00
Shipping Outside US, add $15	
Florida residents, add 6% sales tax	
TOTAL DUE (US funds **ONLY**)	

Name: _____

Address: _____

City: _____ State/Zip _____

Area Code/Phone No.: _____

Form of Payment: ❑ Check ❑ Money Order
❑ Purchase Order (Institutions Only) ❑ MasterCard ❑VISA

Credit Card # _____

Expiration Date _____

Signature _____

Mail Order to: BARMARRAE BOOKS, INC.
3017 NW 62nd Terrace
Gainesville, FL 32606

Phone Order to: 1-888-276-7780 or
1- 352-378-5554
Fax Order to: 1-352-378-1441